GW00633227

ARTHRITIS SURGERY

Arthritis
Surgery

LEONARD MARMOR, M.D., F.A.C.S.

Attending Surgeon, St. John's Hospital, Santa Monica, California
Lecturer, Prosthetics Education Project
University of California at Los Angeles Medical Center

LEA & FEBIGER·1976·PHILADELPHIA

Library of Congress Cataloging in Publication Data

Marmor, Leonard.
    Arthritis surgery.
    Published in 1967 under title: Surgery of rheumatoid arthritis.
    Includes index.
    1. Arthritis deformans—Surgery.   2. Arthritis—Surgery.
I. Title.   [DNLM: 1. Arthritis, Rheumatoid—Surgery.
2. Arthritis—Surgery.   WE346 M352s]
RD686.M36   1976   617'.472   75-45362
ISBN 0-8121-0537-0

Published in Great Britain by Henry Kimpton Publishers, London

Printed in the United States of America

To My Dear Wife
Caryl
With Love

Some men see things as they are and say why,
I dream of things that never were and
say why not.

GEORGE BERNARD SHAW

Preface

Rheumatoid arthritis has continued to be the leading cause of destruction of joints and has disrupted the lives of hundreds of thousands of patients and their families. However, because of the progress made in the treatment of rheumatoid arthritis, as well as other forms of arthritis, it has been decided to change the title of the book *Surgery of Rheumatoid Arthritis*, which was published in 1967, to *Arthritis Surgery*. The great advances in joint replacement, as well as in other surgical procedures for arthritis, have prompted the broader span of this book.

A change has also been made in the format of the book. Surgical procedures will not be presented if they are not being utilized in arthritis surgery. The previous edition included various operations that were being performed or could be performed on a particular joint. The basic material in this text incorporates the ideas of many men with my own work to present the surgical treatment as clearly as possible.

This book is dedicated to the sufferers from arthritis the world over whose courage and understanding have inspired those who work with them, and whose cooperation has contributed so much to the advancement of medical knowledge. The sine qua non is the mo-tivated patient. Many of the surgical procedures depend upon the cooperation of the patient to exercise and move the joints postoperatively, and therefore motivation plays a great role in the successful result. A good deal has been said about the psychosomatic aspects of rheumatoid arthritis, and it is my opinion that it is not a "personality" that produces the rheumatoid patient, but that the personality is created by the increasing deformities of the disease and the physician's attitude that nothing can be done. Such a grim outlook would depress anyone. Once the patient has been offered help by the surgeon, the patient's personality frequently changes and his depression disappears.

There has been controversy in the medical profession about the role of surgery in the treatment of arthritis. In the past, poorly performed operative procedures or the wrong choice of operation has led to adverse results. However, carefully selected operations for particularly well-motivated patients can give excellent results and allow many patients who have been in wheelchairs for years to get up and walk. The reconstruction of joints of the upper extremities often will allow the patient to feed himself and take care of other personal needs, thus reducing his burden upon the family and rehabilitation personnel. Surgery should be thought of as an adjunct to medical treatment and not a treatment by itself.

The long-term results of surgery for rheumatoid and various other types of arthritis are beginning to be reported, and the results have remained good. In rheumatoid arthritis the recurrence rate has not been as high as was anticipated.

The development of the total hip replacement by John Charnley and McKee-Farrar has revolutionized the treatment of hip disease in the arthritic patient. The acceptance by the body of a total joint replacement cemented into place with methyl methacrylate has made possible rapid rehabilitation of these patients. The success of the total hip replacement stimulated the development of the total knee joint replacement. Probably other total joint replacements will become available in the future.

With the passage of time, arthritis surgery will begin to play a greater role in the work of the orthopaedic surgeon. It will be important that he knows the proper procedure and how to do it when the occasion arises.

I would like to express my appreciation for the encouragement in writing this book which has been given to me by Mr. Edward Wickland and Miss Isabelle Clouser of Lea & Febiger. I am also very grateful to my secretaries—Marlene Walshin, Janet Auerbach, and Laurie Tsurutani—who have spent long hours in typing this text and helping to organize the material. I would like to give credit to Joel Schechter who provided many of the illustrations that have added greatly to this presentation. I am especially grateful to my wife, Caryl, who has sacrificed so much to allow me to complete this book and has given me so much encouragement.

LEONARD MARMOR, M.D.

Los Angeles, California

Contents

1 | Rheumatoid Arthritis

Rheumatoid arthritis has been one of the most crippling and painful diseases affecting mankind because of its numerous manifestations and involvement of multiple joints. The earliest examples of arthritis were noted in the ape man two million years ago and have also been seen in the fossils of the vertebrate skeleton of the platycarpus. The disease was first described 1500 years B.C. in the early Egyptian papyrus rolls, and later the Romans built numerous baths throughout their empire to treat arthritic patients. This disease has been one of medical science's greatest puzzles. The name was coined in 1849 by an English physician, Garrod, who recognized the difference between rheumatoid arthritis and rheumatic fever. In 1941 the term *rheumatoid arthritis* was accepted and defined as a systemic disease affecting primarily connective tissue. Although lesions may be widespread, the predominant clinical finding is joint inflammation and deformity. The disease tends to be chronic and progressive, producing characteristic deformities of the extremities (Fig. 1-1).

It was originally believed that 12 million people are affected by arthritis in the United States alone and that one million are disabled by the disease. A new survey reveals that 20,450,000

people in the United States suffer from rheumatic diseases. Arthritis and rheumatism are second only to heart disease as a cause of chronic limitation of normal activity. The number of days lost from work because of this disease is estimated to be about 27 million days a year. The cost of these diseases to the patients and to the government is estimated to be $4,171,000,000 annually and amounts to 65,800,000 bed days. The rehabilitation of patients with rheumatoid arthritis and associated diseases medically is a tremendous problem, and the surgical reconstruction of the deformities is an even greater problem. The number of physicians specially trained to combat this problem is less than 2,000. The number of surgeons specifically trained to correct these deformities is probably less than several hundred. Even if the cause of the disease and its cure were found today, an overwhelming number of patients would still require reconstruction of their deformities.

The rheumatic diseases consist of a large number of illnesses that are grouped together because of joint symptoms. A classification has been established by the American Rheumatism Association (Table 1-1). Although many of the conditions mentioned in the classification may respond to surgical ther-

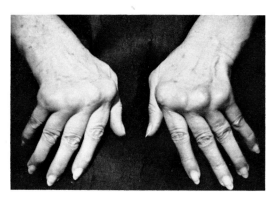

FIG. 1-1 An illustration of the chronic and progressive deformities of the hands produced by rheumatoid arthritis. Notice the symmetrical involvement of the hands with dislocations of the metacarpal-phalangeal joints and ulnar drift.

apy, the main emphasis in this book will be directed towards rheumatoid arthritis and osteoarthritis.

It is important that the surgeon and internist work together in the care of the patient with rheumatoid arthritis. Complete total care of the patient frequently will require the services of a physical therapist, an occupational therapist, and an orthotist. Therefore, a multidisciplinary approach is often of great value.

The surgeon must use his knowledge as a physician to understand and recognize the medical problems of the rheumatoid patient in order to treat the patient intelligently. He must know the various drugs that are used by the internist for the care of the patient and their effects which may play a role in the pre- or postoperative care of his patient. Therefore, a brief review of the total picture of rheumatoid arthritis is indicated before surgical treatment is discussed.

Etiology

The exact etiology of rheumatoid arthritis is unknown at the present time. A number of causes have been suggested, but at the present the prevalent theory is that it is an autoimmune disease. Ehrlich and Morgenroth at the beginning of this century first recognized that the living animal would not form antibodies which would be harmful to its own tissue. Burnet and Fenner attributed this ability as the capacity of distinguishing between "self" and "not self" and termed this "self recognition." This phenomenon is of basic importance in understanding the autoimmune theory.

The formation of organ-specific autoantibodies by human beings therefore is a remarkable process, but not surprising from an immunologic standpoint. It has been demonstrated by animal experiments that organ-specific antibodies may be formed. Patients with rheumatoid arthritis produce an antibody-like factor called the rheumatoid factor, which is a macroglobulin capable of reacting with gamma globulin of various species. The final explanation in this disease has not been reached, but recent studies have indicated that such an abnormality of the immune mechanism may be genetically conditioned. Lawrence has stated that "rheumatoid arthritis may be precipitated by some common respiratory infections, but the most severe forms apparently depend upon a genetically determined predisposition." Only two of the rheumatoid factors that are commonly seen in patients with rheumatoid arthritis are routinely tested for. One reacts in the sheep cell agglutination test and one in the latex fixation and bentonite flocculation tests. The proportion of positive tests in different populations varies from 1 percent to as much as 9 percent. Rheumatoid arthritis tends to develop in 20 percent and eventually probably in a higher percentage of people with a positive rheumatoid factor test. The disease develops in only a few of the seronegative persons. It is believed the evidence indicates that rheumatoid factor may have an environmental cause.

Table 1-1 *AHA Nomenclature and Classification of Arthritis and Rheumatism (Tentative)*

I. Polyarthritis of unknown etiology
  A. Rheumatoid arthritis
  B. Juvenile rheumatoid arthritis (Still's disease)
  C. Ankylosing spondylitis
  D. Psoriatic arthritis
  E. Reiter's syndrome
  F. Others

II. "Connective tissue" disorders
  A. Systemic lupus erythematosus
  B. Polyarteritis nodosa
  C. Scleroderma (progressive systemic sclerosis)
  D. Polymyositis and dermatomyositis
  E. Others

III. Rheumatic fever

IV. Degenerative joint disease (osteoarthritis, osteoarthrosis)
  A. Primary
  B. Secondary

V. Nonarticular rheumatism
  A. Fibrositis
  B. Intervertebral disc and low back syndromes
  C. Myositis and myalgia
  D. Tendinitis and peritendinitis (bursitis)
  E. Tenosynovitis
  F. Fasciitis
  G. Carpal tunnel syndrome
  H. Others
  (See also shoulder-hand syndrome, VIII. E.)

VI. Diseases with which arthritis is frequently associated
  A. Sarcoidosis
  B. Relapsing polychondritis
  C. Henoch-Schönlein syndrome
  D. Ulcerative colitis
  E. Regional ileitis
  F. Whipple's disease
  G. Sjögren's syndrome
  H. Familial Mediterranean fever

  I. Others
  (See also psoriatic arthritis, I. D.)

VII. Associated with known infectious agents
  A. Bacterial
    1. Brucella
    2. Gonococcus
    3. Mycobacterium tuberculosis
    4. Pneumococcus
    5. Salmonella
    6. Staphylococcus
    7. Streptobacillus moniliformis (Haverhill fever)
    8. Treponema pallidum (syphilis)
    9. Treponema pertenue (yaws)
    10. Others
  B. Rickettsial
  C. Viral
  D. Fungal
  E. Parasitic
  (See also rheumatic fever, III.)

VIII. Traumatic and/or neurogenic disorders
  A. Traumatic arthritis (viz, the result of direct trauma)
  B. Lues (tertiary syphilis)
  C. Diabetes
  D. Syringomyelia
  E. Shoulder-hand syndrome
  F. Mechanical derangement of joints
  G. Others
  (See also degenerative joint disease, IV.; carpal tunnel syndrome, V. G.)

IX. Associated with known biochemical or endocrine abnormalities
  A. Gout
  B. Ochronosis
  C. Hemophilia
  D. Hemoglobinopathies (eg, sickle cell disease)
  E. Agammaglobulinemia
  F. Gaucher's disease
  G. Hyperparathyroidism
  H. Acromegaly
  I. Hypothyroidism
  J. Scurvy (hypovitaminosis C)
  K. Xanthoma tuberosum

  L. Others
  (See also multiple myeloma, X. G.; Hurler's syndrome, XII. C.)

X. Tumor and tumor-like conditions
  A. Synovioma
  B. Pigmented villonodular synovitis
  C. Giant cell tumor of tendon sheath
  D. Primary juxta-articular bone tumors
  E. Metastatic
  F. Leukemia
  G. Multiple myeloma
  H. Benign tumors of articular tissue
  I. Others
  (See also hypertrophic osteoarthropathy, XIII. G.)

XI. Allergy and drug reactions
  A. Arthritis due to specific allergens (eg, serum sickness)
  B. Arthritis due to drugs (eg, hydralazine syndrome)
  C. Others

XII. Inherited and congenital disorders
  A. Marfan's syndrome
  B. Ehlers-Danlos syndrome
  C. Hurler's syndrome
  D. Congenital hip dysplasia
  E. Morquio's disease
  F. Others

XIII. Miscellaneous disorders
  A. Amyloidosis
  B. Aseptic necrosis of bone
  C. Behçet's syndrome
  D. Chondrocalcinosis (pseudogout)
  E. Erythema multiforme (Stevens-Johnson syndrome)
  F. Erythema nodosum
  G. Hypertrophic osteoarthropathy
  H. Juvenile osteochondritis
  I. Osteochondritis dissecans
  J. Reticulohistiocytosis of joints (lipoid dermato-arthritis)
  K. Tietze's disease
  L. Others

3

Recent evidence tends to support the theory that rheumatoid arthritis may be produced by a virus. The clinical aspects of the disease have suggested the possibility of an infection with a virus, bacteria, or other infectious agent; yet no agent has been found. The development of the "slow-virus theory" and the reports of slow-virus diseases with specific target organs have raised the possibility that rheumatoid arthritis also may be due to a slow virus. The triggering of acute exacerbations of inflammation by stress, the latency and periodicity, and its localization in the joints all suggest a specific etiologic agent such as a slow virus. Warren et al. have published a number of reports on an active agent that could be transmitted from human rheumatoid arthritis tissue to mice. These experiments demonstrate the presence of an active transmissible agent producing an acute response as well as long-term chronic effects involving the articular structures in mice. Mellors suggested that it is not unreasonable that an organotrophic virus could change or modify the immunogenic activity involving the lymphoid cells and could transform them into autoaggressive cells. Another fact tending to support the virus theory is that if a virus is already in a cell, another virus cannot enter this cell. Cells taken from a patient with rheumatoid arthritis and grown in tissue culture will not accept a virus, a fact suggesting that there may already be a virus within the cell.

Pathology

The primary pathologic change in rheumatoid arthritis is an acute, nonspecific synovitis. It is generally agreed that the primary lesion occurs either in the small blood vessels or in the ground substance of the synovium. The basic disease process is a rheumatoid synovitis with secondary changes in the joint structures as the disease progresses. The changes occurring in the synovium are inflammatory in nature and consist of edema, vascular congestion, lymphocytic infiltration, and exudation of fibrin (Fig. 1-2A). The synovial lining, which is usually a single layer in thickness, becomes greatly hypertrophied and thickened (Fig. 1-2B). The thickened synovium is thrown into villous folds with proliferative granulation tissue. The swelling of the synovium tends to distend the joint, thus stretching the capsule and collateral ligaments and

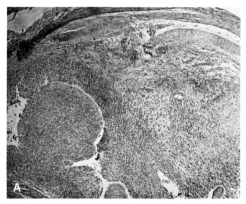

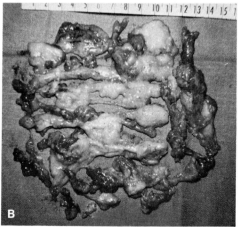

FIG. 1-2 Arthritic changes in the synovial layer. A. Photomicrograph showing invasion of lymphocytes and inflammatory cells. B. Photograph showing hypertrophy and a massive amount of thickening.

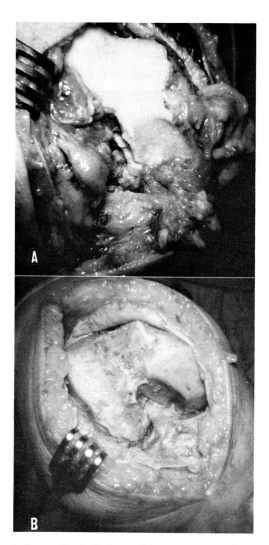

FIG. 1-3 Surgical views of the synovium in rheumatoid arthritis. A. Synovial tissue growing over the articular cartilage as pannus. B. After removal of pannus and synovium from another patient. Notice the loss of articular cartilage of the joint with only raw bone remaining. The cruciate ligaments are still intact and have not been destroyed by the disease.

interfering with normal joint motion. This process is most evident in the active stage of the disease in joints of the fingers and knees.

As the process progresses, the synovium becomes more aggressive and invasive, growing over the articular cartilage as a sheet of pannus (Fig. 1-3). It

can also erode the subchondral bone, destroying the overlying articular cartilage. The massive synovial thickening eventually interferes with the extension of the joint by mechanically blocking it, and the consequent muscle spasm associated with the inflammatory component leads to the development of flexion contractures. The inflammatory response with swelling, heat, redness, and destruction produces a great deal of the patient's pain. The pain and inevitable decreased use combined with the inflammatory disease produce osteoporosis of the bones adjacent to the joint. Enzymes released from the lymphocytes cause destruction of the articular cartilage. The joints can be completely destroyed by the synovial tissue, resulting in fibrous ankylosis (Fig. 1-4). In some cases the

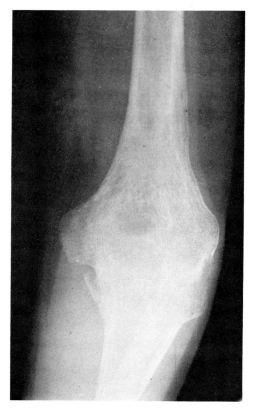

FIG. 1-4 Roentgenogram showing ankylosis in an elbow joint that has been completely destroyed and fused by the disease process.

fibrous tissue may be replaced by osseous tissue so that the joint is completely obliterated.

Since tendon sheaths and bursae contain synovial membranes, characteristic changes may also occur in them during periods of rheumatoid inflammation (Fig. 1-5). The bursal tissue may become so inflamed that fluid collects and the bursal tissue itself is thickened. The synovial proliferation can directly invade the tendinous structures to interfere with their nutrition and to cause their rupture.

Prior to the latter part of 1948, little information appeared in the medical literature in regard to rupture of the tendons due to rheumatoid arthritis. Ruptures of tendons were probably not recognized because of the severe deformities and resultant loss of function produced by the disease.

Nodules are also characteristic of rheumatoid disease and are located subcutaneously. They are found frequently on the forearm in the region of the olecranon and tend to occur over pressure areas (Fig. 1-6). Due to cellular necrosis, they tend to have a central area

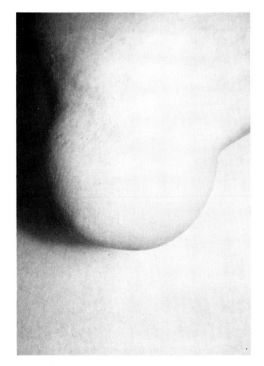

FIG. 1-6   An olecranon nodule characteristic of rheumatoid arthritis.

of fibrinoid tissue surrounded by a zone of large cells arranged in rows called "palisades."

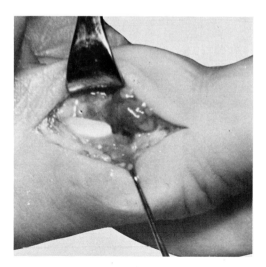

FIG. 1-5   Incision in a finger, revealing synovial involvement of the flexor tendon sheath.

Diagnosis

Rheumatoid arthritis is a common disorder that is three times more prevalent in women than in men. It tends to occur at any age but is more often seen in the young and the middle-aged person. It is extremely important to make a correct diagnosis of the type of arthritis one is dealing with and to determine whether it is rheumatoid arthritis. Diagnostic error can often lead to severe disasters.

Decker has stated that four salient points may be gathered in the workup of a patient with suspected rheumatoid arthritis, one from the history, two from the examination, and another from the laboratory. Although these will not establish the diagnosis, they are very suggestive of the disease. The fact obtained from the history is morning stiffness, or gelling, which is a common finding in rheumatoid arthritis. This sensation should last at least 15 minutes after arising. On the physical examination, the finding of polyarthritis is important. Two or more joints should show the classic signs of inflammation with swelling, increased heat, and tenderness (Fig. 1-7A). The second point in the physical examination is the symmetrical aspect of the disease (Fig. 1-7B). The laboratory fact would be the finding of an elevated sedimentation rate.

Grades of Diagnosis

Criteria for the diagnosis of rheumatoid arthritis were drawn up by the American Rheumatism Association. Four grades of diagnosis can be determined: classical, definite, probable, or possible rheumatoid arthritis. A number of variants of rheumatoid disease exist.

Classical Rheumatoid Arthritis

Classical rheumatoid arthritis may be diagnosed only if 7 of the following 11 criteria are present and if the total duration of joint symptoms, including swelling, has been continuous for at least 6 weeks.

1. Morning stiffness.

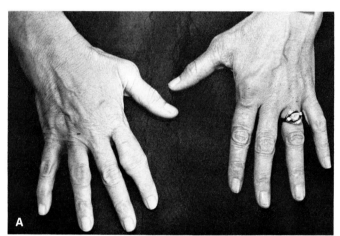

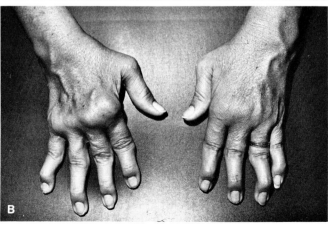

FIG. 1-7 Classic signs of rheumatoid arthritis. A. Swelling of the proximal interphalangeal joint of the right index finger and the metacarpal-phalangeal joint of the thumb. Swelling of the right wrist and loss of the superficial veins are also obvious. B. Symmetrical involvement of both hands with typical deformities that produce dislocations of the metacarpal-phalangeal joints and swan-neck deformities of the fingers.

2. Pain on motion or tenderness in at least one joint.
3. Swelling (soft tissue thickening or fluid—not bony overgrowth alone) in at least one joint, continuously, for not less than 6 weeks.
4. Swelling of at least one other joint (any interval free of joint symptoms between the episodes of involvement may not be more than 3 months).
5. Symmetrical joint swelling with simultaneous involvement of the same joint on both sides of the body (bilateral involvement of proximal interphalangeal, meta-carpal-phalangeal, or metatarsal-phalangeal joints is acceptable without absolute symmetry). Distal interphalangeal joint involvement will not satisfy this criterion.
6. Subcutaneous nodules over bony prominences or extensor surfaces or in juxta-articular regions.
7. Roentgenographic changes typical of rheumatoid arthritis (which must include at least bony decalcification localized to or greatest around the involved joints and not just degenerative changes). Degenerative changes alone, however, do not exclude the diagnosis of rheumatoid arthritis.
8. Positive reaction to sheep cell agglutination test. (Any modification will suffice that does not give more than 5 percent of positive results in non-rheumatoid control subjects.)
9. Poor mucin precipitate from synovial fluid.
10. Characteristic histologic changes in synovial membrane with three or more of the following: marked villous hypertrophy; proliferation of superficial synovial cells often with palisading; infiltration of chronic inflammatory cells (lymphocytes or plasma cells predominating) with tendency to form "lymphoid nodules"; deposition of compact fibrin, either on the surface or interstitially; foci of cell necrosis.
11. Characteristic histologic changes in nodules: granulomatous foci with central zones of cell necrosis surrounded by proliferated fixed cells, and peripheral fibrosis and chronic inflammatory cell infiltration, predominantly perivascular.

Definite Rheumatoid Arthritis

This diagnosis calls for at least five of the above criteria with a total duration of joint symptoms, including swelling, for a continuous period of at least 6 weeks.

Probable Rheumatoid Arthritis

This diagnosis requires at least three of the above criteria and a total duration of joint symptoms of at least 4 weeks.

Possible Rheumatoid Arthritis

This diagnosis requires two of the following criteria and total duration of joint symptoms of at least 3 weeks:

1. Morning stiffness.
2. Tenderness or pain on motion with history of recurrence or persistence for 3 weeks.
3. History or observation of joint swelling.
4. Subcutaneous nodules.
5. Elevated sedimentation rate or C-reactive protein.
6. Iritis.

Anatomic Stages

Steinbrocker has described various anatomic stages for classifying patients with rheumatoid arthritis. There are four stages of the disease, and this classification system is often used to compare various series of patients (Table 1-2).

Clinical Features

In its clinical picture, rheumatoid arthritis may be quite varied in its severity and in its joint involvement. The earliest complaints of the patient with rheumatoid arthritis are joint pain, stiffness, fatiguability, and weakness. The usual onset is insidious, and the course is slowly progressive but may be interspersed with periods of improvement and exacerbations. The rate of progression may vary considerably:

Intermittent. The disease flares up and then enters remission for a long time, followed by a relapse and remission again. The disease may also continue on without complete remission and then flare up again (stair-step type).

Chronic Progressive. In 85 percent of the patients the disease flares up, then smolders but definitely progresses.

Single Flare-up. The disease has no recurrence.

Fulminating. The disease progresses to severe disability and death.

Most cases of rheumatoid arthritis in adults are polyarticular, and the disease tends to involve the small joints of the hands and feet. The joints are likely to be involved symmetrically, and frequently the patient complains of morning stiffness. The important diagnostic features of rheumatoid arthritis are:

1. A slowly progressing polyarthritis with great tendency for symmetrical involvement of joints.
2. Fusiform, soft tissue type of joint swelling during the early years of the disease.
3. Early morning stiffness.
4. Development of typical deformities such as ulnar deviation of the fingers in later years.
5. Typical rheumatoid subcutaneous nodules.
6. Positive reaction to test for rheumatoid factor.

Table 1-2 *Steinbrocker's Anatomic Stages*

Stage I. Early
* *1. No destructive changes roentgenologically.
2. Roentgenologic evidence of osteoporosis may be present.

Stage II. Moderate
* *1. Roentgenologic evidence of osteoporosis, with or without slight bone destruction; slight cartilage destruction may be present.
* *2. No joint deformities, although limitation of joint mobility may be present.
3. Adjacent muscle atrophy.
4. Extra-articular soft tissue lesions, such as nodules and tenovaginitis, may be present.

Stage III. Severe
* *1. Roentgenologic evidence of cartilage and bone destruction, in addition to osteoporosis.
* *2. Joint deformity, such as subluxation, ulnar deviation or hyperextension, without fibrous or bony ankylosis.
3. Extensive muscle atrophy.
4. Extra-articular soft tissue lesions, such as nodules and tenovaginitis, may be present.

Stage IV. Terminal
* *1. Fibrous or bony ankylosis.
2. Criteria of stage III.

*These criteria must be present to permit classification of a patient in any particular stage or grade.

Laboratory Findings

The patient with active rheumatoid arthritis will have an elevated sedimentation rate and may have hypochromic anemia. A diagnosis of active rheumatoid arthritis in the absence of an elevated sedimentation rate is uncommon.

The various serologic tests for arthritis may also be positive and be an aid in diagnosis. The rheumatoid factor test can be obtained and is of value, but it should be noted that in a high percentage of patients a negative test does not rule out rheumatoid arthritis. The rheumatoid factor is present in 70 to 80 percent of the patients with classical or definite rheumatoid arthritis.

If there is fluid within the joint, aspiration is indicated for analysis of the fluid (Table 1-3). The synovial fluid should be examined for appearance, viscosity, white and red blood cells, mucin clotting, bacteria, and rheumatoid factor.

Appearance. The color and clarity of the synovial fluid are aids to diagnosis. The normal fluid is straw-colored or lighter. In osteoarthritis it will be yellow to amber and clear. Cloudy synovial fluid with a greenish tinge is indicative of rheumatoid arthritis. In gout the fluid will be milky white.

Viscosity. One test of viscosity is the "sink" test in which a sample of synovial fluid is dripped slowly from a syringe. In osteoarthritis the fluid strings out as much as 3 inches; in rheumatoid arthritis, it drops rapidly like water. Another test is to place a drop of synovial fluid on the thumb and touch it with the index finger. When the fingers are separated, the fluid produces a string up to 2 inches before breaking if the viscosity is normal.

Cell Counts. Cells must be counted quickly to avoid clotting of fibrin. Do not use ordinary white blood cell diluent but physiologic saline solution (0.9 percent). If the fluid is bloody, use hypertonic saline solution (0.3 percent) to take out the red blood cells. Count in a regular whole blood counting chamber.

Mucin Clot. Synovial fluid added to acetic acid produces a clot. For the Ropes test, add a few drops of fluid to about 20 cc of 5 percent acetic acid in a beaker. Allow a minute for the clot to form and then shake the beaker. A good clot is seen in osteoarthritis—a firm ropy mass that does not fragment on shaking. In rheumatoid arthritis a poor clot, tending to break up into flakes, is formed.

Culture. The fluid should be cultured for tuberculosis bacilli and pyrogens. A differential diagnosis may be suggested by the synovial fluid.

Immunologic Tests. The joint fluid can be tested for rheumatoid factor, using the latex fixation test. The sensitized sheep cell agglutination test may also be of value in detecting rheumatoid factor. Complement may also be tested for in joint fluid. The synovial fluid levels of complement tend to be low in rheumatoid arthritis.

Roentgenograms

Early in rheumatoid arthritis roentgenograms of the joints are of little diagnostic value, but they are of value if the disease has been present for a period of time because of their characteristic findings. In the early stages of the disease the radiologic findings may be variable and nonspecific (Fig. 1-8). The disease may affect any joint but has a predilection for the smaller joints of the hands, wrists, and feet. Its progression is usually symmetrical, although one side may be affected earlier than the other. The cervical spine may also be involved, especially in the upper region.

Soft tissue changes tend to produce swelling about the ulnar head and the finger joints, but can involve any of the tendon sheaths.

Osteoporosis is characteristic of rheumatoid arthritis and tends to involve the bones adjacent to the joint (Fig. 1-9).

Periosteal elevation and bone formation are observed at times adjacent to the involved joints or at tendon insertions. These are early signs of the disease and may be due to inflammation of the syn-

Table 1-3 *Synovial Fluid Analysis in Arthritis*

	Appearance	Viscosity	Cell Count	Mucin Clot	Urate Crystals	Cartilage Fibers	Bacteria	Rheumatoid Factor
Normal	Straw-clear	High	200–600 WBC 25% Neutrophils	Good	0	0	0	0
Traumatic arthritis	Cloudy Yellow-bloody	High	Many RBC 2000 WBC 30% Neutrophils	Good	0	0 or +	0	0
Osteoarthritis	Yellow Clear	High	1000± WBC 20% Neutrophils	Good	0	++	0	0
Rheumatic fever	Yellow Slightly cloudy	Low	10,000± WBC 50% Neutrophils	Good	0	0	0	0
Rheumatoid arthritis	Yellow to green Cloudy	Low	15,000± WBC 65% Neutrophils	Poor	0	0	0	0 or +
Gout	Yellow to milky Cloudy	Low	12,000± WBC 60% Neutrophils	Poor	+	0	0	0
Septic arthritis	Bloody Cloudy	Low	80,000± WBC 90% Neutrophils	Poor	0	0	+	0
Tuberculous arthritis	Yellow Cloudy	Low	25,000± WBC 50–60% Neutrophils	Poor	0	0	+	0

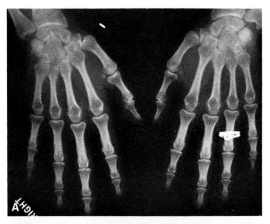

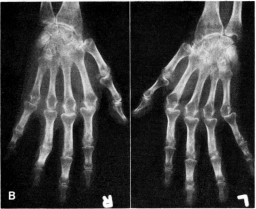

FIG. 1-8 Roentgenograms of hands of young woman with rheumatoid arthritis. A. April, 1964. Radiologic findings are nonspecific. B. April, 1974. Signs of advanced rheumatoid arthritis are ulnar drift, loss of the joint space at the metacarpal-phalangeal joints, thickening of the periosteum of the phalanges and metacarpals, and involvement of the proximal interphalangeal joints. The wrist joints also reveal cystic formation in the radius.

the subchondral bone (Fig. 1-10). The lesions may have sharp margins and appear punched out, simulating gout (Fig. 1-11). They tend to occur most often in rheumatoid arthritis at certain sites, such as the radial side of the metacarpal head, the ulnar styloid, and the navicular as well as the calcaneus near the Achilles bursa (Fig. 1-12). Punched-out lesions at the base of the phalanx are also common.

In far-advanced cases the joint surfaces will reveal sclerosis of the bone due to loss of the articular cartilage. Rheumatoid arthritis is the most common cause of multiple dislocations of the metacarpal-phalangeal joints (Fig. 1-13) and destruction of joints.

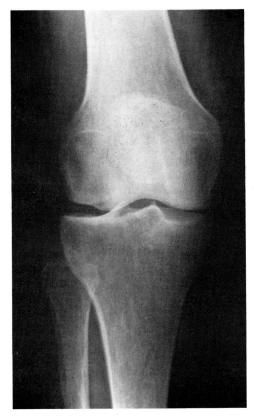

FIG. 1-9 Roentgenogram of the knee revealing osteoporosis of the tibia, thinning of the cortical margins, and changes in the lateral femoral condyle. Early subchondral change is also noted on the medial femoral condyle and the tibial plateau.

ovium and capsule where these structures attach to the periosteum. This type of linear new bone formation is not observed in osteoarthritis.

Bone erosion is the most definitive radiologic sign, and it implies the removal of bone substance. This tends to occur in rheumatoid arthritis at the joint margin where the articular cartilage ends and the synovial lining begins. This erosion is due to the pannus growing over the surface of the cartilage and into

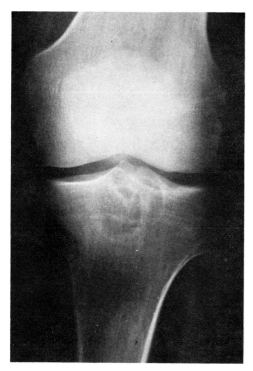

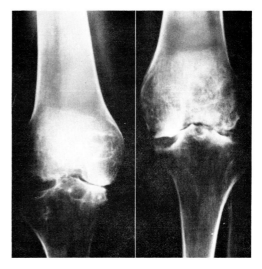

FIG. 1-11 Roentgenograms revealing destruction of both knees due to rheumatoid arthritis. Multiple punched-out lesions and erosions of the subchondral bone are evident, as is loss of joint space.

FIG. 1-10 Roentgenogram revealing erosion and cystic formation in the adjacent bony surfaces of knee joint. A large cyst has developed in the proximal tibia due to synovial invasion.

Differential Diagnosis

Some of the common diseases that should be differentiated from rheumatoid arthritis are the following:

Osteoarthritis
Tuberculosis of joints
Rheumatic fever
Infectious arthritis
Gout
Traumatic arthritis
Lupus erythematosus

The most common diagnostic problem is distinguishing between osteoarthritis and rheumatoid arthritis. Osteoarthritis usually occurs in patients over the age of 45 who are generally overweight and most often tends to involve the weight-bearing joints. In the hands, the distal interphalangeal joints are most commonly involved in osteoarthritis as compared to the metacarpal phalangeal joints in rheumatoid arthritis (Fig. 1-14).

Loss of the joint space due to destruction of the articular cartilage is frequently observed in rheumatoid arthritis. In contrast to osteoarthritis in which the one area of the joint which bears the most stress is most affected, generally the entire joint surface is involved (Fig. 1-15). The earliest sign of rheumatoid arthritis is the loss of a fine line of compact subchondral bone.

Variants of Rheumatoid Arthritis

A number of variants of rheumatoid disease exist.

Juvenile rheumatoid arthritis—also called Still's disease. This condition is essentially rheumatoid arthritis in a child, but it has several characteristics that are different from the adult disease. Spinal involvement and growth disturbances are common, as well as an absence of the rheumatoid factor.

Felty's syndrome—rheumatoid arthri-

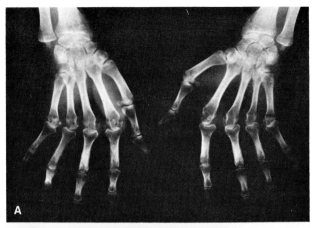

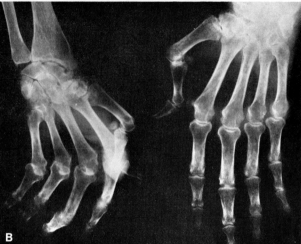

FIG. 1-12 Roentgenograms revealing changes in hands due to rheumatoid arthritis. A. Typical destruction of the radial side of the metacarpal. There are ulnar drift and loss of the joint space at the metacarpal-phalangeal joints and adjacent osteoporosis. B. Punched-out lesions in the navicular, as well as the base of the thumb, in the right hand. Destruction of the carpal bones is seen in the left wrist.

tis associated with hypersplenism, leukopenia, thrombocytopenia, and anemia.

Palindromic rheumatism—often a migrating polyarthritis with acute attacks of hydrathrosis, usually involving the large joints. Frequent remissions with rheumatoid factor absent.

Caplan's syndrome—a variant of rheumatoid arthritis associated with lung lesions.

Sjögren's syndrome (or Sicca syndrome)—rheumatoid arthritis with involvement of the eyes, nose, and tracheal tree which suffer from a lack of secretions.

Rheumatoid vasculitis—rheumatoid arthritis with a severe polyarthritis, thrombosis, gangrene, and high titers of rheumatoid factor.

Arthritis and agammaglobulinemia—rheumatoid arthritis associated with a complete lack of gamma globulin.

Psoriatic arthritis—believed by many to be a variant of rheumatoid arthritis in patients with psoriasis (Fig. 1-16). Psoriasis is often associated with arthritis and tends to involve the distal interphalangeal joints more often than the proximal.

Rheumatoid Spondylitis (or Marie-

Strümpel disease)—believed to be a different syndrome and not a variant of rheumatoid arthritis. It is ten times more common in young males than in women and tends to involve primarily the spine and sacroiliac joints. At times it may involve the large proximal joints of the body but not the peripheral joints such as the hands and feet. Both the spine and the thorax may become completely rigid.

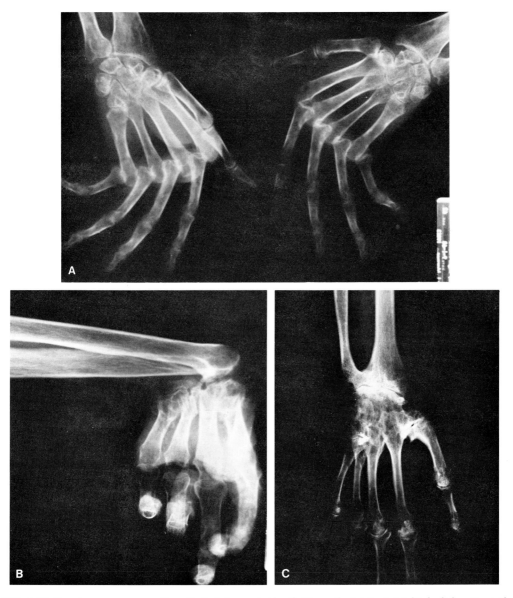

FIG. 1-13 Roentgenograms revealing effect of rheumatoid arthritis on the joints. A. Multiple dislocations of the metacarpal-phalangeal joints. Osteoporosis with thinning of the cortex, cystic changes within the metacarpal and phalangeal bones, and ulnar drift are obvious. B. Severe destruction of the joint. The carpal bones have disintegrated and disappeared, leaving the wrist flail. C. Spontaneous fusion of the carpal bones. Note the synostosis of the radius and ulna.

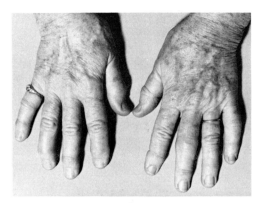

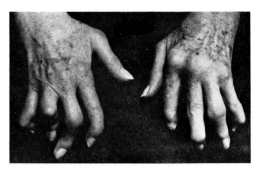

FIG. 1-16 Typical psoriatic changes in the nails with rheumatoid arthritis of the hands. Ulnar drift tends to occur with involvement of the metacarpal-phalangeal joint as seen in the left hand.

FIG. 1-14 Photograph of hands of patient with osteoarthritis. Note involvement of the distal interphalangeal joints with minimal involvement of the proximal interphalangeal joints, Heberden's nodes on the distal interphalangeal joints, and swelling of the middle and fifth fingers of the left hand.

Bibliography

Berens, D. L., et al.: Roentgen changes in early rheumatoid arthritis. Radiology, 82:645, 1964.

Berkson, D. A., and Pearson, C. M.: Laboratory procedures. J. Am. Phys. Ther. Ass., 44:699, 1964.

Bywaters, E. G. L.: The early radiological signs of rheumatoid arthritis. Bull. Rheum. Dis., 11:231, 1960.

Cracchiolo, A. III, and Barnett, E. V.: The role of immunological tests in routine synovial fluid analysis. J. Bone Joint Surg., 54-A:828, 1972.

Decker, J. L.: Rheumatoid arthritis. Clin. Trends in Rheumatology, 2:1, 1971.

Ferguson, A. B.: Roentgenographic features of rheumatoid arthritis. J. Bone Joint Surg., 18:297, 1936.

Freyberg, R. H.: Differential diagnosis of arthritis. Postgraduate Med., 51:8, 1972.

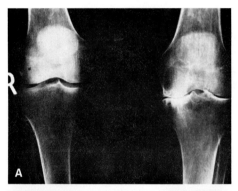

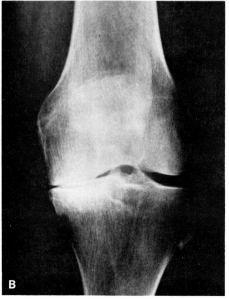

FIG. 1-15 Roentgenograms revealing loss of joint space. A. Rheumatoid arthritis. Observe loss of space on both sides of the left knee joint and the early development of a varus deformity. B. Osteoarthritis. Narrowing of the medial joint space involving the medial compartment of the knee with an essentially normal lateral compartment is typical.

Kodama, T.: Some clinical aspects of rheumatoid arthritis. Acta Med. Okayama, *13*:137, 1959.

Kulka, J. P., et al.: Early joint lesions of rheumatoid arthritis. Arch. Pathol. (Chicago), *59*:129, 1955.

Lawrence, J. S.: Genetics of rheumatoid factor and rheumatoid arthritis. Clin. Exp. Immunol., *2*:769, 1967.

Martel, W.: The pattern of rheumatoid arthritis in the hand and wrist. Radiol. Clin. North Am., *2*:221, 1964.

Mellors, R. C.: Virus-like agent. Bull. Rheum. Dis., *17*:429, 1966.

Ropes, M. W., and Bauer, W.: Synovial Fluid Changes in Joint Disease. Cambridge, Harvard University Press, 1953.

Seth-Smith, D. W.: The differential diagnosis of rheumatic conditions by radiology. Rheumatism, *15*:44, 1959.

Soila, P., and Oka, M.: Roentgen manifestations of senile rheumatoid arthritis. Acta Rheum. Scand., *5*:206, 1959.

Warren, S. L., et al.: An active agent from human rheumatoid arthritis which is transmissible in mice. Arch. Intern. Med., *124*:629, 1969.

Zvaifler, N. J., and Martinez, M. M.: Antinuclear factors and chronic articular inflammation. Clin. Exp. Immunol., *8*:271, 1971.

2 | Osteoarthritis

Osteoarthritis is a degenerative disease of the joints and is related to the destruction of the articular cartilage. It existed in prehistoric man and was noted in the American Indian prior to the arrival of the white man. Examination of skeletons from a study in Alabama revealed that spinal osteoarthritis was present in the young population that did heavy work. Approximately 40 million Americans have radiologic evidence of osteoarthritis and approximately 5 percent of the persons above 50 years of age also have symptoms of osteoarthritis. Although osteoarthritis is a common disease, it is one that has not received much attention in regard to the surgical correction of deformities and relief of pain.

In the past, conservative therapy was generally the method of choice, but with the rapid advances in orthopaedic surgery, treatment has changed quite rapidly. The clinical symptoms, radiologic findings, and treatment for osteoarthritis of each joint will be discussed in more detail later in the book.

Etiology

Osteoarthritis has various causes, and it has been customary to divide the disease into idiopathic (primary) and secondary types. Degeneration of a previously normal joint is spoken of as idiopathic disease.

The classification of various forms of osteoarthritis has been confusing because many studies were done at post mortem when the disease was inactive. Stecher studied the various types of Heberden's nodes and has distinguished between traumatic and idiopathic forms of osteoarthritis. He believes that osteoarthritis is a disease that appears clinically in one joint or a pair of joints and that osteoarthritis occurring in several joints is unrelated and not a generalized disease.

There is no evidence that the changes in the primary and secondary osteoarthritis are in any way different from each other, and all degenerative changes appear to be related as part of the same process. It is believed by some that obesity, trauma, and microtrauma may be possible causative factors, and by others that osteoarthritis may be due to genetic factors. Often there is a family history of arthritis. Stecher and others stated that certain structural factors may lead to alteration in the degradation of enzymes and also in the rate of poly-saccharide synthesis. It is no longer believed that "wear-and-tear" or the aging process is the only factor in the etiology of osteoarthritis.

Pathology

The essential feature of osteoarthritis is a breakdown and loss of the articular cartilage. The earliest gross changes observed in a joint are minute ulcera-tions in the hyaline cartilage that pri-marily affect the intercellular matrix. Erosions develop in the cartilage and extend to the osteocartilaginous border, and fragments of cartilage often break loose. Since hyaline cartilage does not have the ability to regenerate, loss of the cartilage leads to exposure of the bone which eventually becomes sclerotic from pressure (Fig. 2-1).

Osteoarthritis in some stages can be extremely erosive, destroying the joints and producing severe pain in the hand (see Chapter 8). This type of disease is called erosive osteoarthritis because of the prominent early osteophyte forma-tion, cartilage destruction, and juxta-articular erosion.

Gross examination of knee joints of people over 40 years of age frequently reveals loss of the smooth glistening appearance of the articular cartilage. Chondromalacia is often observed and is associated with fibrillation. At the bony

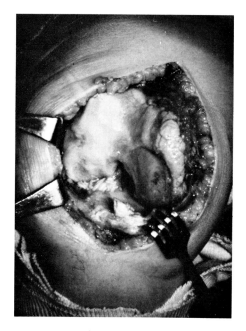

FIG. 2-1 Surgical view of knee joint illustrating the destruction of the articular cartilage in osteo-arthritis. The medial compartment has been eroded down to sclerotic bone with large osteophyte for-mations along the medial condyle. The lateral compartment shows evidence of loss of the articu-lar cartilage in small areas.

margin one frequently sees proliferative changes leading to the formation of osteophytes. These are believed to be attempts at repair of the degenerated articular surface. Early in osteoarthritis the synovial tissue may have an inflam-matory component (Fig. 2-2), but late in the disease the synovium is usually atrophic. This type of activity often can be confused with active rheumatoid disease.

At the histologic level, a loss of matrix staining is noted, which is be-lieved due to the escape of mucopoly-saccharide and the appearance of multi-ple groups of cartilage cells in the deep layers. The mechanism of this disintegra-tion is not known at the present time and is under investigation. In the marrow cavity beneath the subchondral bone hypervascularization occurs, and there

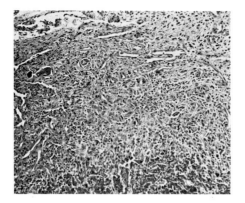

FIG. 2-2 Microscopic appearance of synovial tissue in a patient with active synovitis due to osteoarthritis.

is proliferation of fibrous tissue. The blood vessels may penetrate the subchondral bone and extend into the cartilage. Two processes go on in this area of the joint: one is loss of bony substance leading to cyst formation, and the other is deposition of bone beneath the worn-out cartilage to produce sclerosis and increase the density of the bone. These two phenomena result in the usual radiologic changes seen in osteoarthritis, namely, bone sclerosis and cyst formation (Fig. 2-3).

It has been suggested that each joint may have its own pattern of degenera-

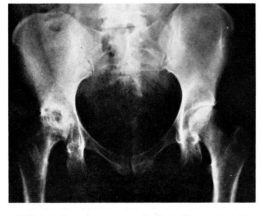

FIG. 2-3 Roentgenogram of pelvis illustrating sclerosis and cystic formation involving the acetabulum and the femoral head of the right hip.

tion and that degenerative changes begin in particular regions of the cartilage and then undergo a certain sequence of changes.

Diagnosis

The clinical picture of osteoarthritis may vary in severity and in the joints that are involved. The symptoms of osteoarthritis are generally local in character. Occasionally some patients may have multiple joint complaints, but these are unusual. Degenerative changes tend to begin early in life, but the patient is usually not aware of the symptoms for many years until the articular cartilage destruction is far advanced. About the age of 45, symptoms make their first appearance. The onset is gradual, and the patient complains of stiffness, aching, and crepitation in the joint. Some patients have acute inflammatory episodes that are accompanied by severe pain, increased heat in the joint, and swelling. These episodes tend to occur frequently in the knee joint and may not be associated with any history of trauma. Heberden's nodes may often become extremely painful during their formation (Fig. 2-4). Most patients tend to overlook the minor changes and complaints until the stiffness and pain become so annoying that they interfere with normal joint function. The most important symptom of this disease, therefore, is pain that occurs with use and is relieved by rest. The pain generally is aching in character and is rarely intense or severe, until the disease process has been present for many years. The patient will often complain of stiffness, especially after sitting, and may have difficulty taking the first few steps. This stiffness tends to decrease with use and does not persist as

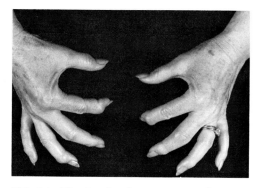

FIG. 2-4 The hands of a woman with osteoarthritis involving the distal interphalangeal joints and producing Heberden's nodes.

long as it does in rheumatoid patients who have a gelling component.

A generalized form of osteoarthritis also exists in some patients with involvement of the cervical spine, wrists, hands, hips, knees, and often the first metatarsal-phalangeal joint (Fig. 2-5). Not all of the joints may be involved, nor may they all be symptomatic at the same time. There is also no correlation between the radiologic appearance of severe degenerative disease and the patient's symptoms. Patients whose roentgenograms reveal minimal involvement may have severe symptoms.

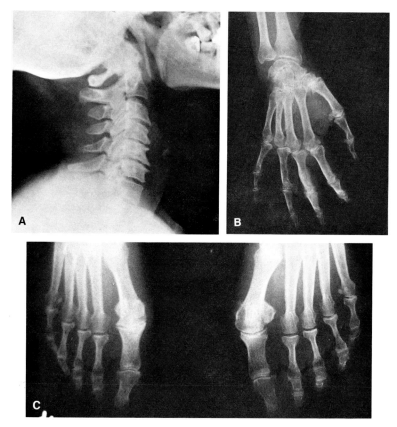

FIG. 2-5 Roentgenograms illustrating generalized osteoarthritis with involvement of multiple areas in the body. A. Advanced osteoarthritis of the cervical spine. B. Osteoarthritis in the carpal-metacarpal joint of the thumb, the distal interphalangeal joints, and the proximal joints of the hand. C. Osteoarthritis in the great toe joints with evidence of advanced disease in the metatarsal phalangeal joints simulating bunion formation.

Laboratory Findings

Laboratory tests for the patient with osteoarthritis generally are negative. The complete blood count usually is normal, and there is no evidence of anemia as is commonly found with rheumatoid arthritis. The sedimentation rate is within normal limits unless the patient has an associated disease. The serologic tests are generally normal and are of no aid in the diagnosis of osteoarthritis, except for ruling out other diseases. The rheumatoid factor is usually absent in these patients.

Aspiration of joint fluid for analysis may be of some value, especially in ruling out septic arthritis or tuberculosis. The fluid generally appears clear or slightly yellow in color and has a high viscosity. The white blood cell count is usually 1,000 and is not as high as that seen in rheumatoid arthritis, gout, or septic arthritis. The mucin clot is good as compared to the poorer one obtained in rheumatoid arthritis.

Roentgenograms

Very early in osteoarthritis, the radiologic findings may be normal or nonspecific. Although the disease may affect any joint, it has a predilection for the weight-bearing joints such as the hips, knees, cervical spine, and lumbar spine. The principal change that is seen in osteoarthritis of a joint is narrowing of the joint space and loss of the articular cartilage. One must be extremely careful in evaluating the x-ray films for osteoarthritis. It is difficult to see joint narrowing early, especially in the weight-bearing joint, unless the roentgenogram is taken with the patient in a standing position with weight applied to the joint (Fig. 2-6). Much of the joint space will disappear when weight is applied to the knee joint. In the diagnosis of osteoarthritis it may be advisable to take

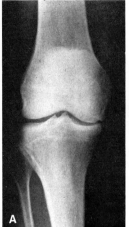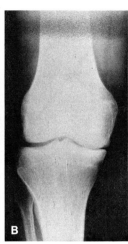

FIG. 2-6 Roentgenograms of a knee joint of a patient with early arthritis. A. Appearance when patient was not standing. A small osteophyte and erosion can be seen on the medial femoral condyle. B. Appearance when the patient was standing. Note the narrowing of the joint space indicating a loss of the articular cartilage.

roentgenograms of the hips or knees with the patient in a standing or weight-bearing position to obtain a more critical evaluation of the patient's joints.

The radiologic features tend to vary with the particular joints involved. The principal joint changes in osteoarthritis are bony sclerosis, osteophyte formation, marginal lipping, and bone cysts (Fig. 2-7). Osteoporosis of the bone adjacent

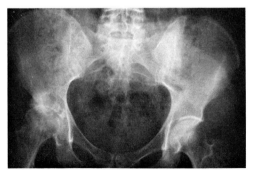

FIG. 2-7 Roentgenogram of the hip joint revealing typical findings in advanced osteoarthritis: loss of joint space, sclerosis of the adjacent bone, and cystic formation. Osteophyte formation along the acetabulum is also visible.

Table 2-1 *Osteoarthritis: Major Diagnostic Criteria*

Age:	**(Spontaneous disease)** Middle and old age.
	(Secondary to joint trauma/defects) Any age.
Major Sites:	Hips, knees, terminal (sometimes also proximal) interphalangeal joints, lumbar and cervical spine.
Symptoms:	Joint pain on motion; subsidence of pain with rest. Pain is seldom intense (except in advanced hip disease).
	Joint stiffness; is associated with resting in a fixed position. It is quickly relieved by normal activity.
	Grating sensations in affected joint.
	No constitutional symptoms. (Such symptoms are present in rheumatoid arthritis.)
	(Hip/spine) Pain may be localized or referred to the extremities.
	(Other joints) Pain is usually localized. Heberden's nodes are usually painless.
Signs:	Affected joint may appear normal.
	Joint enlargements are hard, may be slightly tender.
	Crepitus may be present.
	Joint effusion is uncommon; it is most likely to occur with knee involvement.
	Flexion and deviation deformities of fingers occur with Heberden's nodes; flexion/adduction/external rotation deformity of leg occurs with advanced osteoarthritis of the hip.
	No subcutaneous nodules (which may be present in established rheumatoid arthritis).
Laboratory Tests:	No specific tests. (In contrast to possible findings in rheumatoid arthritis: erythrocyte sedimentation rate is usually normal; anemia is usually absent; rheumatoid factors are not present; mucin test is normal or near normal.)
Roentgenogram:	Positive findings may be present in absence of clinical disease—and clinical onset may antedate positive findings.
	(Initial finding) Narrowed articular space.
	(Subsequent findings) Eburnation, osteophytes, marginal lipping, bone cysts.

to the joint is not commonly seen in osteoarthritis, but is more common in rheumatoid arthritis and infectious diseases involving the joint. Aseptic necrosis and collapse of the joint may be seen in far-advanced osteoarthritis, but can be associated with other diseases.

Differential Diagnosis

The differential diagnosis of osteoarthritis from rheumatoid arthritis and other diseases is suggested by the age of the patient, the onset of the disease, and the characteristic roentgenograms. There are no specific diagnostic criteria for osteoarthritis as there are for rheumatoid arthritis, but the characteristic radiologic picture and absence of positive laboratory tests for rheumatoid arthritis and other collagen diseases help to confirm the diagnosis of osteoarthritis (Table 2-1).

Bibliography

Chamberlain, E. B., and Taft, R. B.: Ancient arthritis. Radiology, *30:*761, 1938.

Collins, D. H.: The pathology of osteoarthritis. Br. J. Rheumat., 1:248, 1939.

Ehrlich, G. E.: Inflammatory osteoarthritis. I. The clinical syndromes. J. Chronic Dis., *25:*317, 1972.

Kellgren, J. H.: Osteoarthrosis. Arthritis Rheum., *8:*568, 1965.

Kellgren, J. H., Lawrence, J. F., and Bier, F.: Genetic factors in generalized osteoarthrosis. Ann. Rheum. Dis., 22:237, 1963.

Landells, J. W.: The bone cysts of osteoarthritis. J. Bone Joint Surg., 35-B:643, 1963.

Mankin, H. J.: Biochemical and metabolic aspects of osteoarthritis. Orthop. Clin. North Am., 2:19, 1971.

Radin, E. L., Parker, H. G., and Paul, I. L.: Pattern of degenerative arthritis: Preferential involvement of distal finger-joints. Lancet, 1:377, 1971.

Stecher, R. M.: Heredity of osteoarthritis. Arch. Phys. Med., *46:*178, 1965.

3 | Medical Treatment

A multidisciplinary approach is necessary for the treatment of rheumatoid or other forms of arthritis because effective therapy involves several medical specialties. Careful education of the patient will aid greatly in obtaining successful results. The patient should be informed about his disease and the method of treatment.

In both rheumatoid arthritis and osteoarthritis, it is important for the physician to take a strong and pleasant but positive attitude toward the treatment of the patient. This attitude will reassure the patient and instill in him the confidence that is necessary for the management of a chronic disease. It is important for the physician to realize that the patient listens carefully to every word about the prognosis. He may forget about the use of aspirin, rest, or heat, but if he is told that he must learn to live with his disease and will be unable to lead a normal life, he will be greatly disturbed. Emotional factors do play a role in therapy, but much of this problem can be alleviated by intelligent counsel from the physician.

Rheumatoid Arthritis

Since at present there is no specific therapy to cure rheumatoid arthritis, a realistic goal must be selected for each patient. It is reasonable to try to decrease the inflammation, to prevent deformity, and to maintain function. Although no curative therapy is available and the eventual course of the disease may be predetermined, one has only to see a neglected patient to realize the importance of medical supervision and care. The patient must be informed about the unpredictable course of his disease, however, and must realize that it will take time to arrive at a suitable, individualized program of therapy.

Nonspecific Management

Rest is one of the basic factors in the treatment, but it should not be total or prolonged thereby seriously hampering

25

joint function. A regular plan of general exercises should be encouraged. Exercises to prevent or reduce flexion deformities are of value. To maintain a full range of motion it is essential that the extensor muscles be developed. Muscle strength should be improved by isometric exercises; exercises to improve the patterns of motion, or "proprioceptive neuromuscular facilitation," are also of value.

Diet has frequently been mentioned in the care of rheumatoid arthritis patients, but it has never been proved to be of any specific value. The patient should receive an adequate diet with calcium-containing foods, vitamins, and high-protein content.

Climate will not cure or generally improve the patient with rheumatoid arthritis. The dry, hot climate of the desert country seems to make the patient feel a little better. A move should not be recommended primarily for the climate, since pulling up his "roots" may place additional burdens on the patient.

Anemia, which may be hypochromic due to an iron deficiency, may also be present in patients with chronic rheumatoid arthritis. Ordinarily the anemia is normochromic and will not respond to iron therapy. A trial of iron, however, is certainly indicated. The surgeon should be cognizant that most chronic rheumatoid patients have anemia, but this should not delay surgical therapy when indicated unless the anemia is severe and blood loss is anticipated. In some patients an enlarged spleen may be associated with a low white blood count. Even though the count may be below 5,000, these patients will respond to the stress of surgery, and the white count will become normal. Infection has not been a problem in these patients.

Drug Therapy

Medications for the arthritic patient should be selected with care, and potentially hazardous drugs should be avoided, if possible. Drugs should be used to decrease the inflammatory process and to relieve pain. Aspirin should be the mainstay of treatment. Other drugs may be added to control the symptoms of rheumatoid arthritis and may be used along with the aspirin rather than in place of it.

Analgesic Drugs

The best drug available at the present is *aspirin* or sodium salicylate. Salicylates are relatively safe and inexpensive and provide some relief of the pain associated with arthritis. They have been shown by Fremont-Smith and Bayles to exert an objectively demonstrable anti-inflammatory effect when given in large doses on a regular schedule to rheumatoid patients. Aspirin should be administered to the point of toxic symptoms, and then the dosage should be reduced to a lower level and continued at this level for an indefinite period. A minimal dose is about 12 tablets of 0.3 gm daily.

Delayed-release aspirin has been developed to decrease the early morning stiffness of the patient. The patient may take the delayed-release tablet upon retiring. The aspirin will be released during sleep to maintain a blood level until morning, thus relieving some of the early morning stiffness.

Aspirin does have a toxicity that is not insignificant. The main complications are gastrointestinal bleeding, tinnitus, and hearing loss. It is contraindicated in patients with a history of proven peptic ulcer, gastrointestinal bleeding, or allergy to salicylates.

Ibuprofen (Motrin) is a new drug that has been released for relief of the painful symptoms of rheumatoid arthritis and may eventually find a place in the treatment of the rheumatoid patient. The drug has been compared to aspirin and is better tolerated in patients who have a gastrointestinal intolerance to aspirin. Ibuprofen can be administered to patients with gastrointestinal disease, but in some patients it may cause gastrointestinal distress or occasional bleeding. The drug has been reasonably effective in certain patients, but one should not expect all the patients to have a dramatic response.

The suggested dosage is 300 to 400 mg three or four times a day. Depending upon the response of the patient, the dosage may be lowered or raised. The total daily dosage should not exceed 2,400 mg, and it is better to maintain the patient on the lowest dose that gives symptomatic relief. The drug may be taken at mealtime, but it is not necessary to take the medication with food.

Adverse reactions have been noted, especially gastrointestinal discomfort, occasional gastrointestinal bleeding, and dizziness.

Other analgesic drugs may be used along with aspirin to relieve the pain of rheumatoid arthritis. Dextropropoxyphene (Darvon) has been a valuable drug for certain patients. The relief of pain obtained from this drug varies with each patient, but in some patients it can be of great benefit in relief of chronic pain. Codeine can be used in small doses to aid in control of severe symptoms and can be used at night to provide the patient with a comfortable night's sleep. It is wiser to prescribe small doses of codeine for the patient than to allow large doses of steroids to control pain. Great care, however, should be exercised in the use of narcotics to avoid addiction.

Anti-inflammatory Drugs

Patients who do not respond to the basic therapeutic plan pose a problem, since there is no general agreement as to what drugs should be added to the therapy. With the advent of cortisone a new era of medical care of the arthritic patient evolved. As experience with the steroid drugs accumulated, however, it became apparent that the side effects were extremely harmful to the patient. Therefore other anti-inflammatory drugs were developed, namely, oxyphenbutazone and indomethacin.

Oxphenbutazone (Tandearil) is related to butazolidin and has been used with success in the rheumatoid patient. It may be added as an adjunct to the salicylate therapy or in place of it. The usual dosage is 400 mg given daily divided into three or four doses after meals to prevent gastric disturbance. If a response is obtained in one week, the dosage may be reduced to a maintenance level of 100 to 200 mg daily. Because a few cases of agranulocytosis have been reported, a white cell count should be obtained at weekly intervals for one month and then bimonthly or monthly while the patient is taking the drug.

Indomethacin (Indocin) has been found effective in patients with rheumatoid arthritis and usually produces a significant decrease of pain and stiffness within 48 hours, but, if no response is noted, administration of this drug should be continued for one month before concluding that it is of no benefit, since a delayed response may occur. If a response does occur, the dosage of the aspirin or steroid given concomitantly may be reduced.

The dosage of indomethacin is 25 mg given two or three times a day. If the response is not adequate, the daily dosage should be increased by 25 mg at weekly intervals until a satisfactory response is obtained, or until a dosage of 150 to 200 mg a day is reached. If adverse reactions develop as the dosage is increased, the dosage should be decreased to a tolerated level and maintained for three to four weeks.

Indomethacin and oxyphenbutazone

are both potent anti-inflammatory drugs. Neither should be considered a simple analgesic to be administered casually. Patients must be evaluated carefully and supervised closely by the physician.

Oxyphenbutazone and indomethacin are contraindicated in patients with peptic ulcer, ulcerative colitis, or gastrointestinal disease because of their irritating effect on the gastrointestinal tract. Central nervous system effects, headache, blurred vision, edema, and dizziness have been reported with indomethacin administration.

Antimalarial Drugs

During World War II the antimalarial drugs, quinine and quinacrine, were replaced by synthetic compounds which seemed to have a beneficial effect in patients having rheumatoid arthritis. In the past 5 years, ocular changes have been described. These drugs are slowly excreted and accumulate in the body so that improvement does not occur until after 1 to 3 months' therapy. The problem is whether to use antimalarials which produce a moderate beneficial effect but in rare instances an irreversible retinopathy. These drugs should be prescribed with caution.

Of the various antimalarials available, the chloroquines have shown a definite but mild antirheumatic effect. The most popular chloroquine derivative is Plaquenil, which appears to be less toxic than Aralen, a chloroquine phosphate. The usual initial dosage is 400 to 600 mg daily; the maintenance dosage is 200 to 400 mg daily. Contraindications for the use of chloroquines are liver, kidney, or lung disease.

Corticosteroids

In 1949, when Hench and his associates described their dramatic results in rheumatoid arthritis, there was a tremendous enthusiasm for the use of steroids. It soon became evident that the steroids did not prevent the progression of the disease. These agents should not be employed until the conservative regimen has failed.

There are a number of important considerations in the use of corticosteroids systemically. These drugs should not be used as an initial agent in the treatment of the patient with rheumatoid arthritis, and they should be part of a generalized program of management for a particular patient. Conservative therapy should be given a thorough trial, and only after failure to achieve a satisfactory result should steroids be considered. The patient should be advised of the risks and problems associated with prolonged corticosteroid treatment. The following are indications for the systemic use of corticosteroids in rheumatoid arthritis:

1. Patients with severe rheumatoid arthritis that has not responded to a more conservative program.
2. Severe rheumatoid vasculitis.
3. Patients unable to continue their occupations or daily activities because of their arthritis.
4. Patients who have recently received corticosteroids and are undergoing operation or stress.

Prednisone and prednisolone were the first man-made corticosteroids that possessed increased anti-inflammatory response and reduced the tendency for retention of sodium and loss of potassium seen with naturally occurring corticosteroids. Prednisone and prednisolone, which are analogs of cortisone and cortisol, are two similar compounds that differ in chemical structure from the basic steroid only in the presence of a double bond between carbons 1 and 2. The majority of other steroid compounds available today have increased potency per milligram, but have no therapeutic advantage over prednisone, the steroid most frequently tolerated for a long period.

The dosage for prednisone is 10 mg or less daily. The initial dosage should be low—5 to 10 mg divided into two to four doses. Steroids tend to reduce pain and may prevent the need for narcotics in severe cases of rheumatoid arthritis. Care must be exercised, however, to prevent the patient from greatly increasing the dose for pain relief. A large number of complications have occurred with prolonged therapy.

Corticosteroids would be contraindicated for patients with a history of peptic ulcer, diabetes mellitus, psychiatric disturbances, severe osteoporosis, or tuberculosis.

Intra-articular Injections

Hollander and his associates in 1951 described the intrasynovial injections of inflamed arthritic joints. Since that time they have reported over 250,000 steroid injections into more than 8,000 patients. When corticosteroids are injected into joints, tendon sheaths, and the bursae of patients with rheumatoid arthritis, the response in relief of symptoms has been generally favorable. Local injections may obviate the use of oral steroids in the conservative program if only a few joints are severely affected.

The average duration of improvement in a joint will vary with the type and dosage of medication used. There have been many analogs of hydrocortisone which have been developed for intra-articular use in the past few years. Hollander has used triamcinolone hexacetonide in 500 patients with an average duration of palliation twice as long as that for any other steroid suspension. When we have used a combination of triamcinolone diacetate and triamcinolone hexacetonide, we have noted prolonged relief of symptoms following intra-articular injection. Relief has been obtained for 6 weeks and longer with this combination. The average dose has consisted of 1 cc of each drug in the larger joints. The indications for intra-articular injection of corticosteroids would therefore be as an adjunct to the conservative treatment of rheumatoid arthritis to control severely painful joints. It should be pointed out that this is only a palliative treatment for rheumatoid arthritis.

Contraindication to the local use of corticosteroids is infection in or about the joint. If the patient has no improvement from the injections, one should then consider this a contraindication to further injections. However, failure can also be due to the fact that the needle has not entered the joint space of the involved area. It is interesting to note on exploring a joint surgically that deposits of cortisone that have not been absorbed still remain in the capsule and surrounding tissue of the joint or in the ligaments. One way to be sure that the injection has reached the joint is first to inject lidocaine (Xylocaine) into the joint along with the steroids. If the patient has immediate relief of pain, one can assume that the steroids have reached the correct joint space.

If a joint remains swollen despite adequate medical therapy and local injections of steroids, surgical intervention should then be considered.

Alkylating Agents

In 1960 Vainio and Julkunen reported the use of nitrogen mustard intra-articularly for rheumatoid arthritis with an effective result in mild cases. Flatt reported that thiotepa injected into finger joints affected with rheumatoid arthritis also resulted in some clinical improvement. Howes and Jarvis injected 15 mg thiotepa powder dissolved in 3 ml sterile saline solution into 9 knee joints.

Improvement was observed clinically in all of the knee joints.

We have been using a combination of thiotepa and steroids since 1967 with dramatic results in chronic synovitis due to rheumatoid disease. Based upon the work of Arthur Brooks, we have used repeated injections of this combination at weekly intervals for a series of three injections. Our results utilizing multiple injections in this manner have improved, especially in injections of the knee joints. The results are better in patients who have no gross evidence of destruction or mechanical disruption of the joint. The dosage level that has been used for knee joints consists of 7 to 10 mg thiotepa and 40 mg of prednisolone (Hydeltra-TBA). The joint is prepared with an antiseptic solution, and under sterile technique the joint is aspirated of all fluid and then injected with 5 cc lidocaine (Xylocaine) followed by 2 cc prednisolone (Hydeltra-TBA) combined with 1 cc thiotepa. Thiotepa comes in a vial as a powder and is mixed with 2 cc sterile saline solution. Once it has been mixed, it must be kept refrigerated. If not used after 5 days, it should be discarded. The same combination may be used in smaller dosages to treat the elbow, shoulders, hip, or other joints as necessary. There have been no systemic adverse effects to this type of dosage if it is given at weekly intervals for 3 weeks. Prolonged improvement has been noted in patients. Synovitis has decreased, and symptoms have disappeared for as long as 6 months and even up to one year in certain cases. It is certainly worthwhile to consider the use of the various alkylating agents for patients who are not candidates for synovectomy or for a palliative procedure until synovectomy can be considered to arrest the disease.

Gold Therapy

The use of gold compounds in the treatment of rheumatoid arthritis has been known for over 40 years. Gold therapy has been the center of a great deal of controversy, but its popularity has been steadily increasing with the knowledge that has been gained clinically over the past 20 years.

The exact way in which gold produces a therapeutic result in rheumatoid arthritis is not known at the present time. Gold apparently tends to suppress rheumatoid arthritis and control the activity of the disease. Since gold does not repair joints, it is important to employ the drug during the active stage of rheumatoid arthritis. It can arrest the disease, preventing further destructive changes if the patient responds to the medication.

There is no firm rule for gold therapy, and one must be cognizant of the potential toxic effect of this drug. A more conservative program should be carried out first, and, if the patient does not respond to this, then gold therapy can be considered. It is hard to decide when to use gold in preference to corticosteroids. Gold has been administered to the patient with active disease that cannot be controlled and in whom multiple joints are becoming swollen and involved. When steroids are contraindicated because of a peptic ulcer, diabetes mellitus, or tuberculosis, gold may be the treatment of choice. Toxicity in gold therapy is fairly high and may be extremely serious. A severe dermititis may develop with involvement of the mouth and tongue. Nephritis, as well as blood dyscrasias, can also be produced by gold. The incidence of this toxicity can vary from 4 percent to 55 percent. In a large series toxic reactions were noted in 32 percent of the patients. At the first evidence of gold toxicity the drug should be discontinued.

The gold compound most commonly used has been Myochrysine, which is 50 percent gold in a soluble crystalline compound. The dosage schedule in an average adult consists of weekly intramuscular injections of a soluble compound of gold. The first injection is 10 mg, the second injection is 25 mg, and the third injection is 50 mg, which is continued for approximately 20 injections. If improvement occurs during this period of time, instead of discontinuing treatment it is preferred to continue with a maintenance dosage to prevent relapse. Injections of 50 mg may be given at 2-week intervals and continued for four injections at which time 50 mg can be given at 3-week intervals for four injections. Following this regimen, if the patient is doing well, 50 mg can be given at monthly intervals for several years. The concept of a maintenance dosage has developed in recent years and appears to be much better than giving a short course of twenty injections and repeating it at a later date.

Gold therapy is contraindicated for the patient who has had previous severe toxicity to gold or other heavy metals.

Improvement from gold therapy occurs slowly, and the patient should be informed of this prior to the institution of treatment. Effective therapy will decrease inflammation, lessen pain, and improve function. This form of therapy is not advised for other types of arthritis.

Physical Therapy

Physical therapy has an important place in the treatment of arthritis and is part of the total treatment and rehabilitation program. It offers a safe and effective way to relieve pain, increase circulation, improve function, relax muscles, and improve the range of motion and strength of affected joints. The proper utilization of physical therapy requires that the patient be motivated to continue therapy at home, as well as under the supervision of the therapist. The physician must know how to utilize physical therapy and also work with a knowledgeable therapist who is reassuring to the patient. Therapy can produce a limited amount of improvement in patients with severe destructive arthritis of their joints which limits them in carrying out their exercise due to pain in these joints. This type of patient will benefit greatly from physical therapy after surgical correction rather than before. It is important to point out that physical therapy may prevent the development of flexion contractures but in general will not prevent the advance of rheumatoid destruction.

The main objectives of physical therapy in arthritis are to help relieve the symptoms, prevent or correct deformities, and improve function.

Almost every form of physical therapy has been recommended in the treatment of arthritis, especially in other countries such as Japan, Germany, Russia, and France. The most commonly used modalities are heat, massage, hydrotherapy, and exercise.

Heat

Heat has been recommended for relief of pain in the arthritic patient since early medical history first was recorded. It is probably the most widely used treatment for arthritis and varies greatly in each country, as well as among physicians. The use of heat varies in regard to frequency, duration, type, and the intensity of heat. The local physiologic responses to heat are dilatation of the blood vessels, perspiration, and hyperemia. In addition to its analgesic properties, heat can relax muscles and with the increased circulation improve local nutrition.

Heat may be applied either as moist or dry heat, depending upon the modality available. Moist heat may be applied as hot fomentations that can consist of heavy Turkish towels at about 115° Farenheit or as Hydrocollator packs which maintain heat for 30 to 60 minutes. These hot packs are of great value in the treatment of acutely painful joints. A hot tub bath, a whirlpool, or the Hubbard tank may also be of value in limbering up arthritic patients.

Some patients prefer dry heat such as a heat lamp, but great care should be taken that the skin is not burned from the use of this type of energy. Diathermy and ultrasound have been used widely for the treatment of arthritis. These forms of heat tend to penetrate much deeper than the superficial heat lamp and can be of value where deep heating is required. They should not be used when metal implants are present in the patient.

Cold Packs

Cold packs have been utilized in the treatment of arthritis and bring about local effects. Cold produces cutaneous vasoconstriction, decreases cellular activity, and tends to relieve pain. In some patients who have acutely inflamed joints, the cold produces a soothing effect and tends to decrease the local tissue swelling.

Massage

Massage, which also dates back to the early days of medical history, has been used frequently in the treatment of arthritis. The personal contact between the patient and the therapist through the "laying on of hands" brings a sense of well being. Massage will stimulate sensory nerve endings and produce muscle relaxation and reflex vasodilatation. Pressure is usually given in a perpendicular manner in the direction of the long axis of the limb. One should always massage toward the trunk to help empty the venous and lymphatic channels. The movements should be slow and rhythmic and should not cause pain or discomfort. Massage may be used in rheumatoid arthritis in patients with extensive articular changes around the knees, shoulders, and hips, as well as in cervical arthritis and in elderly patients as a substitute for exercise.

Exercise

Exercise when used intelligently is the most important aspect of physical therapy. The program for complete treatment of the arthritis patient should always include exercise periods. Prolonged bed rest is bad for the arthritis patient and often leads to weakness and fatigue with atrophy of the muscles. Therapeutic exercise will aid in preserving the range of motion in the affected joints as well as in preventing muscular atrophy. Active exercise is far superior to passive, since muscle contractions are physiologic. Passive exercise in which the therapist moves the part and the patient does nothing but relax can be an aid in maintaining joint motion, but it will not contribute to the development of muscular strength. Isometric muscular contractions or muscle setting does not require the motion of the joint and can be utilized when a joint is painful or the leg is encased in a cast. It is much more advantageous to repeat these exercises frequently than to perform them once a day.

Therapeutic exercises can reduce muscular stiffness and maintain the functions of the joints even when the patient is at rest and relatively inactive. Watkins in the Department of Physical Medicine at the Massachusetts General Hospital recommends the exercise program in Table 3-1. Each patient need not do every exercise listed in this chart, but exercises can be selected according to the specific joints involved. When exercises are combined with other modalities such as heat, hydrotherapy, and massage, patients may be made much more comfortable with arthritis and can maintain a good range of motion in their joints without the development

Table 3-1 *Exercises for Arthritic Patients*

General Instructions. The proper amount of exercise and rest is essential in the treatment of most patients with arthritis. The purpose of properly performed exercise is to (a) increase the range of motion in the affected joint, (b) strengthen the muscles moving the joint, and (c) *PREVENT DEFORMITY.*

Specific exercises for each patient are to be taught and supervised by a physical therapist; the patient will then repeat exercises daily as instructed. Although details will vary for each individual depending upon the severity of the illness, the following general rules should be applied to all exercises for maximum benefit:

1. After learning the motions to be performed, begin with only one or two repetitions of each exercise and repeat two to four times daily as ordered. Every few days, when possible, gradually increase the number of repetitions of each exercise to a maximum of 10 repetitions.

2. Rest should follow each series of exercises. As improvement occurs, the rest periods will be shorter and exercise periods longer.

3. All exercise movements should be done *slowly, carefully* and *forcefully.* Each active movement should be done through as great a range of motion as is possible.

4. An increase in pain or excessive fatigue that lasts for more than 2 hours following exercise indicates that the exercise has been too strenuous, and fewer repetitions should be performed at the next exercise session.

5. Other physical therapeutic procedures such as local use of heat, hydrotherapy, and massage are often prescribed to facilitate exercise.

Shoulders
1. Supine position with elbows comfortably bent, abduct the arms to shoulder level. (*Do not allow scapular or clavicular motion.*)
2. Now from position of abduction externally rotate as far as possible. (*Point hands to head of bed.*)
3. Then internally rotate as far as possible (*point hands to foot of bed*) and return to starting position.
4. Place each palm or forearm on top of head, then bring elbows together in front and back to sides.
5. With elbows straight at sides lift arms forward and up over head to extreme elevation.
6. Use pulleys as instructed.

Elbows
1. Fully and forcefully flex and extend.
2. Repeat above exercise with hand alternately in pronation and supination.
3. Add resistance of weights to exercise 1 as instructed.

Wrists
1. With elbow flexed and fingers relaxed completely extend wrist.
2. Now fully flex wrist.
3. With elbows flexed fully supinate.
4. Now fully pronate.
5. Do radial deviation (*lateral movement towards thumb*).

Fingers
1. Make a tight fist.
2. Fully extend fingers and spread apart.
3. With distal joints of fingers relaxed fully extend at proximal joints (*metacarpal-phalangeal*).
4. Full radial deviation of thumb, then move finger in same direction individually.

Table 3-1 *Exercises for Arthritic Patients (Continued)*

	5. Oppose thumb to each finger tip, opening hand as wide as possible between each movement.
	6. Gentle assisted stretching of contractures as specified.

Neck
1. Recumbent: flatten cervical spine, chin down and in.
2. Rotate head to left and right.
3. Flex neck laterally, chin straight ahead.
4. Head traction as instructed: _____ minutes, _____ pounds.

Jaw
1. Open jaw fully.
2. Full lateral motion to both sides.
3. Protrude jaw forcefully.

Upper back
1. Lying with small towel under mid-spine, extend back against bed with knees flexed.
2. Breathe deeply with prolonged inspiration.
3. Breathe deeply against sandbag on chest.
4. Breathe deeply while stretching ribs with hands.

Low back
1. Gluteal setting. Forcefully tighten buttocks and pinch together.
2. Contract lower abdominal wall bringing pelvis up slightly.
3. Alternate straight leg raising with feet in dorsiflexion.
4. With hands behind head lift head and shoulders off bed.
5. Lying face down, raise head and shoulders off bed with back muscles.

Hips
1. Abduction in internal rotation:
   a. With knees straight and toes pointing slightly together, spread legs laterally.
   b. Standing, raise one leg, then the other, as far laterally as possible.
2. Internal rotation:
   a. Rotate entire extremity inward (*toes pointing together*).
   b. Standing, feet 12 inches apart, turn foot and leg inward and outward.
3. Fully flex the hips and knees alternating each leg.
4. Extension:
   a. Lying face down, lift thigh off bed.
   b. Standing with trunk stationary, move thigh backwards.
5. Stationary bicycle riding.

Knees
1. Extension:
   a. With pillow under knees lift heels till knees are straight without hip motion.
   b. Quadriceps setting.
   c. Sitting on edge of support, straighten leg.
   d. Repeat with weights on feet as instructed.
2. Lying face down, fully bend knee.
3. Lying face up with hips flexed, flex and extend knees as though riding bicycle.
4. Standing: mark time with full hip and knee flexion.
5. Bicycle riding as instructed.

Ankles and feet
1. Full dorsiflexion and slight inversion.
2. Repeat with toes curled downward.
3. Circling motions of ankle through dorsiflexion, inversion, plantar flexion, and eversion.

Watkins, A. L.: Therapeutic exercise in rheumatoid arthritis. Courtesy Arthritis Rheum., 2: 21, 1959.

of contractures. Good muscle tone will certainly be a valuable aid in speeding the recovery of the patient undergoing reconstructive procedures.

Splints and Braces

Some joint deformities that are apt to develop in rheumatoid arthritis can be prevented or decreased by proper protection with splints during the acute stage. Splinting is of value in relieving pain, reducing inflammation through rest, in preventing the development of contractures, and improving function. Splinting is not effective in every joint and is not always necessary. The joints that respond best to splinting are the hands, wrists, knees, ankles, neck, back, and feet. Splinting of the elbows, hips, and shoulders has not been of value in the treatment of arthritis. In the treatment of the patient with rheumatoid arthritis the joints should not be splinted for long periods of time without being put through a range of motion. Generally speaking, joints should be put through a daily range of motion to avoid contractures. It is important, however, not to force patients through a range of motion if the joint is extremely painful. Immobilization is safe in general unless a surgical procedure has been performed within the joint. If a joint is kept immobilized or splinted after an operation, contractures can develop and loss of motion will occur. Even though the patient is immobilized, it is possible to continue with isometric or muscle-setting exercises.

Plaster has been one of the most widely employed materials for making simple splints; however, the development of the thermolabile plastics has made it possible to make lightweight plastic splints. Heating the plastic in hot water allows it to be cut with scissors and molded into any shape, which it will retain as it cools. Many physical ther-apists are competent at making various types of braces and should be encouraged to aid the surgeon in making splints, especially for the hand and wrist.

In the chronic stage of rheumatoid arthritis, bracing and splinting have less to offer because, once a deformity has developed, a brace or splint cannot be expected to correct it. In the past, plaster splints and casts were used to wedge out flexion contractures that developed from muscle spasm. If the contracture is only due to muscle spasm, rest would tend to decrease the deformity and the joint would slowly straighten out by itself. However, if the contracture is due to bony irregularities in the joint itself, splinting and bracing and plaster correction will not correct the deformity. Wedging casts may do more damage than good to the joint. Forcing a knee joint, for instance, into extension by wedging a plaster cast tends to compress the soft bone, leading to deformity of the joint surfaces. More recent advances have shown that early synovectomy will prevent progressive destruction of the joint by relieving the pain and relaxing the muscle spasm, therefore alleviating the flexion contracture.

When the neck is involved in rheumatoid arthritis, instability of the cervical spine and excess motion at the atlantoaxial joint occasionally may lead to neurologic symptoms. Most frequently, however, the patient will complain of excruciating neck pain without neurologic findings. A collar may be used to support the neck and relieve a good deal of the patient's symptoms. In severe cases a cervical brace with shoulder support (four-poster) can be utilized to relieve the symptoms rapidly. Heavy cervical traction is not recommended for the rheumatoid arthritis patient, especially with involvement of the upper cervical spine.

The hand and wrist may be protected by a lightweight molded cast to maintain extension in the wrist. It may be worn as a night splint or during the day when the patient is using the extremity. The functional hand braces have not been able to prevent deformities despite their continual use by the patient. The disease will usually progress within the finger joints, gradually leading to deformity when the brace is removed.

Osteoarthritis

At the present time since the etiology of osteoarthritis is not definitely known and the disease cannot be prevented, treatment at the best is symptomatic rather than specific. The treatment in many respects is similar to that for rheumatoid arthritis, except that osteoarthritis is a much less agressive disease and is not systemic. The patient should be reassured that the disease is mainly a wearing out of the articular cartilage and that a cancer or tumor is not producing his symptoms. It is important to point out to the patient that if conservative management does fail to relieve his symptoms and if they do warrant more aggressive therapy, surgery can offer a good deal of relief and return of function. The great advances that have been made in orthopaedic surgery recently in joint implantation have opened new vistas for the arthritic patient.

Nonspecific Management

Rest should be one of the basic factors in the treatment of the patient with osteoarthritis. Every effort should be made to reduce the load upon the joint that is symptomatic. Excessive use can accelerate the degeneration within the joint and increase the patient's symptoms. A patient with osteoarthritis of the hip or knee should be encouraged to preserve the joint by avoiding prolonged use such as taking long hikes or walking. It is better to preserve the joints by limiting this type of activity. The use of a cane in hip disease will considerably reduce the load upon the painful joint and will prolong its use. Complete bed rest is not recommended in osteoarthritis, and it is important that some of the rest periods be taken in the prone as well as the supine position. This will prevent the development of hip contractures which tend to increase the patient's disability and produce functional shortening of the extremity. Isometric *exercises* should be encouraged to maintain muscle strength. *Hydrotherapy* is of definite value in the lower extremity to maintain a good range of motion.

Many types of "fad" diets, as well as the use of vitamin E and other health foods, have been suggested in the past. At the present time no clinical evidence supports any form of diet as a therapeutic aid in the treatment of osteoarthritis. It is important, however, for obese patients to lose weight to reduce the stress upon their weight-bearing joints. Many patients with osteoarthritis of the hip or knee will be overweight and never seem to be able to lose weight despite the increasing symptoms from their arthritic joint. Weight reduction is of value in alleviating their symptoms, as well as in aiding the surgeon in the surgical correction of these deformities. The patient, however, should receive an adequate diet with calcium-containing foods, vitamins, and a high protein content.

Drug Therapy

Many patients with osteoarthritis may be managed without drug therapy for long periods of time following the onset of their disease. It is important to avoid the use of potentially hazardous drugs in osteoarthritis because it is not as destructive a disease as rheumatoid arthritis. The use of systemic cortisone should be avoided in the management of the patient with osteoarthritis because the cortisone drugs tend to suppress inflammatory reactions. Generally in osteoarthritis the articular cartilage, not the synovium, is involved. The local injection of steroids into an osteoarthritic joint often can bring dramatic relief. This type of steroid therapy is recommended, and only the systemic type of oral or intramuscular injection of corticosteroids should be avoided. It is important to remember that drug therapy does not cure the disease and cannot replace the destroyed articular cartilage. In many cases it can relieve the pain and allow the patient to be more active. The side effects of the more potent anti-inflammatory drugs should be weighed against the symptoms of the patient to determine whether steroids should be utilized in that particular case.

Analgesics

Aspirin still remains one of the best drugs available for the treatment of osteoarthritis, as it does in rheumatoid arthritis. Aspirin or acetylsalicylic acid is an anti-inflammatory drug, as well as an analgesic drug. The proper use of aspirin, however, requires that the patient understand the problems associated with aspirin therapy. It is important to realize that aspirin is excreted rapidly in the urinary tract, and therefore a high dose must be given frequently to maintain an effective blood level. Ten grains of aspirin every 4 to 6 hours will often produce a therapeutic effect. If symptoms are not relieved by this dosage and the patient can tolerate a higher level of aspirin therapy, the dosage can be increased to three or four 5-grain aspirins at a time. If tinnitus or loss of hearing should develop, the aspirin level can be lowered until these symptoms disappear.

Many patients cannot tolerate aspirin in this dosage due to gastric upset and indigestion. Therefore, buffered aspirin or enteric-coated aspirin is of value. In some patients, aspirin can cause bleeding due to its effect on the platelets, and therefore it may have to be discontinued. In certain extremely sensitive patients, aspirin will produce bleeding into the joint with minimal trauma. If gross blood is aspirated from a joint, one should at least consider aspirin as a cause in the patient who has been on heavy dosages of aspirin. The use of ibuprofen (Motrin) as a substitute for aspirin has been discussed on page 26.

Other medications can be added to the aspirin program. Darvon, 65 mg, gives excellent relief of symptoms in many patients. Minimal side effects have been noted with the use of this drug combined with large doses of aspirin. Small doses of codeine may also be used in patients with severe pain, but the stronger narcotics should be avoided in chronic cases to prevent addiction. One should not be afraid to give small doses of codeine to the severely arthritic patient in the older age group who cannot tolerate surgery or who has other contraindications such as failure of the cardiovascular system or general health.

Anti-inflammatory Drugs

Several anti-inflammatory drugs can be utilized in osteoarthritis. Their basic effect is on the inflammatory process taking place in the synovial tissue. In the far advanced case with marked sclerosis of the joint evident on a roentgenogram, one finds very little evidence of active synovial inflammation. Our experience with anti-inflammatory drugs is that they are most useful in the early case of acute osteoarthritis.

Oxyphenbutazone (Tandearil) and phenbutazone (Butazolidin) have been widely used in the management of osteo-arthritis. One of these drugs may be added to the salicylate therapy or in place of it. The usual dosage is 400 mg divided into doses of 100 mg four times a day. This is maintained approximately 5 to 7 days, at which time the dosage is decreased to 100 mg twice a day. Since some cases of aplastic anemia have been reported, the white blood cell count should be checked weekly for approx-imately one month, then bimonthly or monthly while the patient is taking the drug. If the white blood cell count drops below normal, the drug should be dis-continued immediately. It is important to stress to the patient that the original loading dosage is necessary and that the maintenance dosage must be faithfully carried out to maintain the proper blood level in order to obtain a satisfactory result. A history of peptic ulcer would be a contraindication to the use of this drug. Occasionally, rapid increase of weight due to the retention of fluid is seen while the patient is on this drug. As soon as the drug is stopped, the patient will have diuresis.

Indomethacin (Indocin) has received a great deal of attention in the treatment of the patient with osteoarthritis. The effectiveness of this drug varies with the patient, and although there have been many reports of excellent results with the use of indomethacin in osteoarthritis, each case will have to be evaluated on its own merits. On stopping the indometha-cin, a number of patients have noted an increase in their symptoms; the drug was of value in their particular cases. A number of side effects have been re-ported with the use of this drug, and the physician should be aware of them when prescribing the medication. The most frequent side reactions to watch for are gastrointestinal disturbance, gastro-intestinal bleeding, headaches, and dizziness.

It is suggested that the patient be started on 25 mg indomethacin at lunch and 25 mg with dinner. Taking the med-ication with food tends to minimize the gastric disturbances. Gradually the do-sage may be increased to 75 mg up to a maximum of 150 mg daily. If the patient does not respond to the dosage within several weeks, it is unusual to see a pronounced effect later on.

Physical Therapy

Physical therapy can be utilized in the treatment of osteoarthritis to relieve pain and stiffness and to improve the range of motion in the involved joint. It is not a cure for the disease, but as in rheumatoid arthritis it can benefit the patient with acute symptoms.

Probably the most effective form of therapy for relieving pain is heat, which relaxes the muscle spasm. Heat can be applied as a Hydrocollator pack, an electric heating pad, or diathermy. Gen-erally, a program at home rather than in the office of the physician or the ther-apist is much less expensive, and the patient is more likely to follow through with the treatment. Hot packs may be purchased inexpensively and used at home for long periods of time without having to be replaced. When the hands are involved, paraffin wax baths or hot water baths are of great value. Massage with the heat can aid in the relief of muscle spasm. Frequently a good deal of the patient's pain is due to the spasm rather than the irritation within the joint. Isometric exercises are much more valu-able than exercises that put stress upon the joint.

In the cervical spine, heat massage and cervical traction not to exceed 7 pounds of static pull can often give a considerable amount of relief for the patient. Range of motion exercises are not stressed as vigorously in osteo-arthritis because frequently nature will attempt to stiffen a joint to relieve the symptoms. This is especially true in the cervical spine, and it is not recommended to force motion or to manipulate the neck to continue a full range of motion. The development of a good posture is much more important.

Bibliography

Rheumatoid Arthritis

Bagnall, A. W.: Value of chloroquine in rheumatoid arthritis. Can. Med. Assoc. J., *77*:182, 1957.

Baker, F.: Rheumatoid arthritis, present day physical therapy. Calif. Med., *92*:330, 1960.

Bayles, T. B.: Gold salt therapy in rheumatoid arthritis. Med. Clin. North Am., *45*:1230, 1961.

Bayles, T. B.: Hypertrophic arthritis (degenerative joint disease). Med. Clin. North Am., *34*:1435, 1950.

Bennett, G. A., Waine, H., and Bauer, W.: Changes in the Knee Joint at Various Ages. New York, The Commonwealth Fund, 1942.

Bollet, A. J.: An essay on the biology of osteoarthritis. Arthritis Rheum., *12*:152, 1969.

Bollet, A. J.: Stimulation of protein-chondroitin sulfate synthesis by normal and ostearthritic articular cartilage. Arthritis Rheum., *11*:663, 1968.

Brooks, A.: Personal communication.

Clark, G. M.: New drugs in rheumatic disease. Arthritis Rheum., *5*:415, 1962.

Currey, H. L. F.: Intra-articular Thio-tepa in rheumatoid arthritis. Ann. Rheum. Dis., *24*:388, 1965.

Duthie, J. J. R.: Management of rheumatoid arthritis. Manit. Med. Rev., *42*:432, 1962.

Flatt, A.: Intra-articular Thio-tepa in rheumatoid disease of the hands. Rheumatism, *18*:70, 1960.

Fremont-Smith, K., and Bayles, T. B.: Sali-cylate therapy in rheumatoid arthritis. J.A.M.A., *192*:1133, 1965.

Gristina, A. G., Pace, N. A., Kantor, T. G., and Thompson, W. A. L.: Intra-articular Thio-tepa compared with depomedrol and procaine in the treatment of arthritis. J. Bone Joint Surg., *52*-A:1603, 1970.

Hartung, E. F.: The non-specific management of rheumatoid arthritis. Bull. Rheum. Dis., *15*:366, 1965.

Hollander, J. L.: The local effects of compound F (hydrocortisone) injected into joints. Bull. Rheum. Dis., *2*:3, 1951.

Hollander, J. L., Editor: Arthritis and Allied Conditions, 6th ed. Philadelphia, Lea & Febiger, 1960.

Hollander, J. L.: An attempt to rationalize therapy of rheumatic disease. Ann. N.Y. Acad. Sci., *86*:1129, 1960.

Hollander, J. L., and McCarty, D. J.: Arthritis, 8th ed. Philadelphia, Lea & Febiger, 1972.

Howes, R. G., and Jarvis, B.: The effects of intra-articular Thio-tepa on synovial fluids. Arthritis Rheum., *8*:495, 1965.

Hume, R., Currie, W. J. C., and Tennant, M.: Anemia of rheumatoid arthritis and iron therapy. Ann. Rheum. Dis., *24*:451, 1965.

Kelly, M.: The correction and prevention of deformity in rheumatoid arthritis. Can. Med. Assoc. J., *81*:827, 1959.

Knott, M.: Neuromuscular facilitation in the treatment of rheumatoid arthritis. J. Am. Phys. Ther. Assoc., *44*:737, 1964.

Knott, M., and Voss, D. E.: Proprioceptive Neuromuscular Facilitation: Patterns and Techniques. New York, Paul B. Hoeber, Inc., 1956.

Lockie, L. M.: Steroid therapy in rheumatoid arthritis. J.A.M.A., *170*:1063, 1959.

Lugiato, P. E.: Arthritis deformans of the hip joint and its pathologic histology. J. Bone Joint Surg., *30*-A:895, 1948.

Martin, G. M., Lowman, E. W., and Kammerer, W. H.: Physical medicine in rheumatoid arthritis. Arthritis Rheum., *6*:177, 1963.

McEwen, C.: The management of rheumatoid arthritis. Manit. Med. Rev., *44*:545, 1964.

McEwen, C.: Management of rheumatoid arthritis. Mod. Treat., *1*:1171, 1964.

Percy, J. S., Stephenson, P., and Thompson, M.: Indomethacin in the treatment of rheumatic diseases. Ann. Rheum. Dis., *23*:226, 1964.

Peter, J. B., Pearson, C. M., and Marmor, L.: Erosive osteoarthritis of the hands. Arthritis Rheum., *9*:365, 1966.

Primer on the Rheumatic Disease, 5 ed., J.A.M.A., *171*:1205, 1959.

Rhinelander, F. W.: The effectiveness of splinting and bracing on rheumatoid arthritis. Arthritis Rheum., *2*:270, 1959.

Rotstein, J.: Simple Splinting; Philadelphia, W. B. Saunders Co., 1965.

Scherbel, A. L., and Harrison, J. W.: Chemotherapy in rheumatoid arthritis. Postgrad. Med., *26*:857, 1959.

Seltzer, C. C.: Anthropometry and arthritis. Medicine, *22*:163, 1943.

Short, C. L., and Bauer, W.: The course of rheumatoid arthritis in patients receiving simple medical and orthopaedic measures. N. Engl. J. Med., *238*:142, 1948.

Smith, R. T.: Effective antirheumatoid gold therapy. A.I.R., *6*:60, 1963.

Smyth, C. J.: Indomethacin in rheumatoid arthritis. Arthritis Rheum., *8*:921, 1965.

Stecher, R. M.: Heberden's nodes: the incidence of hypertrophic arthritis of the fingers. J.A.M.A., *115*:2024, 1940.

Stecher, R. M.: Heberden's nodes—heredity in hypertrophic arthritis of the finger joints. Am. J. Med. Sci., *201*:801, 1941.

Steinbrocker, O., and Argyros, T. G.: Phenyl-butazone as a therapeutic agent in rheumatic diseases. Arthritis Rheum., *3*:368, 1960.

Stolzer, B. L., et al.: Intra-articular injections of adrenocorticosteroids in patients with arthritis. Pa. Med. J., *65*:911, 1962.

Ungar, G., Damgaard, E., and Hummel, F. P.: Action of salicylates and related drugs on inflammation. Am. J. Physiol., *171*:545, 1952.

Vainio, K., and Julkunen, M.: Intra-articular nitrogen mustard treatment of rheumatoid arthritis. Acta Rheum. Scand., *6*:25, 1960.

Wanka, J., et al.: Indomethacin in rheumatic diseases. Ann. Rheum. Dis., *23*:218, 1964.

Watkins, A. L.: Therapeutic exercise in rheumatoid arthritis. Arthritis Rheum., *2*:21, 1959.

Wood, P. H. N.: Salicylates. Bull. Rheum. Dis., *13*:297, 1963.

Zuckner, J., et al.: Evaluation of intra-articular Thio-tepa in rheumatoid arthritis. Ann. Rheum. Dis., *25*:178, 1966.

Osteoarthritis

Howell, D. S., et al.: A comprehensive regimen for osteoarthritis. Med. Clin. North Am., *55*:457, 1971.

Nebo, F.: Drug therapy for osteoarthritis of the spine. Rheumatism, *20*:67, 1964.

Stillman, J. S.: Medical management of osteoarthritis. Postgrad. Med., *51*:44, 1972.

Ungar, G., Damgaard, E., and Hummel, F. P.: Action of salicylates and related drugs on inflammation. Am. J. Physiol., *171*:545, 1952.

Wood, P. H. N.: Salicylates. Bull. Rheum. Dis., *13*:297, 1963.

4 | Surgical Treatment

The team approach in the treatment of arthritis has led to early consultation between the internist and the orthopaedist. No longer are surgical procedures considered the last resort to be used only for patients with severe destruction in their joints. More and more the surgical treatment of both rheumatoid arthritis and osteoarthritis is being considered one of the forms of therapy to be used along with medical therapy.

Specific details about surgical correction of rheumatoid and osteoarthritis deformities will be discussed in chapters relating to specific joints. In this chapter some general principles will be considered.

One of the most important factors in the outcome of the surgery, besides the skill of the surgeon, is the cooperation of the patient. In general, the patient who is forced into the operation by the physician or the family is a poor risk. Flatt has stated that, "It is pointless to try to sell a patient an operation; the long-term results are far too uncertain to justify any pressure being exerted." One of the best methods of encouraging patients is to have them meet other patients who have

had surgery. An excellent way to do this is to have a physical therapy clinic in which all the rheumatoid patients gather for pre- and postoperative care. The recalcitrant patient will soon be demanding surgery after seeing the other patients. It is extremely important to gain the cooperation of the patient before operation because his postoperative course will then be much smoother and the result will be better.

If the patient is in generally good health, despite his age, surgery can be performed with the expectation of a reasonable result. Older patients who have had arthritis for a long time are used to having pain and therefore usually are cooperative and will work hard postoperatively. The young patient often gives the most problems because of a low pain threshold and resistance to moving the joints.

The risks connected with operative therapy have been decreased considerably by modern anesthesia, excellent control of the patient's pre- and postoperative care, as well as the combined approach of an internist and a surgeon managing the patient during the hospital stay.

Rheumatoid Arthritis

The development of cortisone and other drugs, which alleviate the patient's pain and were thought to prevent the progression of the disease, held back the use of surgical treatment in the rheumatoid patient. Since it has become evident, however, that the disease progresses despite adequate medical therapy, surgery is finding its proper place. Surgery is not a cure but it is an excellent adjunct to the care of the patient and will relieve the patient's pain and correct his deformities.

Rheumatoid arthritis can be compared to appendicitis in the early 1900's when McBurney advocated removal of the appendix before it ruptured and the patient died. This was contrary to most medical thinking at that time, although it later proved to be correct. Today the same type of thinking prevails against the early surgical treatment of rheumatoid disease to prevent future deformities of the hand. Riordan has stated that "the orthopaedic surgeon has a well-defined role in the treatment of the rheumatoid patient. The arthritic process is a continuing one and in most cases, there comes a time when despite the best medical treatment joint damage occurs. Mechanical deformities cannot be improved with medication, and it remains for the orthopaedic surgeon to offer relief and the restoration of function. Too often, however, the orthopaedic surgeon does not see the arthritic until the involved joints have begun to deteriorate, or have deteriorated to such an extent that only a salvage procedure can be done. This is truly unfortunate, for orthopaedic surgery has much to offer in the early stages of the disease

when musculoskeletal damage seems imminent."

The surgical treatment of rheumatoid arthritis cannot cure rheumatoid disease but should be considered as one of the forms of therapy to be utilized along with the medical treatment. Frequently surgery is called a radical method of therapy and is delayed as long as possible. But with the passage of time, the severe deformities have continued to develop despite medical treatment, and it is becoming more evident that it is more "radical" to be "conservative" in the treatment of progressive rheumatoid disease (Fig. 4-1). When medical and nonsurgical orthopaedic care has proved to be ineffective in the early cases or when advancing destruction of the joint is evident, surgery should be considered. It used to be thought impossible to operate upon rheumatoid patients during the active stage of the disease, since it was believed that they would have exacerbation of their disease process. This has not been the general experience, however, and the surgeon need not wait for the disease to be "burned out."

Smith-Petersen, Aufranc, and Larson in 1943 were early proponents of surgery during the active phase of the disease, and although they met with: "Wait until the acute condition quiets down"; "Don't operate during the acute stage," their concept of early surgery has stood the test of time. These statements are still heard today more than three decades later. Smith-Petersen and associates stated, "The point that we are most anxious to bring home is early surgical treatment before destruction of the joint is too far advanced to allow maximum benefit from the operation." The conservative approach of rest may relieve pain and slow the disease process, but it is usually not successful in preserving function. The attitude of putting one joint to rest often jeopardizes the func-

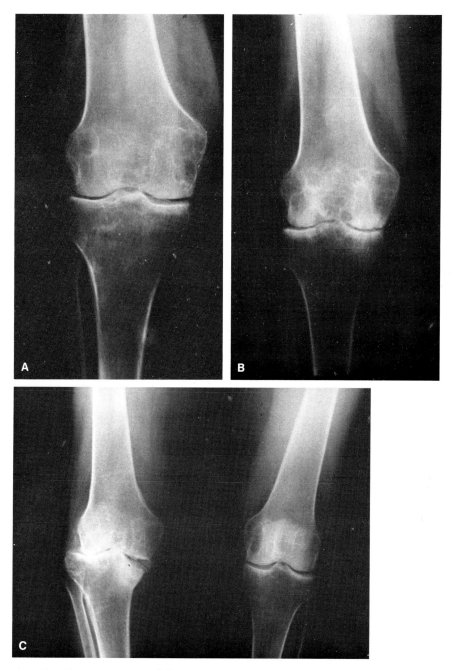

FIG. 4-1 A series of roentgenograms of the knees of a patient who was treated conservatively for rheumatoid arthritis. A. January 23, 1968. A reasonably good joint space with cyst formation taking place in the femoral condyles. Osteoporosis is evident. B. March 10, 1970. Increased cyst formation with narrowing of the joint space and beginning erosion of the articular margin due to pannus formation. C. July 24, 1972. Destruction of the tibial plateau with subluxation of the femur on the tibia.

tion of other joints, and then the treatment becomes questionable.

The operative procedures for rheumatoid arthritis can be divided into several categories. Surgery may be performed prophylactically to prevent progression and destruction of the disease within the joint when medical therapy has been unable to control the synovitis with drugs (Fig. 4-2). Surgery may also be considered for the patient with partial loss of function and pain when there is evidence of advanced changes. And finally, a salvage procedure may rehabilitate the patient with severe destruction of the joint (Fig. 4-3).

In the past there was much debate about the value of surgery in rheumatoid arthritis, but the world literature on this subject now contains numerous articles that substantiate the value of surgery in

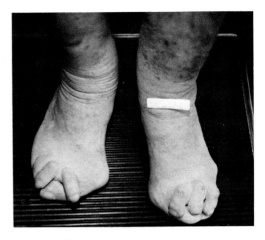

FIG. 4-3 Photograph of forefeet of patient with severe deformities due to rheumatoid arthritis.

rheumatoid arthritis. At the Rheumatism Foundation Hospital in Heinola, Finland, more than 1,000 operations are performed each year. The risks connected with operative therapy, as compared to conservative treatment, often have been overexaggerated in the past. The use of toxic drugs and steroids, for example, carries with it a number of serious complications. Many patients on steroids have had gastric hemorrhages and required gastrectomies to prevent death. Our experience, as well as that of other surgeons, has shown that there is less risk from surgery than from the more toxic drugs now being used. In our series of over 1,600 patients, there has not been a mortality due to the surgery (Table 4-1). Many patients with advanced rheumatoid arthritis are on corticosteroid therapy, but their surgical wounds will heal despite the steroids. The surgeon need not fear that cortisone therapy will prevent wound healing. We have had some difficulty with patients on large dosages of steroids, but the wounds heal extremely well despite thin, parchment-like skin. At the time of surgery it is wise to pad the legs of the patient with this type of skin, using soft roll or other protective bandages.

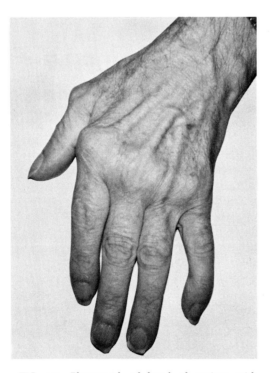

FIG. 4-2 Photograph of hand of patient with active proliferating synovitis due to rheumatoid arthritis. Despite adequate medical therapy, deformity is increasing, and surgery is indicated.

Table 4-1 *Operative Cases*

Shoulders	12
Elbows	50
Wrists	144
Hands	432
Hips	165
Knees	352
Ankles	8
Feet	416
TOTAL	1,629
Mortality	0

Since rheumatoid arthritis is a systemic disease that tends to progress despite adequate treatment, one must mention to the patient the possibility of recurrence of the deformity, as well as of the disease within the joint. The proper education of the patient about his disease and realistic expectations from surgery is important for a successful result. The patient should never be promised a normal joint, but only one that will be reasonably comfortable and perhaps improve the function. It is important to stress that the result will depend more than 50 percent upon the cooperation of the patient postoperatively to exercise and move the joint. A successful result is dependent upon an active, well-educated patient who cooperates fully.

One of the most important aspects of surgery for rheumatoid arthritis is determining the proper approach to a patient's deformities. The orthopaedic surgeon must, with the patient's aid, decide where to operate on the patient who has severe disease with multiple joint involvement. This decision is often difficult for the inexperienced surgeon when a patient with multiple joint contractures and involvement of the upper and lower extremities is brought into his office in a wheelchair. At first the situation may appear to be hopeless, but with careful evaluation of the patient's desires, one can arrive at a reasonable approach to the problem. In the severely

disabled patient, one should evaluate whether it would be feasible to try to make the patient ambulatory. Reconstruction requiring hip replacements, knee replacements, triple arthrodeses, ankle fusions, and surgery of the forefoot might be overwhelming because of the age of the patient and the family situation. This type of patient may be better off in a specialized hospital for treatment of arthritis patients. However, if the feasibility of making the patient ambulatory is small, one should then concentrate on restoration of the upper extremities to aid the patient in feeding and taking care of himself.

The shoulder, elbows, wrists, and hands should be evaluated in regard to the simplest procedures to improve function of the extremity. For the patient who is poorly motivated it is often wise to perform an operation that requires little effort by the patient to regain function. This will give the surgeon a baseline as to what kind of cooperation he will have when he attempts operations that require more active participation by the patient. For instance, excision of the ulnar head or radial head to improve pronation and supination requires little effort by the patient, and the results generally are good for relieving pain and improving function. If the patient does cooperate well, then an arthroplasty of the hand could be done at a future date. This is a valuable concept to keep in mind when dealing with a new patient.

Generally the wrist and elbow are operated upon first or in combination with the hand. If a wrist fusion is anticipated, it is wise to carry this out before doing the arthroplasty of the hand because of the postoperative swelling and the chance of developing stiffness in the fingers if the procedures are all done at one time. In the beginning it is preferable to do small procedures and not combine many procedures at one time because of the swelling that one often encounters in these patients. As the surgeon becomes more familiar with his operating speed and the procedures for various operations, combinations may then be put together, such as excision of the ulnar head, arthrodesis of the metacarpal-phalangeal joint of the thumb, and arthroplasty of the metacarpal-phalangeal joints of the hand.

Prior to the development of the total joint replacement, evaluation of the lower extremities was a difficult problem. The total hip replacement opened up new avenues for salvaging the hip joint of many severely disabled patients. In the past, before the development of a suitable total knee replacement, the surgeon would usually concentrate on trying to preserve or restore knee function because a good replacement for the knee joint was not available. Replacement of the knee joint has now become possible. In general, we have been correcting the knees first, then considering the hips, and finally the feet and ankles.

Indications for Surgery

In the past the indications for surgery varied greatly with the different arthritis centers of the country and the world because of lack of uniformity. However, with the passage of time and the accumulation of experience, the general consensus about surgery is that surgical treatment for some joints is indicated for prophylaxis and for rehabilitation, as follows:

Progressive Synovitis. If the patient has progressive, severe synovitis that does not respond to medical therapy, a synovectomy can be considered as a modality of treatment (Fig. 4-2).

Deformities. Salvage procedures can rehabilitate some patients with severe destruction of the joint (Fig. 4-3).

Loss of Function and Pain. Surgical procedures may be considered for the patient with partial loss of function and

pain when there is roentgenographic evidence of bony destruction and erosion, with or without narrowing of the joint space (Fig. 4-4).

Tenosynovitis or Bursitis. Early surgical removal of the synovium about the tendon can prevent attrition and rupture of the tendon. The severe pain of bursitis may also be relieved by the surgical excision of the inflamed bursa (Fig. 4-5).

Pain. Constant severe pain in a joint or tendon sheath can be relieved by surgery. Early synovectomy may prevent advancing destruction and also prevent the excessive use of steroids and narcotics by the patient.

Faulty Alignment. Valgus or varus deformities of the knee joint can be corrected by osteotomy of the tibia or femur, as well as by joint replacement. Flexion contractures of the knee and hip may also be corrected by surgical procedures that will improve the patient's ability to ambulate (Fig. 4-6).

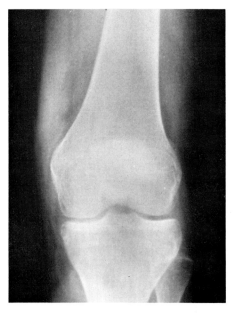

FIG. 4-4 Roentgenogram of the left knee of a young woman with active rheumatoid synovitis with slight narrowing of the joint space and beginning erosions at the articular margins. Synovectomy should be considered for this type of patient.

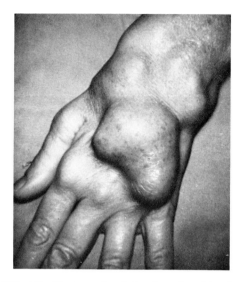

FIG. 4-5 Photograph of hand and wrist of a patient with severe synovial disease involving the dorsum.

Tendon Ruptures. Rupture of an important tendon of the hand or leg may require surgical correction to restore function (Fig. 4-7).

Nerve Compression. Entrapment of an important nerve by rheumatoid swelling can produce severe pain as well as neurologic loss of motor and sensory function. This is most common at the wrist and the carpal tunnel but also can occur at the elbow and ankle.

Stiffness of Joints. Loss of joint motion may severely handicap a patient. Ankylosis of both elbow joints can prevent a patient from taking care of most of his daily needs such as eating. Drifting of the fingers and dislocations with stiffness may prevent the patient from grasping and holding articles in his hand. Arthroplasty can be of great value in this type of patient (Fig. 4-8).

Contraindications

The main contraindication for surgery in a patient with rheumatoid arthritis is lack of motivation. This is stressed again because of the difficulties en-

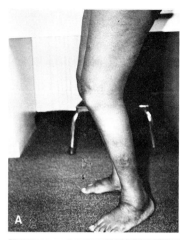

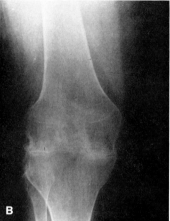

FIG. 4-6 A. Photograph of young woman with severe flexion deformities of both knee joints. B. Roentgenogram of the knee joint, showing destruction of the joint surface with fibrous ankylosis.

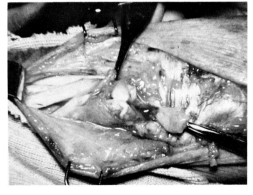

FIG. 4-7 Illustration of the dorsum of the wrist revealing a proliferative synovitis with rupture of the common extensor tendons of the wrist.

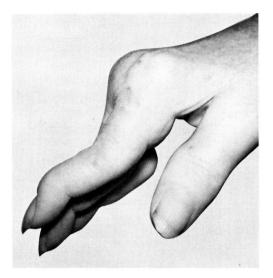

FIG. 4-8 Photograph of the typical Swan neck deformities of the fingers with dislocation of the metacarpal-phalangeal joint. This type of stiff hand is extremely inefficient, and surgery can restore function.

countered with this type of patient. It is an accepted fact that if a patient lacks strong motivation and a desire to cooperate with the postoperative rehabilitation, almost any reconstructive procedure is doomed from the start. Cooperation may be difficult to obtain from the patient with a poor home situation.

A second major contraindication for surgery in the rheumatoid arthritis patient is the patient with severe generalized disease that is extremely active and involves most joints. This type of patient will do poorly unless his active disease can be controlled by medical therapy. Synovectomy in this type of young patient frequently is doomed to failure, as the disease may recur within a short time. The result in the fulminating type of disease is disappointing to both the patient and the surgeon.

The patient in the older age group who has adapted to severe deformities often is best left with the fixed deformities. For instance, the patient with severe flexion deformities of the hips at 90° and with the knees dislocated and flexed 90° is better off in the wheelchair. Trying to reconstruct all of these joints would be unrealistic. Vainio feels that many patients with juvenile rheumatoid arthritis do amazingly well with their handicapped hands and other deformities. If they are gainfully employed, it is unwise to consider reconstruction of these joints.

The patient with severe amyloidosis generally, because of the short life expectancy, should not be considered for major reconstructive surgery. Minor procedures, however, may be carried out to aid in the rehabilitation of these patients when necessary.

Prognosis

Results to be gained from surgical procedures in rheumatoid arthritic patients depend upon many factors. The most important are the correct selection of the operation to be performed and the ability of the surgeon to perform this operation. Frequently a reasonably performed procedure in a patient who is extremely well motivated can lead to an excellent result. A well-performed operation carried out in a patient with minimal motivation will often lead to a poor or an average result. Other factors of importance are the extent of destruction of the articular cartilage within the joint, the general health of the patient, the number of joints involved, the extensiveness of the disease, and finally, the degree of fixed deformity of the tissues about the joint. It is important to realize that for the severely handicapped patient, a small increase in useful function is extremely important and gratifying. Although patients frequently state that they are not interested in cosmetic improvement, surgery is a tremendous psychologic lift, and the cosmetic improvement often is high on the list of their postoperative satisfaction. It is well recognized that surgery is performed mainly for the improvement of function and the relief of pain, but it is stressed that the cosmetic improvement should not be overlooked, especially in women who are terribly ashamed of their hands. Such women will not volunteer this information unless you specifically ask but will hide their hands in their laps or beneath their coats when you are taking the history or talking to them. In addition to lifting the patient's spirits and personality, the most dramatic change in the majority of cases has been the relief of pain following surgery. Both the patient and the surgeon are satisfied with the results.

Preoperative Preparation

The rheumatoid arthritic patient should have a complete medical evaluation prior to admission to the hospital. Many of these patients who have been on steroids for a long period of time may have developed diabetes, anemia, or ulcer symptoms which should be taken care of prior to operation. Many have a chronic anemia that cannot be corrected by iron therapy. It is not unusual to have a patient admitted with a hemoglobin of 9 to 9.5 grams. This should in no way deter the anesthetist from giving anesthesia to these patients. Although the majority of patients with rheumatoid arthritis are anemic, these patients have withstood surgical procedures very well. It is important to point out also that patients with Felty's syndrome often have a low white blood cell count of 2,000 or less. These patients, however, respond well to surgery, and infection has not been a major problem with this syndrome.

It is important in evaluating a patient for surgery to inquire carefully whether the patient has had any cortisone or one of its derivatives during the year prior to surgery. Unless one mentions some of

the drugs such as prednisone or some of the trade names, the patient will not realize he is taking cortisone. If the patient is going to have a general or spinal anesthesia, no matter how minor the operation to be performed, it is advisable to give a booster dose of steroids to aid in the stress situation. We have used Solucortef in over 500 cases without any complications. In 500 more recent cases, we have used Solumedrol to prepare our patients for surgery. The major reason for changing has been that Solumedrol costs less. Usually the patient is given 40 mg of Solumedrol intramuscularly the night before surgery and then 40 mg intravenously during the operation. The night of the operation the patient receives an additional 40 mg of Solumedrol intramuscularly. The day after operation he receives 20 mg of Solumedrol intramuscularly in the morning, and 20 mg in the evening and then resumes his routine oral medications. On the second postoperative day, the patient receives 20 mg of Solumedrol intramuscularly in the morning and 20 mg in the evening and then returns to his original preoperative routine.

We have found it advisable to discuss the operation thoroughly with the patient, explaining what is going to be done and what can be expected in the postoperative period. Whenever possible, the patient is seen preoperatively by the physical therapist for evaluation in regard to the use of crutches, modes of ambulation, and exercises to be performed postoperatively. This evaluation is advantageous, as the patient then realizes who the therapist is and is not confronted after the operation with a stranger insisting that the patient perform certain exercises and get out of bed. Whenever possible, patients who will have to use crutches postoperatively should be seen by the physical therapist as an outpatient to receive training in the use of crutches. This preoperative preparation speeds the postoperative recovery and makes it much easier for the patient. It is easier to learn how to use crutches before the operation than it is after the operation has been performed.

In the evaluation of the patient, it is advisable also to check the cervical range of motion and the ability to open the mouth because often rheumatoid arthritis will involve the cervical spine and the temporomandibular joint. If the patient has difficulty opening his mouth, as well as stiffness of the cervical spine, the problems with anesthesia rise precipitously. Therefore, whenever possible, one would consider a regional block rather than a general anesthesia in this type of patient. Many patients with rheumatoid arthritis have involvement of the upper cervical spine and have a subluxation of C1 on C2. If the patient gives a history of having a good deal of difficulty with his neck, roentgenograms are certainly worthwhile having preoperatively in flexion and extension to determine whether there is a subluxation of C1 on C2. These patients should be handled carefully on the way to the operating room, during the operative procedure, and postoperatively. Frequently a soft collar or some other form of cervical fixation is advised when these patients are being transported and being operated upon. The surgeon should advise the anesthetist of this problem preoperatively so that proper care can be instituted.

Since many rheumatoid arthritis patients have thin skin, preoperative preparation of the skin must be handled with care. Many of these patients should not be shaved because thin skin can easily be stripped from the extremity by an inexperienced aide. Vigorous scrubbing of the skin is also contraindicated in some patients with parchment-like skin. The use of plastic adherent drapes during the operative procedure is contraindicated because the skin may be torn when the drapes are removed. Many of these pitfalls can be avoided by careful planning. Once the skin is damaged or ulcerated, it may take months to heal.

Postoperative Management

Any of the usual postoperative complications may occur in the rheumatoid patient, but in general these patients respond extremely well to surgery. It is important to stress early mobilization, and the patient should be ambulatory or placed in a wheelchair as soon as possible after the operation. Active isometric exercises, deep breathing exercises, and exercises to increase range of motion of the joints will prevent many of the complications of prolonged bed rest in rheumatoid arthritis patients. Whenever possible on the night of the operation it is advisable to split any dressings down to the skin to relieve the pressure from swelling and tight bandages. It is surprising how releasing the hand or foot will relieve pain postoperatively. The use of ice bags and elevation where possible also tends to reduce swelling and relieve the patient's discomfort. Narcotics are generally not required after the second or third day by most patients. Early discharge is utilized to get patients out of the hospital as soon as possible and back into their home environments if there are suitable home situations.

Complications

One of the most common complications in the patient with severe rheumatoid arthritis is the slow healing of the skin. Frequently the skin is extremely thin from steroid therapy and tends to tear when being sutured. However, healing will occur with a minimal amount of scar in most cases. Adhesive tape and dressings should be kept off the skin whenever possible to prevent further injury.

Infection has not been a major problem in rheumatoid arthritic patients despite the use of cortisone and other drugs like azathioprine (Imuran) and cyclophosphamide (Cytoxan) that tend to depress the white cell count. When infection does occur, culture and sensitivity studies should be carried out and the proper antibiotic therapy should be instituted. Cortisone therapy should be maintained to aid the patient in meeting the stress of the situation. It is important to be sure that the steroid therapy is maintained postoperatively and to place the patient back on his original dosage of cortisone. Frequently it is possible to decrease the steroids slowly once the painful joints have been corrected by surgery.

Phlebitis and pulmonary emboli are reasonably rare in rheumatoid arthritis. In our series of over 1,600 cases there has not been a death due to a pulmonary embolus. These patients frequently take large doses of aspirin which does have an effect upon the platelets and prevents them from coagulating and producing thrombosis. For many of our patients who are not on aspirin, salicylate therapy is instituted one week preoperatively with 10 gr of aspirin four times a day. This therapy is continued postoperatively until the patient is ambulatory. Recently there have been several approaches to the prevention of postoperative thrombosis and pulmonary emboli. The most simple and the safest approach so far has been described by Sharnoff and DeBlasio. At midnight prior to surgery 10,000 units of heparin sodium are given subcutaneously, then 2,500 units are given subcutaneously following the operation, and the same amount every 6 hours until the patient is fully ambulatory. Heparin used at this dosage level will not produce postoperative hemorrhage or problems in the surgical patient. However, some recent reports contradict Sharnoff and DeBlasio's findings.

Urinary tract infection is common in the elderly female with rheumatoid arthritis. When symptoms occur, a sample of urine should be cultured, and appropriate antibiotic therapy should be started. In total joint implant patients, cultures are obtained preoperatively and if there is a growth of over 100,000 colonies, antibiotic therapy is started immediately to treat the urinary problem. Catheterization should be avoided whenever possible in both the male and female patient.

Osteoarthritis

Osteoarthritis is a common degenerative disease of the joints that can be treated by surgery when conservative treatment fails. However, it is surprising how often the patient is advised by the physician to learn to live with the disease because nothing can be done to correct the problem. This is no longer a valid statement. Much can be done to relieve the patient's symptoms and to restore function. Surgery should be considered as a method of treatment for osteoarthritis when conservative management has failed or when the patient is developing fixed deformities and losing joint function (Fig. 4-9).

The surgical treatment of osteoarthritis differs from the treatment of rheumatoid arthritis because, in many cases, the operation is definitive and tends to correct or alleviate the arthritis. The operative procedures generally are performed not to prevent progression of the disease but to relieve the patient of severe pain or to restore function where it has been lost due to contractures,

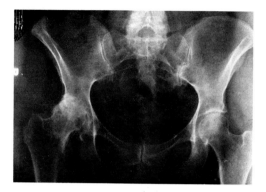

FIG. 4-9 Roentgenogram revealing advanced osteoarthritis of the right hip with loss of joint space and beginning subluxation. The patient was treated by total hip replacement.

fibrous ankylosis, or deformity of the articular surface of the joint.

Since osteoarthritis is not a systemic disease that tends to progress in various joints or to recur, the possibility of recurrence of the deformity is much less in osteoarthritis than in rheumatoid arthritis. As in rheumatoid arthritis, it is important to stress to the patient that the result will depend on his cooperation and that surgery is only 50 percent of the result; the rest is exercise and cooperation.

The evaluation of the osteoarthritic patient for surgery is much easier than that for the rheumatoid patient. Generally, only one or two joints are involved in the osteoarthritic patient. It is unusual to have multiple joints to correct and since osteoarthritis is not a progressive disease, it is much easier to arrive at a method of surgical correction. If the patient has bilateral hip disease, the most painful or deformed hip can be selected first to give the patient relief. Often the patient will make the decision for the surgeon and state which hip he prefers having operated upon. If the hip and knee on the same side are involved with arthritis, then it is probably better to do the hip first and wait until it is well healed and there is no chance of dislocation before considering knee surgery. There is no contraindication to doing the

knee first and the hip second and it would depend upon the preference of the patient as well as that of the surgeon. It is important to be sure that the patient's symptoms are not being referred to the knee from the hip. If radiologic and clinical examinations reveal disease in both joints, frequently the injection of lidocaine (Xylocaine) into one of the joints will give relief. If the pain is being referred from the hip joint, injection of Xylocaine into the hip will relieve the knee pain very quickly. If it does not relieve the knee pain, one must be sure that the injection was into the hip. If it was, then the pain in the knee is a separate entity and should be handled as such.

Indications for Surgery

Age is not a contraindication to surgery so long as the patient is in reasonably good health. The tendency has been to procrastinate and tell the patient to wait, or to think that a patient is too old when he is in his 60's. However, patients with osteoarthritis have a life expectancy well into their 70's or longer and continue to be restricted in their activities because of pain. Many patients have stated they would rather be dead than suffer the severe pain when trying to walk with a diseased hip or knee. These patients either are forced into wheelchairs and become burdens on their families because they are unable to take care of themselves or end up in nursing homes completely disabled because they cannot walk. Therefore, surgery in osteoarthritis should be performed when the indications for it exist. The development of the total joint replacement has opened up new vistas in the treatment of the aged person. Function can be restored to a joint even when it has been restricted for decades. Older patients who have had the disease for a long time are generally cooperative and will work harder postoperatively because the pain from the surgical incision is much less than their arthritic pain.

The major indication for surgery in osteoarthritis is pain. These patients suffer a tremendous amount of pain and limitation of function, especially in the weight-bearing joints. Flexion contractures, joint deformities, and ankylosis of the joint are other indications for surgical intervention. Any combination of these may exist with severe pain. The major indications for surgery for osteoarthritis in the various joints are as follows:

Shoulder. Pain is often the most common symptom of osteoarthritis in the glenohumeral joint. Several prosthetic devices are available for replacement of the articular surface of the humerus and will be discussed in Chapter 5. The acromioclavicular joint often produces symptoms of pain due to osteoarthritis involving the articular surfaces. Excision of the distal end of the clavicle will often relieve the symptoms.

Elbow. The elbow joint is subjected to a good deal of trauma from labor and sports injuries, leading to osteoarthritis and traumatic arthritis. Pain and loss of function frequently occur when the radial head is involved. Excision of the radial head and replacement with a Silastic prosthesis tends to improve motion and relieve the pain.

Wrist. Fracture of the navicular bone frequently produces arthritis of the wrist joint involving the articular surface of the radius and the navicular. Replacement of the navicular with a Silastic prosthesis has given encouraging results. Severe degenerative changes of the wrist joint can be treated by fusion of the wrist, but relief of pain is accomplished by loss of wrist motion. Localized disease of the wrist tends to occur also, producing osteoarthritis between the navicular and the trapezium (greater multangular), (Fig. 4-10). The patient will often have pain upon using the wrist and

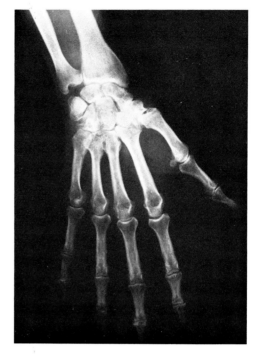

FIG. 4-10 Roentgenogram revealing loss of the joint space between the navicular and the trapezium.

trying to pinch with the thumb. It easily can be confused with arthritis of the carpal-metacarpal joint of the thumb which produces similar symptoms. Intercarpal fusion has been utilized for local carpal arthritis, and replacement of the carpal-metacarpal joint of the thumb with a Silastic trapezium has given good results (Fig. 4-11).

Hand. The hand and fingers are often involved with osteoarthritis. Heberden's nodes tend to occur at the distal interphalangeal joints, producing pain and deformities (Fig. 4-12). If the joints become unstable, function is lost in pinching. Arthrodesis of the distal interphalangeal joint is a reasonable operation to relieve the patient's pain, but it is accomplished by a loss of motion at this joint. The interphalangeal joints may also be involved in osteoarthritis, and a type of erosive disease of these joints can produce severe destruction of the hand.

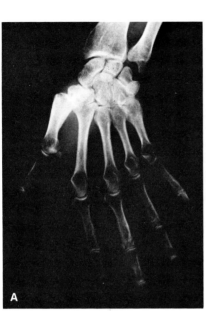
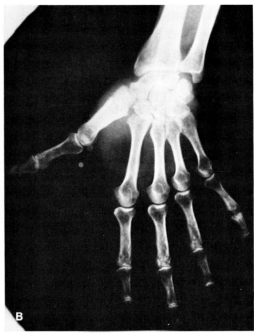

FIG. 4-11   A. Roentgenogram of patient's hand revealing advanced osteoarthritis of the carpal-metacarpal joint of the thumb with cystic formation. B. Roentgenogram after replacement of the trapezium with a Silastic prosthesis.

The erosive type of disease can often be confused with rheumatoid arthritis, but it is limited to the finger joints and the carpal-metacarpal joint of the thumb. In contrast to rheumatoid arthritis the metacarpal-phalangeal joints are gener-ally not involved in this disease (Fig. 4-13). Arthrodesis tends to give excellent results in the proximal interphalangeal joints, and occasionally a Swanson Silastic prosthesis can be used in selected cases.

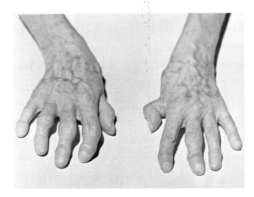

FIG. 4-12   Photograph of hands of patient with advanced Heberden's nodes and involvement of the proximal interphalangeal joint as well as the carpal-metacarpal joints of the thumb. Hyper-extension deformities are developing at the meta-carpal-phalangeal joints.

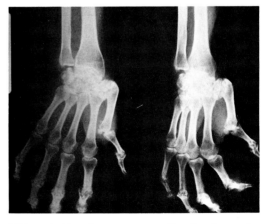

FIG. 4-13   Roentgenogram revealing involvement of the proximal and distal interphalangeal joints with severe deformities of the wrist and the thumb.

Hips. Both hips may be involved in osteoarthritis because the hips are weight-bearing joints. The treatment of osteoarthritis of the hip has been revolutionized by the work of Charnley and McKee. The development of a total hip implant has made it much easier to rehabilitate the older patient with bilateral hip disease. In the past arthrodesis or cup arthroplasty entailed prolonged hospitalization and required some patients to walk with crutches for years. The replacement with a total hip has allowed the patient to bear full weight in 6 weeks or less in most cases, and the success rate has been as high as 95 percent or more in some series. In contrast to this, the success rate for hip fusion is about 60 percent because of pseudoarthroses, and that for cup arthroplasty is about the same (Fig. 4-14). The number of excellent results for the cup arthroplasty will never equal those for the total hip replacement.

Knee. The knee joint is commonly involved in osteoarthritis and has been a great problem for the orthopaedic surgeon, as well as for the patient (Fig. 4-15). Osteotomy of the tibia and fibula in unilateral compartment disease has been of value in aiding many patients with osteoarthritis. However, it is a great problem for the elderly patient to tolerate the cast and the prolonged inactivity. The development of total knee replacements in the past few years is beginning to approach that of the total hip, and it is hoped the knee replacement will become the procedure of choice for elderly patients. The Marmor Modular knee system allows unilateral compartment replacement in patients with osteoarthritis when there is a varus or valgus deformity with loss of articular cartilage on one side of the joint only.

The tibial plateau prosthesis (MacIntosh) has not proved helpful for the patient with a varus or valgus deformity because of extreme pressure

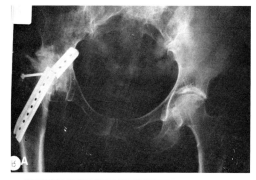

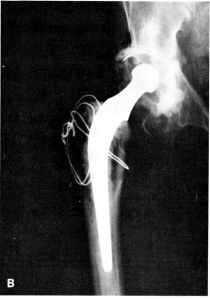

FIG. 4-14 Roentgenograms of right hip of patient with osteoarthritis. A. Arthrodesis performed 17 years ago. Note evidence of nonunion and fracture through the Z-nail. B. After total hip replacement.

placed upon the femoral condyle on that side (Fig. 4-16).

Ankle. The ankle joint is seldom involved primarily with osteoarthritis, but tends to be secondarily involved due to trauma. Destruction of the articular cartilage will produce aching, pain, swelling, and stiffness of the joint. Arthrodesis of the ankle joint is still an excellent operation in selected cases. At the present time arthroplasty of the ankle joint can be considered instead of arthrodesis.

Foot. The foot is composed of a num-

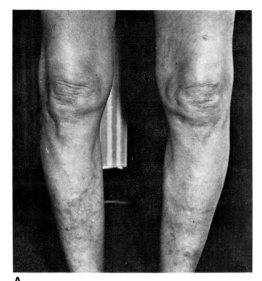

A

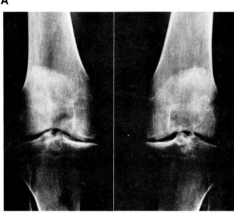

B

FIG. 4-15 A. Photograph of legs of patient with osteoarthritis in both knee joints that is producing increasing pain and inability to walk. Note the varus deformities. B. Roentgenogram revealing moderate involvement of the medial compartments of both joints.

ber of joints, any one of of which may develop osteoarthritis; however, certain joints are involved more frequently. Probably in the order of frequency, the first metatarsal-phalangeal joint is involved more often than any other joint in the foot. Osteoarthritis of this joint may occur with involvement of the hands, knees, and neck. The involvement of the metatarsal-phalangeal joint tends to be bilateral, but one side may be more symptomatic than the other. The patient

will complain of pain and gradual loss of joint motion, resulting in severe cases in a hallux rigidus. The Keller arthroplasty can be utilized in these patients, and recently a Silastic rubber replacement has been developed by Swanson to replace the excised base of the phalanx to prevent shortening of the great toe. Arthrodesis of the metatarsal-phalangeal joint has been proposed by some, but it is not the procedure of choice generally in osteoarthritis.

The talar-navicular joint, as well as the talar-calcaneal (subtalar) joint, is also involved occasionally in osteo-arthritis. The patient will often have severe pain in the ankle or foot, but it may be hard to localize the site of the patient's pain, except by palpation of the area and the use of the roentgenogram (Fig. 4-17). Arthrodesis of the joint will often give dramatic relief of the patient's symptoms.

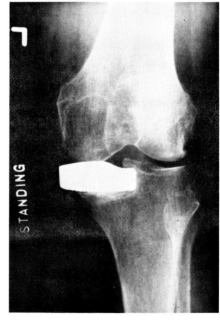

STANDING

FIG. 4-16 Roentgenogram of tibial plateau prosthesis (MacIntosh). Increased pressure on the femoral condyle generally results in a return of pain.

Neck. The neck is frequently involved in osteoarthritis and most persons beyond the age of 35 years will show some degenerative changes of the apophyseal joints or the joints of Luschka. The most frequent site of degenerative change in the neck is the C5–C6 disk space (Fig. 4-18). Pain and stiffness of the neck are generally the presenting complaint, but occasionally there are characteristic radiation syndromes into the shoulder, the upper back, and especially the superior border of the scapula. The pain may often have a burning or searing character, especially if associated with irritation of the cervical nerve roots. The majority of patients will respond generally to conservative therapy, but occasionally anterior or posterior spinal fusion can dramatically relieve the patient's complaints when conservative therapy fails.

Lumbar Spine. The lumbar spine is

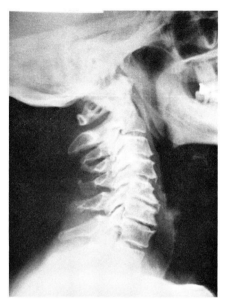

FIG. 4-18 Roentgenogram showing typical degenerative arthritis of C5–C6 and C6–C7 disk spaces. Osteophyte formation is present with loss of the disk height.

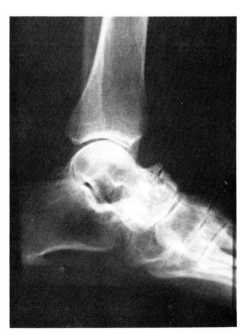

FIG. 4-17 Roentgenogram revealing localized talar-navicular arthritis with osteophyte formation at the dorsum of the joint. This is a common site for osteophyte formation.

prone to the development of osteoarthritis. It is probably related to man's erect position which places additional stress upon the lumbosacral and the apophyseal joints of the lumbar spine. Increasing lordosis with poor muscular tone increases the wear on these joints. The patient will often develop an aching low back pain which becomes constant in contrast to the severe excruciating pain produced by a herniated disk. Conservative therapy will often relieve most of the patients of their symptoms. When there is advanced osteoarthritis of the lumbosacral joint, spinal fusion can be considered to relieve the patient's pain.

Contraindications

The main contraindication for surgery in the patient with osteoarthritis is poor general health. If the risks of surgery are greater because of the general systemic condition of the patient, surgical correction may be contraindicated.

The patient must be made fully aware of all of the complications that can occur, and the so-called informed consent must be obtained to prevent any misunderstanding if such a patient is operated upon. The patient with cardiac failure or diabetes presents even more of a problem and should be carefully evaluated before considering surgery.

Preoperative Preparation

The osteoarthritic patient in the older age group who has not had a complete medical evaluation in the past 6 months should be seen by his internist prior to admission to the hospital. Many of these patients will have other disease that will delay surgery or cause a cancellation at the time of admission to the hospital if not taken care of beforehand.

It is wise to delve into the medications that the patient is taking at the present time or has taken within the past year. It is surprising how many patients have been or are on cortisone or one of its derivatives for osteoarthritis. It is felt that steroids should not be utilized orally or by injection other than into a joint as a form of treatment for osteoarthritis. In the advanced osteoarthritic patient, steroids do not relieve the symptoms and are of limited value in the treatment of the disease.

It is also wise to discuss the operation thoroughly with the elderly patient and his or her family. The patient who is well informed about preoperative, postoperative, and surgical procedures will be able to cooperate much better and will be less fearful of the outcome. The entire hospital course will be much smoother. If the patient is going to have to use crutches or a walker postoperatively, it is advantageous to have the therapist see the patient and train him in the use of the crutches or the walker before the operation is scheduled. The elderly patient, once he has mastered the use of crutches, can be mobilized postoperatively very easily. It is more difficult for the patient to learn how to use crutches after the operation, and for the older patient the pickup walker may be a better choice than crutches.

Postoperative Management

Any of the usual postoperative complications may occur in the osteoarthritic patient, but in general these patients will respond well to surgery. Since many of these patients are elderly, it is important to stress early mobilization, and they should be ambulated as soon as possible after the operation or up in a wheelchair. Ice bags and elevation of the upper extremity tend to reduce swelling and relieve the patient's discomfort. Whenever possible, the night of the operation the dressings should be split down to the skin to relieve pressure from swelling and tight bandages. Narcotics should be used with discrimination in the elderly patient, and small doses are frequently all that are necessary. Early discharge is utilized to get the patients out of the hospital as soon as possible and back into their home environments, as it is less disrupting to their psyches.

Complications

Phlebitis and pulmonary emboli are serious complications occurring more frequently in the osteoarthritic patient than in the rheumatoid patient. We have tended to use aspirin as an anticoagulant in our osteoarthritic patients if they are not on it preoperatively. In many of our cases salicylate therapy is instituted one week preoperatively with 10 gr of aspirin four times a day. This therapy is continued postoperatively until the patient is ambulatory. The most simple and safe approach to the prevention of postoperative thrombosis and pulmonary emboli is the administration of Heparin sodium as advocated by Sharnoff and DeBlasio (page 51).

Urinary tract infection is common in the elderly patient with osteoarthritis. Postoperative catheterization of the male frequently leads to cystitis and complications. If an elderly male has a history of prostatic disease, it is advisable to obtain a urologic consultation and have the prostate problem treated first. If it is not taken care of preoperatively, cathetherization postoperatively will lead to edema of the urethra with subsequent infection of the bladder and possible septicemia. In some cases, emergency prostatectomy will have to be considered before the catheter can be removed. Treatment of urinary tract infections is extremely important before total joint implantations, and cultures of the urine should be obtained before the operation, especially in the female. If there is a growth of over 100,000 colonies, antibiotic therapy should be started to treat the urinary infection. A urinary tract infection is a complication that can lead to severe problems if it is not treated.

Bibliography

Rheumatoid Arthritis

Badgley, C. E.: The orthopedic treatment of arthritis. Am. Acad. Orthop. Surgeons, Lect., 5:314, 1948.

Bickel, W. H.: Cortisone and ACTH in orthopaedic surgery. Am. Acad. Orthop. Surgeons, Lect., 8:85, 1951.

Conaty, J. P., and Nickel, V.: Functional incapacitation in rheumatoid arthritis: a rehabilitation challenge. J. Bone Joint Surg., 53-A:624, 1971.

Cregan, J. C. F.: Indications for surgical inter-vention in rheumatoid arthritis of the wrist and hand. Ann. Rheum. Dis., 18:29, 1959.

Law, W. A.: Surgical treatment of rheumatic diseases. J. Bone Joint Surg., 34-B:215, 1952.

Marmor, L.: Surgical treatment of chronic arthritis. Mod. Therapy, 1:1313, 1964.

Mathews, R. S., et al.: Pre-operative evaluation of patients with rheumatoid arthritis. South. Med. J., 64:138, 1971.

Mercer, W.: The surgery of rheumatoid arthritis. Bull. Hosp. Joint Dis., 15:101, 1954.

Reveno, W. S., and Firnschild, P. G.: Pre-operative and postoperative steroid therapy. Surg. Clin. North Am., 39:1691, 1959.

Schneewind, J. H., and Cole, W. H.: Steroid therapy in surgical patients. J.A.M.A., 170:1411, 1959.

Sharnoff, J. G., and DeBlasio, G.: Prevention of fatal postoperative thromboembolism by heparin prophylaxis. Lancet, 2:1006, 1971.

Short, C. L., Bauer, W., and Reynolds, W. E.: Rheumatoid Arthritis. Cambridge, Harvard University Press, 1957.

Smith-Peterson, M. N., Aufranc, O. E., and Larson, C. B.: Useful surgical procedures for rheumatoid arthritis involving joints of the upper extremity. Arch. Surg., 46:764, 1943.

Swanson, A. B.: The need for early treatment of the rheumatoid hand. J. Mich. Med. Soc., 60:348, 1961.

Vainio, K.: Surgery in rheumatoid arthritis. Manit. Med. Rev., 44:548, 1964.

Vainio, K., and Pulkki, T.: Surgical treatment of arthritis mutilans. Ann. Chir. Gynaecol. Fenn., 48:361, 1959.

Wilkinson, M. C., and Lowry, J. H.: Synovectomy for rheumatoid arthritis. J. Bone Joint Surg., 47-B:482, 1965.

Wilson, P. D.: Reconstructive surgery of arthritis. Rheumatic Diseases, American Rheumatism Association. Philadelphia, W. B. Saunders Co., 1952.

Osteoarthritis

Charnley, J.: Arthroplasty of the hip: A new operation. Lancet, 1:1129, 1961.

French, B.: The surgical approach to osteo-arthritis. Br. J. Clin. Pract., *13*:622, 1959.

Kelikin, H., et al.: Surgical endeavors in arthritis. Clin. Orthop., *14*:121, 1959.

Marmor, L.: Surgery for osteoarthritis. Geriatrics, *27*:89, 1972.

Marmor, L.: Surgery of osteoarthritis. Semin. Arthritis Rheum., *2*:117, 1972.

McKee, G. K., and Watson-Farrar, J.: Replacement of arthritic hips by the McKee-Farrar prosthesis. J. Bone Joint Surg., *48B*:245, 1966.

Anatomy

Arthritis of the shoulder joint can produce a great deal of discomfort for the patient and interfere with his ability to perform his daily activities as well as with his sleep. Rheumatoid arthritis is a much more common cause of destruction of the shoulder joint than osteoarthritis. In rheumatoid arthritis, both shoulders may be involved, in contrast to osteoarthritis where frequently only one shoulder is involved. Trauma related to the patient's occupation or an accident may accelerate the development of osteoarthritis in the shoulder joint.

Pain is the major complaint that brings the patient to the doctor, especially when it interferes with sleep. Because of the numerous joints and bursae in the shoulder girdle, the exact diagnosis of the patient's complaint requires careful evaluation of the clinical findings and roentgenograms.

A knowledge of anatomy is extremely important in order to determine the basis of the patient's symptoms and to arrive at a correct diagnosis. The shoulder joint and pectoral girdle consist of four separate articulations: the glenohumeral, acromioclavicular, sternoclavicular, and scapulothoracic or thoracoscapular (Fig. 5-1).

The glenohumeral, or true shoulder joint, is essentially a ball-and-socket joint surrounded by an articular capsule lined with synovial membrane. The large humeral head articulates with the glenoid cavity which is increased in depth by the fibrocartilaginous glenoidal labrum. The humeral head has about three times the articular surface of the glenoid, and the shallow glenoid cavity therefore allows a wide range of motion in all directions except on abduction when the greater tuberosity strikes the acromion process.

The synovium tends to surround the joint within the articular capsule and also follows the biceps tendon as it passes beneath the transverse humeral ligament in the bicipital groove (Fig. 5-2).

The bursae in the region of the shoulder joint are numerous. A large bursa is located between the deltoid muscle and the capsule but does not

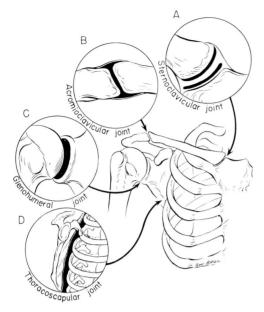

FIG. 5-1 The four separate articulations of the shoulder. A. Sternoclavicular joint. B. Acromioclavicular joint. C. Glenohumeral joint. D. Scapulothoracic joint. (From DePalma, A. F.: Surgery of the Shoulder, 2nd ed. Philadelphia, J. B. Lippincott Co., 1973.)

communicate with the joint. The subscapular bursa, which lies between the capsule of the joint and the subscapular tendon, communicates with the joint through an opening in the front of the capsule. Several other bursae are located about the shoulder in various relationships to the muscles about the joint.

Functionally, the shoulder joint is mobile and depends on its ligaments, capsule, and muscle tone for stability and prevention of dislocation. The capsule of the shoulder joint is quite redundant and has a large surface area with a capacity of approximately 20 cc. The anterior aspect of the capsule is reinforced by the superior, middle, and inferior glenohumeral ligaments, which tend to extend from the supraglenoid tubercle of the scapula to the humerus. The capsule is also reinforced by the coracohumeral ligament, which extends from the greater and lesser tuberosity to

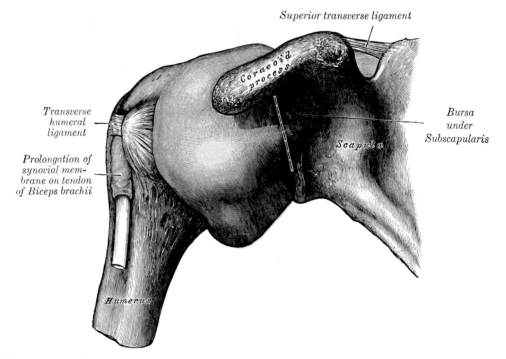

FIG. 5-2 Synovial membrane lining the articular capsule of the shoulder joint (distended). Anterior aspect. (From Gray's Anatomy of the Human Body, 29th ed. C. M. Goss, editor. Philadelphia, Lea & Febiger, 1973.)

the coracoid process. The capsule, supraspinatus tendon, and the coracohumeral ligament are all blended together across the front of the joint. It is believed that when these fibers become inflamed and shortened they contribute to fixation of the joint in internal rotation. The capsule is also reinforced by the short rotator muscles, which insert distal to the articular surface of the humerus. These tendons, which form the rotator cuff, blend with the capsule, reinforcing it. On the anterior surface the subscapularis tendon is located, blending with the capsule. On the superior aspect is the supraspinatus, and on the posterior aspect are the infraspinatus and teres minor.

The motion of the shoulder joint is dependent upon the relationship of the humerus and the scapula. During the first 30° of abduction and the first 60° of flexion, the scapula is usually stabilized, and motion takes place in the glenohumeral joint. During the remainder of the range of motion, there is a continuous simultaneous movement of the scapula and humerus in a ratio of two humeral movements to one of the scapula. The glenohumeral joint alone allows approximately 120° of abduction, and the remainder of the 60° of abduction is supplied by the scapula, rotating on the chest wall.

The nerve supply to the shoulder joint is supplied by the suprascapular, axillary, radial, and lateral anterior thoracic nerves. The suprascapular nerve supplies motor fibers to the supraspinatus and infraspinatus muscles and passes beneath the transverse scapular ligament in the suprascapular notch. The axillary nerve supplies the deltoid muscle and the teres minor. The trapezius muscle is supplied by the spinal accessory nerve, and the subscapularis receives its innervation from the upper and lower subscapular nerves from the brachial plexus.

Physical and Radiologic Examinations

Physical examination of the patient is similar for rheumatoid arthritis and for osteoarthritis. Careful physical examination combined with radiologic examination may accurately localize the site of the disease.

Inspection

Inspection of the shoulder joint may reveal localized swelling over the acromioclavicular joint, the anterior aspect of the shoulder, or the entire shoulder itself. Synovial effusion in the joint will produce a diffuse, broad swelling involving both the anterior and posterior aspects of the shoulder joint. Rupture of the biceps tendon may occur when synovial disease interferes with nutrition to the long head. This rupture will be noticed as a round swelling located in the anterior lateral aspect of the arm and tends to move with contraction of the biceps against resistance (Fig. 5-3).

Palpation

Palpation of the shoulder may often give valuable information. Tenderness along the bicipital groove may indicate a tenosynovitis of the biceps tendon. If the tendon can be rolled under the finger, one may palpate a thickness or enlargement of the long head of the biceps. Localized tenderness over the anterior aspect of the shoulder with the arm in external rotation often will indicate a tendinitis involving the supraspinatus tendon (Fig. 5-4). This is a common location of calcific deposits. Tenderness over the anterior superior aspect of the

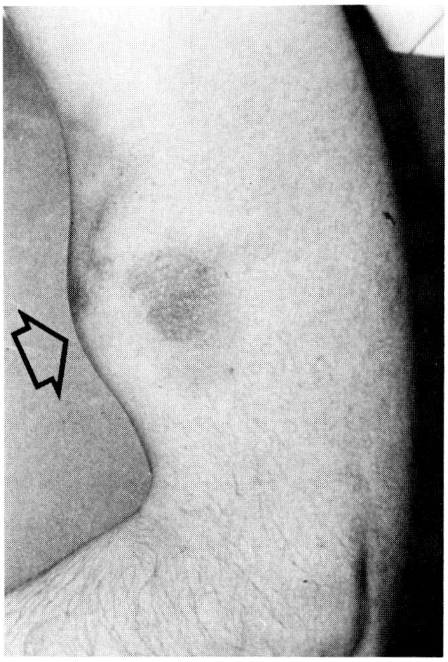

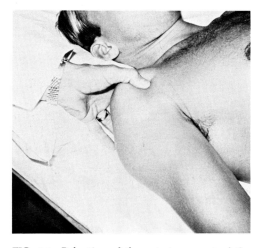

FIG. 5-3 Arm of patient with recent rupture of the biceps tendon (arrow).

shoulder lateral to the acromion process is often indicative of a subacromial bursitis.

Biceps Subluxation Test

Subluxation of the biceps tendon can also produce a chronic bicipital tendinitis. For the bicipital subluxation test the patient raises his arm over his head with the elbow flexed. This motion allows the biceps tendon to fall into the bicipital groove, and then the arm is brought down to 90° of abduction in external rotation. In the final maneuver, the arm is internally rotated, and the forearm is pronated while the examiner maintains a finger on the bicipital tendon in the groove. In a positive test a click will result as the biceps tendon slides out of the bicipital groove, and the patient may also complain of pain at that instant (Fig. 5-5).

Rotator Cuff Tests

Ruptures of the rotator cuff occur frequently in rheumatoid arthritis, and the various rotator cuff tests, numbered with Roman numerals I, II, and III, may help to determine whether a cuff tear is present.

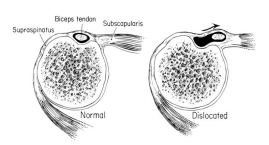

FIG. 5-5 Diagrams of a cross section of the biceps tendon. Left, normal position with the tendon lying in the anterior groove of the humerus and covered by a synovial sheath. Right, distended. (From Marmor, L.: The painful shoulder. Am. Fam. Physician, 1:1, 75, 1970.)

FIG. 5-4 Palpation of the anterior aspect of the shoulder joint to localize an area of tenderness associated with a calcific deposit in the supraspinatus tendon.

Rotator Cuff Test I. The patient is asked to abduct or raise the arm over the head. If the patient cannot actively raise his arm, the examiner passively abducts the arm and asks the patient to hold it up. The test is positive if the patient cannot actively raise the arm over his head but can maintain it there after it has been elevated by the examiner. This is indicative of a rupture of the rotator cuff. If the patient cannot maintain the abduction, a paralysis of the deltoid muscle or a fracture of the humerus should be suspected, especially if there is a history of trauma.

Rotator Cuff Test II. The patient's arm is abducted to 90° and the forearm is placed at 90° with the shoulder in full internal rotation. The examiner pushes down on the elbow in an effort to place stress on the shoulder cuff. Then the shoulder is placed in full external rotation, and the arm is pushed downward by the examiner to place the stress on the anterior aspect of the rotator cuff. The test is positive if the patient reports pain and is unable to maintain the abduction against the force of the examiner's hand. Pain alone is not a positive test. In this manner, small ruptures or tears in the rotator cuff may be detected by the examiner.

Rotator Cuff Test III. The patient is examined sitting down and relaxed (Fig. 5-6). The examiner supports the patient's flexed elbow in one hand, and with his other hand he palpates the humeral head. With the hand supporting the elbow, the examiner rotates the humerus internally and externally to move various parts of the rotator cuff to a position beneath the examiner's fingers. It is important to have the patient's deltoid muscle relaxed by supporting the arm. With careful palpation, frequently one can feel the defect in the cuff and palpate directly to the humeral head. The test is positive if the examiner can palpate a defect in the rotator cuff.

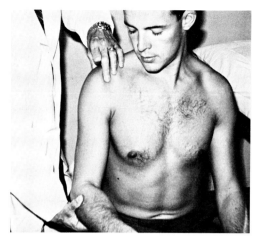

FIG. 5-6 Position for detecting a tear in the rotator cuff by test III. Note the patient's arm is supported to relax the deltoid muscle, and the examiner is rotating the forearm while he palpates the shoulder. (From Marmor, L.: The painful shoulder. Am. Fam. Physician, 1:1, 75, 1970.)

Range of Motion

The range of motion of the shoulder is also tested in the various directions, both actively and passively. Abduction or elevation of the arm, internal and external rotation, and flexion and extension should be tested. Frequently abduction and external rotation are lost early in rheumatoid disease.

Roentgenograms

Roentgenograms of the shoulder joint can be of great value in determining the pathologic condition within the joint. Anteroposterior and lateral views, as well as x-ray films of internal and external rotation, will often aid in diagnosis of shoulder problems. In selected cases arthrograms are also helpful in detecting a rupture of the shoulder cuff.

Osteoarthritis tends to produce sclerotic changes in the humeral head with osteophyte formation and loss of the joint space (Fig. 5-7). Osteoporosis, cyst formation, and erosions of the joint

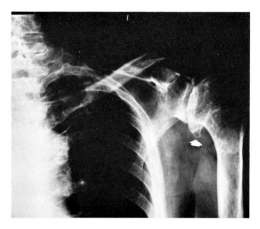

FIG. 5-7 Roentgenogram showing large osteophytes on the lower aspect of the humeral head (arrow). These are typical of osteoarthritis.

margins, which are usually seen in roentgenograms of patients with rheumatoid arthritis, are rarely seen in osteoarthritis.

Rheumatoid Arthritis

Rheumatoid arthritis may affect both shoulders, but not necessarily to the same degree (Fig. 5-8). Pain, stiffness, and deformity of the shoulder can be produced by local disease within the shoulder joint or be secondary to immobilization produced by rheumatoid disease in other parts of the upper extremity. The shoulder is frequently found to be involved along with the elbow, wrist, hand, and often the opposite shoulder. It is quite unusual to have rheumatoid arthritis start primarily in the shoulder joint. The disability of the shoulder usually develops gradually in rheumatoid arthritis and occurs late in the course of the disease.

The presenting symptom of rheumatoid arthritis involving the shoulder usually is mild aching or limitation of motion. Gradually there will be an increasing loss of abduction and external rotation with the development of pain and disability. Since there are many bursae and articulations about the shoulder, there are many potential sites in which symptoms may originate from rheumatoid arthritis. The subdeltoid bursa, when seriously diseased, can destroy the supraspinatus tendon by pressure, necrosis, and invasion (Fig. 5-9). A frequent cause of limitation in shoulder joint motion is disease involving the subacromial bursa or the acromioclavicular joint.

Early in the course of the disease, the synovial tissue in and about the shoulder joint may become involved. This synovitis can produce pain and limitation of motion, and it is difficult at times to determine whether the involvement is in the subacromial bursa, biceps tendon, or the glenohumeral joint.

Subdeltoid Bursitis

The subdeltoid or the subacromial bursa is often involved in rheumatoid arthritis, and, characteristically, the patient will complain of chronic shoulder pain (Fig. 5-9). The bursa becomes inflamed and thickened due to the proliferation of the synovium. The synovium may be thrown up into large villous folds which will produce crepitation in the shoulder joint (Fig. 5-10). The patient may often complain of a grating sensation on abduction or internal rotation of the shoulder. The clinical features generally consist of severe pain in the shoulder on abduction or internal rotation of the arm. Pain is often referred to the insertion of the deltoid muscle, and the patient will complain of a constant aching in the arm (Fig. 5-11). The pain of bursitis about the shoulder is almost never referred below the elbow, in contrast to cervical arthritis where the pain

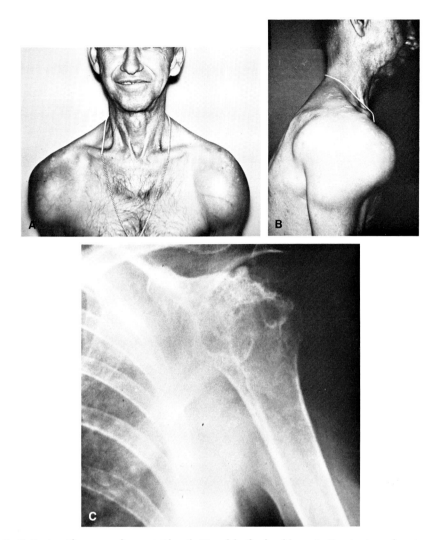

FIG. 5-8 Patient with severe rheumatoid arthritis of both shoulders. A. Front view, showing synovial swelling. B. Lateral view of the shoulder showing massive anterior swelling and posterior swelling due to destruction of the shoulder joint. C. Roentgenogram revealing destruction of the humeral head and involvement of the glenoid cavity.

will radiate down the arm into the wrist or hand. Frequently the pain is increased at night when the patient is lying in bed relaxed and may prevent him from falling asleep. Roentgenograms of the shoulder may reveal rheumatoid arthritis involving the glenohumeral joint, but if only the bursa is involved no bony abnormalities will be noted, even though the patient has conspicuous crepitation and pain on motion of the shoulder.

Conservative Treatment

The treatment of an acute subdeltoid bursitis generally can be conservative with immobilization of the arm in a sling and cold applications to ease pain. The best way to localize the area if local injections are to be utilized is to have the patient lying down on the back, relaxed, with the arms slightly abducted and the palms upward. Careful palpation with

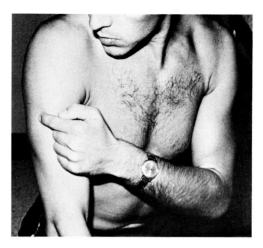

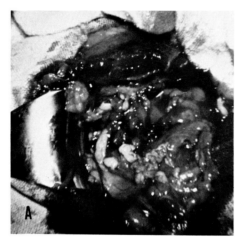

FIG. 5-9 The subdeltoid bursa. (From Duthie, R. B., and Ferguson, A. B. Jr.: Mercer's Orthopaedic Surgery, 7th ed. Baltimore, The Williams & Wilkins Co., 1973. By permission of Edward Arnold (Publishers) Ltd., London.)

FIG. 5-11 Patient indicating pain in the region of the insertion of the deltoid muscle. (From Marmor, L.: The painful shoulder. Am. Fam. Physician, 1:1, 75, 1970.)

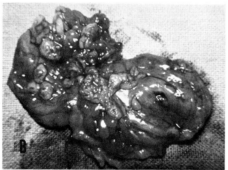

FIG. 5-10 Rheumatoid arthritis of the subdeltoid bursa. A. Anterior approach to the shoulder joint revealing fungating synovial tissue protruding up from the subdeltoid area. B. Subdeltoid bursa after excision from the subdeltoid area.

the finger will generally localize the area, which can be extremely small, to the anterior aspect of the shoulder joint. Occasionally there can be involvement slightly more lateral near the acromion process, and palpation will help to determine this. After localization, the area can often be marked with the end of a swab stick, leaving a small indentation in the skin. The area is prepared with an antiseptic solution, and under sterile technique approximately 5 cc of lidocaine (Xylocaine) combined with an intra-articular steroid in the same syringe may be injected into the localized area over the anterior aspect of the shoulder joint. The needle should be advanced and retracted a number of times while injecting the solution. The patient should experience immediate relief of his symptoms, and if this does occur one can be sure that the steroids are in the right place. It is wise to caution the patient that a severe inflammatory reaction can occur that night, and that ice and local analgesics are of value. Occasionally an injection will have to be repeated in a week or two if symptoms have not been relieved because the area of involvement has not been accurately palpated at the time of injection or there are several areas. It is advantageous to check carefully prior to the injection to be sure that the patient has not moved from the time the area was marked with the applicator stick.

Excision

When the symptoms are severe and do not respond to local injections, excision of the bursa may be necessary to relieve the symptoms and improve the function of the shoulder. In late cases the bursa can erode through the shoulder cuff and the joint capsule to produce a tear of the supraspinatus or infraspinatus tendon.

Rotator Cuff Calcific Tendinitis

One of the most frequent causes of shoulder pain is a calcium deposit in the supraspinatus or infraspinatus tendon. This condition is often called a subdeltoid bursitis in error. Although the symptoms are identical in many respects, the lesion is in the tendon and not in the bursa. Occasionally when the calcific deposit ruptures from the tendon into the subdeltoid bursa, severe pain can develop and both structures may be involved.

The symptoms may be acute or may pursue a chronic, aching course with stiffness and limitation of shoulder motion. The pain often is described at the insertion of the deltoid muscle on the lateral aspect of the arm, and in acute cases may be unbearable. This type of symptom is unusual with rheumatoid arthritis involving the glenohumeral joint and should suggest an acute calcific deposit. Limitation of abduction and internal rotation is quite common when the supraspinatus tendon is involved.

Calcium deposits occur in the tendinous portion of the muscles of the

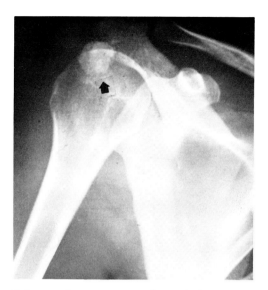

FIG. 5-12 Roentgenogram taken with the patient's arm in internal rotation. A large calcific deposit is indicated by the arrow.

rotator cuff near their insertion into the greater tuberosity of the humerus. The lesions may be best demonstrated by roentgenograms taken in internal and external rotation of the shoulder (Fig. 5-12). If a deposit is seen best in a roentgenogram made during an internal rotation, it is located in the infraspinatus tendon; if it is seen best during external rotation, it is located in the supraspinatus tendon. These deposits can be quite large or can exist as faint streaks running parallel to the fibers of the tendon or muscle they lie in. If the calcification appears cloudy with a round border, it is probably an acute deposit and quite liquefied. If, however, the lesion appears to be quite dense and has irregular margins, it has probably been there for a period of time and is usually quite thick like heavy cheese.

Conservative Treatment

The calcium deposit, if symptom producing, may be localized by palpating the shoulder with the patient in the supine position similar to that for a

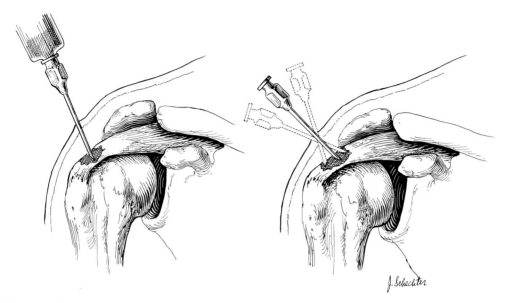

J. Schechter

FIG. 5-13 Illustration of technique for injecting a mixture of Xylocaine and cortisone into a calcific tendinitis of the shoulder. On the right, observe locations of multiple punctures.

subdeltoid bursitis. The time spent in determining the exact location of maximum tenderness may be the difference between success or failure of local injection. A mixture of lidocaine (Xylocaine) and an intra-articular steroid should be injected into the calcium deposit, with multiple puncture holes being made in the deposit (Fig. 5-13).

Excision

In recalcitrant cases, surgical excision of the deposit may be necessary. If, at operation, the tendon is thickened and impinges upon the acromion or the coracoacromial arch, the arch should be sectioned to prevent compression of the tendon on abduction.

Scapulothoracic Bursitis

The scapulothoracic bursa is located near the superior aspect of the scapula between the posterior chest wall and the undersurface of the scapula (Fig. 5-14). This bursa allows the scapula to slide easily over the chest wall and often is a well-defined bursa. It can become inflamed by rheumatoid arthritis or chronic trauma and produce severe pain in the upper back, which is accentuated by use of the arm, especially in such activities as ironing or hammering. The symptoms from scapulothoracic bursitis may be either acute or chronic, persisting for long periods of time without improvement. In the acute case the pain may be excruciating. The patient may complain of radiation of the pain into the neck or shoulder posteriorly, and it can be confused with radiation from the cervical spine downward. However, careful examination of the cervical spine will often rule this out as a source of the patient's complaints.

On examination of the back, local tenderness may be elicited by palpating the chest wall near the superior medial undersurface of the scapula and the rhomboid region while the patient adducts the arm to the other shoulder to move the scapula away from the midline. Frequently the patient will have

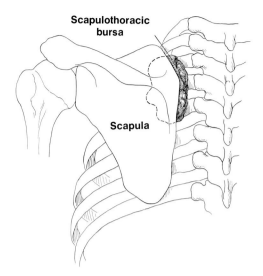

FIG. 5-14 Location of the scapulothoracic bursa. Posterior view.

exquisite tenderness at this site, and in the chronic case the thickened bursa can be palpated or felt to grate under the examiner's finger. If the patient is asked to extend the arm anteriorly as in reaching for an object, one can often feel grating at this site, and the patient may complain of additional pain if the arm is required to lift a weight.

Examination of the range of motion will show a full range of motion without limitation in abduction and internal rotation as is often seen with a calcium deposit in the rotator cuff or a subdeltoid bursitis. Roentgenograms of the involved area are usually negative.

Conservative Treatment

The local injection of the bursa with cortisone or other steroids will frequently relieve or eliminate the patient's symptoms for long periods of time. Recurrences are reasonably frequent and require repeated injections at times. The injection of this area, however, carries a certain amount of risk of a pneumothorax, and this should be kept in mind. Under sterile technique a mixture of lidocaine (Xylocaine) and steroids is combined in a syringe, and the injection is usually given with the patient in a sitting position. The patient is asked to place the arm on the involved side across the chest to pull the scapula out of the way to expose the bursa. The area is carefully prepared with an antiseptic solution, and the examiner wears a sterile glove while palpating the scapulothoracic area to localize the site of severe pain. If it is possible to localize the site of the pain over a rib, this is a good area to inject into to prevent going between the ribs and producing a pneumothorax. The needle should be inserted carefully, only after the patient has exhaled to the the maximum to provide a certain amount of safety. The needle should be inserted in several directions to cover as much of the area as possible, and the solution should be spread through the tissues to give maximum benefit. Immediate relief will generally occur if the proper area has been injected. Again it is wise to caution the patient that a severe reaction may occur the night of the injection, and ice and local analgesics should be prescribed.

Excision

Some surgeons have advised that excision of the superior aspect of the scapula will relieve all symptoms and bring permanent improvement. Excision can be utilized in those cases that do not respond to local injections, but this is rarely required. The bursa is excised along with the superior pole of the scapula.

Suprascapular Nerve Entrapment

The suprascapular nerve, which supplies the infraspinatus and supraspinatus muscles, passes through the suprascapular notch in the spine of the scapula. Entrapment of the nerve at this level can produce pain over the apex of the shoulder or in the scapular region. The pain is often related to abduction of the arm when it is elevated to the horizontal position. This is a good test to perform to determine whether the nerve is trapped in the suprascapular notch. If the test is positive, it is possible to inject local anesthesia into the nerve in the notch. If this injection relieves the patient's symptoms, one can be reasonably sure of an entrapment of the suprascapular nerve.

Conservative Treatment

A local anesthesia and steroids may be injected into the suprascapular nerve in the area of the notch while the patient is seated with the arms at the side and the hands resting on the thighs. A technique suggested by Wertheim and Rovenstine is to bisect the inferior angle of the scapula and draw a line to intersect a line parallel to the upper edge of the spine of the scapula. The upper outer triangle that is formed by the intersection of these lines is bisected, and the injection is made 1.5 cm along this line. After sterile preparation, the needle is directed slightly downward and medial to contact the scapula at the medial side of the base of the coracoid process. The needle is then withdrawn slightly and redirected medially until the notch and nerve are encountered and the patient experiences paresthesia over the apex of the shoulder. Approximately 5 cc lidocaine (Xylocaine) without epinephrine and 1 cc of a local steroid are injected.

Excision

If relief is not permanent, the superior transverse scapular ligament may be removed from where it covers the notch, decompressing the suprascapular nerve.

Bicipital Tenosynovitis

The long head of the biceps tendon arises from the supraglenoid tubercle and passes through the shoulder joint to exit through the bicipital groove tunnel. The tendon is covered by a synovial sheath that is an out-pouching of the joint. A rheumatoid synovitis involving the shoulder joint will produce an inflammation and enlargement of the biceps tendon sheath because it is a continuation of the joint synovium. Therefore bicipital tenosynovitis is extremely common in rheumatoid arthritis.

The patient will complain of shoulder pain, especially on abduction combined with rotation, motions used in combing the hair, putting on a coat, or reaching up on a shelf. The pain is usually dull and aching but accentuated and sharp when the shoulder joint is moved, and the biceps tendon is forced to slide through the inflamed sheath.

On palpating the shoulder, the biceps tendon sheath will be enlarged and tender. It may easily be rolled beneath the examiner's thumb, and this procedure will produce pain.

Routine radiographic study of the shoulder frequently reveals no evidence of disease, but an arthrogram made with a water-soluble contrast medium may demonstrate the disease in the biceps tendon and the joint.

Conservative Treatment

Injection of the biceps tendon sheath with cortisone may relieve the symptoms for long periods of time.

Synovectomy

If symptoms persist, the biceps tendon sheath should be explored, the transverse humeral ligament divided, and the synovium excised. If shoulder symptoms are severe, the glenohumeral joint should be explored, and a synovectomy performed.

Operative Technique. The shoulder may be approached through a deltopectoral incision (Fig. 5-15). The cephalic vein is ligated if necessary, and the interval developed between the pectoralis major and the deltoid muscles. The biceps tendon may be visualized without releasing the clavicular portion of the deltoid (Fig. 5-16). The humeral ligament is divided, and the synovium excised from the sheath. If the tendon appears frayed, a drill hole is made in the humerus at the distal end of the bicipital groove; the biceps tendon is divided at

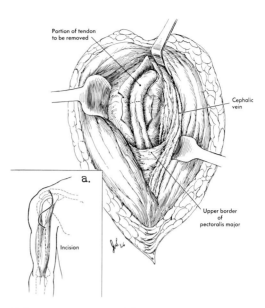

FIG. **5-16** Exposure of the anterior aspect of the shoulder to show the biceps tendon. Insert illustrates the position for the incision.

the capsule, and the distal end is placed into the hole and sutured in place. The transverse humeral ligament is sewn over the tendon (Fig. 5-17). It is not necessary to remove the intra-articular portion of the biceps tendon.

Complications. In chronic cases of bicipital tenosynovitis, the long head of the biceps tendon may rupture from attrition. This can occur with minimal trauma or spontaneously. The patient will often have slight discomfort and note the development of ecchymosis and a mass in the arm. The mass will be noted to move on contraction of the biceps tendon. Repair generally is not indicated in the older patient, but if the patient is extremely active, the biceps tendon can be resutured to the transverse humeral ligament or into a hole drilled in the humerus at this level. Resuturing will improve the cosmetic appearance of the arm but will leave a scar.

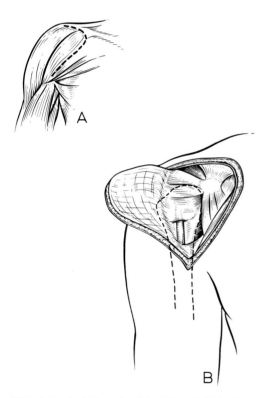

FIG. **5-15** A deltopectoral incision. A. Skin incision. B. Exposure of the entire shoulder. It is not always necessary to turn the deltoid back as far posteriorly as illustrated for most shoulder operations in the arthritic patient.

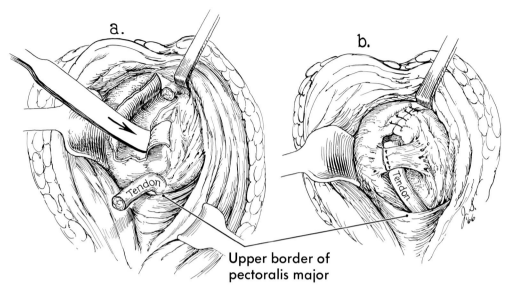

Upper border of
pectoralis major

FIG. 5-17 Exposure of the anterior aspect of the shoulder. A trough or drill hole in the bicipital groove for insertion of the biceps tendon (a). The transverse humeral ligament sutured over the tendon for further fixation (b).

Glenohumeral Synovitis

Rheumatoid arthritis in the glenohumeral joint can result in a chronic proliferative synovitis. The disease process is similar to that seen in other joints with rheumatoid arthritis, and it can be bilateral. The chronic synovitis gradually leads to destruction of the articular surface of the humeral head, resulting in an irregular surface that produces severe grating and limitation of motion (Fig. 5-18). The patient will have a gradual insidious loss of motion, and pain will become more chronic and constant as the disease process continues. Acute proliferative synovitis can lead to distension of the capsule with effusion and swelling of the shoulder joint. The patient will continue to compensate for a loss of motion as long as he can reach the top of his head or his face. However, with progression of the disease, the pain continues to increase and the limitation of function becomes greater. The patient will usually be more concerned with the limitation of function or the deformities that are developing in the hands, wrists, or elbows, and only secondarily will complain about the shoulder. However, careful clinical examination will often reveal the limitation of motion that has developed in the shoulders of these patients.

Roentgenograms of the shoulder will

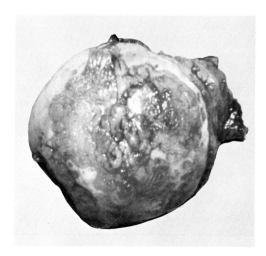

FIG. 5-18 Erosion of the articular surface of the humeral head by the synovial pannus.

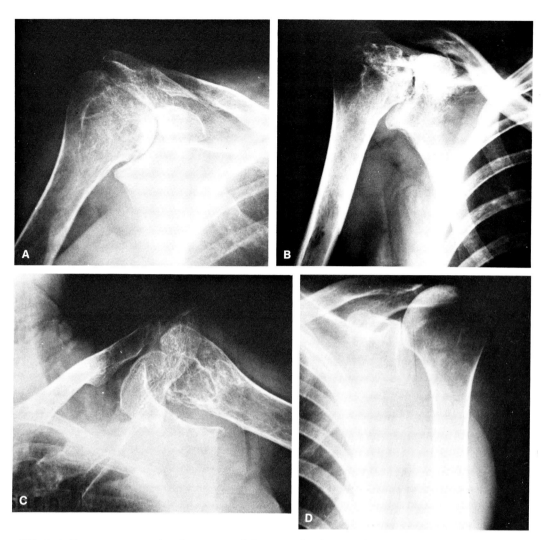

FIG. 5-19 Roentgenograms of various stages of rheumatoid arthritis in the shoulder. A. Osteoporosis and narrowing of the glenohumeral joint characteristic of the early stage. B. Extensive destruction of the articular surface and beginning destruction of the humeral head and the glenoid cavity evident in advanced rheumatoid arthritis. C. Complete destruction of the humeral head and glenoid cavity occurring in late rheumatoid disease. Note the severe cyst formation and osteoporosis. D. Subluxation of the humeral head upward out of the glenoid cavity after rupture of the shoulder cuff.

reveal all stages of articular destruction. Early in the disease, osteoporosis and narrowing of the joint space may be noted (Fig. 5-19). Gradually, erosions will develop along the articular margins of the humerus and glenoid cavity (Fig. 5-19B). As the destruction proceeds, all stages of loss of the humeral head can be noted with almost complete destruction of the humeral head and even erosions of the edge of the glenoid cavity into the surgical neck of the humerus (Fig. 5-19C). If the shoulder cuff has been destroyed by the rheumatoid process, the humerus will tend to sublux upward, out of the glenoid cavity (Fig. 5-19D). This is a characteristic finding when the rotator cuff has been destroyed and can be a contraindication to some surgical procedures.

Conservative Treatment

Although rheumatoid arthritis may involve the shoulder joints in a number of patients, surgical treatment is not indicated often in the early stage of the disease because other procedures take precedence in restoring the patient's function. In many cases, even with radiologic evidence of destruction within the joint, local injection of the joint can bring prolonged relief of the patient's symptoms and should be considered as the primary treatment in disease of the shoulder. The use of intra-articular steroids and lidocaine (Xylocaine) has given excellent relief in many patients for prolonged periods. The injection is given with the patient either in the supine position with the arm at his side or in a sitting position with the arm relaxed, hanging at the side of the body. Under sterile precautions, the area should be prepared, and then the surgeon can palpate the coracoid process and the greater tuberosity as landmarks for his injection. The needle is advanced until either the humeral head is struck or the glenoid region of the scapula, proceeding from the anterior surface of the shoulder. If the needle is advanced either medially or laterally until it drops into the shoulder joint, the fluid will be injected with ease. Aspiration in those joints that are filled with joint fluid will definitely indicate the proper area of injection. If the joint has been reached, the Xylocaine will bring immediate relief, and the patient will be able to tell the surgeon with confidence that the joint has been injected. If there is any doubt, the joint should be injected again prior to letting the patient leave the office; otherwise relief will not be obtained. Both shoulders may be injected at the same time if they are involved.

Synovectomy

If roentgenograms shows evidence of an active synovitis with rapid progression of degeneration within the joint, synovectomy should be considered early to prevent further destruction. If the roentgenograms reveal extensive destruction of the joint or if at the time of synovectomy there is noticeable articular destruction of the humeral head, replacement of the articular surface of the humerus with a metal prosthesis is indicated. Usually the glenoid cavity maintains its integrity. Several types of prostheses are available at the present time: (1) Neer prosthesis and (2) HJB prosthesis (Fig. 5-20). Several total joint replacements now coming into vogue use a high density polyethylene socket for the glenoid cavity and a metal humeral head with the stem to be inserted down the humeral shaft. Fixation with methylmethacrylate is often necessary to maintain the correct alignment of the total shoulder components.

The patient with active synovitis with progressive disease and roentgenographic evidence of early destruction taking place within the shoulder joint is a candidate for synovectomy if conservative measures have failed or if the disease is progressive. If the roentgenogram shows subluxation of the humerus upward with more than half the head above the glenoid labrum, one should not consider a synovectomy because the cuff has been badly destroyed by the disease process and the head will continue to migrate upward, producing a poor result. A chemical synovectomy with thiotepa can be considered to see if this will control the synovitis in those patients who do not desire surgery. The best regimen is three injections at 7 to 10 days apart. One cc of thiotepa is injected with 2 cc of steroids and Xylocaine into the shoulder joint. In some cases dramatic relief from symptoms and decrease of the synovitis may occur.

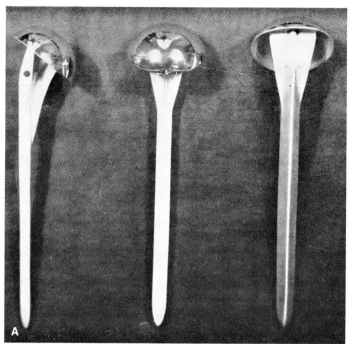

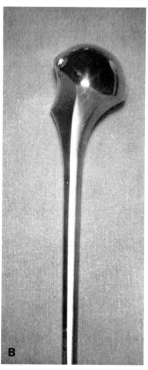

FIG. 5-20 Shoulder prostheses for replacement of the articular surface of the humerus. A. Neer prosthesis. The small, medium, and large models are shown inside, front, and back, respectively. Size refers to thickness of the shaft. (From Neer, C. S.: Articular replacement for the humeral head. J. Bone Joint Surg., *37-A*:215, 1955.) B. The HJB prosthesis.

However, if the disease process does not respond or there is continued evidence of destruction taking place, synovectomy should be considered strongly.

Operative Technique. The anterior approach should be used, and the interval between the deltoid and the pectoralis major muscle is developed (Fig. 5-21). The deltoid is detached from the clavicle and the acromion, if necessary, to obtain exposure. However, in most arthritic patients whose deltoid muscles are not well developed, this is not necessary. The tendinous portions of the coracobrachialis and the short head of the biceps muscle close to the coracoid process are incised, leaving the muscle fibers intact. Care should be exercised to prevent bleeding from the circumflex vessels located at the inferior border of the subscapularis tendon. This incision allows better exposure without having to osteotomize the coracoid process. The

subscapularis tendon is visualized across the anterior aspect of the joint, and the arm is externally rotated to put the subscapularis tendon on stretch. The lower border of the tendon is marked by several vessels, and care should be exercised not to damage these when dividing the subscapularis tendon close to the insertion into the lesser tuberosity. Several sutures may be placed in the subscapularis tendon before it is completely divided to prevent retraction and difficulty in repair.

The capsule of the joint can be separated from the tendon and opened separately in some cases to expose the synovial tissue. Most of the synovial tissue should be excised from the joint with a rongeur or a pituitary forceps. The articular margins can be curetted to remove all of the synovial tissue that is invading the subchondral bone. It is possible to sublux or dislocate the head

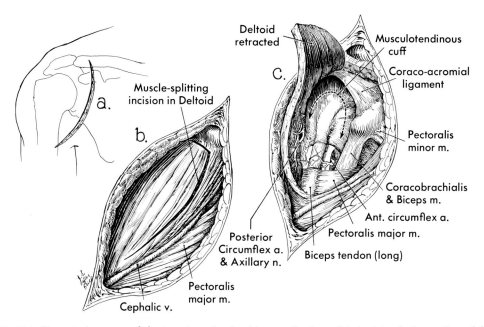

FIG. 5-21 The anterior approach for insertion of a shoulder prosthesis. a, Skin incision. b, Separation of the deltoid muscle from the cephalic vein and pectoralis major muscle. c, The upper end has been detached from the clavicle, an unnecessary procedure when the muscle is fairly atrophic. Retraction of the deltoid to expose the subscapularis tendon.

anteriorly out of the joint and remove all of the synovial tissue from the posterior aspect of the joint.

When all of the synovial tissue has been removed, the head should be reduced and the capsular tissue should be repaired with a nonabsorbable suture. The subscapularis tendon is then resutured to the portion of the tendon that was left attached to the lesser tuberosity. The tendinous portion of the coracobrachialis and the short head of the biceps tendon are resutured, and the wound is allowed to fall together. If the deltoid has been removed, it should be resutured to the clavicle and acromion process. A Velpeau dressing is applied, and the arm is immobilized for approximately 5 days, at which time pendulum exercises are instituted.

Arthroplasty

The replacement of the articular surface of the humeral head is indicated in rheumatoid arthritis when there is extensive destruction of the joint surface. Frequently in roentgenograms one will see distinct pathologic changes involving the humeral head, but the glenoid cavity often maintains its integrity (Fig. 5-22). The condition of the glenoid cavity is extremely important when considering the replacement of the humeral head alone. Arthroplasty is also indicated when, at the time of synovectomy, the articular destruction is far advanced in the humeral head and success cannot be anticipated without replacement. The patient should be informed of this possibility prior to considering a synovectomy. Replacement of the shoulder joint without repair of the shoulder cuff results in dislocation of the humeral head upward. If the roentgenogram reveals preoperatively that the humeral head is subluxed upward or dislocated, arthroplasty generally is not indicated, as it will tend to fail, and total joint replace-

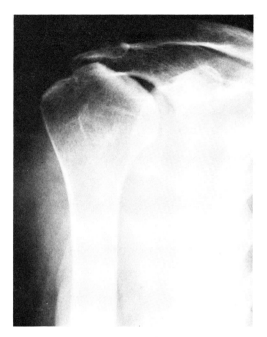

FIG. 5-22 Roentgenogram of shoulder revealing pathologic changes in the humeral head. Usually the glenoid cavity maintains its integrity.

ment should be considered. However, in most situations excellent results can be anticipated with just the articular replacement of the humeral head. Pain relief can be quite dramatic, and improved function is often obtained.

Operative Technique. The anterior approach similar to that for a synovectomy is used in an arthroplasty (Fig. 5-23), and a synovectomy is performed first. The short head of the biceps tendon and the coracobrachialis tendon are partially divided to increase the anterior exposure of the shoulder. The subscapularis tendon is divided, and stay sutures are placed through the tendon to prevent retraction. After removal of the synovial tissue, the articular surface of the humeral head is removed at the anatomic neck with a broad osteotome to expose the glenoid cavity. This cut is made at an angle of 35° of retroversion (Fig. 5-24). The medullary canal of the humerus is

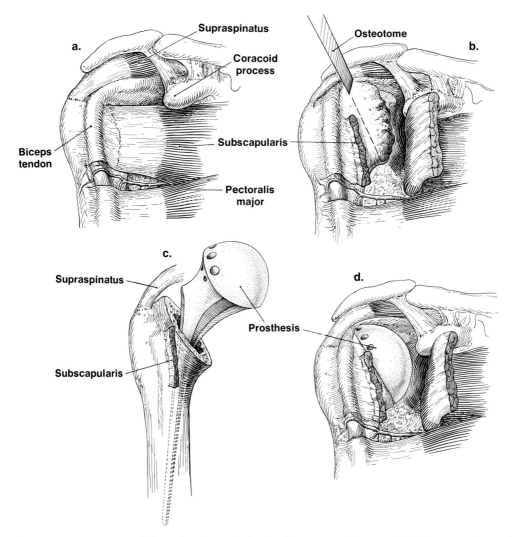

FIG. 5-23 Anterior approach for arthroplasty of the shoulder. a, Visualization of the biceps tendon and the subscapularis muscle. The dotted line represents the incision in the suprascapularis tendon. b, The osteotome retroverted at 35° for removal of humeral head and exposure of the glenoid cavity. c, Insertion of the humeral head prosthesis down the shaft of the humerus. d, The head of the prosthesis impacted down to fit nicely onto the surgical neck without disrupting any of the attachments of the rotator cuff.

opened with a curette and enlarged to accept the prosthetic stem.

In the patient with advanced osteoporosis, the Neer prosthesis should be utilized because of its light construction. The HJB prosthesis is quite heavy, and although it tends to impact well, weight can be a consideration in the osteoporotic patient. To date, we have not cemented the prosthesis in place, although cementing could be considered if loosening is a problem. This complication has not been noted in any of our cases.

The proper size of stem should be selected to fit the canal, and the prosthesis should be inserted in 30° to 45° of retroversion, using the bicipital groove as the anterior landmark. The prosthesis is impacted down the shaft until its head rests firmly and snugly on the anatomic

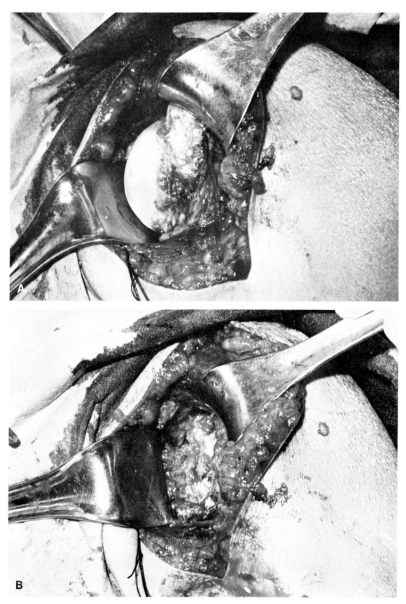

FIG. 5-24 Surgical views of the left shoulder of a patient. A. Deltoid retracted upward and laterally and the subscapularis medially to expose humeral head. B. Exposure of glenoid cavity and synovial tissue after removal of the humeral head.

neck (Figs. 5-23D; 5-25), and the shoulder is then reduced. The capsule and sub-scapularis tendon are repaired with heavy sutures to prevent dislocation, and the deltoid is sutured back into place if it has been removed.

A Velpeau dressing is applied to im-mobilize the arm. The patient usually can be discharged on the fifth or sixth postoperative day, ambulatory, and is kept immobilized in the Velpeau ban-dage for 5 days. At the end of this time the dressing is changed, and the patient is started on pendulum exercises to re-gain motion. The arm should be pro-tected in a sling and swathe for 3 weeks further when not exercising, and then the patient can be started on an active therapy program to regain further motion. Results of this type of surgery in the rheumatoid arthritis patient have been gratifying, and the shoulders reconstructed have not deteriorated with the passage of time. The longest follow-up is over 9 years.

In one patient whose humeral head was subluxed upward preoperatively, after arthroplasty of the shoulder there was a tendency for the prosthesis to ride upward because of rupture of the rotator cuff. Many humeral heads will sublux upward a short distance, but if the cuff is destroyed rather than stretched, the humeral head will begin to ride under the acromion process and produce pain on motion (Fig. 5-26). Removal of the acromion process is not indicated because the head will continue to sublux upward and function will be lost. It is in

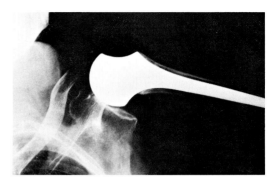

FIG. 5-26 Roentgenogram showing the humeral head abutting against the acromion and subluxing upward.

this type of case that salvage may be obtained with a total joint replacement.

Total Joint Replacement

Total joint replacement is still in its infancy in the restoration of shoulder function. However, with the improvement in technique and the development of new devices, this may become the procedure of choice after the failure of synovectomy or in advanced disease. In many cases prosthetic arthroplasty alone does not suffice, and the results could be improved with total joint replacement. Replacement of the head alone usually will not restore a full range of motion, and often only 90° of abduction can be obtained.

The Stanmore total shoulder replacement, which was developed in England, has been used in over 25 patients with rheumatoid arthritis who had severely disabling pain and no glenohumeral movement. It has been reported that almost full rotation, 90° of flexion and abduction, improvement of function, and relief of pain have been obtained with the Stanmore replacement. The device consists of a metal socket to replace the glenoid cavity and a prosthetic stem to replace the humeral head (Fig. 5-27).

An experimental device developed at

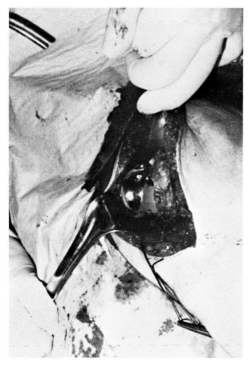

FIG. 5-25 Surgical view of the prosthesis inserted into the medullary canal.

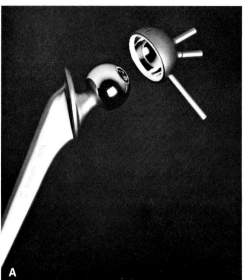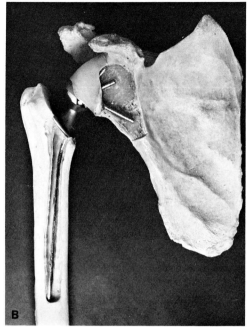

FIG. 5-27 A. The Stanmore total shoulder replacement for patients with severe disease of the glenohumeral joint. B. Specimen illustrating the implantation of the total shoulder joint. (Courtesy Zimmer Orthopaedic Ltd.)

the Mayo Clinic consists of a plastic glenoid socket which snaps into a metal humeral head that is inserted into the humeral shaft.

Shoulder replacement should become a valuable technique in the years to come.

Arthrodesis

Arthrodesis is seldom indicated in the rheumatoid patient because of generalized involvement of most of the joints in the upper limbs. Immobilization in a cast is of concern because it interferes with function of the other joints.

Acromioclavicular Arthritis

The acromioclavicular joint is formed by the articulation of the acromion process of the scapula and the distal end of the clavicle. Integrity is maintained by the weak capsular liga-ments and the strong coracoclavicular ligaments, the conoid and trapezoid (Fig. 5-28). The ligaments are arranged to allow the clavicle to rotate as the shoulder is elevated.

The articular capsule may be distended by synovial proliferation in rheumatoid arthritis. If swelling is acute enough, a prominence may be obvious over the joint. The patient complains of shoulder pain which is aggravated by use of the arm. It may be difficult to distinguish these symptoms from those originating in the glenohumeral joint.

On physical examination, tenderness may be marked over the acromioclavicular joint. A good test is to have the patient place his hand from the involved side on the opposite shoulder. A slight pressure on the elbow adducting the arm will accentuate the pain by compressing the acromioclavicular joint.

Roentgenograms of the shoulder joint may reveal evidence of narrowing of the

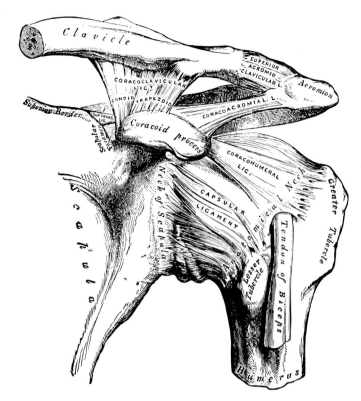

FIG. 5-28 The acromioclavicular joint with the weak capsular ligaments and the conoid and trapezoid ligaments. (From Gray's Anatomy of the Human Body, 29th ed. C. M. Goss, editor. Philadelphia, Lea & Febiger, 1973.)

acromioclavicular joint with small osteophytes (Fig. 5-29).

Conservative Treatment

The local injection of Xylocaine and cortisone into the acromioclavicular joint often will provide dramatic relief of the symptoms.

Resection

If the symptoms are severe and recurrent, however, resection of the distal end of the clavicle is indicated.

Operative Technique. The lateral end of the clavicle is exposed through a short curved incision. The acromioclavicular joint is exposed and the lateral 1 inch of the clavicle is stripped subperiosteally.

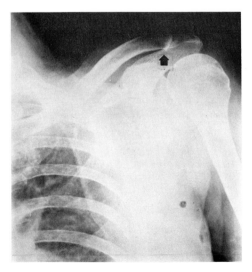

FIG. 5-29 Roentgenogram of the acromioclavicular joint revealing arthritic involvement (arrow).

After the clavicle has been divided lateral to the conoid and trapezoid ligaments, the distal end is removed. The end of the clavicle is covered with the periosteum, and the incision closed. The arm is protected in a sling for comfort, and early motion is instituted.

Sternoclavicular Joint Disorders

The sternoclavicular joint is formed by the articular surface of the sternal portion of the clavicle, the sternum, and the cartilage of the first rib. An intra-articular disk divides the joint into two compartments (Fig. 5-30). The stability of the joint is due to the costoclavicular ligament.

Although this joint takes part in every motion of the shoulder girdle, it is generally asymptomatic. The most common complaint related to the sternoclavicular joint is a painless swelling (Fig. 5-31). Rheumatoid changes accompanied by swelling and pain that can be quite uncomfortable may also develop in this joint.

Conservative Treatment

A local injection of cortisone will alleviate the pain and can be of value in decreasing synovial proliferation in the sternoclavicular joint.

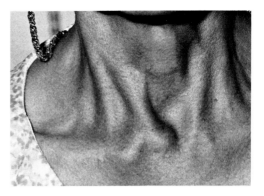

FIG. 5-31 Photograph of patient with swelling at the sternoclavicular joint.

Resection

In severe chronic cases of rheumatoid arthritis in the sternoclavicular joint, the clavicle can be resected. A 2-inch incision is made over the proximal clavicle, and the proximal 1 inch of the clavicle is resected. The periosteum should be sutured over the medial end of the clavicle (Fig. 5-32).

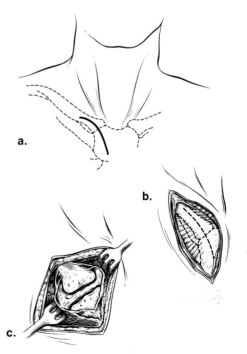

FIG. 5-32 The operative approach to the sternoclavicular joint. a, Skin incision. b, Incision of capsule and periosteum. c, Exposure of the joint.

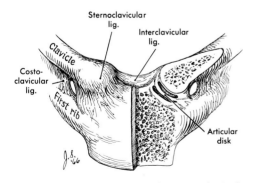

FIG. 5-30 Coronal section of the sternoclavicular joint revealing the articular disk that divides the joint.

Osteoarthritis

Patients with osteoarthritis of the shoulder joint are seldom seen in the early stages of the disease because of the minimal symptoms. Elderly patients often have advanced disease of the shoulders (Fig. 5-33). The presenting complaint generally is severe pain with loss of motion. The patient should be examined carefully to rule out acromioclavicular arthritis which is very common in the elderly patient and can be confused with osteoarthritis of the glenohumeral joint.

The various conditions that were described in rheumatoid arthritis are often associated with or seen with osteoarthritis. Subdeltoid or subacromial bursitis can occur in the patient with osteoarthritis but is generally not related to the disease process at all. The types of bursitis that were described in the section on rheumatoid arthritis are not associated with osteoarthritis which is a degenerative process within the joint itself.

Glenohumeral Joint Destruction

Osteoarthritis of the glenohumeral joint is a result of wearing out of the articular cartilage. Severe grating and limitation of rotation are seen with this problem. Abduction can produce a severe crunching and grating sound as the rough articular surface of the humeral head rubs against the irregular glenoid surface.

Conservative Treatment

Osteoarthritis of the shoulder joint can be treated in a number of patients by local injection of steroids. The mixture of lidocaine (Xylocaine) and a local steroid can give quite a bit of relief to the patient with involvement in this joint.

Arthroplasty

If conservative treatment does not give satisfactory results or if, in time, this fails, surgical intervention can be of value. The operation of choice is replacement of the humeral head with the Neer or the HJB prosthesis. This operation is described in the section on rheu-

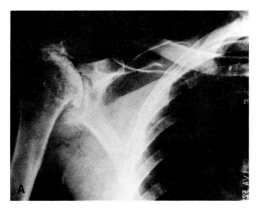 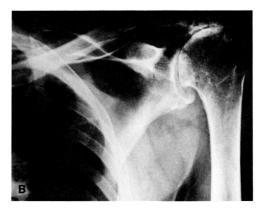

FIG. 5-33 Roentgenograms of elderly patient with severe osteoarthritis. A. Sclerosis and loss of the joint space in the right shoulder joint are obvious. Rotator cuff appears also to be damaged, as there is subluxation upward of the humeral head. B. Advanced disease in the left shoulder with sclerosis between the humeral head and the acromion. This would indicate that the shoulder cuff has been destroyed, allowing the head to subluxate upward.

matoid arthritis (page 79). Replacement of the articular surface in patients with a good shoulder cuff can improve the range of motion and also relieve the patient of severe pain (Fig. 5-34).

Acromioclavicular Joint Destruction

Osteoarthritis of the acromioclavicular joint occurs frequently in the elderly patient or in patients who have suffered an injury to the shoulder joint from a previous acromioclavicular separation. The patient will complain of pain in the region of the shoulder, and at times it is difficult to evaluate the exact site of the patient's complaint. Careful examination will often reveal some swelling in the area of the acromioclavicular joint and local tenderness. Adducting the arm across to the opposite shoulder tends to increase the pain by compressing the acromioclavicular joint, reproducing all of the symptoms (Fig. 5-35).

The roentgenogram may demonstrate narrowing of the acromioclavicular joint with small spurs projecting from the margins of the joint. If the glenohumeral

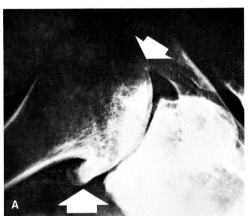

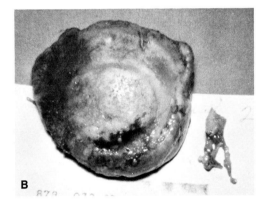

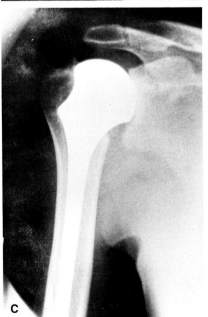

FIG. 5-34 Arthroplasty of the osteoarthritic shoulder. A. Roentgenogram of shoulder of 63-year-old man, revealing advanced osteoarthritis with loss of joint space and osteophyte formation. B. Humeral head removed. Note sclerosis and indentation where the glenoid cavity was rubbing against the surface of the humeral head. C. Roentgenogram showing prosthesis in place.

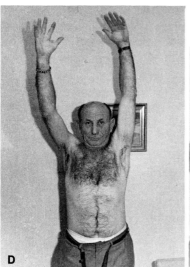
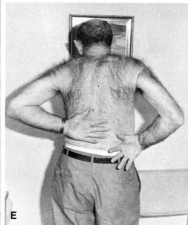
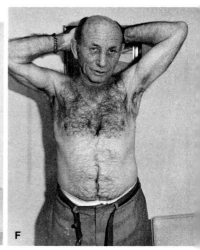

FIG. 5-34 (continued) D–F. Photographs of patient 7 years after the operation: D, abduction that is possible in the right shoulder; E, slight limitation of internal rotation, as compared to the normal side; F, almost complete external rotation with freedom from pain.

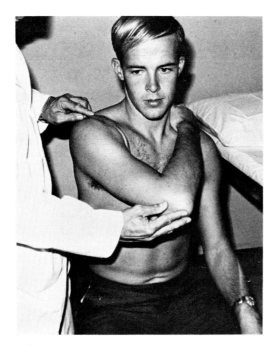

FIG. 5-35 Test for acromioclavicular arthritis. The patient places his hand on the opposite shoulder, and the examiner pushes on the elbow, compressing the acromioclavicular joint to elicit pain. (From Marmor, L.: The painful shoulder. Am. Fam. Physician, 1:1, 75, 1970.)

joint appears normal, this observation tends to support the diagnosis considerably. A good therapeutic test is to inject the acromioclavicular joint with Xylocaine and see if it relieves the patient's symptoms immediately.

Conservative Treatment

The use of a local steroid with the Xylocaine can often give prolonged relief of the patient's symptoms. The best way to do this is to use a 21 gauge needle and proceed along the edge of the clavicle until the needle falls into the small joint space and then the medication may be injected. Only a small quantity of fluid can be injected, so small quantities should be used with a 1 or 2 cc syringe.

Mumford Resection

In the patient with intractable symptoms, the operation of choice is to excise one inch of the clavicle lateral to the coracoclavicular ligaments (Fig. 5-36).

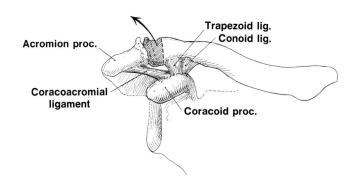

Acromion proc.

Trapezoid lig.
Conoid lig.

Coracoacromial ligament

Coracoid proc.

FIG. 5-36 Excision of the clavical distal to the coracoclavicular ligament (conoid and trapezoid ligaments) to relieve symptoms of painful acromioclavicular arthritis.

This is the Mumford operation, and it can bring prolonged relief if an adequate resection is carried out. The removal of the distal end of the clavicle tends to prevent rubbing of the surfaces of the acromion against the clavicle, and the patient will be relieved of the symptoms produced by the osteoarthritis. It is not advisable to resect proximal to the coracoclavicular ligaments because the clavicle will then protrude upward and produce an obvious deformity.

Bibliography

Rheumatoid Arthritis

Codman, E. A.: The Shoulder. Boston, Thomas Todd Co., 1934.

DePalma, A. F.: Surgical approaches to the region of the shoulder joint. Clin. Orthop., 20:163, 1961.

DePalma, A. F., and Snedden, H. E.: Shoulder joint. In Surgery of Arthritis, R. A. Milch, editor. Baltimore, The Williams & Wilkins Co., 1964, p. 85.

Hitchcock, H. H., and Bechtol, C. O.: Painful shoulder: observations of the role of the long head of the biceps. J. Bone Joint Surg., 30-A:263, 1948.

Inman, V. T., Saunders, J. B., and Abbott, L. C.: Observations on the shoulder joint. J. Bone Joint Surg., 26:1, 1944.

Lucas, D. B.: Biomechanics of the shoulder joint. Arch. Surg., 107:425, 1973.

McLaughlin, H. L.: The "frozen shoulder." Clin. Orthop., 20:126, 1961.

Mosely, H. F.: Shoulder Lesions. Springfield, Ill., Charles C Thomas, 1945.

Neer, C. S.: Articular replacement for the humeral head. J. Bone Joint Surg., 37-A:215, 1955.

Neer, C. S.: Degenerative lesions of the proximal humeral articular surface. Clin. Orthop., 20:116, 1961.

Neviaser, J. S.: Surgical approaches to the shoulder. Clin. Orthop., 91:34, 1973.

Schrager, V. L.: Tenosynovitis of the long head of the biceps humeri. Surg. Gynecol. Obstet., 66:785, 1938.

Wertheim, H. M., and Rovenstine, E. A.: Suprascapular nerve block. Anesthesiology, 2:541, 1941.

Osteoarthritis

Barton, N. J.: Arthrodesis of the shoulder for degenerative conditions. J. Bone Joint Surg., 54-A:1759, 1972.

Bremner, R. A.: Monarticular, non-infective subacute arthritis of the sternoclavicular joint. J. Bone Joint Surg., 41-B:749–753, 1959.

DePalma, A. F., and Snedden, H. E.: Shoulder joint. In Surgery of Arthritis, R. A. Milch, editor. Baltimore, The Williams & Wilkins Co., 1964, p. 94.

Marmor, L.: The painful shoulder. Amer. Family Phys. G. P., 1:75–82, 1970.

Neer, C. S.: Replacement arthroplasty for glenohumeral osteoarthritis. J. Bone Joint Surg., *56-A*:1, 1974.

Neer, C. S.: Articular replacement for the humeral head. Bone Joint Surg., *37-A*:215, 1955.

Neer, C. S.: Degenerative lesions of the proximal humeral articular surface. Clin. Orthop., *20*:116, 1961.

Olsson, O.: Degenerative changes of the shoulder joint and their connection with shoulder pain. Acta Chir. Scand. (Suppl.), *181*:99, 1953.

6 | The Elbow

Arthritis does not involve the elbow joint as frequently as it does the hand, wrist, or foot. When it does, however, it can become symptomatic, resulting in a loss of function and at times in severe disability. Involvement of both elbow joints that limits motion can completely disable a patient by interfering with his daily activities of living. If both elbows are stiff at about 90°, the patient cannot take care of his personal hygiene nor feed himself. When severely disabled patients are asked what they desire the most, the majority would reply they desire the ability to feed themselves.

Rheumatoid arthritis can produce severe destruction of the elbow joints leaving very little bone for reconstruction. Osteoarthritis, in contrast, tends to produce a loss of the joint space with sclerosis of the adjacent bone.

Anatomy

The elbow joint is essentially three joints functioning together rather than simply a hinge joint. These joints are the radio-humeral, the radioulnar, and the humeroulnar. The articular surface of the humerus is divided into two main portions by the trochlear ridge. The lateral aspect, called the capitulum, articulates with the radial head, and the medial side, called the trochlea, articulates with the ulna. The ulna contains a semicircular trochlear notch that contains the olecranon process and the coronoid process. This notch forms the hinge joint for the elbow and articulates with the trochlea of the humerus.

The rounded head of the radius articulates with the distal surface of the capitulum and also with the side of the ulna forming the proximal radioulnar joint. On rotation of the forearm, the rounded radial head slides against the lateral side of the ulna.

The synovial membrane of the elbow joint is extensive. It reaches from the margin of the articular surface of the humerus and lines the coronoid, radial, and olecranon fossa. The capsule of the elbow joint is relaxed anteriorly and posteriorly to allow easy movement of the elbow joint. On the medial and lateral side of the joint are strong collateral ligaments which add stability. The annular ligament passes around the neck of the radius and tends to hold the radius from moving away from the ulna on rotation of the forearm (Fig. 6-1).

Since the distal radioulnar joint is extremely important in the pronation and supination of the forearm, it is included in the anatomy of the elbow. The distal end of the ulna is bulbous and has a small styloid process that extends from the medial posterior surface of the arm. There is a fibrocartilaginous disk that is in contact with the radius and the ulna. The distal radioulnar joint acts as a pivot. As the radius rotates around the ulna, the fibrocartilaginous disk rotates with the radius, sliding over the distal surface of the ulna. The synovial cavity involving the distal radioulnar joint usually does not communicate with the wrist joint unless the rheumatoid disease has been severely active and has resulted in destruction of the joint capsule.

The nerve supply of the elbow joint proper is derived from the median, radial, ulnar, and musculocutaneous nerves.

A large, subcutaneous bursa between the skin and the undersurface of the olecranon process can become involved in rheumatoid arthritis, resulting in symptoms.

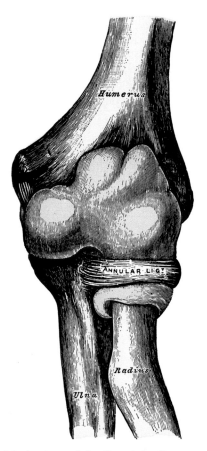
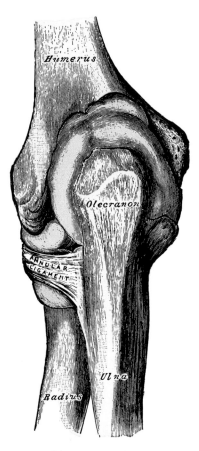

FIG. 6-1 Anatomy of the elbow joint illustrating the synovial tissue within the joint. The annular ligament encloses the neck of the radius and holds it in place. A. Anterior aspect. B. Posterior aspect. (From Gray's Anatomy of the Human Body, 29th ed. C. M. Goss, editor. Philadelphia, Lea & Febiger, 1973.)

Function of the Elbow Joint

The basic functional requirement of the elbow is to allow the hand to reach the face and the perineum for eating and personal hygiene. Generally, if the shoulder is not severely arthritic, loss of motion in the elbow joint and forearm can easily be compensated for by substitution of other motions by the patient. Rotation of the shoulder joint is utilized to substitute for loss of pronation and supination. Loss of supination occurs frequently in rheumatoid arthritis. If the shoulder is involved, the patient is unable to receive anything into the palm of the hand and is severely disabled. Loss of supination in both wrists will mean that women will be unable to receive coins or change in their hands and must have it deposited into their purses. Bilateral involvement also prevents opening doors and jars, turning a key in a lock, and many other daily activities of living. The normal range of elbow motion is from 0° of extension to 145° of flexion (180 to 35). In certain persons, hyperextension is possible, but this is rare in rheumatoid arthritis because of the early development of flexion contractures. Pronation and supination usually allow 90° of motion.

the region of the radial head. Synovial effusion can be detected by palpating and obtaining the following landmarks: (1) radial head, (2) olecranon tip, and (3) lateral epicondyle. These points form a triangle, the center of which should be soft and not distended if there is no effusion of the elbow joint. When disease is present with synovial swelling, a thickness or bulge can be palpated in this area. The radial head is best determined by having the patient pronate and supinate the forearm, if possible, as the examiner feels the rotation of the radial head. Tenderness directly over the radial head may indicate osteoarthritis. Palpation will also reveal rheumatoid nodules which are often located on the olecranon and forearm. These usually occur where there is pressure and can be multiple. The olecranon bursa may become thickened due to synovial hyperplasia or a collection of fluid within the bursa. Palpation of the lateral epicondyle is also important in determining whether epicondylitis is present. The ulnar nerve can be palpated in the groove behind the medial epicondyle, and if tender may reveal the presence of a neuritis. The range of active motion should be recorded in flexion, extension, pronation, and supination.

Physical Examination

The elbow joint is generally included as part of the complete examination of the upper extremity. The shoulder should be examined along with the wrist and hand when evaluating the elbow. The normal contour should be examined for evidence of an effusion within the joint which will be noted as a swelling near

Roentgenograms

Roentgenograms of the elbow joint are of value in the diagnosis of arthritis of the elbow. They should be obtained from both the anteroposterior and the lateral views. Usually by the time the patient has developed persistent symptoms involving the elbow joint, changes due to the disease process will be visible in roentgenograms (Fig. 6-2). In both rheumatoid arthritis and osteoarthritis

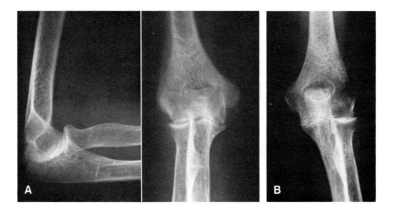

FIG. 6-2 Roentgenograms of advanced joint changes when symptoms arise in the elbow joint. A. Lateral view (left) and anterior view (right) revealing narrowing of the joint surface with beginning erosion along the olecranon surface. B. Gradual loss of the joint space and beginning deformities of the radial head as rheumatoid disease progresses.

there may be a narrowing of the joint space between the capitulum and the radial head because of loss of articular cartilage. Deformities or irregularities may be observed in the radial head. Erosion of the articular margins along the medial side of the joint is characteristic of rheumatoid arthritis, but not of osteoarthritis. Sclerosis and irritation are much more common than osteoporosis in osteoarthritis involving the elbow joint (Fig. 6-3).

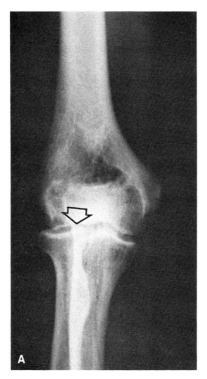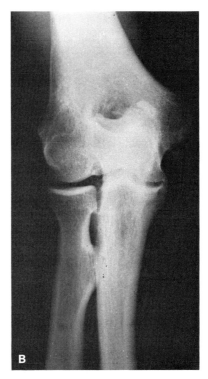

FIG. 6-3 Roentgenograms of early osteoarthritis of the elbow. A. Narrowing of the joint space between the capitulum and the radial head (arrow) due to loss of the articular cartilage. B. Sclerosis and osteophyte formation between the trochlea and ulna.

Rheumatoid Arthritis

Early in the course of rheumatoid arthritis the patient will complain of pain and swelling of the elbow joint with limitation of motion. The first objective signs are swelling of the synovial tissue and effusion within the joint, resulting in a bulging of the lateral aspect of the elbow adjacent to the radial head (Fig. 6-4). This results in loss of motion with limitations of flexion, extension, pronation, and supination. There is a tendency for exacerbations of the symptoms in the elbow with long periods of improvement between.

In evaluating the elbow joint of a patient with rheumatoid arthritis, it is important to consider the functions of both the distal radioulnar joint and the shoulder joint. Frequently in rheumatoid arthritis the wrist is involved early, and advanced disease of the radioulnar joint may lead to limitations of pronation and supination that will not be relieved by simple excision of the radial head (Fig. 6-5). Deformity of the radial head itself, which is common in rheumatoid arthritis, also can result in limitation of pronation and supination. The destruction of the trochlear notch is usually due to erosion from the disease process, and erosion can also produce a medial osteophyte. This will be visible on the medial side of the trochlea as a ridge (Fig. 6-6). Gross destruction of the elbow joint may take place as the disease process continues, resulting in loss of the lower end of the humerus and settling into the trochlear notch (Fig. 6-7).

Nerve entrapment about the elbow joint occurs occasionally. It may simulate a tendon rupture. Although it is rare, one should consider this condition when the patient has definite paresthesias in the hand or muscle weakness. Several authors have noted that the ulnar nerve and the posterior interosseus nerve, which is a branch of the radial nerve, have been involved in entrapment syndromes.

Severe involvement of the elbow joint with loss of motion can result in fibrous ankylosis or bony fusion of the elbow joint. Bilateral involvement with loss of motion can severely disable the patient, preventing him from being self-sufficient (Fig. 6-8).

Conservative Treatment

In treating the elbow joint, if symptoms are not too severe and the roentgenograms show minimal destruction or irregularity of the radial head or elbow joint, conservative therapy should be utilized. This consists of aspiration of the elbow joint and the injection of a corticosteroid into the joint through the lateral aspect. The landmarks for injection of the elbow joint are the lateral condyle of the humerus, the tip of the olecranon, and the radial head. When the elbow joint is flexed approximately

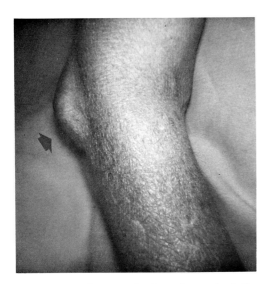

FIG. 6-4 Swelling on the lateral aspect of the elbow (arrow), the first objective sign of rheumatoid arthritis.

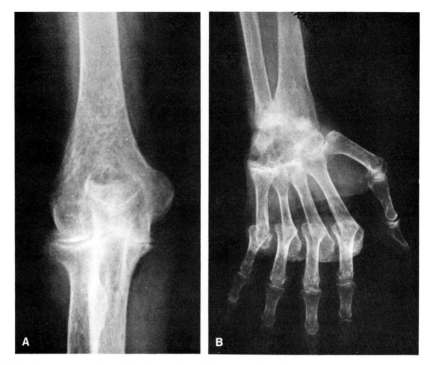

FIG. 6-5 Roentgenograms for evaluating extent of rheumatoid arthritis in a patient who exhibited loss of pronation and supination. A. Elbow joint. Evidences of advanced disease are loss of joint space, sclerosis, and spur formation on the medial aspect of the joint. The radial head is deformed. B. Wrist. Involvement of distal radioulnar joint was the cause of the limitation in range of motion. There is spontaneous fusion of the carpal bones.

90°, these three points will form a triangle within which is a soft area leading directly to the elbow joint. If the joint is swollen, the forearm should be rotated while the examiner is palpating the radial head to outline the site of injection. This is the easiest approach to the elbow joint and the most satisfactory. The area should be thoroughly prepared with an antiseptic solution. Under sterile technique the needle is inserted carefully into the soft area of the elbow joint, and the joint is aspirated. Approximately 2 cc of lidocaine (Xylocaine) and 1 cc of the corticosteroids should be mixed in the syringe and injected into the elbow joint. Relief of pain is generally quite satisfactory, and the injection may be repeated if symptoms warrant in 3 to 6 weeks.

Synovectomy and Excision of the Radial and Ulnar Heads

The two major indications for surgery in the elbow have been pain, limitation of motion, or both symptoms combined. The patient with symptoms severe enough to have surgery performed on the elbow usually has extensive involvement of the radial head and the joint surfaces. The major cause for surgery in our series has been pain that has not responded to conservative treatment. The youngest patient was 18 years of age and the oldest, 65. The average age for elbow surgery was 43 years. The average length of arthritis symptoms was 14 years, the shortest was 2 years, and the longest, 27 years prior to surgery. In certain situations, synovectomy of the elbow joint can be carried out without

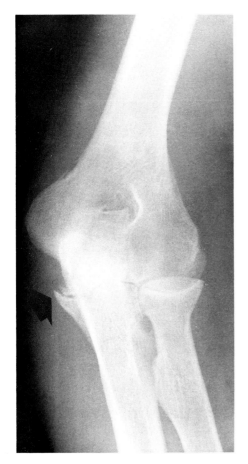

FIG. 6-6 Roentgenogram in which a bony prominence or ridge (arrow) is obvious along the subchondral margin of the olecranon.

excision of the radial head, but when there are deformity of the radial head and chronic synovitis, the combined approach of synovectomy and excision of the radial head is indicated. However, before any surgical procedure is considered on the elbow joint, it is important to evaluate the distal radioulnar joint and the wrist. Deformity of both the radial head and the distal radioulnar joint can prevent pronation and supination. Excision of the radial head alone will not correct the situation, and the ulnar head must be removed before the patient can be advised that the range of motion will be improved postoperatively. The patient with long-standing rheumatoid arthritis will have accepted the loss of function and will not realize that something can be done to aid in regaining pronation and supination. If the distal radioulnar joint is not involved and only the radial head is affected, an improvement of supination and pronation can be expected by excision of the radial head. The combined procedure of excision of the radial head and the ulnar head when both joints are involved will also improve function of the forearm. The relief of pain and the improvement of function observed in these patients make synovectomy and excision of the radial head a valuable procedure in the treatment of the patient with rheumatoid arthritis. The long-term follow-up of these patients over 7 years after surgery revealed that the initial good results in regard to pain relief, increased joint motion, and improved function were retained and did not deteriorate with the passage of time (Fig. 6-9). Therefore one can predict that if the patient has an initial good result it will persist (Fig. 6-10).

It is important to point out that the radial head should not be removed in a growing child when the epiphysis is open, since it contributes to the growth of the radius. Removal of the proximal radial epiphysis produces a severe deformity due to continued growth of the ulna and shortening of the radius.

Operative Technique. The operation is performed under a tourniquet placed high up on the arm to give adequate exposure of the area. A posterolateral approach to the joint is utilized, as it is simple and gives adequate exposure. Internal fixation is not required as in the transolecranon approach described by Inglis, Ranawat, and Straub (Fig. 6-11). Many of the complications associated with that approach can be avoided by the posterolateral approach and excision of the radial head.

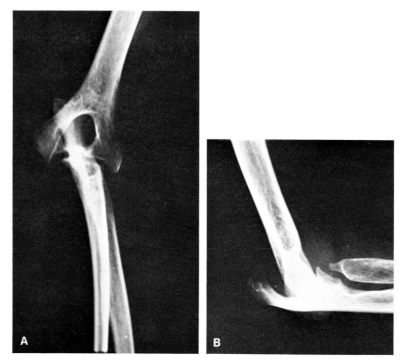

FIG. 6-7 Roentgenograms of the elbow joint of a 28-year-old woman with advanced rheumatoid disease. A. Anteroposterior view. The trochlea and the capitulum have been destroyed. B. Lateral view. The olecranon and the radial head have also been destroyed.

The incision is started on the lateral condyle and carried distally over the radial head toward the ulna (Fig. 6-12). The plane between the anconeus and the extensor carpi ulnaris muscles is developed to expose the capsule of the elbow joint. The capsule is opened and the radial head is exposed. In very active cases the synovial tissue will bulge from the joint and will have to be removed before adequate exposure of the head is possible. The incision in the capsule should not go beyond the radial neck to prevent injury to the supinator branch of the radial nerve. The neck of the radius is exposed, and holes are placed across it at the level of the excision with a small drill (Fig. 6-12B). The drill holes mark the line for excision of the radial head with a small osteotome (Fig. 6-12C). Instead of the drill holes, it is also possible to use an air drill with a cutting tool or a small power saw to remove the radial head at the neck. Once the head has been removed, adequate visualization of the entire joint is possible, and the joint may be rocked open by adduction of the forearm. The joint is inspected, and the synovial tissue within the joint is removed with a small rongeur and a curette. Usually a good deal of synovium will be found anteriorly under the capsule, and care should be exercised to prevent damage to the median nerve and the brachial vessels. By rocking open the joint, one can also remove the synovium from the posterior recesses of the joint and curette off any pannus formation. The sharp spicules of bone remaining on the radial neck should be removed with a rongeur and may be smoothed with a power reamer or rasp if so desired.

A Swanson Silastic radial head may be inserted to maintain both the length

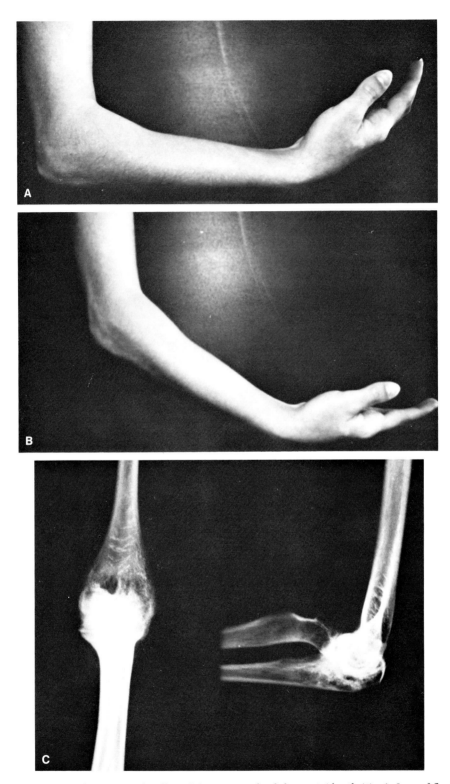

FIG. 6-8 Limitation of motion in the elbow joint as a result of rheumatoid arthritis. A. Loss of flexion. B. The maximum extension possible. C. Roentgenograms revealing involvement of the elbow joint (left) and blocking of flexion by the radial head (right).

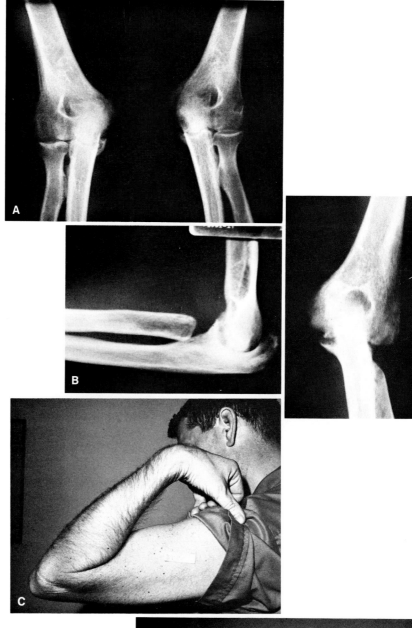

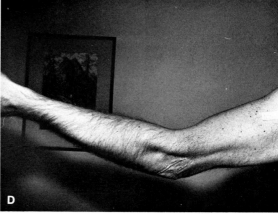

FIG. 6-9 Follow-up of a patient after resection of the radial head and synovectomy of the elbow joint. A. Roentgenogram before the operation in 1966, showing rheumatoid disease in the elbow joint. B. Roentgenograms 9 years after the operation. Lateral (left) and anterior (right) views. C. Photograph showing excellent flexion with no pain. D. Photograph showing some limitation of extension, which is extremely common in rheumatoid arthritis of the elbow.

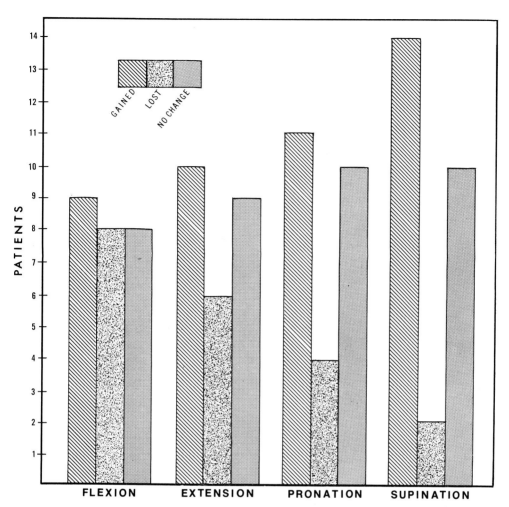

FIG. 6-10 Graph showing the range of motion obtained postoperatively by 19 patients after excision of the radial head and synovectomy of the elbow joint. Six of the patients had bilateral surgical procedures.

of the radius and the normal relationship of the radioulnar joint at the elbow (Fig. 6-13). At this stage of the operation after removal of the bony spicules from the radial neck, a drill hole is made down the medullary cavity with a reamer or broach. The prosthesis is available in various sizes (Fig. 6-14). When the proper size has been selected, the permanent prosthesis is inserted with its stem down the medullary cavity and its head slipped into the elbow joint. To prevent tearing the Silastic, sharp instruments should be avoided.

The joint is thoroughly irrigated with saline solution, then the capsule is repaired, and the muscles are approximated. The subcutaneous tissue and skin are also repaired, and a bulky soft compressive dressing is applied from the forearm to the midarm. Postoperatively the patients are instructed to start flexion-extension and pronation-supination exercises on the first day. The bulky pressure dressing is removed on the third day to allow further motion, and the patients are allowed to go home on the fifth postoperative day. A plaster

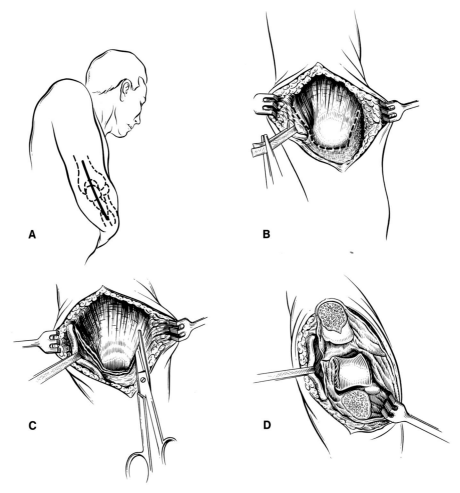

FIG. 6-11 Posterior approach to the elbow joint (transolecranon approach). A. Skin incision. B. The ulnar nerve isolated and pulled out of the way with a tape. The dotted line illustrates the incision through the tendon of the triceps. C. Division of the tendon with scissors. D. Transection of the olecranon with the triceps tendon attached. (Redrawn from Campbell's Operative Orthopaedics, 5th ed. A. H. Grenshaw, editor. St. Louis, C. V. Mosby, 1971.)

cast or splint is not recommended. The patient should be advised to exercise the shoulder and raise the arm over the head at least once a day to prevent the development of a stiff shoulder. A good range of motion may be anticipated (Fig. 6-15).

Results. Pronation and supination may not be improved by excision of the radial head alone if the distal radioulnar joint is involved. When there is involvement of the distal joint, surgery should be performed at the same time to remove the ulnar head (see Chapter 7). Contrac-

ture of the interosseous ligament between the radius and ulna has not been a problem in developing increased pronation and supination. The patient must exercise vigorously to regain pronation and supination and must be taught to fix the elbow at the side of the body to prevent internal and external rotation of the shoulder from substituting for the forearm motion. Gradual stretching by the patient with a therapist or a member of the patient's family will result in increased pronation and supination. Symp-

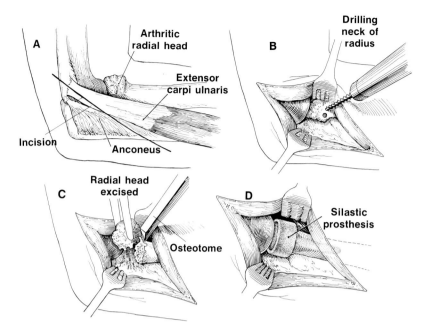

FIG. 6-12 Technique for synovectomy and excision of the radial head. A. Posterolateral approach to the elbow joint. B. Drill holes placed across the radial neck. C. Removing the radial head with an osteotome. D. Silastic prosthesis inserted into the radius to replace the radial head.

toms may persist for up to 6 weeks as the joint heals.

Complications. Medial osteophytes due to arthritic changes may be present within the joint. A large osteophyte may extend from the trochlea and another from the olecranon, producing symp-

toms on the medial aspect of the joint motion. These osteophytes plus erosions of the synovial tissue through the capsule can also produce an ulnar neuritis or nerve palsy (Fig. 6-6). When symptoms due to the osteophytes persist, a medial incision to remove these osteo-

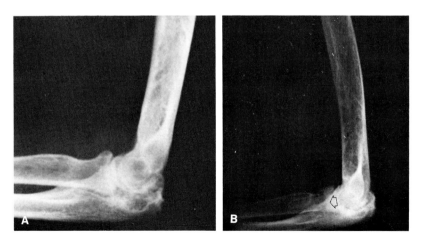

FIG. 6-13 Lateral roentgenograms of left elbow of a patient. A. Before excision of the radial head and synovectomy. Signs of severe rheumatoid arthritis are evident. B. After the operation. The Silastic radial head is indicated by the arrow.

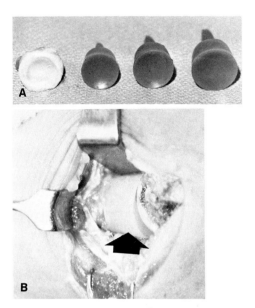

FIG. 6-14 Silastic replacement for radial head of elbow. A. Trial prostheses placed beside the radial head (left) that has been removed from the patient. B. Surgical view of Silastic prosthesis (arrow) inserted into the elbow joint.

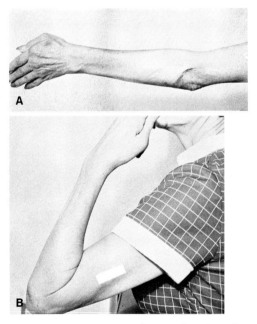

FIG. 6-15 Demonstration of range of motion after radial head replacement illustrated in Figures 6-11 and 6-12. The patient's pronation and supination were normal. A. Extension is slightly limited. B. Flexion of the elbow is excellent.

phytes may be made when the radial head is excised. Care must be exercised to protect the ulnar nerve which is located just posterior to the osteophyte.

The distal radioulnar joint is excised after closure of the elbow incision without releasing the tourniquet. A 2-inch incision running parallel to the shaft of the ulna is made over the distal ulna at the ulnar head. It is important to look for the dorsal sensory branch of the ulnar nerve which passes superficially just distal to the ulnar styloid and which can be easily divided in this area. The extensor carpi ulnaris tendon is retracted laterally out of the way, and the extensor retinaculum is opened and retracted to expose the ulnar head. The extensor digiti quinti tendon should also be retracted medially to prevent injury. The periosteum is incised over the distal ulna and stripped from the shaft for about 1 to 2 cm proximally. Drill holes are placed across the shaft at the proximal end of the exposed ulna and an osteotome is used to divide the ulna between 1 to 2 cm from the styloid process. The ulnar head is then removed by sharp dissection from the muscular attachment and periosteum, and all synovial tissue in the area should be removed from the joint with a rongeur. Both the radial portion of the radioulnar joint and the articular surface of the lunate can be visualized in the distal aspect of the incision. The distal end of the ulnar shaft is smoothed with a rongeur and rasp or with a power reamer to remove any sharp spicules. The shaft is then depressed with an instrument such as a hemostat, and the periosteum is resutured over the top of it to prevent the ulna from riding dorsally postoperatively. The retinaculum is also repaired, and the incision is closed. Postoperative care is exactly the same, whether the ulnar head is removed at the time of radial head excision or not.

Arthroplasty

Rheumatoid arthritis in the elbow joint may at times progress to ankylosis (Fig. 6-16). When this occurs, the joint becomes painless. If the position of the elbow is about 130° with 25° of pronation, this may be satisfactory if the dominant elbow joint is normal. If both joints are ankylosed, however, or have limited motion, this may be totally unaccept-able. It is important that one hand be able to reach the face for eating and the other below the waist for toilet care. This need must be considered in planning the range of motion in an arthroplasty of the elbow and is one of the main reasons to consider an arthroplasty rather than an arthrodesis in disease of the elbow. Also, stability of the elbow is not as necessary as stability in the lower

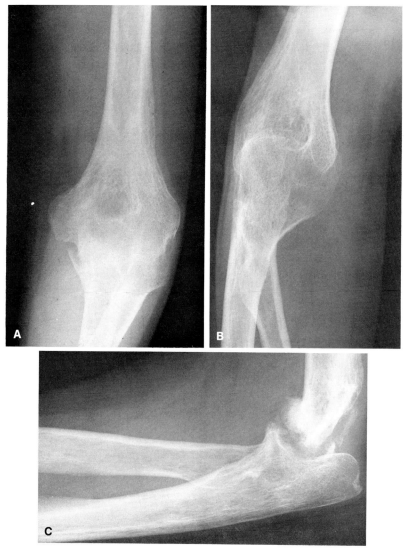

FIG. 6-16 Roentgenograms before and after arthroplasty for ankylosis of the elbow joint in full extension. A. Anterior view before operation. B. Lateral view before operation. C. Lateral view 10 years after arthroplasty of the distal end of the elbow.

limbs where the body weight must be supported.

Since there is a tendency toward ankylosis following surgery, postoperative traction and the interposition of fascia lata or other material to cover the raw bony surfaces are of value.

Operative Technique. The elbow joint may be exposed from the lateral or the posterior approach in performing an arthroplasty.

The lateral approach may be performed under tourniquet control. An incision is started 3 inches above the lateral condyle and extended distally 3 inches beyond the radial head. The extensor muscle origin can be removed from the condyle, thus exposing the lateral aspect of the joint capsule. The capsule and collateral ligament are divided to expose the lateral aspect of the joint. The lower articular portion of the humerus is dissected free of adhesions and the capitulum and trochlea are excised so that a single condyle is formed. The radial head is removed at the orbicular ligament to allow rotation of the forearm, and the trochlear notch of the ulna is deepened (Fig. 6-17A, B). At this stage of the operation the previously

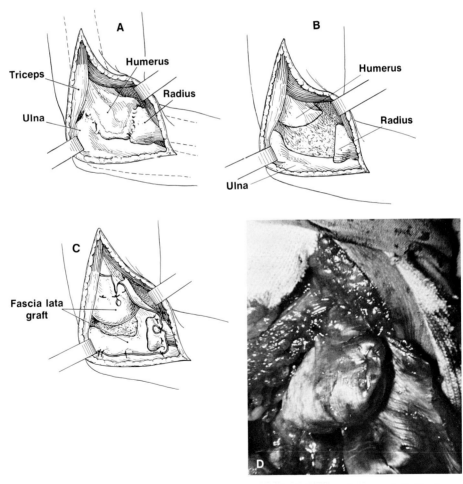

FIG. 6-17 Technique for fascial arthroplasty. A. Exposure as a result of the lateral approach. B. The lower end of the humerus has been removed along with the trochlear notch of the ulna and the radial head. C. Fascia lata taken from the thigh is used to cover the raw surfaces of the bone to prevent ankylosis. D. Surgical view showing the humerus covered by the facia lata and the remainder of the fascia lata to be used as a covering of the radial head and the olecranon notch.

prepared thigh is exposed and a fascia lata graft large enough to cover the raw surfaces of the joint is removed. The fascia is sewn about the lower humerus and folded over the ulna and radius (Fig. 6-17C). The joint is then reduced, and the extensor muscle origin is resutured to the deep fascia or lower humerus.

If the patient has a tendency for ankylosis or has active rheumatoid arthritis, a Steinmann pin should be inserted through the olecranon, care being taken to avoid the ulnar nerve. The procedure is best executed by approaching the ulna from the medial side and pushing the nerve aside. The arm is then placed in overhead traction to maintain distraction and allow early elbow motion (Fig. 6-18).

An alternate method of aftercare is to place the elbow in a posterior, molded splint. It is important to determine the degree of elbow flexion at which to set the splint by the function that will be needed by the patient. Since it is unusual to regain full motion, the appropriate range should be selected. If the hand is to reach the face, 90 degrees or less of flexion would be appropriate. If the hand is to go below the waist, 135 degrees of flexion would be desirable (Fig. 6-19).

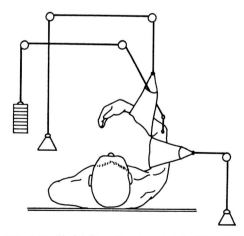

FIG. 6-18 Skeletal traction to maintain distraction of the joint and allow early elbow motion.

The splint may be removed by a therapist in one week so that carefully guarded exercises to increase the range of motion may be performed.

The posterior approach, as described by Campbell, will also give excellent exposure for an elbow arthroplasty (Fig. 6-20A). The skin incision is started 4 inches proximal to the elbow on the posterolateral aspect of the arm and is continued distally for 4 inches. The deep fascia is divided, and the triceps tendon is exposed. A tongue-shaped flap is turned down distally to the olecranon to expose the elbow joint (Fig. 6-20B). The periosteum and the triceps muscle are stripped off the lower humerus, and the joint is freed 6-20C). The remainder of the arthroplasty and aftercare are the same as described previously.

Implant Resection Arthroplasty

A flexible hinge elbow implant developed by Swanson utilizes a Silastic implant to maintain the joint space relationship (Fig. 6-21). The implant, however, does not provide for medial-lateral stability and requires the reconstruction of a strong, ligamentous system around the joint. The indications for this particular implant are (1) ankylosis of the elbow joint due to arthritis or trauma or (2) ankylosis of both elbow joints. The contraindications are (1) children with open epiphyses, (2) infection or inadequate skin over the joint, and (3) severe myositis ossificans.

Operative Technique. The elbow joint can be approached through a posterior, a lateral, or a bilateral incision. The ulnar incision should start approximately 4 inches above the elbow and extend approximately 4 inches below the elbow. The ulnar nerve should be identified, released from the ulnar groove, and retracted out of the way. The flexors are released from the epicondyle, and the joint is opened. Following this, a radial incision is made, using a dorsal-

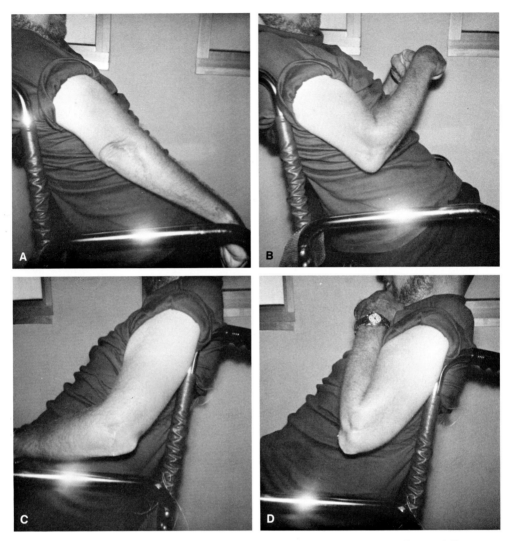

FIG. 6-19 A patient after bilateral arthroplasties of ankylosed elbows. A. The right elbow in full extension. B. Flexion to 90°. This arm is used to take care of his personal hygiene. C. Extension of the left arm. D. Flexion of the left arm which allows the patient to reach his face and feed himself. The patient is 15 years since his fascial arthroplasties.

lateral approach to expose the lateral epicondyle and the radial head along with the distal end of the humerus. At this stage, a synovectomy can be carried out in the rheumatoid patient to remove as much synovium as possible. The distal end of the humerus is exposed subperiosteally and is then transected at the transverse biepicondylar line. The medullary canal, which is often thin in this area, may need to be enlarged with an air drill or a small chisel. The proximal end of the ulna and the olecranon fossa are shaped to receive the thick middle section of the implant. The intramedullary canal of the ulna is opened to receive the stem of the implant. All rough edges should be smoothed to prevent damage to the implant. Three sizes of implants are available, and one should be selected to fit the elbow. If necessary, the radial head may also be removed and replaced with a Silastic radial head.

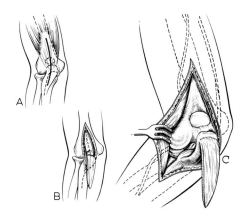

FIG. 6-20 Posterior approach to the elbow joint. A. The skin incision started approximately 4 inches proximal to the elbow on the posterior aspect of the joint. B. A tongue-shaped flap dissected from the triceps and turned distally. C. The entire joint can be dissected out and the ulnar nerve retracted out of the way. (Redrawn from Campbell's Operative Orthopaedics, 5th ed. A. H. Grenshaw, editor. St. Louis, C. V. Mosby, 1971.)

The most important step is the reconstruction of a strong collateral ligament system. A strip of fascia lata, measuring approximately 30 cm in length and 4 cm in width, can be removed with the fascia lata stripper from the opposite thigh. Holes are drilled through the olecranon coronoid process and distal humerus on both sides of the joint. The fascia lata strips are inserted through these holes to reconstruct a collateral ligament. The elbow implant is then inserted, and the

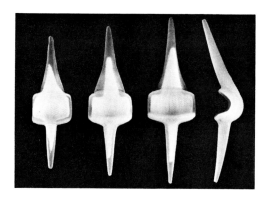

FIG. 6-21 Three different sizes of the Swanson Silastic elbow implant. Lateral view at right.

ends of the fascia lata strips are brought tightly together and sutured to themselves and the surrounding tissues. The ulnar nerve can be transplanted anteriorly, and the wound is closed in layers. Drains are removed from the elbow in 48 hours, and a soft, bulky dressing is used. Traction should be avoided, and the alignment of the humerus and ulna should be checked frequently when dressings are changed. Swanson advises keeping the elbow protected from 4 to 6 weeks. Rotational strains should be avoided for at least 3 months following the surgery.

The results of this type of arthroplasty have been satisfactory for the rheumatoid patient (Fig. 6-22), but this procedure is not avisable in patients who require an elbow that will be of value in heavy, manual labor.

Total Replacement Arthroplasty

The total replacement arthroplasty of the elbow is still under development. Several devices have been tried with varying results. A prosthesis developed by Dee in England can be used in patients with severe instability and bone loss. Dee has also reported using it in patients with ankylosis of the elbow, resulting in better than 90° of useful motion. The problem with all large metal implants is the thin skin in rheumatoid patients, and great care must be exercised in handling the skin flaps in this type of patient.

At the present stage of our knowledge, the total replacement arthroplasty is recommended only as a salvage procedure in severe cases of rheumatoid arthritis for patients with good skin and subcutaneous tissue.

Arthrodesis

Occasionally, arthrodesis may be considered in rheumatoid arthritis of the

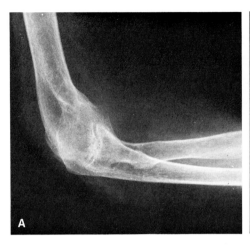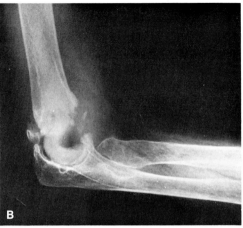

FIG. 6-22 Roentgenograms of the elbow joint. A. Lateral view revealing ankylosis due to rheumatoid arthritis. B. Lateral view after a Swanson Silastic arthroplasty. The prosthesis is visible. (Courtesy of Dr. Alfred Swanson.)

elbow if stability is required, but it is rarely recommended. If the elbow joint is completely destroyed by the arthritic process and a flail, useless joint has resulted, arthrodesis may be necessary.

The elbow joint is not an easy joint on which to perform an arthrodesis; however, patients with rheumatoid arthritis have a greater tendency toward fusion than do normal persons.

If a unilateral fusion is considered, the best position would be 90 to 130 degrees of flexion as desired for best function.

Operative Technique. The posterior or lateral approach as described in the section on arthroplasty may be used. A large iliac cancellous cortical graft is inserted from the humerus into the ulna, and cancellous chips are packed about the denuded joint surfaces (Fig. 6-23). A posterior molded splint is used for several weeks, and then a circular cast is applied.

Rheumatoid Nodules

Nodules are characteristic of rheumatoid arthritis and are generally found over the elbow joint in the subcutaneous tissue on the ulnar side of the forearm. These nodules may coalesce to form one large mass, or they may be small, discrete nodules located along the forearm. At times they may become quite tender and produce symptoms due to pressure when the forearm is rested on a flat surface. They may vary in size from several millimeters to over a centimeter in mass.

Conservative Treatment

If symptoms warrant, the nodules can be injected directly with a small amount

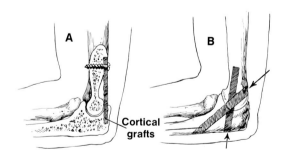

FIG. 6-23 Arthrodesis of the elbow joint. An iliac bone graft may be placed across the humerus into the olecranon for fusion. A. Lateral view revealing a posterior onlay graft. B. Lateral view with cortical grafts inserted through the ulna to the humerus.

of lidocaine (Xylocaine) and local steroids. Occasionally the nodules will disappear with this type of treatment.

Excision

If rheumatoid nodules are persistent and the patient is concerned either about the symptoms or the cosmetic appearance, surgical excision can be considered. There is a great tendency, however, for other nodules to develop in the same area, and the patient should be warned of the possibility of a recurrence of the deformity. Nodules may be removed during another surgical procedure rather than as a separate procedure. However, they can be removed independently, using local anesthesia and carefully excising them from the overlying skin and the subcutaneous tissue. If the defect left by their removal is reasonably large, a small drain can be left in for 24 hours. Remember the location of the ulnar nerve to prevent damage during removal of a nodule.

Olecranon Bursitis

The bursa over the olecranon process frequently becomes involved in a rheumatoid proliferative synovitis with effusion. This large bursa is cosmetically unacceptable to many patients and is extremely tender when the elbow is rested on a hard surface (Fig. 6-24). Trauma frequently will be a cause of olecranon bursitis in addition to the rheumatoid disease. On palpation the bursa is soft. It can be filled with fluid or else with firm, hard rice bodies that may be extremely tender. In chronic cases the thickened bursa will have a grating sensation when it is rolled under the finger.

Conservative Treatment

If the bursa is extremely large and cosmetically unacceptable or if it is

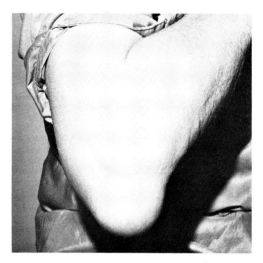

FIG. 6-24 A large bursa in an acute case of olecranon bursitis without a history of trauma.

tender and painful, conservative measures may result in improvement. It is worthwhile to consider them as the first course of treatment. After skin preparation with an antiseptic solution and under sterile precautions, the fluid should be aspirated from the bursa, and corticosteroids should be injected. A compression dressing should be applied for one week to prevent reaccumulation of the fluid and also to avoid infection.

Excision

If the effusion and swelling persist or continue to produce symptoms despite conservative care, surgical excision of the bursal sac may be carried out.

Operative Technique. Under tourniquet control, a transverse incision is made over the enlarged bursa. The bursa should be carefully dissected from the overlying skin and kept intact if possible. Some surgeons will consider injecting methylene blue into the bursa to outline the sac and insure complete removal. On the medial side of the bursa one should be extremely cautious to look for the ulnar nerve, as it may be adherent to a large bursal mass. The triceps tendon will be visible in the base of the incision, and the bursa should be scraped off the tendon. After removal of the bursa, the tourniquet is released and hemostasis is obtained. A small Penrose drain is inserted for 24 hours, and a pressure dressing is applied for 7 days. To prevent separation of the wound, it is wise to use interrupted sutures and remove them only after several weeks when the skin is thoroughly healed.

Complications. Occasionally, chronic ulceration of the olecranon bursa may occur spontaneously with rheumatoid arthritis (Fig. 6-25). The patient will have a large ulceration with healed skin edges with granulation tissue in the base. The best way to handle this condition is to consider complete excision of the bursa and granulation tissue along with the edges of the skin to aid in healing of the incision. The sutures should be left in place a minimum of 3 weeks, as there is a great tendency for the thin skin of the rheumatoid patient to heal slowly and to separate.

Lateral Epicondylitis

Lateral epicondylitis or "tennis elbow" may occur in rheumatoid arthritis and produce symptoms about the elbow joint or in to the forearm. It is believed that the etiologic basis of this condition lies in an inflammation at the origin of the common extensor tendons from the lateral epicondyle of the humerus. Bosworth has suggested that the symptoms are due to an irritation of the orbicular ligament within the elbow joint.

Symptoms may be quite varied in the syndrome. The patient frequently complains of pain in the forearm or about the lateral aspect of the elbow and occasionally only in the forearm. The patient may also complain of a weakness in his grasp and the inability to open a jar or to

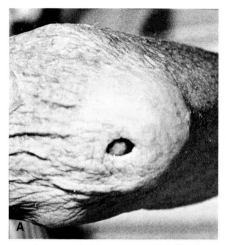

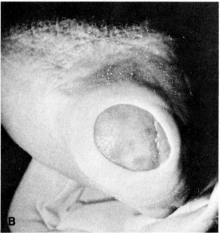

FIG. 6-25 An example of chronic ulceration of the olecranon bursa. A. A small ulceration. B. A large olecranon ulceration with the base filled with granulating tissue and with the skin edges rolled. This developed after surgical resection of the ulcer without prolonged protection of elbow motion.

wring out a washcloth. The patient frequently will point to the lateral condyle as a source of pain and state that he has accidentally struck this area several times in the past. If the patient says that the pain radiates up the arm from the elbow, the condition can be confused with a cervical arthritis or coronary artery disease. At times a physician unfamiliar with this disease process may do an extensive medical workup to try to rule out the latter problems.

On physical examination, the patient will have tenderness over the lateral epicondyle and just distal to it over the conjoined tendon of the extensor muscles. A test for this syndrome is to have the patient extend the wrist and resist forced flexion by the examiner. This maneuver will usually intensify the symptoms considerably. Another test is to shake hands with the patient and ask him to squeeze your hand as hard as possible. This action frequently will reproduce the pain in the area of the epicondyle. The roentgenogram is usually negative, but occasionally a calcium deposit can be visualized in the area of the conjoined tendon.

Conservative Treatment

The patient usually will respond to conservative therapy and the local injection of steroids into the epicondyle. It is wise to mix the steroid with 1 to 2 cc of lidocaine (Xylocaine) and use multiple injections over the tender spot on the epicondyle or conjoined tendon. The patient should be advised to use ice for the first 24 hours on the elbow joint if symptoms arise from the injection, because at times these injections can be extremely painful for the first 12 to 24 hours. In some patients the use of a wrist splint to prevent forced flexion of the wrist will relieve the pull on the extensor tendons and also alleviate the symptoms. Repeated injections may be necessary to relieve the patient completely.

Surgical Treatment

In some cases that are extremely chronic and disabling, surgical procedures may be utilized to relieve the patient. At the time of exploration one generally does not find much evidence of disease in the region of the patient's tenderness. A small 2-inch incision is made over the lateral epicondyle of the humerus, and the conjoined tendon is exposed. The tendon and all muscle attachments are carefully dissected off the lateral condyle and allowed to migrate distally. Occasionally some greyish-white gelatinous material may be found if repeated injections of steroids have been given. Bosworth has advised dividing the orbicular ligament for relief of symptoms. We have utilized this approach along with the stripping of the epicondyle in the more chronic or severe cases, especially if there is tenderness over the radial head. The results of this type of surgery in carefully selected cases have been satisfactory when local injections of steroids have failed.

Medial Epicondylitis

A condition similar to lateral epicondylitis or "tennis elbow" may exist on the medial aspect of the elbow joint at the medial epicondyle. Symptoms develop at the point where the flexor muscles originate. A patient will complain of pain on the medial aspect of the elbow joint with a loss of grip and discomfort on forceful use of the hand. On examination the patient will have localized tenderness over the medial epicondyle. A good test for this condition is to have the patient flex the wrist and resist forced extension. Severe pain during this test is an indication of epicondylitis. The roentgenograms are usually negative for any disease in the area of the epicondyle.

Conservative Treatment

The conservative treatment consists of local injection of the area with steroids and lidocaine (Xylocaine). It is important to advise patients that there may be some numbness in the ulnar nerve following the injection of the local anesthetic and that they should avoid smoking or extremely hot water because of lack of sensation. On injection one should be very careful to stay close to the bone and away from the posterior aspect of the epicondyle so that the nerve is not directly injected.

Surgical Treatment

Surgical release would be indicated in those chronic cases that do not respond to local injections. Entrapment of the ulnar nerve in this region may also simulate an epicondylitis, but the patient will have paresthesias in the hand. Surgical release of the muscles and tendons attached to the epicondyle should be carried out carefully because of the proximity of the ulnar nerve.

Posterior Interosseous Nerve Palsy

The posterior interosseous (or deep radial) nerve passes around the radius and through the supinator muscle to innervate the extensors of the fingers, the thumb extensors, and the thumb abductor. It is suceptible to traction injury where it passes around the radial neck

because of dislocation of the radius or tumors arising locally. The supinator muscle is a common area for a deep lipoma, which can produce a paralysis similar to that seen in synovial hypertrophy due to rheumatoid arthritis (Fig. 6-26A). The hypertrophy of the synovial tissue within the elbow joint frequently destroys the orbicular ligament and distends the joint so that the radial head is dislocated outward (Fig. 6-27). This distension within the joint, combined with the dislocation of the radial head, can produce a traction and stretching of the posterior interosseous nerve, resulting in paralysis and loss of extension of the fingers and thumb. The wrist extensors will not be affected by this palsy, since they are supplied by the radial nerve proximal to the elbow joint and therefore will continue to function (Fig. 6-28). Differential diagnosis must include rupture of the common finger extensors at the wrist, since this will also produce a loss of finger extension even though the posterior interosseous nerve is intact. It may be difficult to tell if the rupture has occurred at the wrist unless there is an

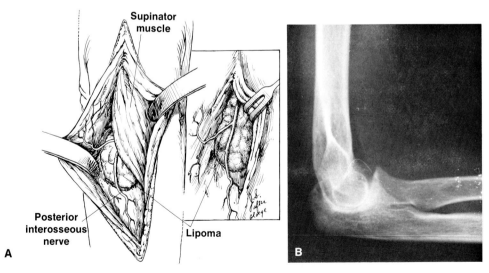

FIG. 6-26 Causes of paralysis of the wrist or hand. A. Deep lipoma beneath the posterior interosseous nerve of the supinator muscle. B. Displacement of the radial head upward because of synovial disease that has destroyed the orbicular ligament of the elbow joint.

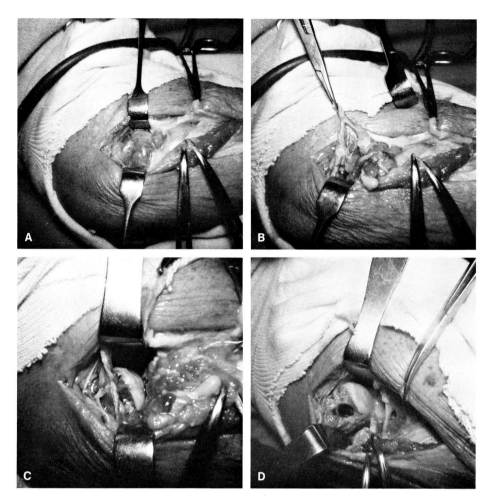

FIG. 6-27 Surgical views of the elbow joint of a patient with posterior interosseous nerve palsy. A. Posterior lateral incision, revealing the synovial proliferation within the joint. B. Villus synovial hyperplasia upon entering the elbow joint. C. Articular changes on the humeral surface seen after removal of some of the synovial tissue. D. Cystic formation in the area of the capitulum of the humerus.

associated extensor tenosynovitis of the wrist or the patient has definitely felt a snap at the wrist joint. Careful examination and palpation will reveal the site of separation of the extensor tendons at the wrist. When there is a doubt, electrical stimulation of the muscles in the forearm can be of value in differentiating the two conditions. If a nerve palsy is present, the fingers will extend with stimulation because the tendons are still intact. If the patient has had the condition for 3 or 4 weeks, an electromyogram can be of value in determining whether the nerve is involved. It should be stressed that tendon rupture at the wrist is far more common than nerve palsy at the elbow.

Treatment

The aim of management of a posterior interosseous nerve palsy at the elbow should be to relieve the traction on the posterior interosseous nerve. The posterior lateral approach to the elbow

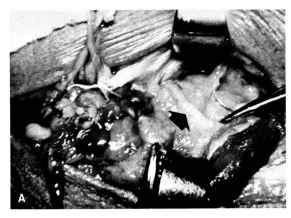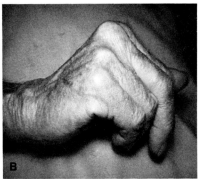

FIG. 6-28 A. Surgical view of the posterior interosseous nerve (arrow) of a patient with paralysis of the finger extensors. The synovial hyperplasia has stretched the nerve. B. Patient illustrating extension of the wrist but loss of extension of the fingers due to supinator palsy from rheumatoid arthritis.

joint should be made, exposing the radial head and neck (Fig. 6-29). The radial head should be excised at the neck, and the synovium should be removed from the joint to relieve the pressure exerted on the posterior interosseous nerve. During the recovery period, a Thomas suspension splint would be of value to prevent stretching of the common extensor digital muscles and the abductors of the thumb by the flexor muscles.

Ulnar Nerve Palsy

Rheumatoid arthritis of the ulnar nerve, though rare, may produce a neu-

ritis either by direct involvement of the nerve with the synovial tissue or by compression in the region of the medial epicondyle because of the capsular swelling (Fig. 6-30). The ulnar nerve is fairly immobile in this area and can be compressed easily by a soft tissue mass. Several cases of compression of the ulnar nerve in this region have been described by the author and others, such as Osborne.

The patient usually will complain of tingling and paresthesias in the fourth and fifth fingers of the hand and in advanced cases, of weakness of the fingers. At times, atrophy of the

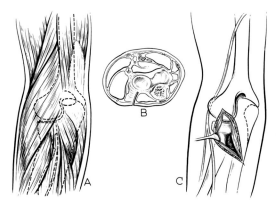

FIG. 6-29 Operative procedures for posterior interosseous palsy. A. Posterior-lateral approach to the elbow joint. B. Transverse sections through the elbow revealing the plane of approach to the radial head. C. Exposure of the radial head and neck through the posterior-lateral approach. (Redrawn from Campbell's Operative Orthopaedics, 5th ed. A. H. Grenshaw, editor. St. Louis, C. V. Mosby, 1971.)

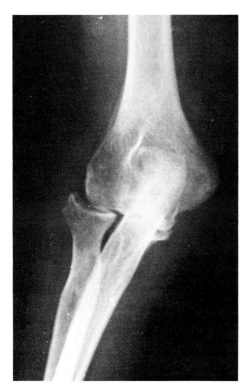

FIG. 6-30 Roentgenogram of the elbow of a patient with an ulnar neuritis due to rheumatoid disease. Subluxation of the radial head and a cubitus valgus deformity are seen. The patient had entrapment of the ulnar nerve because of the synovial tissue protruding from the joint surface.

interossei muscles may be obvious because of long-standing compression. The patient will complain that, on certain motions of the elbow, electric shocks shoot down the arm into the hand.

On examination of the patient, there may be some soft tissue swelling behind the medial epicondyle in the region of the ulnar nerve. Compared to the normal nerve on the opposite elbow, the nerve itself may be thickened due to the irritation. A positive Tinel's sign may be present, and tapping the irritated nerve will produce electric shocks and paresthesias. In order to confirm the diagnosis, nerve conduction studies can be carried out, comparing the normal side to the abnormal to see if there is retardation of the impulse.

Surgical Treatment

The treatment for ulnar nerve palsy requires release of the ulnar nerve behind the elbow and transplantation of it to the subcutaneous tissue in front of the medial epicondyle. The nerve should be freed thoroughly to prevent any binding, especially from the intermuscular septum in the proximal area, and then it should be placed in the subcutaneous tissue which is sutured to prevent the nerve from slipping back behind the elbow joint. The patient will note dramatic relief of the symptoms following surgery, and in most cases anterior transplantation will result in a cure.

Biceps Tendon Rupture

Rupture of the biceps tendon may occur in rheumatoid arthritis, and although it is rare, it should be considered when the patient complains of pain in the shoulder or elbow and has noted a mass in the arm. Rupture may occur at the insertion into the radial tuberosity or in the long head of the biceps in the bicipital groove. Synovial hyperplasia tends to destroy the nutrition of the tendon, weakening it, and then rupture occurs with minimal stress. This may take place spontaneously with little pain or discomfort, and the patient may notice only a mass in the lower arm and some weakness on supination.

Repair of Rupture

It is generally not advisable to undertake a surgical reconstruction to reinsert the tendon when rupture occurs in the region of the radial tuberosity. The tendon is often frayed, and it would be difficult to reach the tuberosity without a fascial graft. Therefore, if surgery is considered, it would be more advisable to suture the biceps tendon to the brachialis tendon. This procedure retains the power of the biceps muscle for elbow flexion but does not improve supination.

The repair may be carried out through an anterior transverse incision in the antecubital space. This will give a cosmetically acceptable scar, and, if more room is required, the incision may be extended vertically at each end for exposure. The lacertus fibrosa should be excised, and the biceps tendon should be sutured to the brachialis tendon with nonabsorbable sutures. A posterior molded splint should be utilized for 4 weeks, and supervised motion should be started to prevent the development of contractures.

If the rupture occurs in the long head of the biceps tendon, repair is not necessary unless the patient is concerned about the cosmetic appearance or the weakness that may be associated with loss of the long head of the biceps. An incision can be made over the bicipital groove. In many patients the long head of the biceps tendon will be found protruding from the shoulder joint. It should be cut off and left attached to the origin on the scapula. The remaining long head that is attached to the biceps muscle can be brought back to the transverse humeral ligament, the tendon can be sutured to the ligament, and a hole can be drilled in the humerus for insertion of the proximal portion. This procedure will anchor the muscle and restore its length and function. Healing should be relatively complete within 6 weeks, and motion should be started reasonably early to regain function (see Chapter 5).

Synovial Cyst

Occasionally in rheumatoid arthritis, a hard, firm mass or cyst may develop in the antecubital space or protrude distally in the forearm. This mass can arise rapidly, is fairly firm, and does not transilluminate. It may simulate a tumor mass, and generally fluid cannot be aspirated from it. This mass is produced by synovial hyperplasia from the elbow joint with protrusion through the capsule as a direct herniation beneath the deep fascia. The cyst can produce symptoms by its mass and the tension on the surrounding structures. It is similar to the popliteal cyst seen in rheumatoid arthritis of the knee (Chapter 10).

Conservative Treatment

The treatment for this condition generally is injection with local steroids either directly into the mass or laterally between the triangle formed by the radial head, the lateral condyle, and the olecranon. Aspiration and injection of the elbow joint with steroids will often resolve the mass. In our experience, it has not been necessary to excise this mass, as it will disappear with subsidence of symptoms.

Osteoarthritis

Osteoarthritis in the elbow joint generally involves the proximal radioulnar joint (Fig. 6-31). It frequently follows trauma and may progress to the humeroulnar joint. The patient usually will note the onset of pain in the area of the elbow and gradual loss of extension and flexion. The synovial membrane is not swollen or thickened as it would be in rheumatoid arthritis. The patient may reveal loss of pronation, supination, flexion, and extension. Bilateral disease is unusual in osteoarthritis.

Conservative Treatment

The patient with osteoarthritis of the elbow joint usually can be treated conservatively for a long period of time.

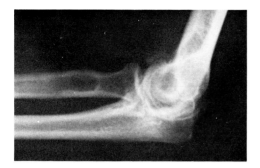

FIG. 6-31 Roentgenogram revealing osteoarthritis of the radioulnar joint.

Avoiding overuse of the elbow joint and using salicylates and various anti-inflammatory drugs will tend to decrease symptoms. If these fail to control the symptoms, local injection of the elbow joint with a corticosteroid through the lateral approach will often relieve the symptoms for prolonged periods of time.

Excision of the Radial Head

The patient with severe symptoms and deformity of the radial head can often be relieved by excision of the radial head (Fig. 6-32). If pronation and supination have been lost, it is important

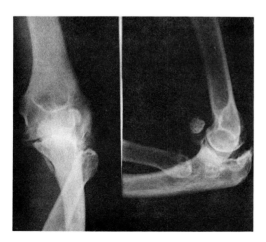

FIG. 6-32 Roentgenograms revealing excision of the radial head. Anterior view (left). Lateral view (right).

to take a roentgenogram of the distal radioulnar joint to be certain that it is not involved in a disease process that could limit these motions. Excision of the radial head will allow pronation and supination and for some patients increase the flexion of the joint. When the roentgenogram reveals a deformity of the radial head, excision is indicated. Extension is rarely gained in severe disease because of contractures of the joint itself.

Operative Technique. The operation is generally performed under a tourniquet which is placed high up on the arm to give adequate exposure of the elbow joint. A posterolateral approach to the joint will give adequate exposure with minimal trauma. The incision starts on the lateral condyle and passes distally over the radial head toward the ulna. The plane between the extensor carpi ulnaris and the anconeus is developed to expose the capsule of the elbow joint. The capsule is opened and the radial head is exposed. It is important not to exceed the limits of the capsule to prevent damage to the supinator branch of the radial nerve which is located distal to the radial neck. The neck of the radius is exposed, and drill holes are placed across it and transected with a small osteotome. The head is then removed, and the remaining neck is smoothed with a rasp. At this stage it is possible either to replace the radial head with a Silastic prosthesis or to leave the neck remaining as it is. If replacement is desired, a broach or reamer is passed down the medullary cavity of the radius, and then the various Silastic prostheses are tried to determine the proper fit. The stem of the prosthesis is slipped down the medullary cavity of the radius, and the head portion is reduced into the joint. When the proper size has been selected, the permanent prosthesis is inserted without the use of sharp instruments to prevent damage to or tearing of the Silastic material which could lead to failure. A tight fit is not necessary to obtain a good result. The capsule is repaired, and the muscles are approximated for closure. A bulky pressure dressing is adequate and is applied from the wrist to the midarm (Fig. 6-12).

Patients should be instructed to start flexion-extension, and pronation-supination exercises on the first postoperative day. The bulky pressure dressing should be removed about the third day to allow further motion of the elbow joint. Patients should be advised to continue this exercise program and also to raise their arms over their heads at least once a day to prevent development of stiff shoulders.

Total Joint Replacement

At the present state of our knowledge, it is not advisable to resect an osteoarthritic elbow joint and replace it with a metallic elbow hinge when the disease is severe. Until more conservative arthroplasties are available, the conservative approach should be carried out. Arthrodesis can still be utilized for relief of pain, or a fascial arthroplasty may give an adequate result. The operative technique for fascial arthroplasty of the elbow was described under arthroplasty for rheumatoid arthritis of the elbow.

Bibliography

Rheumatoid Arthritis

Bosworth, D. M.: The role of the orbicular ligament in tennis elbow. J. Bone Joint Surg., *37-A*:527, 1955.

Campbell, W. C.: Incision for exposure of the elbow joint. Am. J. Surg., *15*:65, 1932.

Chang, L. W., et. al.: Entrapment neuropathy of the posterior interosseous nerve. A complication of rheumatoid arthritis. Arthritis Rheum., *15*:350, 1972.

Chrisman, O. D.: Elbow. Surgery of Arthritis. R. A. Milch, editor Baltimore, The Williams & Wilkins Co., 1964, p. 101.

Chrisman, O. D., and Southwick, W. O.: The experimental production of articular spurs. Arthritis Rheum., *5*:289, 1962.

DeAndrade, J. R., and Casagrande, R. A.: Ulnar nerve entrapment in rheumatoid arthritis. Arthritis Rheum., *8*:294, 1965.

Dee, R.: Total replacement arthroplasty of the elbow for rheumatoid arthritis. J. Bone Joint Surg., *54-B*:88, 1972.

Gellman, M.: Arthrodesis of the elbow. J. Bone Joint Surg., *29*:850, 1949.

Howard, F. M.: Surgical air for arthritis of the hand and elbow. J. Int. Coll. Surg., *33*:336, 1960.

Inglis, A. E., Ranawat, C. S., and Straub, L. R.: Synovectomy and debridement of the elbow in rheumatoid arthritis. J. Bone Joint Surg., *53-A*:625, 1971.

Knight, R. A., and Van Zandt, I. L.: Arthroplasty of the elbow. J. Bone Joint Surg., *34-A*:610, 1952.

Laine, V., and Vainio, K.: Synovectomy of the elbow in early synovectomy in rheumatoid arthritis. Proceedings of the symposium on early synovectomy in rheumatoid arthritis. Amsterdam, April 12 to 15, 1967, pp. 117–118. Edited by W. Hijams, W. D. Paul, and H. Herschel. Amsterdam, Excerpta Medica Foundation, 1969.

Leffert, R. D., et. al: Antecubital cyst in rheumatoid arthritis surgical findings. J. Bone Joint Surg., *54-A*:1555, 1972.

Marmor, L.: Surgery of the rheumatoid elbow. J. Bone Joint Surg., *54-A*:573, 1972.

Millender, L. H., Nalebuff, E. A., and Holdsworth, D. E.: Posterior interosseous nerve syndrome secondary to rheumatoid arthritis. J. Bone Joint Surg., *55-A*:375, 1973.

Mori, M.: Wrist. *In* Surgery of Arthritis. R. A. Milch, editor. Baltimore, The Williams & Wilkins Co., 1964, p. 112.

Osborne, G. V.: The surgical treatment of tardy ulnar neuritis. J. Bone Joint Surg., *39-B*:782, 1957.

Osborne, G. V.: Ulnar neuritis. Post grad. Med. J., *35*:392, 1959.

Robinson, R. F.: Arthrodesis of the wrist. J. Bone Joint Surg., *34-A*:64, 1952.

Silver, C. M., et al.: The diagnosis and surgical treatment of tardy ulnar nerve palsy. J. Int. Coll. Surg., *42*:656, 1964.

Souter, W. A.: Arthroplasty of the elbow with particular reference to metallic hinge arthroplasty in rheumatoid patients. Orthop. Clin. North Am., 4:395, 1973.

Staples, O. S.: Arthrodesis of the elbow joint. J. Bone Joint Surg., *34-A*:207, 1952.

Torgerson, W. R., and Leach, R. E.: Synovectomy of the elbow in rheumatoid arthritis. J. Bone Joint Surg., *52-A*:371, 1970.

Wilson, D. W., et. al.: Synovectomy of the elbow in rheumatoid arthritis. J. Bone Joint Surg., *55-B*:106, 1973.

Osteoarthritis

Barr, J. S., and Eaton, R. G.: Elbow reconstruction with a new prosthesis to replace the distal end of the humerus. J. Bone Joint. Surg., *47-A*:1308, 1965.

Chrisman, O. D.: Elbow. *In* Surgery of Arthritis. R. A. Milch, editor. Baltimore, The Williams & Wilkins Co., 1964.

Swanson, A. B.: Silastic radial head prosthesis. Dow Corning Med. Bull., 51007, 1970.

7 | The Wrist

The wrist, being a complex joint consisting of multiarticulated surfaces, is susceptible to degenerative processes due to disease, overuse, heredity, or trauma. Rheumatoid arthritis occurs more frequently in the wrist joint and its surrounding structures than does osteoarthritis, but osteoarthritis occurs often enough for it to be of concern to the orthopaedic surgeon.

Clayton has stated that the wrist joint was involved initially in 2.7 percent of the patients that he had seen with rheumatoid arthritis and that 95 percent had bilateral involvement (Fig. 7-1). Martel, Hayes, and Duff studied 100 patients with rheumatoid arthritis and reported an incidence of radioulnar diastasis at the wrist in 41 percent of the patients. The wrist joint itself may be affected by a synovitis that includes either the proximal or distal row of joints and the radioulnar joint. Other areas of the wrist that may be affected by a proliferative synovitis resulting in symptoms of pain and swelling are the extensor and flexor tendons.

Osteoarthritic changes in the wrist may follow trauma or overuse. Fractures of the navicular, for example, may lead to traumatic arthritis with avascular necrosis and collapse of the navicular articular surface. Pain in the wrist may be produced by osteoarthritis secondary to idiopathic aseptic necrosis of the lunate bone. Severe pain in the hand is often related to compression of the median nerve because of encroachment of the nerve in the carpal tunnel. Osteoarthritis of the carpal-metacarpal joint will also be considered in this chapter because this joint is extremely important to the function of the hand and the wrist.

Anatomy

The wrist joint is composed of two rows of carpal bones which articulate with each other as well as with the radius and the metacarpals (Fig. 7-2). The radiocarpal joint is a joint which is made up of the distal articulation of the radius, the articular disk between the radius and ulna, and the proximal surface of the navicular and lunate bones. The ulnar head is entirely extra-articular to the carpal bones but does articulate with the side of the distal radius and the articular

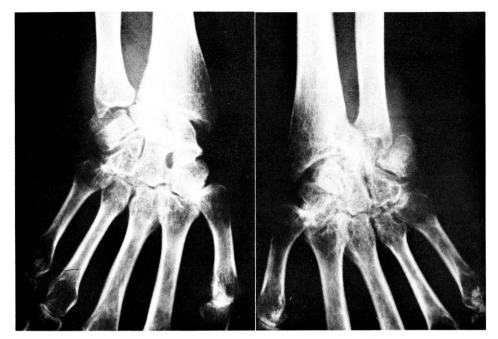

FIG. 7-1 Roentgenogram revealing destruction of the wrist joints with evidence of far-advanced rheumatoid disease involving the distal radioulnar joint on the left. Ulnar subluxation of the wrist is noted in both extremities.

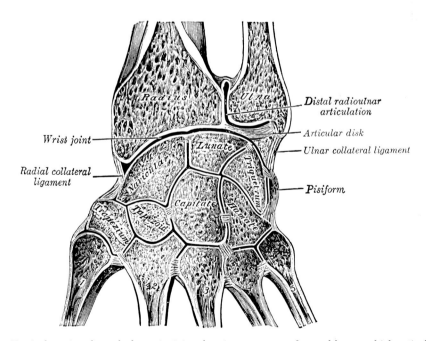

FIG. 7-2 Vertical section through the wrist joint showing two rows of carpal bones which articulate with each other, as well as with the radius and the metacarpals. (From Gray's Anatomy of the Human Body, 29th ed. C. M. Goss, editor. Philadelphia, Lea & Febiger, 1973.)

123

disk. Anatomically various joints of the carpal bones are tightly connected by a series of ligaments and because of their multiple articular surfaces, the vascular supply is tenuous in certain areas.

The fibrocartilaginous articular disk is attached to the styloid process of the ulna and also to the border of the radius (Fig. 7-3). It tends to form a smooth articular surface with the radius and is attached to the capsule of the wrist joint. This disk is an important part of the distal end of the ulna and, when intact, tends to maintain the stability of the distal radioulnar joint (Fig. 7-3). The synovial lining surrounds this joint as well as the carpal joints.

The dorsal carpal ligament extends from the ulna across the dorsal surface of the wrist to the radial side of the radius and the ligament tends to form isolated compartments for the extensor tendons of the fingers and wrist (Fig. 7-4). Because this ligament tends to prevent the tendons from bowstringing, they will be subjected to severe pressure when the distal end of the ulna subluxes upward in rheumatoid disease.

The carpal bones form a tunnel covered by the volar carpal ligament through which the flexor tendons and the median nerve pass into the hand (Fig. 7-5). The ulnar nerve passes superficial to the carpal tunnel and generally is free

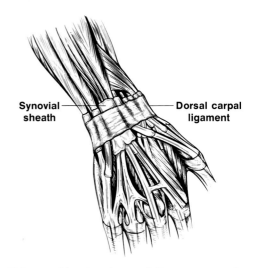

FIG. 7-4 The dorsal carpal ligament extending across the wrist to form isolated compartments for the extensor tendons.

from pressure in this region. However, arthritic changes may result in compression of the nerve. The flexor tendons at the wrist are enclosed in the synovial lined tendon sheath which can become involved with rheumatoid disease. The extensor tendons are also surrounded by a tendon sheath at the wrist, extending for a short distance proximal and distal to the carpal ligament. The wrist joint proper is surrounded by a strong capsule, reinforced by numerous ligaments. The synovial cavity of the radial-carpal joint communicates with the

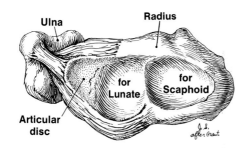

FIG. 7-3 The articular disk located between the radius and the ulna and separating the ulna from the wrist joint. (Redrawn from Grant's Atlas of Anatomy. Baltimore, The Williams & Wilkins Co., 1972.)

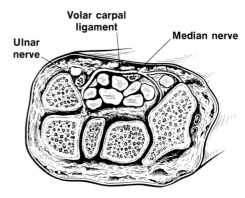

FIG. 7-5 A transverse section through the wrist in the middle of the carpal tunnel.

intercarpal joints of the wrist but is excluded from the distal radioulnar joint by the articular disk and capsule.

The carpal-metacarpal joint, or basal joint of the thumb, is a double saddle joint that works in two planes. Because of its anatomic structure the joint allows flexion, extension, abduction, adduction, rotation, and a combination of motions called circumduction.

The wrist joint allows flexion and extension, as well as radial and ulnar deviation, and is the key joint for proper function and balance of the hand and fingers. It is necessary to have a stable wrist in a proper position of function to allow strong finger function. Extension of the fingers is most powerful when the wrist is in a slightly flexed or neutral position.

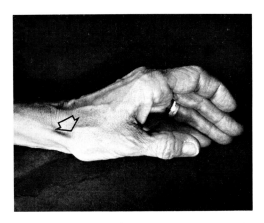

FIG. 7-6 Localized swelling at the base of the thumb (arrow) typical of osteoarthritis of the carpal-metacarpal joint.

Physical Examination

Physical examination of the wrist is important in localizing the site of arthritis. Inspection may reveal subluxation of the carpal-metacarpal joint of the thumb with swelling localized to this joint (Fig. 7-6). A typical deformity of severe osteoarthritis of the carpal-metacarpal joint results in the thumb being adducted with hyperextension of the metacarpal-phalangeal joint and flexion of the interphalangeal joint (Fig. 7-7). Osteoarthritis of the carpal bones can result in some apparent thickening of the wrist joint. The swelling usually is not as noticeable as that in rheumatoid arthritis.

Swelling of the extensor or flexor tendons, as well as involvement of the radioulnar joint at the wrist, is an indication of rheumatoid arthritis. Prom-

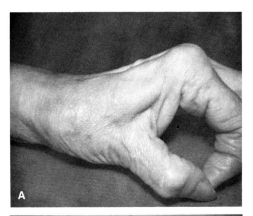
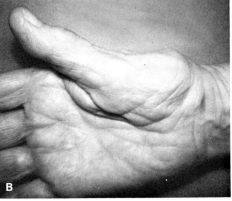

FIG. 7-7 An adduction contracture of the thumb with severe hyperextension of the metacarpal-phalangeal joint. A. Lateral view. B. Volar view.

inence of the ulnar head and swelling may be noted as the ulnar head subluxes upward (Fig. 7-8). Isolated swelling of the extensor carpi ulnaris tendon sheath may also occur early in rheumatoid arthritis of the wrist.

Palpation of the wrist may help to determine sites of localized tenderness and swelling, and on pronation and supination definite crepitation or grating may be noted when there is rheumatoid arthritis in the radioulnar joint. Crepitation at the carpal-metacarpal joint can often be palpated when there is advanced osteoarthritis at the base of the thumb. The grinding test is also positive in arthritis of the thumb and is performed by compressing the metacarpal against the trapezium and rotating the thumb. This will produce grating and increased pain. The navicular, when involved will have the tendency to produce pain on the radial side of the wrist, and palpation in the anatomic snuffbox may reveal tenderness.

Increased local heat is another indication of acute rheumatoid arthritis, as well as of other disease. A test for Tinel's sign should also be carried out to determine if there is tenderness over the median nerve in the carpal tunnel.

The range of motion should be determined for flexion, extension, pronation, and supination. The wrist usually can extend from a neutral position to approximately 65°, and it can flex to approximately 70°. Pronation should go from neutral to 90°, and supination from neutral to 90°. It is important to be sure that the patient is holding the elbow fixed against the trunk to prevent external and internal rotation of the shoulder to compensate for pronation and supination. Loss of motion may help to localize the site of the disease process.

Loss of pronation and supination may also be due to involvement of the proximal radioulnar joint, and the elbow should always be examined for tenderness, deformity of the radial head, and crepitation to rule out elbow disease as a cause of loss of pronation and supination (see Chapter 6).

Rheumatoid Arthritis

Rheumatoid arthritis in the wrist tends to come on early in the course of the disease in most patients. Pain in the wrist may even be the presenting complaint with the onset of the disease process. Early in the course of disease conservative therapy should be utilized to treat these patients. The two major problems encountered at the wrist are (1) synovitis involving the distal radioulnar joint or the carpal joints themselves, and (2) a synovitis involving the extensor and flexor tendons about the wrist (Fig. 7-9). The local injection of steroids frequently will control symptoms for prolonged periods of time, and occasionally a splint may be used to protect the wrist and relieve the symptoms. The splint should

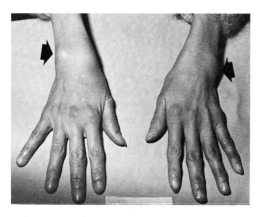

FIG. 7-8 Hands and wrists of patient with rheumatoid arthritis in both wrist joints. The prominent ulnar heads (arrows) are caused by synovial swelling and subluxation.

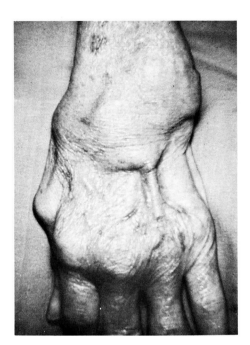

FIG. 7-9 Hand of patient with swelling in the synovial sheaths that extends to the termination of the extensor sheath on the dorsum of the hand.

immobilize the wrist and hand in a position of function of approximately 20° to 30° of extension, leaving the finger joints free. The splint may be made of molded plaster which can be wrapped on with a 2-inch Ace bandage. Commercially available splints have a metal insert that can be removed for laundering and Velcro straps to hold them in place.

Physical therapy at times can relieve some of the aching associated with rheumatoid arthritis. Heat may be applied with a heating pad or a small Hydrocollator pack.

Distal Radioulnar Joint Disease

The distal radioulnar joint often is involved early in rheumatoid arthritis. The synovial tissue lining the joint tends to become thickened and inflamed. This active proliferative synovitis may

be confined only to the radioulnar joint, or it may involve the carpal joints as well. This soft tissue swelling may be observed on the roentgenogram before other signs of rheumatoid arthritis are evident (Fig. 7-10A). The persistent synovial swelling tends to stretch the ligaments, producing laxity and resultant subluxation or dislocation of the ulnar head upward (Fig. 7-10B). Erosion of the ulnar head itself is produced by the proliferative synovitis that destroys the

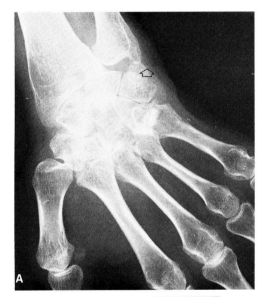

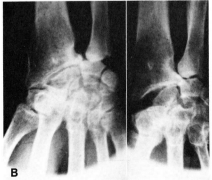

FIG. 7-10 Roentgenograms of wrist of patient with rheumatoid arthritis. A. Soft tissue swelling (arrow). Destruction of the carpal bones is also evident. B. Displacement of the distal end of the ulna by soft tissue swelling that has forced the ulnar head dorsally. Note erosion of radius.

articular cartilage and disrupts the triangular fibrocartilage located between the radius and the ulna (Fig. 7-11).

Disruption of the radioulnar joint produces pain and limits motion mechanically by blocking pronation and supination. The patient will complain of pain in the region of the middle of the wrist joint and will experience difficulty in turning the wrist, as in opening doors and in using a key in a lock. Direct pressure on the ulnar head is painful, and grating and crepitation may be palpated. The ulnar head can be subluxed

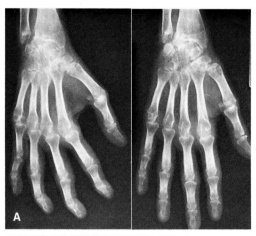

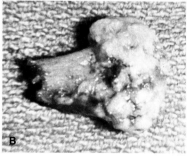

FIG. 7-11 Erosion of the ulnar head produced by proliferative synovitis. A. Roentgenograms revealing destruction of the ulnar heads and of the triangular fibrocartilage located between the distal ends of the radius and the ulna of both wrists. Note also the cystic changes in the base of the metacarpal of the thumb and the fifth metacarpal head. B. Photograph of ulnar head after removal from a patient. Note destruction of the articular surface due to synovial tissue invasion.

easily by grasping it between the examiner's thumb and fingers. If it is compressed against the radius on pronation and supination, the patient will have increased pain and difficulty in using the hand. At times the patient may also complain of locking and catching of the wrist as the triangular cartilage becomes caught between the radius and ulna. The loss of rotation is gradual, and the patient may not realize the amount of disability because he can substitute by internal and external rotation of the shoulder.

Radiologic signs of rheumatoid arthritis involving the distal radioulnar joint consist of (1) erosion and destruction of the distal ulna, (2) synovial soft tissue swelling about the joint, (3) osteoporosis, (4) the scallop sign in advanced disease (Fig. 7-12).

Conservative Treatment

The radioulnar joint may be injected locally with steroids to produce temporary relief in many patients. The injection of 3 cc lidocaine (Xylocaine) combined with 1 cc of a long-acting steroid into the space between the radius and the ulna at the wrist in the region of the triangular cartilage will often give dramatic relief. It is important to be sure the injection is inserted into the correct area between the radius and ulna, or symptoms will persist after the injection. The injection is often an excellent diagnostic test in advanced cases because if the patient's symptoms in the wrist are relieved by the injection, this is an excellent indication that surgery would be of value.

Resection of the Distal Ulna
The Darrach Procedure

The indications for resection of the distal ulna are (1) persistent pain in the region of the distal radioulnar joint, (2)

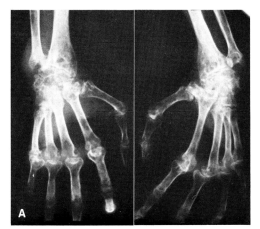

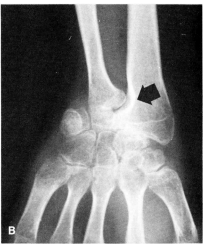

FIG. 7-12 Roentgenograms revealing signs of rheumatoid arthritis in the distal radioulnar joint. A. Severe osteoporosis and cystic formation. B. Scallop sign (arrow) from erosion of the ulnar head. Note the displacement of the carpal bones on the radius, a common sign of advanced rheumatoid disease in the wrist.

subluxation or dislocation of the distal ulna with limited motion and pain, (3) involvement of the extensor tendons with or without rupture, and (4) the scallop sign (Fig. 7-12B).

Resection of the distal end of the ulna, first reported in 1880 by Moore, was popularized by Darrach in 1912. The operation was originally performed for traumatic disruption of the distal radio-ulnar joint. In recent years it has been utilized in rheumatoid arthritis by

Smith-Petersen, Aufranc, and Larson. The procedure has also been utilized as part of the technique of wrist fusion to allow pronation and supination. Reports have been published by Bäckdahl, Clayton, Cracchiolo and Marmor, Flatt, Rana and Taylor, and Vaughan-Jackson.

Operative Technique. The operation is generally performed in a bloodless field. A tourniquet is applied, and after the extremity is wrapped with an Esmarch bandage the tourniquet is inflated. A 2-inch lateral incision is made over the distal ulnar head, and the subcutaneous tissue is retracted carefully to avoid injury to the dorsal sensory branch of the ulnar nerve. The nerve is generally encountered in the distal end of the incision and about one finger breadth from the end of the ulnar head. The dorsal carpal ligament is incised over the ulnar head and proximal for 1 inch to expose the shaft. Care should be exercised to prevent damage to the extensor carpi ulnaris tendon, which is retracted toward the ulnar side, and the extensor digiti quinti, which is retracted toward the radial side. The incision is carried down to the periosteum which is then elevated with a periosteal elevator to remove the attachment of the pronator muscle from the shaft of the distal ulna.

A number of small drill holes are placed across the ulnar shaft approximately $\frac{3}{4}$ inch from the styloid process and the ulna is divided with an osteotome (Fig. 7-13A,B). This can also be accomplished using a power saw or a Hall air drill. The distal end of the ulna is then retracted upward and distally, and the soft tissue and ligaments are dissected off the ulnar styloid process (Fig. 7-13C). The remaining end of the ulnar shaft is smoothed either with a rongeur and rasped or with a power tool using a cup reamer to remove any sharp fragments. It is important to be sure that the remaining ulna does not abut or touch the side of the radius where the

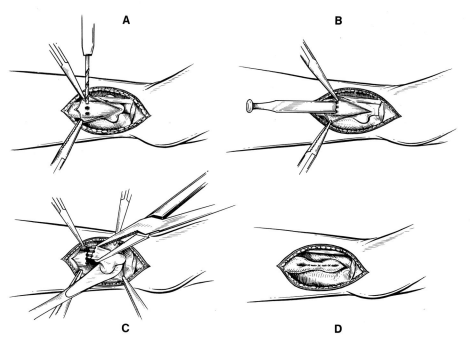

FIG. 7-13 Surgical procedure for resection of the distal ulna. A. Holes drilled across the ulnar shaft approximately ¾ inch from the end of the ulna. B. Division of the ulna with an osteotome. C. Excision of the distal end of the ulna from the styloid ligaments. D. Periosteum resutured over the distal end of the ulnar shaft to prevent it from riding upward. (Redrawn from Campbell's Operative Orthopaedics, 5th ed. A. H. Grenshaw, editor. St. Louis, C. V. Mosby, 1971.)

ulnar head had been in contact. Otherwise symptoms will remain following the surgical procedure. All excess synovium should be removed from the joint and from the portion of the wrist that can be visualized. At this stage the lunate is often visible in the incision and at times the navicular if the wrist has drifted toward the ulnar side.

The periosteum is then resutured over the distal end of the ulna to hold it in place to prevent a deformity postoperatively (Fig. 7-13D). The capsule is also closed, and then the dorsal carpal ligament is repaired. A light compressive dressing is applied without a plaster splint, and the tourniquet is released. The patient is advised to exercise from the first day following the surgery and to expect symptoms to last at least 6 weeks after the operation until a new capsule has formed over the ulna.

It is important to check the radial head prior to performing surgery to remove the ulnar head, since the radial head is frequently involved in rheumatoid arthritis and may be a cause of limitation of the forearm rotation. The radial head may be excised at the same time as the ulnar head if desired. (see Chapter 6).

Excision of the ulnar head may also be combined with excision of the synovial tissue in the extensor tendon sheaths if they are involved.

Results. The results of excision of the ulnar head have been consistently good in most series that have been followed for a long time. In Rana and Taylor's series of 86 wrists suffering from rheumatoid arthritis, the pain was relieved in 93 percent, and full rotation was restored in 87 percent of the patients.

It is important to realize the excision

of the ulnar head usually does not contribute to ulnar subluxation of the wrist. In many cases it is obvious that ulnar subluxation has already occurred prior to removal of the ulnar head and that it does not increase dramatically when the ulnar head is excised (Fig. 7-14). The ulnar head in general has no contact with the carpal bones. Therefore an attempt to preserve some of the distal end of the ulna seems to be unnecessary.

A Silastic ulnar head has been designed for replacement of the ulnar head that has been resected in arthritic patients. However, there is a tendency for the prosthesis to migrate out of the medullary shaft, and it can protrude upward, causing a deformity at the distal end of the ulna. If the ulnar shaft is smoothed with a rasp or power tool, as suggested, the Silastic prosthesis is generally not required at this site.

Carpal Joint Disease

Rheumatoid arthritis may involve the radiocarpal as well as carpal joints. The synovial disease occurs with proliferation and erosion of the articular surfaces of the carpal bones. It is of interest that despite the amount of articular change noted in the roentgenograms of patients with rheumatoid arthritis of the wrist, the most frequent cause of severe pain is involvement of the radioulnar joint rather than of the carpal joints (Fig. 7-15). The carpal joint disease will lead to chronic aching but will not limit the ability to pronate and supinate or to open a door or turn a key. When the radioulnar joint is destroyed by rheumatoid arthritis, the ulna tends to catch on the carpal bones, as well as on the radius, and pronation and supination will be limited.

Two types of disease process seem to occur in the rheumatoid wrist. One is gradual spontaneous fusion of the wrist joint with loss of motion, and the other is destruction of the carpal bones with subluxation both ulnarward and volarward resulting in a totally unstable wrist. As the disease progresses, the wrist becomes more painful and a gradual flexion deformity develops. In addition to spontaneous fusion with resultant stiffness and erosion, deformities usually associated with rheumatoid arthritis of the intercarpal and radiocarpal joints include ulnar drift of the carpal bones on the radius, with or without radial deviation of the hand, volar subluxation of the carpal bones on the ulna with absorption of the proximal carpal row, and occasional ulnar and volar dislocation of the hand from the radius associated with or

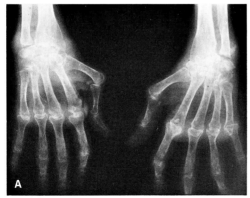
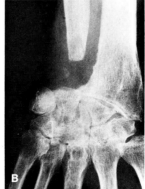

FIG. 7-14 Roentgenograms revealing subluxation of the wrist. A. Before excision of the ulnar head. B. After excision of the ulnar head.

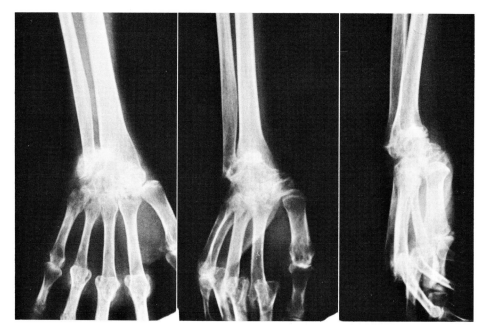

FIG. 7-15 Roentgenograms illustrating destruction of the radioulnar joint and severe involvement of the carpal bones.

without extensor tendon rupture. Severe disease of this type involving the wrist joint results in loss of stability associated with serious loss of hand function (Fig. 7-16).

Conservative Treatment

The wrist joint lends itself to conservative management by protective splinting in a position of function to prevent the development of a flexion contracture. Splinting of the wrist aids considerably in preventing deformities, and either a cockup splint or a lightweight plastic splint with Velcro straps may be used to give active extension of the wrist during the day. Splinting of the wrist will often relieve the patient's pain and improve the function of the hand by giving increased stability and transferring the power of the finger extensors from the wrist to the hand.

Synovectomy of the Wrist

In the past, patients were not referred to the surgeon until the disease was extremely advanced and destruction of the wrist joint was extensive. Therefore, much of the literature still recommends arthrodesis for the treatment of late destructive rheumatoid arthritis of the wrist. As experience has developed with the treatment of rheumatoid arthritis at earlier stages, however, there are indications that a synovectomy of the wrist is worthwhile in the acute or subacute disease. Frequently the patient will also have involvement of the distal radioulnar joint as well as an extensor tenosynovitis. In this case, synovectomy of the wrist can be combined with synovectomy of the extensor tendons and excision of the ulnar head. For many years Mori has advocated synovectomy of the wrist joint for rheumatoid arthritis. It is a little more difficult to do a synovectomy of the wrist joint than other larger joints because of the anatomy involved. The surgeon should also be aware that in performing a synovectomy of the wrist joint, some motion can be lost, and the patient should be advised of this. In those patients with roentgenographic evidence of destruction and subluxation

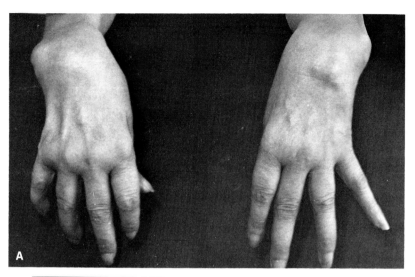

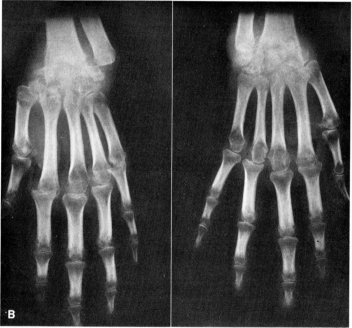

FIG. 7-16   Bilateral rheumatoid arthritis of the wrist joints. A. Photograph showing deformities due to destruction of the carpal joints and extensor tendons and dislocation of the carpal bones from the radius. B. Roentgenograms revealing destruction of the carpal bones with erosion into the radius by the synovial tissue.

in the wrist joint, the procedure is still of value. Straub and Ranawat describe it as a dorsal wrist stabilization. For some patients it can be substituted for arthrodesis and can give a reasonably stable wrist with minimal discomfort. The indications for this procedure are (1) painful synovitis of the wrist joint with a reasonable range of motion, (2) subluxation with pain and weakness of grip, and (3) bilateral disease of the wrist when one wrist has been fused and it is necessary to maintain one wrist with some range of flexion and extension to allow the patient to take care of personal hygiene.

Operative Technique. Under tourniquet control a semilinear dorsal incision is made over the wrist joint (Fig. 7-17). It has been found that the S-shaped or the L-shaped incision tends to give problems with skin healing at the corners of the S or L. The superficial sensory branch of the radial nerve at the wrist should be visualized, as well as the dorsal sensory branch of the ulnar nerve that passes just distal to the ulnar head in the subcutaneous tissue. After these nerves have been visualized, the extensor tendons may be inspected. If the extensor tendons are surrounded by active synovial disease, the tendon sheaths are opened by turning back the dorsal retinaculum, opening each compartment, and clearing the synovial tissue from the tendons themselves. Care must be exercised not to divide the extensor tendons, especially the extensor digiti quinti and the long extensor of the thumb as it passes around Lister's tubercle. The extensor retinaculum should be preserved at its radial side if possible so that it may be laid down beneath the extensor tendons

and over the top of the wrist joint. If the ulnar head is involved, it should be resected at this stage as described previously for ulnar head resection. The dorsal capsule of the wrist is then reflected from the carpal bones and the distal end of the radius, and its attachment is preserved for later repair.

A small rongeur is used to perform a synovectomy of the wrist joint. Usually the synovium will bulge from the wrist joint if the synovitis is very active. All of the synovial tissue is carefully cleaned out and any that remains is curetted, but no attempt should be made to remove the articular cartilage or bone from the carpal area, or spontaneous fusion may occur. The carpal ligament and capsule are resutured, and the extensor retinaculum is placed underneath the extensor tendons and sutured to the capsule of the wrist joint and the distal radius to give further ligamentous reconstruction to protect the extensor tendons from disease involving the carpal bones (Fig. 7-18). If subluxation is present, stabilization can be obtained with Kirschner

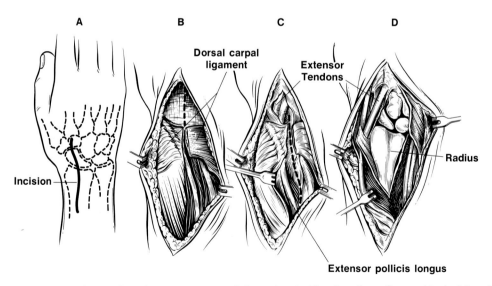

FIG. 7-17 Surgical procedure for synovectomy of the wrist. A. The dorsal semilinear skin incision. B. Visualization of the superficial sensory branch of the radial nerve and division of the dorsal carpal ligament. C. Retraction of the extensor tendons to open the capsule of the wrist and expose the carpal bones. D. Exposure of the carpal bones to excise synovial tissue between the bones. The periosteum has been stripped from the distal end of the radius. (Redrawn from Campbell's Operative Orthopaedics, 5th ed. A. H. Grenshaw, editor. St. Louis, C. V. Mosby, 1971.)

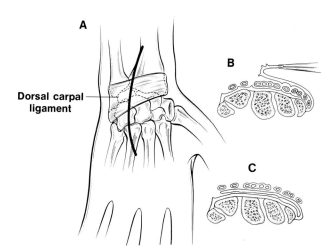

FIG. 7-18 Surgical procedure for synovectomy of the wrist. A. Skin incision. B. Removing the dorsal ligament from the extensor tendons. C. The dorsal ligament placed beneath the extensor tendons. (Redrawn from Flatt, A. E.: The Care of the Rheumatoid Hand, 3rd ed. St. Louis, C. V. Mosby, 1974.)

Dorsal carpal ligament

wires drilled from the radius into the carpal bones and the metacarpals. A bulky pressure dressing is applied with a volar plaster splint for support, but the finger joints are left free for motion to prevent postoperative stiffness. Elevation and ice bags are recommended because of the frequent swelling seen postoperatively. Splitting the dressing the evening of the operation will relieve a great deal of pain.

Postoperative Management. Post operative management consists of early exercise of the fingers, as well as flexion and extension of the elbow joint and shoulder to prevent adhesions and loss of motion. When synovectomy of the wrist alone has been carried out without stabilization with Kirschner wires, the plaster splint should be removed and replaced daily after one week for exercise to prevent stiffness of the wrist joint and loss of motion. In those cases with subluxation and the use of crossed Kirschner wires, some loss of motion will occur if the wires are left in place for 4 to 6 weeks. However, an adequate range of motion for daily activities usually will remain, and the patient will be relieved of the severe preoperative discomfort and pain. Straub and Ranawat in their series noted that a loss of motion would occur in wrists that had an arc of motion of 30° or less preoperatively and that these often would go on to fusion. If the patient had a preoperative arc of motion ranging between 35 to 110°, there would be a loss of 30° or more of the preoperative range of motion.

Arthrodesis

Arthrodesis of the wrist joint has been the classic procedure for treatment of the severely painful joint that has been destroyed by rheumatoid disease. The usual indications for surgical intervention, therefore, are severe pain with destruction of the joint, gross instability, and severe flexion deformity (Fig. 7-19). Although the flexion-extension motion of the wrist is abolished by this procedure, pronation and supination are retained and movement of the finger joints is improved. A number of methods have

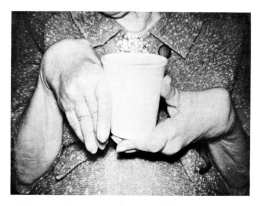

FIG. 7-19 Patient with severe flexion deformity that limits the function of the wrist.

been described for arthrodesis of the wrist, but essentially the basis is a bone graft from the radius into the second and third metacarpals with the hand in the proper position for the individual patient's functional requirements. In patients with a severe flexion deformity and dislocation of the wrist volarward, it is often necessary to excise a portion of the proximal row of the carpal bones to allow for better positioning of the wrist joint (Fig. 7-20).

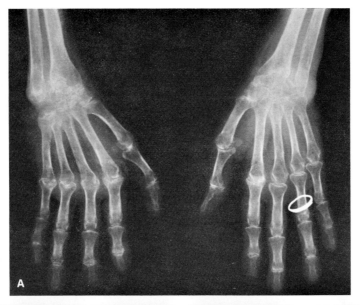

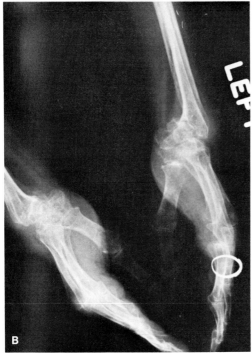

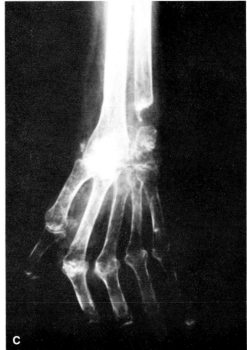

FIG. 7-20. (See page 137 for legend.)

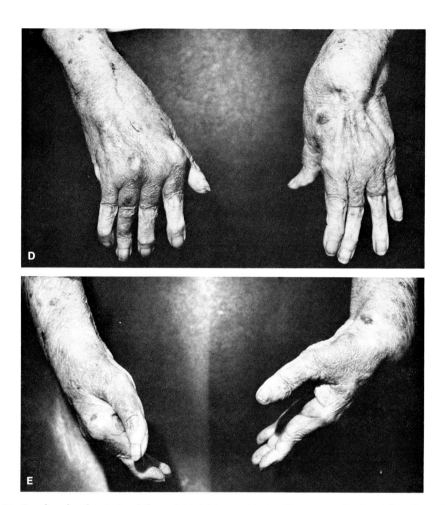

FIG. 7-20 Results of arthrodesis of the wrist joint in a patient with a severe flexion deformity and volar dislocation. A. Roentgenogram revealing dislocation of carpal bones beneath the radius to the volar side. B. Lateral view. C. Roentgenogram after arthrodesis with excision of the ulnar head and placement of a bone graft from the radius into the second metacarpal. D. Photograph showing the right wrist arthrodesed in a neutral position. Despite parchment-like skin, healing of the incision is good. Tenting over the distal radius, which can lead to tendon rupture, is seen in the left hand. E. Lateral view revealing position of the right wrist and dislocation of the left. Extension has been lost in the left wrist.

It is important to consider the position of arthrodesis of a wrist joint, especially if both wrists are involved and surgery is contemplated to correct these deformities. In general, it is not advisable to fuse the wrist in a position of function, but it is better to consider placing the dominant hand in a neutral or slightly extended position. The opposite wrist should be fused in flexion to allow for personal hygiene and other activities of daily living. If both wrists are fused in extension, the patient will have great difficulty in buttoning his clothes and his personal hygiene. Severe deformities can be corrected by arthrodesis even when the carpal bones have been completely destroyed (Fig. 7-21). Function of the hands can be improved by inserting the distal end of the radius into the metacarpals for stability.

Operative Technique. Arthrodesis is usually performed under tourniquet control, and a dorsal incision 3 to 4 inches in

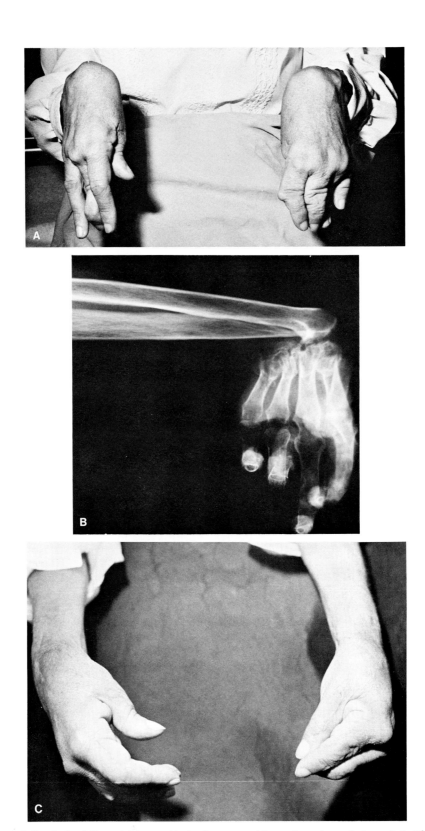

FIG. 7-21 Arthrodesis of the wrist in a patient whose carpal bones have been destroyed. A. Photograph before arthrodesis showing flipper-like appearance of hands. B. Roentgenogram revealing complete distruction of the wrist joint. C. Photograph after successful fusion of the metacarpals to the radius. The right wrist has been placed in slight flexion to allow for personal hygiene, and the left has been placed in a neutral position.

length is made over the wrist joint and onto the back of the hand. A linear or slightly curved incision is made through the skin and subcutaneous tissue. The extensor tendons should be cleaned of any active synovial disease and retracted out of the way, and as suggested by Clayton, the dorsal carpal ligament should be preserved. The ulnar head should be resected and retained, as it can often be used as a bone graft from the radius into the metacarpals (Fig. 7-22). The capsule and ligaments are then elevated from the carpal bones and radius, exposing the carpus. All the synovium is removed from the joint with a small rongeur, and at this stage if the proximal row is dislocated beneath the radius, it should be removed with the rongeur carefully. These portions of carpal bones can be used as bone grafts later. Removal of the proximal row will often allow the wrist to be brought back in position against the distal radius. The basic principle is to obtain a solid fusion from the distal radius into the second and third metacarpal.

The bone graft can be utilized in several ways. It is possible to cut a slot in the distal radius and a trough through the carpal bones to a slot cut in the base of the second and third metacarpals. If bone bank material is available, a piece of cancellous iliac or rib can be cut to lock into place between the radius and the metacarpals (Fig. 7-23). If this type of bone is not available and the proximal row has been excised, frequently the distal end of the ulna that has been removed can be reshaped and impacted into the distal radius and into the slot cut in the second and third metacarpals to give adequate fixation of the wrist (Fig. 7-24). If this is not possible, a sliding graft can be obtained from the dorsal surface of the distal radius and inserted into the second and third metacarpals. The portions of the carpal bone that have been removed from the proximal row can then be packed around the distal radius and the second and third metacarpals.

In general, the rheumatoid arthritic patient's wrist fuses quite readily following almost any type of arthrodesis. The wrist may be fixed internally with several crossed Kirschner wires that are left subcutaneously for easy removal. To avoid injury to the median nerve, care must be exercised not to drill the wire into the carpal tunnel area. The carpal ligaments and capsule are resutured over the graft when possible, and the extensor retinaculum is sutured over the grafts and beneath the extensor tendons to protect them. The periosteum and soft tissue should be resutured around the distal end of the ulna to hold it in place. A soft dressing and either plaster splints or a loose cast are applied from the wrist

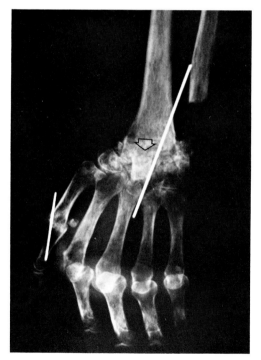

FIG. 7-22 Roentgenogram of a patient who has undergone arthrodesis of the wrist and the metacarpal-phalangeal joint of the thumb. The ulnar head has been removed and used as a bone graft from the radius to the third metacarpal (arrow).

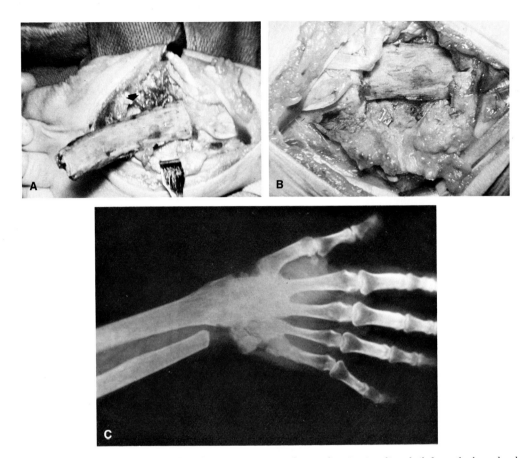

FIG. 7-23 Procedure for a bone graft in the wrist. A. Surgical view showing irradiated rib from the bone bank being inserted into the third metacarpal. The trough in the third metacarpal is visible (arrow). B. Surgical view after the bone graft has been cut to fit and has been inserted from the distal radius into the third metacarpal to serve as a strut for fusion of the wrist. C. Roentgenogram showing solid fusion.

to above the elbow. If internal fixation has been adequate, the cast may be applied only to the elbow. It is important to split the cast at the time of surgery and to elevate the arm and apply ice bags postoperatively to prevent the swelling that often occurs following a wrist fusion. The wrist should be protected approximately 9 weeks to allow union to occur. If a long arm cast has been used originally, it should be changed to a molded short plaster cast in 4 weeks, and at 8 weeks the wrist can be protected with just a volar plaster splint. The Kirschner wires should be removed in 4 weeks or sooner if infection develops around them.

At times a wrist fusion can be combined with arthrodesis of the metacarpophalangeal joint of the thumb or of several fingers (Fig. 7-25). It is advisable, however, to perform an arthrodesis of the wrist prior to reconstruction of the hand by arthroplasty.

Arthroplasty

The function of the hand is greatly aided when wrist motion can be preserved. This becomes even more important when the hand is severely disabled by rheumatoid arthritis. Swanson has reported on a flexible implant arthroplasty of the wrist. The experience that

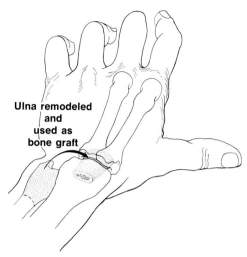

FIG. 7-24 Schematic drawing showing reshaped distal end of the ulna used as a bone graft.

he gained from the development of a finger joint implant led to the concept of a flexible intramedullary stemmed hinged implant for the wrist joint to maintain an adequate joint space and alignment of the wrist. The major indications for this type of arthroplasty are instability of the wrist due to subluxation or dislocation of the radiocarpal joint and stiffness or loss of movement in the wrist. The Silastic prosthesis is available in five different sizes and contains a Dacron reinforcement for greater strength.

The results obtained by Swanson have been satisfactory. If failure does

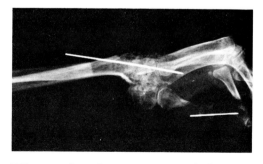

FIG. 7-25 Lateral roentgenogram of the wrist showing the ulnar graft extending from the distal radius into the metacarpals as well as arthrodesis of the metacarpal-phalangeal joint of the thumb.

occur, one can always consider arthrodesis as a salvage procedure.

Operative Technique. The wrist is approached under tourniquet control, using a straight or slightly curved incision over the dorsum of the wrist. A synovectomy is carried out similar to that in arthrodesis of the wrist or wrist stabilization procedures.

The capsule and ligaments are preserved for later reconstruction of the wrist. The proximal row of carpal bones is often subluxed or dislocated toward the volar side beneath the radius. These bones should be resected carefully with a rongeur. After resection of the proximal row, the radiocarpal subluxation should be reduced. The distal end of the radius is squared off, and with a broach or drill a trough or tunnel is made into the medullary canal of the radius. The distal stem of the implant passes through the capitate bone into the medullary canal of the third metacarpal. If necessary, the ulnar head can be removed at this stage. The proximal stem of the wrist joint implant is inserted into the radius, and the distal stem is slipped into the capitate and the third metacarpal bones. The capsule and ligaments are then repaired, and the wrist is tested to be sure that adequate motion is present and that the bone is not impinging. The extensor retinaculum may be placed underneath the extensor tendons and over the wrist joint for further support as in a wrist stabilization.

A plaster splint is used postoperatively, and the wrist maintained in a neutral position. A short arm cast is recommended in a neutral position for approximately 4 to 6 weeks to obtain stability with some motion.

Extensor Tenosynovitis

The carpal ligament over the dorsum of the wrist tends to enclose the extensor tendons into a series of six compart-

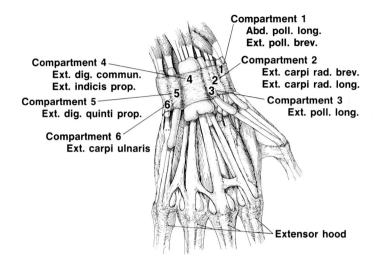

FIG. 7-26   The extensor tendons of the wrist. Dorsal aspect.

ments through which the tendons pass as they cross the wrist (Fig. 7-26). Each compartment has its own synovial sheath which can become affected by rheumatoid synovitis of the wrist. These tendon sheaths surround the extensor tendons from a point proximal to the dorsal ligament of the wrist to approximately the midshaft of the metacarpals.

The first compartment or tunnel contains the abductor pollicis longus and the extensor pollicis brevis tendons. The second compartment contains the extensor carpi radialis longus and brevis tendons to the base of the second and third metacarpals. The third compartment contains the extensor pollicis longus tendon as it passes around Lister's tubercle. The fourth compartment, the largest of the group, contains the common extensor tendons to the fingers and the extensor indicis proprius. The fifth compartment contains the extensor digiti quinti, and the last or sixth compartment contains the extensor carpi ulnaris tendon.

Since rheumatoid arthritis primarily involves the synovial lining of the tendon sheaths, a severe inflammatory change may occur. This synovial proliferation tends to infiltrate the tendons

themselves and to interfere with their proper nutrition (Fig. 7-27). This swelling, which arises on the dorsum of the wrist, is usually obvious to the patient and at times simulates a ganglion. The synovial tissue can protrude proximal to the extensor retinaculum as well as distal to it over the dorsum of the hand. The swelling will be limited to the synovial tendon sheath itself and will follow its anatomic pattern (Fig. 7-28). Since the extensor tenosynovitis is often associated with severe involvement of the ulnar head with dorsal subluxation

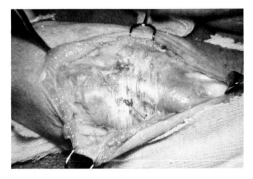

FIG. 7-27   Surgical view of the synovial tissue enclosed by the dorsal carpal ligament. The extensor tendons are just visible under the blunt retractor. Note the proliferation and thickening of the synovial sheaths.

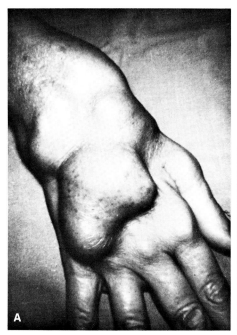
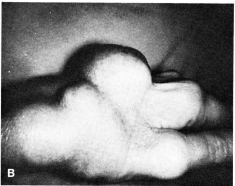

FIG. 7-28 Severe rheumatoid extensor tenosynovitis. A. Dorsal view. The synovitis follows the anatomic pattern of the synovial sheaths. B. Lateral view revealing the swelling of the extensor synovium.

and rough protruding prominences on the ulnar head, rupture of tendons may occur in this region. Direct infiltration of the tendon and interference with its nutrition by the synovitis contributes to the mechanism of tendon rupture. The squeezing of the extensor tendons through the wrist tunnels beneath the dorsal carpal ligament produces a sawing effect and friction, and at times the rough bony spicules of the ulnar head will erode the tendon. Erosion occurs most frequently in the region of the common extensor tendons, which may become attenuated or ruptured beneath the dorsal carpal ligament (Fig. 7-29).

The major indications for surgery for patients with an extensor tenosynovitis are to relieve their pain and deformity and try to prevent rupture of the extensor tendons.

Conservative Treatment

Extensor tenosynovitis can at times be treated conservatively. Patients may

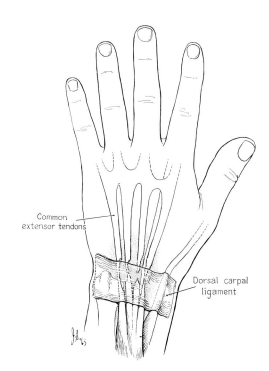

FIG. 7-29 Diagram showing rupture of the common extensor tendons beneath the dorsal carpal ligament.

experience long periods of relief following the local injection of lidocaine (Xylocaine) and a steroid into the sheaths. The swelling will disappear following the injections, but these should not be given repeatedly. If symptoms return after a short period of time, surgical intervention is generally indicated.

Tenosynovectomy

The decision about the operative procedure to be performed depends upon the involvement of the distal radioulnar joint. If the joint is not subluxed clinically, and there is no limitation of pronation or supination, excision of the ulnar head is probably not indicated. Therefore, only a synovectomy of the extensor tendons should be performed. If, however, the roentgenograms reveal involvement of the distal radioulnar joint with subluxation and the patient is having rheumatoid symptoms related to the joint, it should be excised at the same time, and a synovectomy should be performed in the region of the distal end of the ulna where it articulates with the radius.

Operative Technique. Under tourniquet control a semilinear or slightly curved incision is made over the dorsum of the wrist (Fig. 7-30). The subcutaneous tissue is entered, and the radial sensory nerve should be visualized on the radial side of the wrist and the ulnar sensory branch on the ulnar side. These nerves are located in the subcutaneous tissue and can easily be damaged if they are not visualized. Damage to them can result in a painful neuroma and an area of anesthesia on the dorsum of the hand.

Once the nerves have been visualized and retracted out of the way, the synovectomy can be performed. The dorsal retinaculum should be opened over the compartment containing the extensor carpi ulnaris and carefully turned radioward to allow for complete cleaning of the tendon from its synovial tendon sheath. Care should be exercised in tracing the extensor carpi ulnaris distally, as the ulnar sensory branch is close and frequently crosses this tendon in the distal end of the wound. The extensor digiti quinti tendon is next found in the fifth compartment and is lifted out of its tunnel, and the entire area is cleaned of synovial tissue. The extensor retinaculum is carefully kept preserved as much as possible, and the fourth compartment is opened by turning back the retinaculum to expose the common extensor tendons. These are traced both proximally and distally to remove all synovial tissue from both the bed of the tunnel and on the extensor tendons themselves. Then the extensor pollicis longus is found near Lister's tubercle and carefully lifted out and allowed to drift toward the radial side

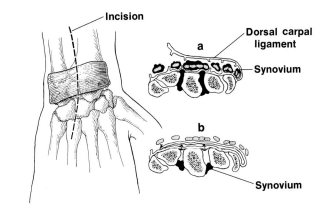

FIG. 7-30 Procedure for tenosynovectomy. Left, semilinear incision over the dorsum of the wrist to expose the dorsal carpal ligament. a. The dorsal carpal ligament dissected off the extensor tendons and turned back to expose the synovial tissue. b. The dorsal carpal ligament folded beneath the extensor tendons to protect them from synovial disease in the wrist. (Redrawn from Flatt, A. E.: The Care of the Rheumatoid Hand, 3rd ed. St. Louis, C. V. Mosby, 1974.)

while the synovial tissue is removed from the tendon itself.

The second compartment containing the wrist extensors is opened and carefully cleaned by turning back the retinaculum. Care should be exercised going proximally, as the abductor pollicis longus and extensor pollicis brevis muscle bellies cross the wrist extensors in the proximal area and can be easily injured. The first compartment containing the thumb tendons lies close to the radial sensory nerve which should be carefully retracted out of the way. If synovitis in the wrist joint is not severe, it is generally not necessary to replace the retinacular ligament beneath the common extensor tendons to protect them from a synovitis of the wrist. The retinaculum can be resutured over the top of the extensor tendons to prevent bowstringing of the extensor tendons. However, if there is synovitis in the wrist joint or the radioulnar joint, it is advisable to suture the dorsal retinaculum beneath the extensor tendons for protection of the tendons. A soft dressing is applied, but plaster immobilization is not necessary.

Results. This type of surgery has relieved symptoms of arthritis and has improved function. Recurrence of tenosynovitis has been reported in a small percentage of patients.

De Quervain's Disease

De Quervain's disease may occur in rheumatoid arthritis and consists of a stenosing tenosynovitis of the abductor pollicis longus and extensor pollicis brevis. These two tendons pass through the first tunnel at the wrist over the radial styloid. Inflammation in this region will severely limit the function of the thumb. The patient usually complains of pain on using the thumb and at times of a lump over the radial styloid. A test described by Finkelstein has been of value in making the diagnosis. The thumb is flexed into the palm of the

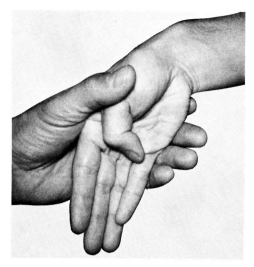

FIG. 7-31 Finkelstein's test for de Quervain's disease. Flexing the thumb into the palm and ulnar deviation of the wrist will accentuate the symptoms.

hand and the wrist is forced into ulnar deviation, reproducing or accentuating the pain (Fig. 7-31).

Treatment

Local injection of the tendon sheath with a steroid and 5 cc lidocaine (Xylocaine) will frequently bring relief. Surgical release is indicated in recurrent or chronic cases that may not respond to local injection because of far-advanced changes in the sheath.

Operative Technique. A transverse incision is made over the radial styloid, and the sensory branch of the radial nerve should be visualized and retracted. The tendon sheath should be incised, and all synovial hypertrophy removed. The area should be inspected to make certain that all the tendons have been released because a number of accessory tendons may be present. To release the tendons it is only necessary to split the sheath and remove as much of the synovium as possible.

Tendon Ruptures

Rupture of the extensor tendons can occur with rheumatoid arthritis.

Vaughan-Jackson in 1959 reported his experiences with rupture of the extensor tendons at the wrist. Since that time numerous papers have been published on this entity. The common extensor tendons and the long extensor tendon of the thumb are most frequently destroyed by rheumatoid disease. The patient usually does not experience pain when the rupture occurs. A pre-existing tenosynovitis would have been present for a period, and often the radioulnar joint is severly involved with rheumatoid disease. The patient will note the inability to extend the fingers and will not realize that the extensor tendons have ruptured.

The patient may still be able to extend the index or the fifth finger because each has an extra tendon that may not have ruptured along with the common extensors. The indicis proprius and the extensor digiti quinti often are not involved. Rupture of the extensor pollicis longus results in loss of extension of the distal phalanx of the thumb (Fig. 7-33). The patient frequently is not concerned about this because it usually is associated with a good deal of arthritic change in the rest of the hand and he can still function as long as the flexor tendon to the distal phalanx is present.

The common site for rupture of the

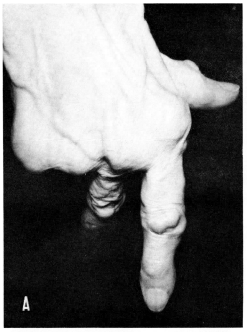

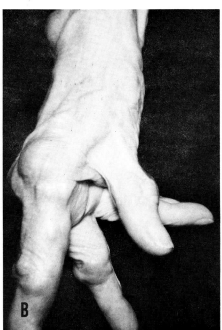

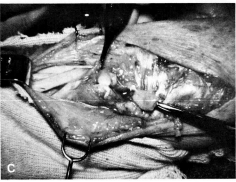

FIG. 7-32 Rupture of the common extensors. A. Dorsal view of the hand. The extensor indicis proprius is still present and allows extension of the index finger. B. Lateral view showing loss of extension in the third, fourth, and fifth fingers. C. Surgical view of rupture of the common extensors and synovial hyperplasia.

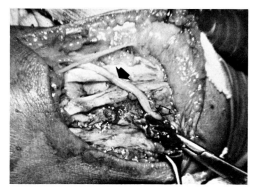

FIG. 7-33 Surgical view of rupture of the extensor pollicis longus (arrows).

extensor tendons at the wrist is beneath the dorsal retinaculum and not at the back of the hand or proximal to the retinaculum (Fig. 7-33). The three basic factors generally responsible for rupture of the extensor tendons of the wrist are (1) a rheumatoid tenosynovitis, (2) pressure from the dorsal retinacular ligament, and (3) erosion by bony spicules from a subluxed or dislocated ulnar head.

Repair and/or Replacement

Repair by end-to-end suture is usually not possible because of the necrotic tendon tissue at the site of the rupture. Repair is usually accomplished by tendon transfer or, in some cases, by a free tendon graft. The common extensors may be repaired by using the extensor carpi radialis longus or brevis (Fig. 7-34). This procedure is better than suturing the common extensors to each other unless only one tendon has ruptured. The extensor pollicis longus usually ruptures at Lister's tubercle and can be repaired by using the extensor indicis proprius. Transferring the extensor pollicis longus tendon from its tunnel toward the radial side of the wrist will also aid in giving better abduction of the thumb postoperatively. If a tendon graft is necessary, the palmaris longus or a long toe extensor tendon can be utilized as a free graft. The necrotic area of the ruptured tendon should be excised, and the graft should be sutured into place with a tendon suture of silk or wire. Generally a pull-out wire is not necessary in this type of repair. In selected situations when the long extensor to the thumb has ruptured and an arthrodesis of the metacarpal-phalangeal joint of the thumb is necessary because of instability, the long extensor tendon can be sutured to the extensor brevis to restore extension of the thumb.

When there have been multiple ruptures of the extensor tendons, a suitable motor tendon may not be available and tendon transfer may not be possible. The flexor digitorum sublimis can be transferred through the interosseous membrane to substitute for the extensor motor power. Usually the use of the fourth and fifth sublimis will give adequate power, and the muscle belly should be pulled through the interosseous membrane to the dorsum of the wrist.

In some cases all the extensor tendons are ruptured and the metacarpal-phalangeal joints are destroyed. Arthrodesis of the metacarpal-phalangeal joints can be carried out as a procedure of choice if the proximal interphalangeal joints are good.

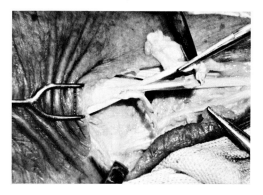

FIG. 7-34 Surgical view showing repair of common extensor tendons by suturing them to the extensor radialis longus and brevis.

Operative Technique. Repair of rupture of the extensor tendons is carried out under tourniquet control. A transverse skin incision can be made over the wrist or a linear incision crossing the wrist joint. A pre-existing tenosynovitis is usually present, and a synovectomy should be carried out. As in the tenosynovectomy of the tendon sheaths the sensory nerves must be protected from damage. The area of tendon rupture will often be stained brown by pigment and will have thinned the tendon in this area considerably, leaving long thin tails. Because it is usually impossible to sew the ends together, the necrotic area should be excised. The proximal portion is usually retracted considerably and cannot be reached for a simple end-to-end suture. The extensor carpi radialis longus can be dissected out of the second compartment and traced down to its insertion on the base of the second metacarpal. As much tendon as possible should be taken with it from the base of the metacarpal to be used as a transfer to the common extensors. The distal portions of the common extensors can be sutured together with 4-0 white silk, and then a common junction can be made with the extensor carpi radialis longus. The pull-out sutures are not necessary, and the tendon of the extensor carpi radialis can be passed through tunnels made in the common extensors and resutured to itself to give excellent fixation. The tendon should be put in tight enough to take up the slack in the extensor tendons and give reasonably good extension of the fingers with the wrist in a neutral position (Fig. 7-35). The extensor carpi ulnaris can also be utilized at times to reconstruct the extensor tendons when they are ruptured.

Rupture of the long extensor of the thumb at Lister's tubercle results in a short distal portion with an attenuated tendon. The extensor indicis proprius can be taken out of the fourth compart-

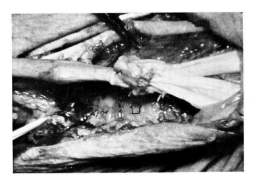

FIG. 7-35 Surgical view showing the common extensor tendons sutured into the wrist extensors (arrow).

ment and brought over and sutured to the distal end of the extensor pollicis longus tendon. The repair should be protected with a plaster splint with the fingers in extension for approximately 2 weeks.

It is important to observe the condition of the metacarpal-phalangeal joints because if they are dislocated in rheumatoid arthritis, full extension will not be possible even with repair of the extensor rupture. The patient may not understand the limitation of motion after the operation unless it is pointed out preoperatively that repair of the tendons will not give full extension.

Flexor Tenosynovitis

The flexor tendons of the wrist as they pass through the carpal tunnel are surrounded by a synovial sheath that can become involved in rheumatoid arthritis (Fig. 7-36). The sheath extends from the forearm proximal to the volar carpal ligament distally into the carpal tunnel and in the fingers may communicate with the synovial sheath of the fifth finger and the thumb. A flexor tendon sheath surrounds the tendons from the distal palmar crease to the distal phalanx. Generally the second, third, and fourth synovial sheaths of the

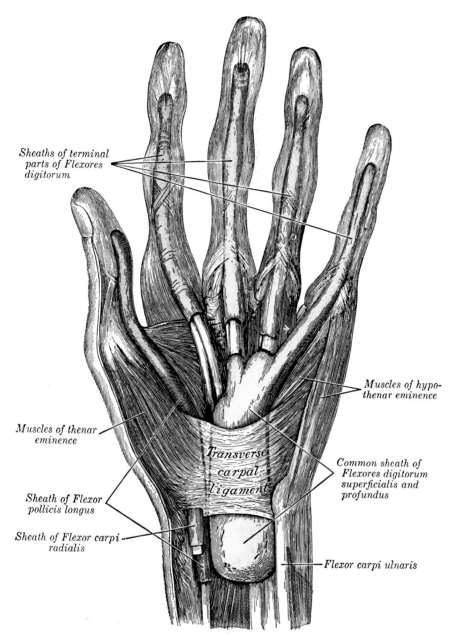

Sheaths of terminal parts of Flexores digitorum

Muscles of hypo-thenar eminence

Muscles of thenar eminence

Transverse carpal ligament

Common sheath of Flexores digitorum superficialis and profundus

Sheath of Flexor pollicis longus

Sheath of Flexor carpi radialis

Flexor carpi ulnaris

FIG. 7-36 The flexor tendons on the palmar aspect of the wrist. They are covered by a synovial sheath in the carpal tunnel. (From Gray's Anatomy of the Human Body, 19th ed. C. M. Goss, editor. Philadelphia, Lea & Febiger, 1973.)

fingers do not communicate with the synovial sheath of the wrist. A severe rheumatoid synovitis developing in the flexor tendon sheaths can produce pain and swelling in the area of the wrist (Fig. 7-37A). This swelling can produce a carpal tunnel syndrome with paresthesias and actual atrophy of the thenar muscles (Fig. 7-37B). A flexor tenosynovitis can also occur simultaneously with severe involvement of the extensors of the wrist.

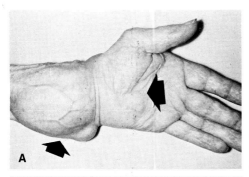

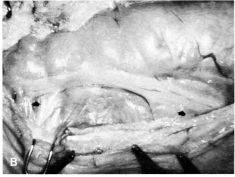

FIG. 7-37 Flexor tenosynovitis. A. Swelling of the wrist and carpal tunnel with protrusion down into the palm of the hand (arrows). B. Surgical view showing compression of the median nerve (arrows) because of swelling of the flexor tendons.

Tenosynovectomy

It is better to limit surgical procedures to either the extensor tendon or to the flexor tendon sheaths rather than to operate on both at the same time. The swelling and interference with the blood supply may produce edema resulting in stiffness of the hand. If the synovial tissue is not removed from the carpal tunnel area, necrosis of the tendons can occur with multiple ruptures, resulting in loss of function and in greater difficulty in restoring use of the hand by late reconstruction.

Operative Technique. An S-type skin incision is made to avoid a vertical incision over the flexor crease of the wrist. The incision generally parallels the thenar base along the crease in the palm, follows this proximally with a slight curve toward the ulnar side, and then passes up along the ulnar border of the forearm to give adequate exposure of the entire area (Fig. 7-38).

The median nerve and its sensory branch to the skin should be isolated carefully, and then the volar carpal ligament should be opened along its ulnar side to avoid damage to the motor branch of the median nerve to the thenar muscles. The flexor tendons then can be visualized quite readily from the proximal portion of the incision in the forearm down through the carpal tunnel into the palm of the hand. Care should be taken not to damage the vascular supply to the hand. Synovial swelling can be quite massive, and there may be numerous rice bodies within the tendon sheaths (Fig. 7-39). The synovial tissue should be dissected off the flexor tendons carefully, the flexor tendons should be lifted out of the carpal tunnel, and then the base of the tunnel should be explored to be sure there is no further disease beneath the flexor tendons (Fig. 7-40).

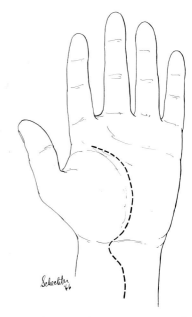

FIG. 7-38 Flexor tendon synovectomy. S-shaped palmar incision.

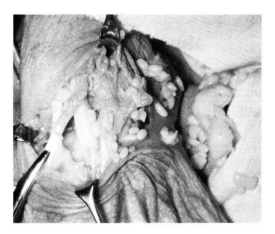

FIG. 7-39 Surgical view showing rice bodies within the tendon sheaths.

The tourniquet is released at completion of the synovectomy and hemostasis is secured. The volar carpal ligament should not be repaired, and the incision is closed with subcutaneous sutures and a skin closure. Postoperatively the patient should be started on early motion of the fingers to prevent stiffness and adhesions of the flexor tendons.

Flexor Tendon Rupture

Persistent active synovitis of the flexor tendons can lead to rupture in the carpal tunnel. Loss of flexion will be-

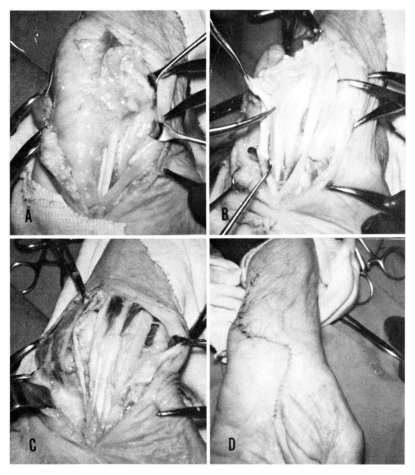

FIG. 7-40 Flexor tenosynovectomy. A. Exposure of the proliferating synovial tissue of the flexor tendon sheaths in the carpal tunnel. B. The synovial tissue being stripped away to expose the flexor tendons. C. Synovial tissue removed to reveal attrition of tendons. D. S-shaped incision sutured.

come apparent, and if multiple ruptures occur, the patient will not be able to use the hand in forceful pinching or grasping motions. However, a single rupture in the flexor digitorum sublimis will not be as obvious to the patient until the profundus tendon in the same finger is lost and flexion is no longer possible. A common area of rupture is the flexor pollicis longus with loss of the ability to pinch with the distal phalanx of the thumb. It is important to diagnose the site of rupture because occasionally the rupture will occur in the flexor tendon in the finger itself where there is synovial hyperplasia due to rheumatoid disease. Advanced stenosing tenosynovitis of the flexor tendons in the hand can also result in loss of flexion and the inability to pinch (see Chapter 8).

Arthrodesis

If only the flexor tendon to the thumb is involved, the rupture can be repaired by arthrodesis of the interphalangeal joint of the thumb. This is a better procedure than trying to reconstruct the flexor pollicis longus tendon in the carpal tunnel. If multiple ruptures have occurred, it is better to explore the entire carpal tunnel and clean out the synovial tissue. No attempt should be made to repair multiple tendon ruptures. Only the flexor pollicis longus and long flexors to the involved fingers should be repaired, and the sublimis should be sacrificed to prevent adhesions and loss of function in the hand. Repair and prolonged immobilization of all the tendons can lead to a stiff hand and a poor result.

Median Nerve Compression or Carpal Tunnel Syndrome

The patient with chronic rheumatoid arthritis frequently has multiple complaints from a variety of deformities and acutely inflamed joints. Destruction of the carpal joints and tenosynovitis of the extensors and flexor tendons about the wrist are characteristic of the disease. Since pain is synonymous with arthritis, the surgeon must be keenly aware of any change in the patient's pain or other symptoms in order to recognize compression of the median nerve in the carpal tunnel (Fig. 7-41).

The anatomy of the carpal tunnel lends itself very readily to compression of the median nerve because of the large amount of synovial tissue which can be affected by rheumatoid disease (Fig. 7-41B). There are multiple causes for compression of the median nerve in the carpal tunnel, and rheumatoid arthritis may be one of them. The median nerve and flexor tendons pass beneath the volar carpal ligament within the carpal tunnel, which is a closed rigid space allowing very little room for swelling. The volar carpal ligament is extremely strong and thick and passes over the top of the median nerve and flexor tendons from the hamate to the navicular bone (Fig. 7-42). Rheumatoid arthritis can produce severe swelling of the synovial sheaths within the carpal tunnel, and the only evidence of this condition, aside from the symptoms of entrapment of the median nerve, will be swelling proximal and distal to the volar carpal ligament. Flexion and extension of the fingers will cause the mass to slide proximal and distal in the volar carpal ligament, an indication that it is synovial tissue.

Operative Technique. The operation is performed under tourniquet control, and the incision is quite similar to that used for a flexor tenosynovitis at the wrist. An S-shaped incision made across the thenar crease will give adequate exposure. It is preferable to a transverse incision which is more cosmetic but tends to limit exposure and can lead to incomplete division of the volar carpal ligament.

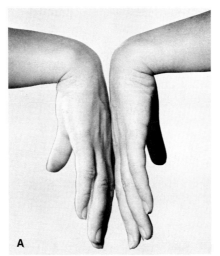

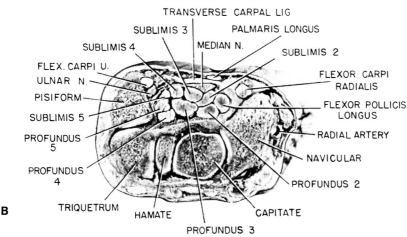

B

TRANSVERSE CARPAL LIG

SUBLIMIS 3   PALMARIS LONGUS

SUBLIMIS 4   MEDIAN N.   SUBLIMIS 2

FLEX. CARPI U.   FLEXOR CARPI RADIALIS

ULNAR N.

PISIFORM   FLEXOR POLLICIS LONGUS

SUBLIMIS 5

PROFUNDUS 5   RADIAL ARTERY

NAVICULAR

PROFUNDUS 4   PROFUNDUS 2

TRIQUETRUM   HAMATE   CAPITATE

PROFUNDUS 3

FIG. 7-41 Carpal tunnel syndrome. A. Flexion test. Pain or parathesia upon flexion is an indication of compression of the median nerve. B. Anatomy of the carpal tunnel. Transverse section across the wrist. (From Robbins, H.: Anatomical study of the median nerve in the carpal tunnel and etiologies of the carpal tunnel syndrome. J. Bone Joint Surg., 45A:953, 1963.)

Since there is often an associated tenosynovitis in rheumatoid arthritis producing a carpal tunnel syndrome, a synovectomy of the flexor tendons should be carried out. At operation the nerve will be observed to be narrowed by the compression and slightly injected and swollen proximal and distal to the carpal ligament. The volar carpal ligament should be divided completely into the palm of the hand on the ulnar side to prevent damage to the motor branch of the median nerve, which is located on the radial side of the median nerve at approximately the level of the base of the thumb when the thumb is fully abducted from the hand (Fig. 7-43A). To prevent a recurrent compression of the nerve, the carpal ligament should not be repaired (Fig. 7-43B).

When there is severe narrowing of the median nerve, neurolysis can be carried out by injecting saline solution carefully into the nerve sheath with a small needle. Curtis and Eversmann have recommended internal neurolysis

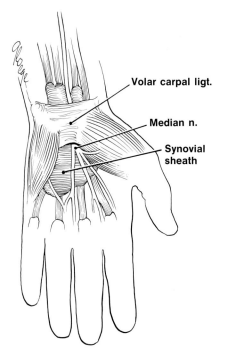

FIG. 7-42 Diagram of the hand showing the volar ligament that encloses the median nerve and flexor tendons in a tight tunnel. (From Marmor, L.: Median nerve compression in arthritis. Arch. Surg., *89*:1008, 1964.)

as an adjunct to the treatment of median nerve compression in the carpal tunnel. Under loupe magnification of 2 to 6 power, the thickened epineurium is opened, and the individual scarred fascicles are released. Each individual fascicle of the nerve is gently teased apart with sharp pointed scissors and a small forceps to relieve any interfascicular scarring. The dorsal aspect of the nerve should remain undisturbed to prevent interference with the microcirculation of the nerve itself.

Results. This procedure may be worthwhile in patients with chronic changes in the nerve and may aid in recovery of sensory and motor function postoperatively. The patient should be encouraged to use the hand after surgery to prevent adhesions and loss of function. In long-standing cases with atrophy of the thenar muscles, recovery of function may be poor and paresthesias can persist for months.

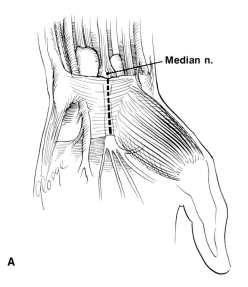

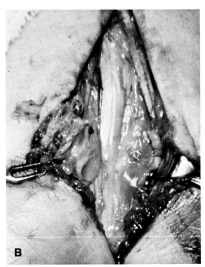

FIG. 7-43 Decompression of the median nerve in the carpal tunnel. A. Division of the entire volar ligament. B. Surgical view at time of release of the volar ligament revealing narrowing and compression with loss of normal vascularity.

Ulnar Nerve Compression

The ulnar nerve at the wrist passes superficially to the transverse carpal ligament, but it tends to lie in a semirigid triangular tunnel that is formed by the volar carpal ligament anteriorly, the pisiform bone, and the flexor carpi ulnaris medially, and the transverse carpal ligament posteriorly.

Proliferation of the synovium within the wrist, edema, or a tenosynovitis of the flexor carpi ulnaris may compromise the ulnar nerve and cause its compression. The symptoms usually consist of pain radiating into the ring finger and the little finger. The pain can be increased by the use of the wrist which contributes to compression of the nerve. Paresthesias may also develop in the ulnar distribution, and occasionally weakness of the intrinsic muscles of the hand may ensue.

Decompression

Surgical release and excision of the synovial tissue will give complete relief of the syndrome. An S-shaped incision will give adequate exposure for division of the volar carpal ligament and exploration of the median and ulnar nerves.

Osteoarthritis

Osteoarthritis in the wrist joint can be localized to a single carpal joint, or else widespread involvement of multiple joints can produce symptoms. The roentgenogram is extremely valuable not only in determining the site of the osteoarthritic process but also in the management of the patient.

Early in the course of osteoarthritic disease when the patient complains of pain, conservative therapy may give excellent results. The local injection of steroids frequently will relieve symptoms for long periods of time. If multiple joints are involved, it is often necessary to insert the needle into the various areas of the wrist joint to relieve the symptoms.

The patient frequently may have no symptoms whatsoever in the wrist joint despite the radiologic evidence of osteoarthritis; however, an injury to the wrist or to another part of the body requiring the use of crutches or a walker can stimulate the onset of symptoms in this joint (Fig. 7-44). This has been noted in patients who have undergone total hip replacement and have to use their arms for support postoperatively. They frequently will blame the insertion of a needle for an intravenous injection into the back of the hand as the cause of their severe complaints in the wrist and hand. However, local injection of the wrist joint with steroids frequently will re-

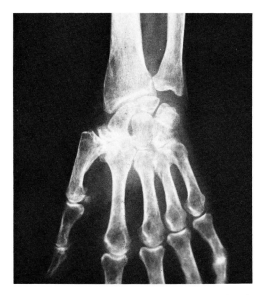

FIG. 7-44 Roentgenogram of a patient with advanced osteoarthritis involving both the carpalmetacarpal joint and the trapezionavicular joint. This patient was asymptomatic until a total hip replacement was carried out, and the patient was required to use crutches.

lieve the symptoms, and as soon as the patient is off the crutches or the walker, the joint will continue to improve. Indomethacin (Indocin) or other anti-inflammatory drugs can be combined with local injections to give prolonged relief. In women the carpal-metacarpal joint of the thumb is commonly affected by osteoarthritis, and both thumbs may be involved simultaneously. Traction on the thumb will tend to open the carpal-metacarpal joint and allow an easier insertion of the needle for local injection (Fig. 7-45). Local steroid injections should be utilized in those patients with the acute onset of pain and minimal roentgenographic changes. Palpation along the thumb toward the proximal base will reveal a prominence at the base of the metacarpal, and the needle should be inserted just proximal to this area. The subluxation of the base of the thumb produces this prominence.

Radioulnar Joint Disease

The distal radioulnar joint can be involved in osteoarthritis due to trauma. Symptoms of arthritis sometimes appear after fractures of the distal radius (Colles) that disrupt the radioulnar joint (Fig. 7-46). The triangular cartilage located between the radius and the ulna also can be disrupted by trauma resulting in pain and limitation of motion on pronation and supination. Tenderness can be palpated at the site of the radioulnar joint, despite the fact that roentgenograms may be normal. Arthrograms have shown that a tear of the triangular fibrocartilage is the cause of symptoms.

Treatment

The radioulnar joint may be injected locally with steroids to produce temporary relief. An excellent therapeutic test

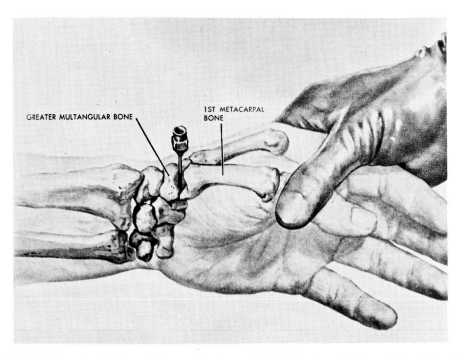

GREATER MULTANGULAR BONE

1ST METACARPAL BONE

FIG. 7-45 Technique for injection of the carpal-metacarpal joint of the thumb. Note position of physician's hand to apply traction on the thumb to open the joint for easier injection in this area.

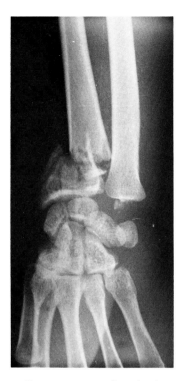

FIG. 7-46 Roentgenogram of patient's wrist revealing comminuted fracture. The radioulnar joint is disrupted, and the triangular fibrocartilage between the radius and the ulna is damaged.

that will often give dramatic relief is to inject 2 to 3 cc lidocaine (Xylocaine) into the area of the triangular cartilage. In patients with specific involvement of the triangular cartilage, local excision of the cartilage can give satisfactory results. If disruption of the radioulnar joint is due to a fracture of the radius with shortening, simple excision of the fibrocartilage generally is not satisfactory. The best procedure in this situation is a resection of the distal ulna, the so-called Darrach procedure. The operation is described in detail in the section on rheumatoid arthritis of the wrist.

Carpal Joint Disease

Osteoarthritis or traumatic arthritis may involve any combination of the carpal bones in the wrist. The two bones most frequently affected in the proximal row are the navicular and the lunate. Fracture of the navicular bone following injuries to the wrist frequently goes on to osteoarthritis of the radial-navicular joint (Fig. 7-47). If this does occur, at times excision of the radial styloid will relieve the patient's symptoms. When excision does not relieve symptoms or if the disease involves the distal end of the navicular or the adjacent carpal bones, the surgeon is then faced with a dilemma if the symptoms are severe.

Many patients with beginning arthritic changes of the navicular bone function extremely well despite the evidence of osteoarthritis in the roentgenograms. In the past, the navicular has been replaced with a metal device but with very limited improvement. Recently a Silastic navicular described by Swanson has given good results in some patients. The proximal row arthrodesis has been uti-

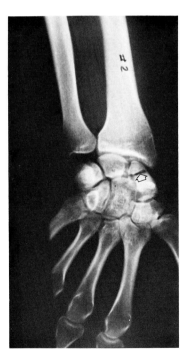

FIG. 7-47 Roentgenogram revealing fracture of the navicular bone (arrow), which can result in osteoarthritis.

lized in some patients, but in general it is not advised because of the loss of function and often increasing involvement in the distal row. Simple excision of the involved bone has not given satisfactory results. In those patients with severe involvement of multiple joints in the wrist, arthrodesis can provide a painless, strong wrist joint.

Navicular Implant Arthroplasty

The indication for a navicular implant in osteoarthritis would be for relief of pain localized to the navicular articular surfaces.

Operative Technique. The surgical approach, as described by Swanson, may be either from the volar or the dorsal lateral surface, and care should be exercised to preserve all the branches of the radial nerve and artery. The preferred incision runs along the anatomic snuffbox, and the joint is approached between the tendons of the extensor pollicis longus and extensor carpi radialis longus. The capsule should be preserved for use in the closure, and careful identification of the navicular should be carried out. Roentgenograms or the image intensifier may be of value.

Fragments of the navicular should be carefully removed, and the correct size of the implant should be determined by fitting it into the space. A left and a right implant are available for each wrist, as well as three different sizes. The implant should fit quite easily into the space left by the navicular bone. A hole is drilled into the trapezium to accept the stem of the Silastic implant. The hole should be drilled at an angle so that the implant will be anatomically oriented. If a satisfactory fit has been obtained, the capsule is repaired with nonabsorbable sutures to provide stability postoperatively. The wrist is placed in a large bulky dressing, and a volar splint is used for approximately one week. Following this, a short-arm cast is applied for 4 to 6 weeks at which time full motion can be resumed.

Lunate Implant Arthroplasty

The lunate implant is recommended for patients with osteoarthritis or traumatic arthritis involving the articulations of the lunate.

Operative Technique. A dorsal approach to the lunate is used. The incision is curved longitudinally over the dorsum. A volar approach is recommended when the lunate is dislocated. The wrist capsule is incised transversely between the third and fourth dorsal compartments and should be preserved for closure. The exposure is carried out between the tendons of the extensor pollicis longus and the extensor digitorum communis. Positive identification of lunate bone should be made by roentgenogram or the image intensifier, if necessary. The lunate should be removed, leaving no pieces behind.

Four implant sizes are available, and the proper size is selected by trial and error. The one selected should be approximately the same size as the lunate bone that has been excised. A small drill or curette is used to make a hole in the triquetrum to accept the stem of the implant. The capsule that has been preserved is carefully closed over the top of the implant to maintain its position. Postoperatively a bulky pressure dressing is used for one week, and then a short-arm cast for 4 to 6 weeks. After 6 to 12 weeks, full activity is possible again.

Carpal-Metacarpal Arthritis

Failure to recognize that the first carpometacarpal joint is damaged by osteoarthritis often leads to erroneous diagnosis (Fig. 7-48). Osteoarthritis of the carpometacarpal joint (trapeziometacarpal) is probably second only in fre-

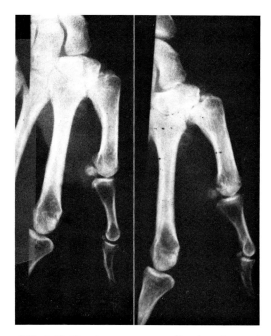

FIG. 7-48 Roentgenogram revealing far advanced osteoarthritis at the base of the thumb and the trapezium.

quency to Heberden's nodes, which are osteophytes at the distal interphalangeal joints associated with osteoarthritis of the hands. The clinical picture of osteoarthritis of the carpometacarpal joint is quite distinctive. A definite tenderness on palpation of the joint is associated with stiffness and pain. The pain at times can be extremely severe and incapacitating and can be confused with de Quervain's disease and less frequently with a flexor tenosynovitis. Crepitation is noted when the metacarpal is rotated against the trapezium, and swelling over the joint may be mistaken for a ganglion. This swelling is due mainly to para-articular spurs, subluxation of the metacarpal base, and synovial proliferation and effusion (Fig. 7-49). Subluxation of the metacarpal proximally and radially results in a squared appearance of the hand (Fig. 7-49B). Atrophy of the thenar muscles occurs because of subluxation and disuse due to pain.

The disease, unless of traumatic origin, is typically bilateral, both clinically and roentgenographically. The disease is much more common in women than in men, approximately 10 to 1. Frequently other members of the patient's family have osteoarthritis of the hands, and there is a tendency for the disease to be prevalent in families.

The roentgenograms generally confirm the diagnosis in the advanced case, and in early disease, a special view may be of value. The patient's forearm is placed flat on the table and fully rotated internally with the dorsal surface of the carpal-metacarpal joint against the roentgenogram film. The distance from the target to film is 30 inches, and the central ray is directed 10° cephalad from the vertical. The roentgenographic features in the carpal-metacarpal osteoarthritis include narrowing of the joint space, osteophyte formation, subchondral sclerosis, para-articular ossicles, radial subluxation of the metacarpal bone, and occasionally juxtaarticular erosions and cysts. This disease can be associated with involvement of other joints in the wrist.

Osteoarthritis of the base of the thumb can result in an adduction contracture of the first metacarpal joint and associated collapse of the thumb into a swan-neck deformity. As the adduction deformity increases, hyperextension of the metacarpal-phalangeal joint of the thumb develops (Fig. 7-50).

Conservative Treatment

Patients with mild symptomatic complaints related to osteoarthritis of the first carpal-metacarpal joint can be treated with aspirin or indomethacin (Indocin) to relieve their symptoms. Injection of the joint also is of value, but generally is transient in benefit. For patients with advanced symptomatic osteoarthritis, surgical intervention may be the procedure of choice.

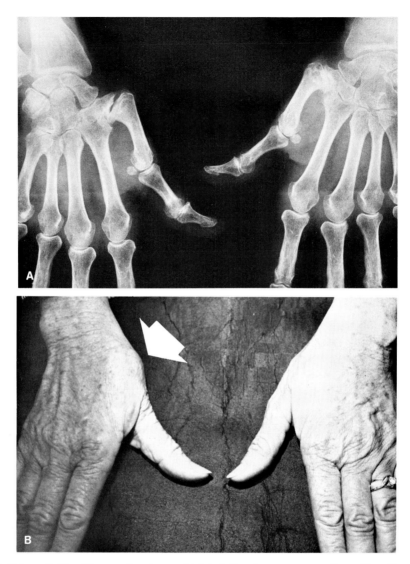

FIG. 7-49 Osteoarthritis of the carpal-metacarpal joint. A. Roentgenogram revealing subluxation of the base of the thumb and erosion of the adjacent joint surfaces. B. Photograph of subluxation (arrow). Note squared appearance of the hand.

Excisional Arthroplasty

Excision of the trapezium can result in excellent mobility with relief of symptoms in a high percentage of the cases. It is important to evaluate the status of the metacarpal-phalangeal joint prior to considering excisional arthroplasty (Fig. 7-51). If the metacarpal-phalangeal joint is normal or has a good range of motion without a hyperexten-sion deformity (Fig. 7-51B), a good result can be expected with excisional arthroplasty (Fig. 7-51C).

Operative Technique. A dorsal lateral incision is made adjacent to the abductor pollicis longus tendon over the carpal-metacarpal joint. The sensory branch of the radial nerve must be protected in this approach (Fig. 7-52). The capsule of the joint is opened and preserved by sharp

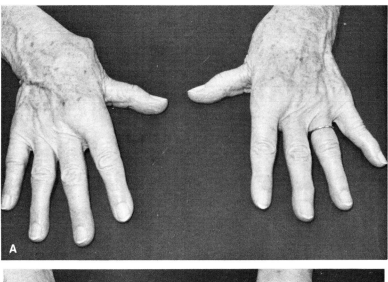

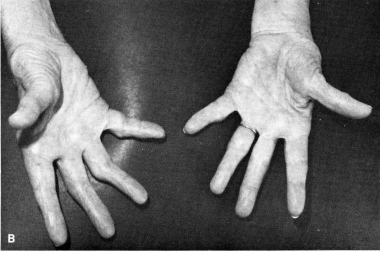

FIG. 7-50 Adduction deformities of the thumb from carpal-metacarpal arthritis. A. Dorsal view of the patient's hands showing fixed hyperextension deformity of the metacarpal-phalangeal joints. B. Volar view of the hand showing the adduction deformity of the thumb with hyperextension at the metacarpal-phalangeal joint.

dissection exposing the trapezium (Fig. 7-53). In the proximal portion of the incision, the dorsal branch of the radial artery should be protected. The trapezium may be removed in pieces by using a rongeur or can be dissected out intact, but the latter is more difficult (Fig. 7-54). All of the fragments of the bone should be removed, and it is important to realize that the trapezium is a large bone that extends a good distance toward the trap-

ezoid. After removal of the trapezium, the defect can be filled with Gelfoam strips or a portion of tendinous graft. The tourniquet is released prior to closure for hemostasis, and the capsule is repaired with 4-0 white silk sutures. The thumb is dressed in a bulky dressing and is maintained in abduction and opposition for approximately 4 weeks.

Results. Long-term results continue to remain excellent. Shortening of the

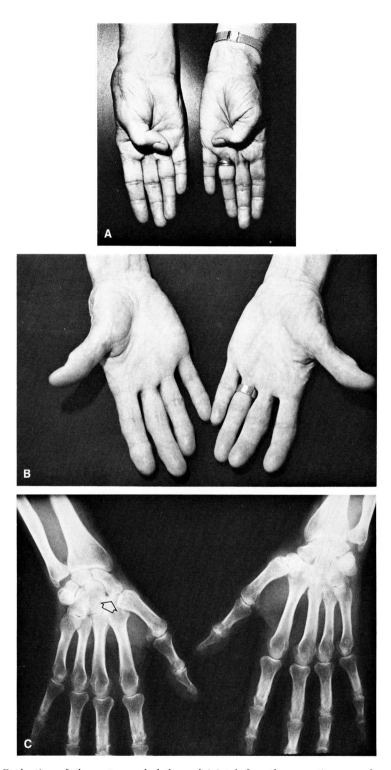

FIG. 7-51 Evaluation of the metacarpal-phalangeal joint before the operative procedure for carpal-metacarpal arthritis. A. Photograph showing hands after replacement of the right trapezium with a Silastic prosthesis. The function of the metacarpal-phalangeal joint is almost normal. This motion prevents subluxation of the prosthesis when there is limited motion of the metacarpal-phalangeal joint. B. Photograph showing hyperextension deformity of the right thumb and beginning adduction of the metacarpal. Surgery would be required on both the metacarpal-phalangeal joint and the carpal-metacarpal joint. C. Roentgenogram of a patient who had an excisional arthroplasty of the right thumb 10 years earlier (arrow). The left wrist shows evidence of carpal-metacarpal arthritis, and the patient has pain.

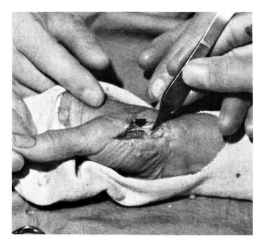

FIG. 7-52 Excisional arthroplasty. Surgical view of a dorsal lateral incision adjacent to the abductor pollicus longus tendon. The sensory branch of the radial nerve must be protected in this approach (arrow).

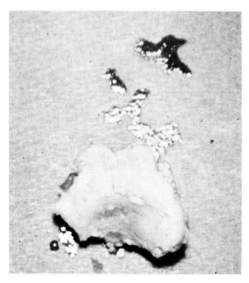

FIG. 7-54 An intact trapezium removed from a patient's wrist. This trapezium reveals loss of the articular cartilage on the concave surface adjacent to the base of the metacarpal.

thumb has not been a problem (Fig. 7-55).

Carpal-Metacarpal Implant Arthroplasty

The Silastic replacement arthroplasty for the trapezium has been developed by Swanson. Five anatomic sizes currently are available for replacement (Fig. 7-56).

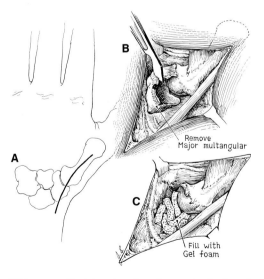

FIG. 7-53 Excisional arthroplasty. A. A dorsal lateral incision over the carpal-metacarpal joint. B. Excision of the trapezium from the joint. C. The defect filled with Gelfoam.

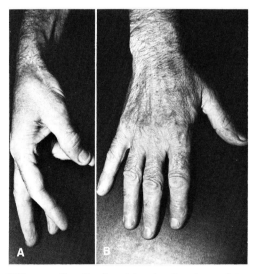

FIG. 7-55 Results of excisional arthroplasty of the right trapezium 10 years earlier. A Lateral view. Excellent function is present and patient has no difficulty touching the fifth finger. B. Dorsal view. The thumb appears normal. See Fig. 7-51C for roentgenogram of this patient.

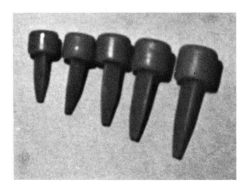

FIG. 7-56 Five sizes of Silastic prostheses for replacement of the trapezium.

Operative Technique. The operative procedure is carried out under tourniquet control. A small straight incision is centered over the trapezium parallel to the extensor pollicis brevis muscle. Branches of the superficial radial nerve should be protected and retracted upward out of the way. The base of the first metacarpal and the carpal-metacarpal joint are carefully identified. The capsule is incised longitudinally and carefully reflected upward. Its attachment to the base of the metacarpal is preserved, as it will be needed to obtain a strong closure. The branch of the radial artery should be carefully retracted proximally off the trapezium. Resection should be carried around the palmar surface of the trapezium to remove all of its attachments. The entire trapezium should be removed with a rongeur (Fig. 7-57). The tendon of the flexor carpal radialis will become visible on the volar surface of the trapezium. The base of the metacarpal is squared off with a rongeur, and a hole is made in the base of the metacarpal with a power tool or a curette.

The trial implant is inserted to determine the size that fits easily into the space left by the resection of the trapezium. The base of the implant should fit properly on the navicular bone. After the proper size has been selected, the permanent implant is carefully inserted

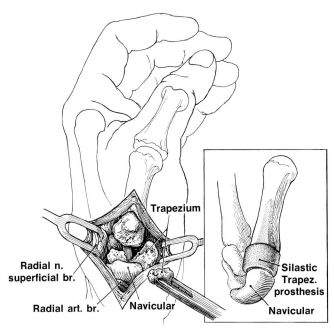

FIG. 7-57 Carpal-metacarpal implant arthroplasty. Excision of trapezium from joint. Note retraction of superficial radial nerve and the radial artery. Inset: Insertion of Silastic prosthesis into medullary canal at base of metacarpal.

into the base of the metacarpal with the collar of the implant against the base of the bone to prevent wobbling (Fig. 7-58).

The capsule should be carefully re-sutured over the base of the thumb and the prosthesis to prevent the prosthesis from subluxating. If the capsule is loose, it should be imbricated; if it is thin, a portion of the flexor carpal radialis or the abductor pollicis longus can be used to reinforce the capsule. There is a tendency, however, for the prosthesis to sublux, but even if subluxation does occur, a good result can be expected post-operatively (Fig. 7-59).

If there is an adduction contracture between the first and second meta-carpals, the origin of the adductor pollicis muscle may be released from the third metacarpal or its tendon may be stripped from the first metacarpal. Hyperextension deformity of the carpophalangeal joint often contributes to the adduction tendency of the metacarpal and causes subluxation of the implant. If the metacarpal-phalangeal joint hyper-extends less than 10°, usually no treatment is necessary. If the metacarpal-phalangeal joint hyperextends from

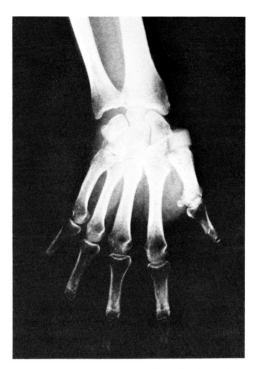

FIG. 7-59 Roentgenogram of patient's wrist 3 years after implant arthroplasty. The Silastic prosthesis is subluxating away from the navicular, but the patient had no complaints.

10° to 20°, a Kirschner wire is placed obliquely across the joint to hold it in 10° of flexion. The wire is removed approximately 4 weeks after operation. If hyperextension is greater than 20°, arthrodesis of the metacarpal joint is indicated (Fig. 7-60). In patients with normal flexion of the metacarpal-phalangeal joint, a capsulotomy is the operation of choice to save the available flexion. If the metacarpal-phalangeal joint has to be fused, it should be placed in 10° of flexion and slight pronation. (See thumb fusions in Chapter 8.)

Postoperatively the hand is placed in a bulky dressing, and the thumb is abducted approximately 40° to 60°. After 3 or 4 days, a navicular-type forearm cast is applied to hold the metacarpal in abduction, but leave the phalanx free. The cast is used from 4 to 6 weeks to allow the capsule to heal. Satisfactory

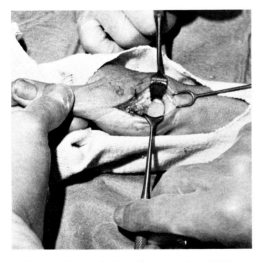

FIG. 7-58 Surgical view after insertion of Silastic implant into base of metacarpal. A good fit has been obtained.

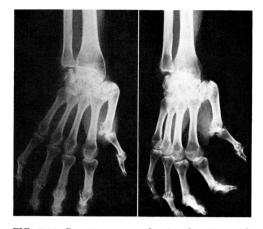

FIG. 7-60 Roentgenogram of wrist of patient with advanced osteoarthritis of the carpal-metacarpal joint with a hyperextension deformity of the metacarpal-phalangeal joint secondary to adduction of the metacarpal.

results have been obtained with this type of arthroplasty.

Arthrodesis

The patient with carpal-metacarpal arthritis can also be aided by arthrodesis. The loss of the carpal-metacarpal joint by fusion still allows a good deal of prehension in the thumb. The thumb, however, will not usually lie in the plane of the palm of the hand because it should be arthrodesed in some abduction. Motion will be gained in the trapezionavicular joint and will compensate somewhat for the loss of motion at the

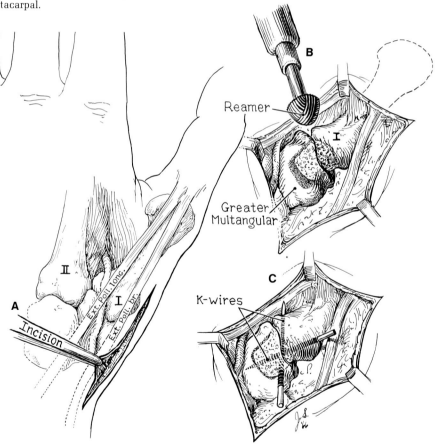

FIG. 7-61 Arthrodesis of the carpal-metacarpal joint for relief of pain due to osteoarthritis. A. The dorsal-lateral incision over the carpal-metacarpal joint parallel to the extensor pollicis brevis. B. Shaping the base of the metacarpal into a rounded ball and the trapezium into a rounded cup. C. Crossed Kirschner wires for fixation of the thumb. (From Marmor, L., and Peter, J. B.: Osteoarthritis of the carpal-metacarpal joint of the thumb. Am. J. Surg., *117*:623, 1969.)

carpal-metacarpal joint. However, the length and strength of the thumb is maintained.

Operative Technique. Arthrodesis of the thumb can be performed successfully with a minimum of effort (Fig. 7-61). An incision is made over the carpal-metacarpal joint on the dorsal lateral surface parallel to the adductor pollicis longus tendon. The radial nerve should be carefully protected in the dorsal flap of the incision, and the capsule of the joint is opened. The dorsal branch of the radial artery should be avoided in the proximal aspect of the incision over the trapezium. The base of the metacarpal is dissected free, and any areas of sclerotic bone, especially from the medial aspect near the trapezoid, are removed with a rongeur. The base of the metacarpal is shaped with a rongeur, and the cartilage and cortex are removed in the form of a ball. A variety of small finger reamers can be used with a power tool to ream the base of the metacarpal into a rounded ball on its surface, and a matching male reamer can be drilled into the trapezoid so that the metacarpal ball will fit into the rounded cup in the trapezoid. The two are fitted together for a good contact, and a single Kirschner wire or crossed Kirschner wires can be drilled across the joint to fix the thumb in abduction and some pronation. The tourniquet should be released at this stage and hemostasis secured.

The wound is closed in layers, and a plaster of paris cast is applied from the distal phalanx to the forearm with the thumb in abduction, pronation, and opposition for approximately 6 weeks. It is important not to immobilize the metacarpophalangeal joint in hyperextension, but it should be fixed in some flexion to prevent subsequent stiffness (Fig. 7-62).

Trapezionavicular Arthritis

Although carpal-metacarpal arthritis is much more common, arthritis can

develop between the navicular and the trapezium as isolated disease. The symptoms generally are the same as those for carpal-metacarpal arthritis. The patient will complain of pain on use of the thumb and swelling in the region of the anatomic snuffbox. Generally crepitation is not present, and the grinding test is also negative. Neither swelling at the base of the thumb nor the square appearance of the hand is noted. The disease may be bilateral or unilateral and can also be associated with carpal-metacarpal arthritis (Fig. 7-63).

Treatment

The patient with moderate symptoms due to osteoarthritis involving the trapezionavicular joint can be treated with salicylates or local injection of the joint. If symptoms are severe, excision of the

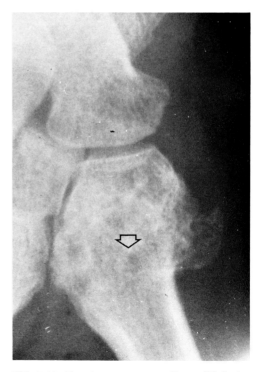

FIG. 7-62 Roentgenogram revealing solid fusion of the base of the metacarpal (arrow) into the trapezium.

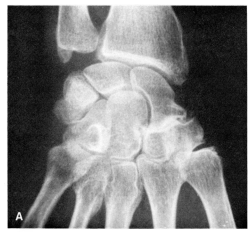

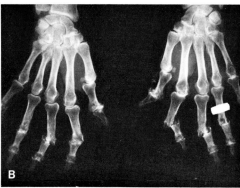

FIG. 7-63 Roentgenograms of wrists of patients with trapezionavicular arthritis. A. Unilateral involvement. B. Bilateral involvement with erosion of the proximal interphalangeal joints.

trapezium can be carried out with or without Silastic replacements.

Operative Technique. The operative technique for trapezionavicular arthritis consists of excision of the trapezium. The various procedures described under carpal-metacarpal arthritis can be utilized in this condition. Arthrodesis of the trapezium to the navicular is not advised for this condition.

Bibliography

Rheumatoid Arthritis

Abbott, L. C., Saunders, J. B., and Bost, F. C.: Arthrodesis of the wrist. J. Bone Joint Surg., 24:883, 1942.

Albright, J. A., and Chase, R. A.: Palmar-shelf arthroplasty of the wrist in rheumatoid arthritis. J. Bone Joint Surg., 52-A:896, 1970.

Bäckdahl, M.: The caput ulnae syndrome in rheumatoid arthritis. A study of the morphology, abnormal anatomy, and clinical picture. Acta Rheum. Scand., Suppl. 5, 1963.

Campbell, R. D., and Straub, L. R.: Surgical considerations for rheumatoid disease in the forearm and wrist. Am. J. Surg., 109:361, 1965.

Carroll, R. E., and Dick, H. M.: Arthrodesis of the wrist in rheumatoid arthritis. J. Bone Joint Surg., 53-A:1365, 1971.

Clayton, M. L.: Surgical treatment at the wrist in rheumatoid arthritis. J. Bone Joint Surg., 47-A:741, 1965.

Cracchiolo, A., III, and Marmor, L.: Resection of distal ulna in rheumatoid arthritis. Arthritis Rheum., 12:415, 1969.

Curtis, R. M., and Eversmann, W. W., Jr.: Internal neurolysis as an adjunct to the treatment of the carpal-tunnel syndrome. J. Bone Joint Surg., 55-A:733, 1973.

Darrach, W., and Dwight, K.: Derangements of inferior radio-ulnar articulations. Proc. N.Y. Acad. Med., Med. Rec., 87:708, 1915.

Dupont, C., et al.: Ulnar-tunnel syndrome at the wrist. J. Bone Joint Surg., 47-A:757, 1965.

Ehrlich, G. E., et al.: Pathogenesis of rupture of extensor tendons at the wrist in rheumatoid arthritis. Arthritis Rheum., 2:332, 1959.

Finkelstein, H.: Stenosing tendovaginitis at the radial styloid process. J. Bone Joint Surg., 30:509, 1930.

Flatt, A. E.: The Care of the Rheumatoid Hand. St. Louis, C. V. Mosby Co., 1963.

Freiberg, R. A., and Weinstein, A.: The scallop sign and spontaneous rupture of the extensor tendons in rheumatoid arthritis. Clin. Orthop., 83:128, 1972.

Haddad, R. J., Jr., and Riordan, D. C.: Arthrodesis of the wrist. J. Bone Joint Surg., 49-A:950, 1967.

Hakstian, R. W., and Tubiana, R.: Ulnar deviation of the fingers. J. Bone Joint Surg., 49-A:299, 1967.

Inglis, A. E., Straub, L. R., and Williams, C. S.: Median neuropathy at the wrist. Clin. Orthop., *83*:48, 1972.

Jacobs, J. H., Hess, E. V., and Beswick, I. P.: Rheumatoid arthritis presenting as tenosynovitis. J. Bone Joint Surg., *39-B*:288, 1957.

Kellgren, J. H., and Ball, J.: Tendon lesions in rheumatoid arthritis. Ann. Rheum. Dis., *9*:48, 1950.

Kessler, I., and Vainio, K.: Posterior (dorsal) synovectomy for rheumatoid involvement of the hand and wrist. J. Bone Joint Surg., *48-A*:1085–1094, 1966.

Marmor, L.: Median nerve compression in rheumatoid arthritis. Arch. Surg., *89*:1008, 1964.

Martel, W., Hayes, J. T., and Duff, J. F.: The pattern of bone erosion in the hand and wrist in rheumatoid arthritis. Radiology, *84*:204, 1965.

Mori, M.: Wrist. *In* Surgery of Arthritis, R. A. Milch, editor. Baltimore, The Williams & Wilkins Co., 1964, p. 112.

McCormack, R. M.: Carpal tunnel syndrome. Surg. Clin. North Am., *40*:517, 1960.

Phalen, G. S.: The carpal-tunnel syndrome. Clin. Orthop., *83*:29, 1972.

Rana, N. A., and Taylor, A. R.: Excision of distal end of the ulna in rheumatoid arthritis. J. Bone Joint Surg., *55-B*:96-105, 1973.

Ranawat, C. S., et al.: Arthrography in the rheumatoid wrist joint. J. Bone Joint Surg., *51-A*:1269, 1969.

Singer, M.: The carpal tunnel syndrome. S. Afr. Med. J., *33*:415, 1959.

Smith-Peterson, M. N., et al.: Useful surgical procedures for rheumatoid arthritis involving joints of the upper extremity. Arch. Surg., *46*:764, 1943.

Sperling, I. L.: Rheumatoid polytendovaginitis. Ann. Rheum. Dis., *9*:43, 1950.

Straub, L. R., and Chitranjan, S. R.: The wrist in rheumatoid arthritis. J. Bone Joint Surg., *51-A*:1-20, 1969.

Straub, L. R., and Ranawat, C. S.: The wrist in rheumatoid arthritis, surgical treatment and results. J. Bone Joint Surg., *51-A*:1, 1969.

Straub, L. R., and Wilson, E. H.: Spontaneous rupture of extensor tendons in the hand associated with rheumatoid arthritis. J. Bone Joint Surg., *38-A*:1208, 1956.

Vainio, K.: Carpal canal syndrome caused by tenosynovitis. Acta Rheum. Scand., *4*:22, 1957.

Vaughan-Jackson, O. J.: Attrition ruptures of tendons as a factor in the production of deformities in the rheumatoid hand. Proc. R. Soc. Med., *52*:132, 1959.

Vaughan-Jackson, O. J.: Rupture of extensor tendons by attrition at the inferior radio-ulnar joint. J. Bone Joint Surg., *30-B*:528, 1948.

Wickstrom, J. K.: Arthrodesis of the wrist. J. Bone Joint Surg., *36-A*:430, 1954.

Osteoarthritis

Aune, S.: Osteoarthritis in the first carpal-metacarpal joint. Acta. Chir. Scand., *190*:449, 1955.

Gervis, W. R.: Excision of the trapezium for osteoarthritis of the trapezio-metacarpal joint. J. Bone Joint Surg., *31-B*:537, 1949.

Goldner, J. L., and Clippinger, F. W.: Excision of greater multangular bone as an adjunct to mobilization of the thumb. J. Bone Joint Surg., *32-A*:267, 1950.

Lassere, C., Paveat, D., and Derennes, R.: Osteoarthritis of the trapezio–metacarpal joint. J. Bone Joint Surg., *31-B*:534, 1949.

Leach, R. E., and Bolten, P. E.: Arthritis of the carpal-metacarpal joint of the thumb. J. Bone Joint Surg., *50-A*:1171, 1968.

Marmor, L., and Peter, J.: Osteoarthritis of the carpal-metacarpal joint of the thumb. Am. J. Surg., *117*:623, 1969.

Michelle, A., Skinner, M. D., and Kreuger, F. T.: Repair and stabilization of the first carpo-metacarpal joint. Am. J. Surg., *79*:348, 1930.

Muller, G. M.: Arthrodesis of the trapezio-metacarpal joint for osteoarthritis. J. Bone Joint Surg., *31-B*:540-542, 1949.

Murley, A. M. G.: Excision of the trapezium in osteoarthritis of the first carpo-metacarpal joint. J. Bone Joint Surg., *42-B*:502, 1960.

Patterson, R.: Carpo-metacarpal arthroplasty of the thumb. J. Bone Joint Surg., *13*:240, 1933.

Peter, J., and Marmor, L.: Osteoarthritis of the first carpal-metacarpal joint. Calif. Med., *109*:116, 1968.

Peterson, H. A., and Lipscomb, P. R.: Intercarpal arthrodesis. Arch. Surg., *95*:127, 1967.

Steindler, A.: Arthritic deformities of the wrist and fingers. J. Bone Joint Surg., *33-A*:849, 1951.

Swanson, A. B.: Arthroplasty in traumatic arthritis of the joints of the hand. Orthop. Clin. North Am., *1*:285, 1970.

Swanson, A. B.: Silicone rubber implants for the replacement of the carpal-scaphoid and lunate bones. Orthop. Clin. North Am., *1*:299, 1970.

8 | The Hand

Arthritis in the hand produces not only pain but also a variety of patterns of severe deformity, depending upon which specific components of the complex mechanism of the hand are involved (Fig. 8-1). Since the deformities are frequently bilateral, there can be a severe loss of function that will prevent the patient from being self-sufficient in his activities of daily living.

The most urgent problem today in the management of the arthritic hand is the education of all concerned with the care of the patient as to the need for early treatment before severe damage has occurred. Early diagnosis of the congenital hip by the medical profession and early surgical treatment have improved the results tremendously. This has been due to the education of the obstetrician, pediatrician, and lay personnel by the orthopaedic surgeon. This same policy should be applied to arthritis in the hand with education of the general practitioner, internist, and rheumatologist in the value of orthopaedic surgery as an adjunct to medical treatment of arthritis deformities of the hand.

At one time a great deal of interest centered upon the use of physical therapy and various splints in the treatment of arthritis of the hand. Several studies using dynamic and rigid splinting to prevent and also to try to correct rheumatoid deformities of the hand were carried out at various centers. It became apparent that splints were not the answer, although splinting may play some role in the preoperative and postoperative care of a patient. When splints are used without any surgical procedures, deformities usually tend to increase because of the destructive process continuing within the joint.

Prior to the 1960's, little had been done to surgically correct these deformities that were one of the major problems of the patient with arthritis in the hands. Much of the previous apathy toward the surgical correction of these deformities was based upon the reluctance of surgeons to operate on hands because of lack of training and experience and because of the fear of interfering with the function that remained. Hand surgery is a specialized area of surgery that requires training in both orthopaedic surgery and plastic procedures. As Brand has so ably stated, "nothing but harm can come of attempts to operate on deformed hands by doctors who lack this training."

171

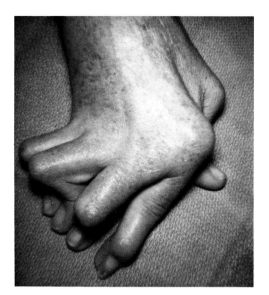

FIG. 8-1 Signs of rheumatoid arthritis in the hand. The patient has severe ulnar drift, boutonnière deformities of the third, fourth, and fifth fingers, and a swan-neck deformity of the index finger. The hand is useless for the activities of daily living.

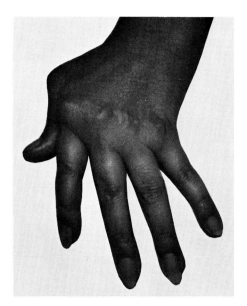

FIG. 8-2 Hand on which a synovectomy was carried out six months earlier, despite the fact that there were dislocations of the metacarpal-phalangeal joints. Recurrence was noted immediately after the original dressing was removed. Patients who have subluxation or dislocation of the metacarpal-phalangeal joints should not have a synovectomy alone.

The surgical care of the hand received great impetus from the experience gained in treating war injuries in World War II. Surgeons with wartime experience began to apply the techniques they had learned to the correction of arthritic deformities of the hand.

Some rheumatologists still rarely consider surgery because of the fear of making the patient worse and because of the failure of earlier surgical attempts (Fig. 8-2). However, as surgeons have gained further experience in correcting arthritic deformities of the hand, the selection of the operation for the particular patient has become much clearer, and the results therefore have improved considerably. It has become apparent that surgery can be divided into prophylactic and reconstructive procedures. In some patients deformities can be prevented; in others patients the deformity can actually be corrected. Either procedure will improve function, despite the stage of the disease.

Anatomy

It is important for the surgeon to have a sound and clear picture of the anatomy of the hand because of the distortion of the normal structures by the rheumatoid disease. The dorsum of the hand is involved more often by rheumatoid disease which disturbs the extensor mechanism. The extensor tendons, which pass across the wrist through fibrous tunnels formed by the dorsal carpal ligament, have a number of oblique and transverse fibers that connect the common extensors (Fig. 8-3). The common extensor tendon enters the extensor hood and passes distally as the central slip to insert at the base of the middle phalanx. The central slip of the common ex-

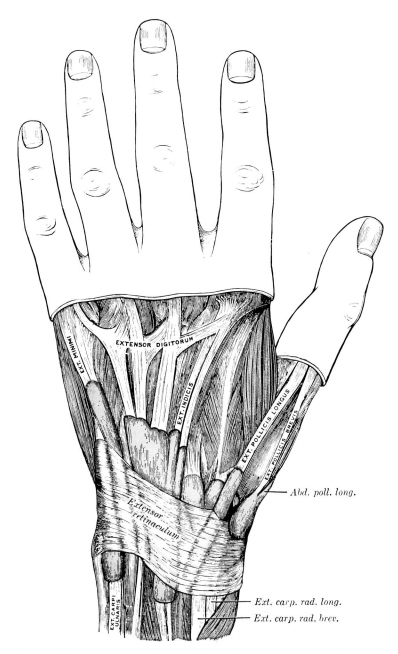

FIG. 8-3 Dorsal view of the wrist showing the synovial tunnels in the dorsal carpal ligament through which the extensor tendons pass. Numerous transverse fibers connect the extensor tendons. (From Gray's Anatomy of the Human Body, 29th ed. C. M. Goss, editor. Philadelphia, Lea & Febiger, 1973.)

tensor tendon is an integral part of the extensor hood covering the metacarpal-phalangeal joint and anchoring the central tendon over the joint by the transverse fibers of the hood. The lateral edges (or lateral bands) of the hood are joined by the tendons of the lumbricals and interossei muscles which insert distally in the dorsal aspect of the base of the distal phalanx (Fig. 8-4). The hood is

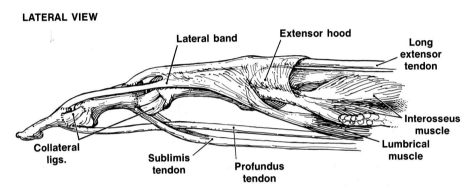

DORSAL VIEW

Triangular lig.

Lateral bands

Extensor hood

Interosseus muscle

Long extensor tendon

Interosseus muscle

Slips of Long. ext. to Lat. band

Interosseus slip to Lat. band

LATERAL VIEW

Lateral band

Extensor hood

Long extensor tendon

Interosseus muscle

Lumbrical muscle

Collateral ligs.

Sublimis tendon

Profundus tendon

FIG. 8-4 Extensor hood. The dorsal view reveals the long extensor tendon inserting on the base of the middle phalanx. The lateral view reveals the thickening of the fibrous slip to from the lateral band which inserts on the base of the distal phalanx. Note also that the lateral bands pass above the axis of the proximal interphalangeal joint.

also composed of a group of oblique fibers which run from the lateral bands to the central slip on each side of the proximal phalanx and which play a role in intrinsic contracture deformity of the finger.

Interossei Muscles

Seven interossei muscles, three volar and four dorsal, arise from the metacarpals. The three volar interossei are inserted into the base of the phalanx and extensor hood of the index (ulnar side), ring (radial), and fifth (radial) fingers (Fig. 8-5). Occasionally a slip of tendon passes to the capsule or directly into the bone. The volar interossei have three functions: (1) flexion of the metacarpalphalangeal joint, (2) extension of the

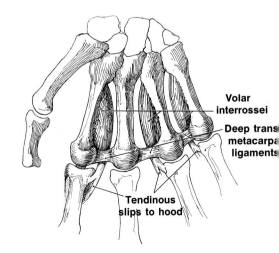

Volar interossei

Deep trans metacarpa ligaments

Tendinous slips to hood

FIG. 8-5 The three volar interossei muscles that arise from the metacarpal shafts of the second, fourth, and fifth metacarpals.

terminal phalanges, and (3) adduction of the fingers toward the third (long) finger. The first volar interosseous muscle, because of its ulnar attachment to the hood, will tend to maintain an ulnar drift deformity.

The four dorsal interossei arise from the dorsal surface of the metacarpals and insert into the base of the phalanx and into the extensor hood (Fig. 8-6). The first dorsal interosseus inserts into the radial side of the index finger and is important in pinching. The second dorsal inserts into the radial side of the third finger. The third and fourth dorsal interossei insert into the ulnar side of the third (long) and of the ring finger contributing to the ulnar drift deformity. The functions of the dorsal interossei are to (1) flex the metacarpal-phalangeal joints, (2) extend the distal phalanges, and (3) abduct the fingers away from the center of the third (long) finger.

Lumbrical Muscles

Four lumbrical muscles arise from the radial side of the flexor digitorum

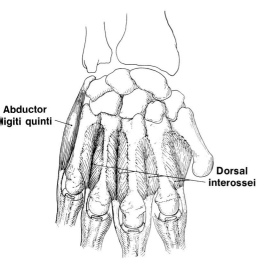

FIG. 8-6 The four dorsal interossei muscles that arise from the dorsal surface of the metacarpal shafts.

profundus tendons (Fig. 8-7). They attach with the interossei tendons to the extensor hood. The functions of the lumbrical muscle appear to be to initiate flexion of the metacarpal-phalangeal joint and to extend the distal phalanges.

The thumb and flexor tendons will be discussed under their appropriate subdivision.

Flexor Tendons

The flexor tendons at the wrist pass through the carpal tunnel and are surrounded by a synovial tendon sheath. The tendons are not covered by a tendon sheath in the palm but develop a separate tendon sheath distal to the palmar crease and extending out into the fingers (Fig. 7-36).

The flexor tendons pass into a thick osseofibrous tunnel and continue into the fingers. These tunnels are formed by the volar surface of the phalanges and by a thick fibrous band that passes over the flexor tendons from the lateral side of the phalanges. At the proximal end of the tunnel over the proximal phalanx, the fibers of the tunnel run transversely and form a strong band called the annular or digital vaginal ligament.

A synovial sheath encloses the flexor tendon within the finger and can become involved in rheumatoid disease. The flexor digitorum sublimis tendon opposite the base of the proximal phalanx, divides into two slips to allow passage of the flexor digitorum profundus tendon (Fig. 8-7). The two slips of the sublimis reunite distally to form a grooved channel for the passage of the profundus tendon. The sublimis tendon finally divides again and inserts into the middle phalanx.

Finger Joints

The metacarpal-phalangeal joint is essentially a ball-and-socket joint which

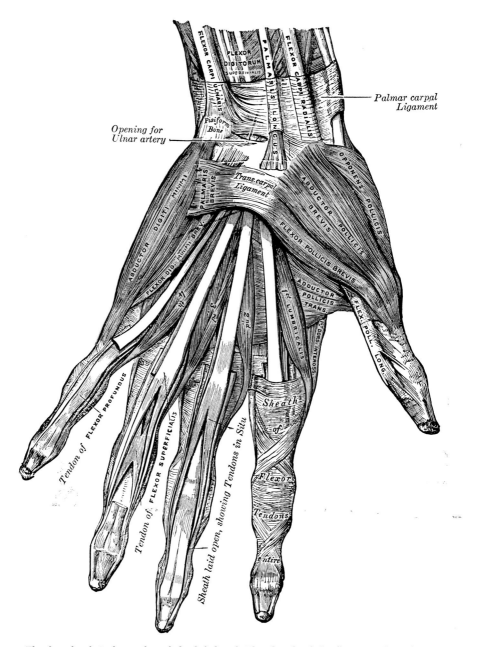

FIG. 8-7 The four lumbrical muscles of the left hand. The sheath of the flexor tendons forms a strong fibrous tunnel within which the sublimis tendon bifurcates. (From Gray's Anatomy of the Human Body, 29th ed. C. M. Goss, editor. Philadelphia, Lea & Febiger, 1973.)

tends to permit motion in several directions. The heads of the metacarpals are narrower on the dorsum than they are on the palmar side to allow for lateral movement of the finger when in full extension because of relaxation of the collateral ligaments. The support to the joint is provided from the collateral ligament located on each side and from the extensor tendon and the thick volar plate which represents the palmar portion of the capsule. The opposing surfaces of the metacarpal head and the base of the proximal phalanx are covered with hyaline cartilage. The joint is lined with a synovial membrane which attaches to the margins of the articular cartilage but is also reflected proximally along the metacarpal neck to form several synovial pouches. The synovial reflection is greatest on the dorsal surface and to a much lesser extent on the ulnar and radial surfaces beneath the collateral ligaments. The volar plate has a cartilaginous deep surface so that only the most proximal part of the volar pouch is formed by a double layer of synovium.

The collateral ligament on each side of the metacarpal-phalangeal joint is extremely important in maintaining the structure of the joint (Fig. 8-8). The two major portions of this collateral ligament are (1) the straplike metacarpal-phalangeal portion that runs from the metacarpal head to the phalanx and (2) the fan-shaped metacarpal-glenoid portion which passes from the metacarpal head to the volar plate.

The metacarpal-glenoid segment of the collateral ligament is known also as the accessory collateral ligament. It acts as a sling for the volar plate, supporting it to the metacarpal. The volar plate is strongly attached to the proximal

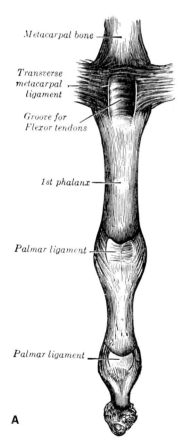
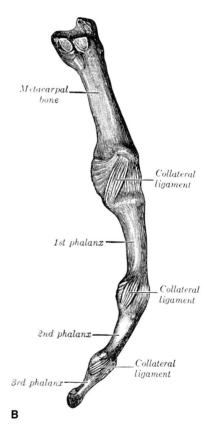

FIG. 8-8 Metacarpal-phalangeal articulation of the finger. A. The volar aspect reveals the thickened volar plate of the joint capsule. B. The ulnar aspect reveals the fan-shaped metacarpal glenoid portion and the strap-like metacarpal-phalangeal portion of the collateral ligament. (From Gray's Anatomy of the Human Body, 29th ed. C. M. Goss, editor. Philadelphia, Lea & Febiger, 1973.)

phalanx distally but has a thin proximal attachment to the metacarpal, and it is reinforced by the metacarpal-glenoid portion of the collateral ligament. The volar plate is continuous on either side of the metacarpal with the adjacent intercapitular ligaments. Proximally at the same point the glenoid fan or accessory collateral ligament inserts into the volar plate along with the proximal flexor retinaculum which controls the position of the long flexor tendons and the transverse fibers of the extensor hood which help to maintain the position of the extensor tendon over the metacarpal head.

The proximal interphalangeal joint, because of its anatomic arrangement, acts in a manner similar to the knee joint. It is primarily a hinge joint maintained by the collateral ligaments, which are extremely thick and broad and maintain its stability. The head of the proximal phalanx actually has two condyles that articulate with the base of the middle phalanx. A synovial lining extends around the periphery of the joint and forms a small pouch that protrudes upward over the superior aspect of the proximal phalanx for a short distance. The central slip of the extensor tendon lies outside of the capsule of the joint and inserts into the base of the middle phalanx on its superior aspect. The proximal interphalangeal joint receives additional stability from the flexor and extensor tendon arrangements that pass the joint.

The distal interphalangeal joint is quite similar in action to the proximal interphalangeal joint and contains a synovial lining. Stability is provided by the collateral ligaments and the insertion of the flexor profundus tendon into the base of the distal phalanx and the extensor tendon into the dorsal aspect of the base of the distal phalanx.

The metacarpal-carpal joint of the thumb anatomically is a saddle-shaped joint which allows a wide range of movement to take place in two axes at right angles to each other. The thumb can be abducted and adducted in the plane of the palm, and it also can be flexed and extended through a plane at right angles to the palm itself. A combination of these motions can produce circumduction simulating a universal joint. For normal function of the hand the first metacarpal must be able to abduct away from the second metacarpal so that a large object can be grasped between the opposed thumb and the fingers. Contracture of the web space between the first and second metacarpals can seriously interfere with the function of the hand. The metacarpalphalangeal joint and the interphalangeal joint of the thumb are similar in their function to the proximal interphalangeal joint of the finger. Stability of the thumb is extremely important in providing a strong pinch as well as normal function of the thumb.

Function

The movements of a person's hands are directed toward serving his social and economic needs. These movements are compound and involve all of the joints and muscles of the hands. Four basic types of grasping function have been described by Brewerton. These consist of precision grasping of small objects, strong grasp of small objects, grasping of objects with handles, and strong grasping of large objects.

The most basic use of the hand consists of applying the tip of the thumb in contact with the tip of a finger to produce prehension. The ability to oppose the thumb to the fingers is extremely important in the function of the hand and supposedly is the reason that man has developed such a high level of intelligence as compared to the ape which does not have prehension. Loss of the thumb usually results in a 50 percent loss in the function of the hand.

The three basic patterns that can be recognized in prehension are (1) tip, (2) lateral, and (3) palmar. Studies carried out by Keller have shown that palmar prehension is utilized the most. This type of pinch uses the thumb opposed to the palmar surface of the second and third fingers.

The versatility of the hand is based upon the mobility of its skeleton. The arrangement of the bones of the hand contribute greatly to its use. The thumb is extremely mobile on the radial border of the hand, and the fourth and fifth fingers and metacarpals are extremely mobile on the ulnar border. The second and third metacarpals are fixed rigidly to the carpal bones, acting as a central pillar for stability of the hand. Flatt contrasts the skeleton of the hand to the mast of a cargo ship and states, "from the mast are slung two mobile borders, the thumb being on the radial side and the ring and little fingers on the ulnar side. The thumb is connected to the mast by intrinsic muscles, and the ulnar fingers by the transverse capitular ligaments." The radial half of the hand generally provides precision in the use of the hand, whereas the ulnar portion provides power and stability in grasp. These patterns of motion are dependent upon the normal function of the skeletal arches of the hand. Rheumatoid disease in general affects the function of the hand by disturbing the normal joints and the intrinsic and extrinsic muscles of the hand (Fig. 8-9).

Physical Examination

The hand of a patient is often a mirror of the patient in miniature. The disease and

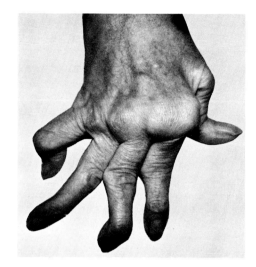

FIG. 8-9 Deformed hand as a result of dislocation of the metacarpal-phalangeal joints and destruction of the intrinsic and extrinsic muscles.

the occupation are often clearly written upon it if the examiner will only look carefully.

Inspection

Careful examination by inspection may often confirm the clinical diagnosis of rheumatoid arthritis or osteoarthritis. In examining the hand it is important also to consider the wrist, as it is the key joint in the function of the hand. Inspection should be carried out of both the extensor and volar aspects of the hand. The extensor tendons should be clearly visible under the skin of the back of the hand of the normal patient. Evidence of an extensor tenosynovitis at the wrist often is a valuable sign of early rheumatoid arthritis (Fig. 8-10). One should not confuse this early swelling, which protrudes either proximal or distal to the extensor retinaculum, as a ganglion.

The fingers should be carefully inspected to determine whether there is any ulnar drift. Atrophy of the first dorsal interosseus muscle is frequently seen in early rheumatoid arthritis. Swelling of the fingers has often been

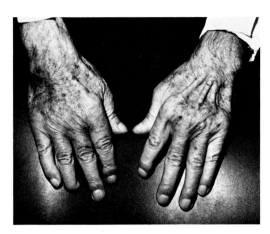

FIG. 8-10 Early rheumatoid arthritis of the hands. Notice the prominence of the extensor tendons on the back of the left hand. Swelling of the right wrist has made the tendons on the back of the right hand almost invisible—an indication of the onset of extensor synovitis. Rheumatoid changes in the metacarpal-phalangeal joints are also beginning.

described as a pathognomic sign of rheumatoid arthritis. The metacarpal-phalangeal joints, which are common sites for rheumatoid disease should be examined for swelling (Fig. 8-11A). The proximal and distal interphalangeal joints may also be involved with swelling in early rheumatoid disease (Fig. 8-11B). Swan-neck deformities, as well as boutonnière deformities, are quite common in advancing rheumatoid disease of the hand. Osteoarthritis is more likely to affect the proximal interphalangeal and distal interphalangeal joints than the metacarpal-phalangeal joints. The carpal-metacarpal joint of the thumb may be deformed and quite obviously enlarged due to osteoarthritis without involvement of the remainder of the hand.

Flexion and extension of the fingers may often demonstrate loss of extension due to rupture of the extensor tendons, without the patient ever realizing this prior to the examination. Ruptures of the extensor tendons of the fifth, fourth, and middle fingers are common (Fig. 8-12).

Loss of extension at the distal interphalangeal joint, the so-called mallet finger, can occur with rheumatoid disease but is not quite as common.

The skin of patients who have had rheumatoid arthritis for a long period of time; especially if they have been taking steroid therapy, will often appear parchment-like with numerous areas of ecchymosis.

The flexor aspect of the hand should also be carefully examined, as it will frequently give a great deal of information. On flexion and extension, synovial

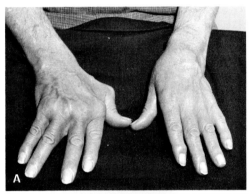

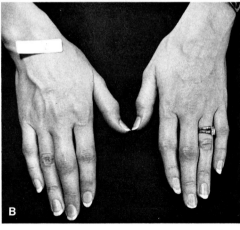

FIG. 8-11 Early signs of rheumatoid arthritis in the hands. A. Moderate ulnar drift and subluxation of the metacarpal-phalangeal joint of the thumb in the right hand and swelling of the extensor tendon sheaths of the left wrist and the distal interphalangeal joint of the index finger of the left hand. B. Symmetrical deformities in the proximal interphalangeal joints, with swelling especially noticeable in the joints of the middle and index fingers.

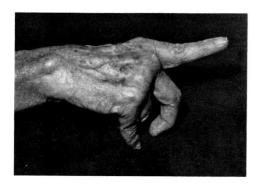

FIG. 8-12 Patient with a rupture of the common extensor tendons but with the indicis proprius intact. The extensor digiti quinti is also ruptured.

swelling can be noted to pass as a moving mass along the flexor tendon beneath the volar carpal ligament. Swelling can be noted both proximal and distal to the volar carpal ligament in severe rheumatoid flexor tenosynovitis (Fig. 8-13). The swelling can extend out into the finger along the flexor tendon sheath and may be very obvious in severe disease. On flexion and extension of the fingers, triggering may occur and the tendon will catch or snap due to a flexor tenosynovitis involving the tendon sheath.

Palpation

After inspection of the hand, the hand and wrist should also be palpated to obtain additional information. Palpation of the finger joints will often give a sensation of synovial thickening and fluid in patients with rheumatoid disease. In contrast, patients with osteoarthritis often will have hard nodules or Heberden's nodes at the distal interphalangeal joints or spurs on the proximal interphalangeal joints. Careful palpation of the dorsum of the hand may reveal the site of a tendon rupture and give an indication of the amount of loss of tendon substance. On the flexor side of the hand, palpation of the flexor tendons in the palm at the distal palmar crease will often reveal a nodular irreg-

ularity when a flexor tenosynovitis is present. Crepitation and crunching may be palpated as the flexor tendon is moved in the tendon sheath. If the nodule is quite large, there will be a loss of active flexion with obvious locking or triggering of the finger in flexion. This can also occur at the site where the profundus tendon passes through the division of the sublimus tendon over the proximal phalanx.

Range of Motion

Loss of motion can be quite insidious and will account for the loss of function. It is important, therefore, in the examination of the patient with arthritis of the hand to record the range of motion of all

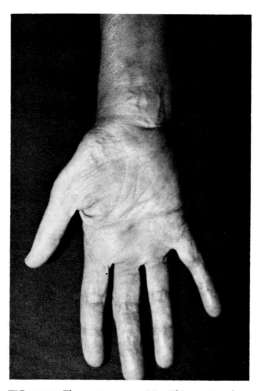

FIG. 8-13 Flexor tenosynovitis. This patient has swelling of the flexor tendon sheaths in the region of the carpal tunnel, as well as swelling in the distal palmar crease in the region of the flexor tendon sheaths.

of the finger joints so that there will be a point of reference for future evaluation. Then it will be possible to determine in future follow-up whether the patient is losing motion. This can often be an indication for surgical intervention. If surgery is carried out, one has a basis for evaluating the improvement in the range of motion of the individual joints that are operated upon.

Starting with the metacarpalphalangeal joints, the examiner should measure the extension and flexion. The average extension in the metacarpalphalangeal joints should be 0°, and flexion of 90° is frequently possible. Unless deformity is present, the proximal interphalangeal joints should ex-

tend to 0° and flex to 100° in the average patient (Fig. 8-14). A distal interphalangeal joint will extend to 0° and flex to 90° when uninvolved. Both hands should be carefully evaluated, and the range of motion should be recorded for future reference. Radial or ulnar deviation of the fingers at any of the individual joints should also be noted. The thumb, in contrast, will abduct from the palm of the hand and the radial side of the index finger approximately 90° in full abduction. It should lie in the plane of the metacarpals. In opposition, the thumb should easily reach the fifth finger without difficulty, touching the tip of the distal phalanx. The metacarpalphalangeal joint will extend to 0° and

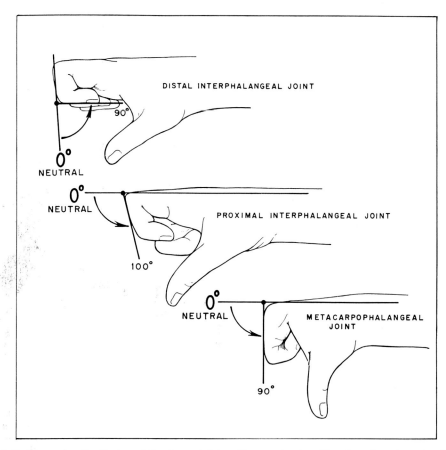

FIG. 8-14 Measuring the flexion of the finger joints with a protractor. (Courtesy American Academy of Orthopaedic Surgeons.)

flex approximately 50° in a normal person. The interphalangeal joint will flex 90° without difficulty and extend to 0°.

Special Tests

In patients with evidence of a possible carpal tunnel syndrome with compression of the median nerve at the wrist, sensory examination should be carried out by using light touch, pinprick, and Tinel's test (Figs. 7-41A; 8-15). Nerve conduction studies and an electromyogram may be of value in determining the diagnosis of median nerve compression.

In some patients with vascular problems, Allen's test can be of value. The examiner compresses the radial and ulnar arteries at the wrist and has the patient close and open the hand rapidly three of four times, forcing the blood out of the hand. On release of either the radial or ulnar artery at the wrist, the

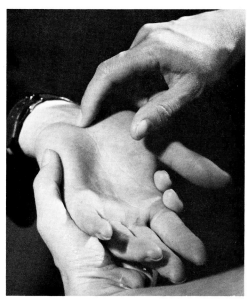

FIG. 8-15 Test for Tinel's sign. The examiner strikes the median nerve at the wrist with his finger to reproduce a sensation of pain or an electric shock.

hand should suddenly flush as the blood rushes into it. If there is vascular disease or interruption of the circulation in either of the arteries, the hand will not fill when the artery is released. Arteriograms can be obtained in selected cases if necessary.

General Observations on Surgical Technique

It is important when considering hand surgery that the proper instruments and equipment are available to compliment the work of a competent surgeon. A tourniquet should be used in order to better visualize the structures that are being operated upon. Bunnell stated that operating without a tourniquet was like trying to operate on the hand in a bottle of ink. The extremities should be wrapped carefully with a Martin bandage, starting from the fingers up to the tourniquet, and then a pneumatic tourniquet should be utilized at the proper pressure of approximately 250 mm of mercury to maintain hemostasis. The tourniquet can be left inflated from 1 1/2 to 2 hours, and most surgical procedures should be planned to finish within that time. Otherwise, it is necessary to release the tourniquet for several minutes to allow flushing of the extremity with oxygen and blood. The longer the tourniquet is left in place, the more edema and discomfort the patient will have postoperatively. Tourniquet paralysis can occur, but this is extremely rare when proper pressure is utilized along with shorter periods of surgery.

Proper instruments should be available, as the large sized orthopaedic instruments are too bulky to use in the hand. Fine hooks, retractors, and forceps are extremely valuable in performing these operations with minimal trauma to the soft tissue. Since many of the finger joints are quite small, it has been found advantageous to use some of the dental instruments for synovectomies of these joints. There are numerous small dental tools that can reach into the crevices beneath the collateral ligaments to remove synovial tissue. These instruments are reasonably inexpensive and a number of instruments of various shapes can be kept available for this type of work.

A power tool is a great advantage for performing some of the procedures required in hand reconstruction. The Hall air drill can be utilized very nicely for performing various arthroplasties and fusions about the hand. The battery-powered drills manufactured by the Mira Company also are helpful for drilling Kirschner wires for finger fusions and for powering reamers and burs for arthrodesis and the Swanson arthroplasty.

Rheumatoid Arthritis

Since rheumatoid arthritis is a systemic disease, the basic changes that occur in the synovium of joints and tendons in other parts of the body will occur in the hand. Thickening of the synovium plus the chronic effusion distends the capsule and supporting ligaments over the dorsum of the fingers and eventually weakens both the capsule and the extensor hood of any joint affected by rheumatoid disease (Fig. 8-16). The volar plate forming the flexor side of the joint is extremely thick and firm and tends to distort very little under pressure. The synovium therefore tends to protrude dorsally in the hand through the metacarpal-phalangeal and the proximal

interphalangeal joints because of the weakened supporting structures in these areas.

The aggressive synovium forms a thickened pannus of a granulomatous tissue that tends to grow over the articular surface and to destroy the articular cartilage. This destruction may occur with minimal deformity of the hand and cannot be ascertained in some cases except by roentgenographic examination (Fig. 8-17). Enzymes that are released from leukocytes within the diseased joint also can attack the synovium and the articular cartilage and lead to the destruction of the joint surface (Fig. 8-18). In advanced rheumatoid disease, stretching and destruction of the joint ligaments with loss of the articular surface, bony erosion, subluxation, and even dislocation of the joints will produce all of the typical rheumatoid deformities.

The deformities seen at the metacarpal-phalangeal joints usually start with an active synovitis. The swelling of the metacarpal-phalangeal joint results in stretching of the transverse fibers of the extensor hood, and as the swelling decreases, the extensor tendon will have a tendency to drift toward the ulnar side (Fig. 8-19). Ulnar drift can occur without subluxation or dislocation of the metacarpal-phalangeal joint. As the disease process continues, subluxation of the metacarpal-phalangeal joint begins to take place. This can be related to tightness of the intrinsic muscles with a development of swan-neck deformities. Continued attempts to flex the proximal interphalangeal joint will result in further subluxation and eventually dislocation of the metacarpal-phalangeal joint (Fig. 8-20).

The extensor tendon crossing the metacarpal-phalangeal joint is loosely bound by the transverse fibers of the extensor hood which attach to the volar plate. The flexor tendons because of

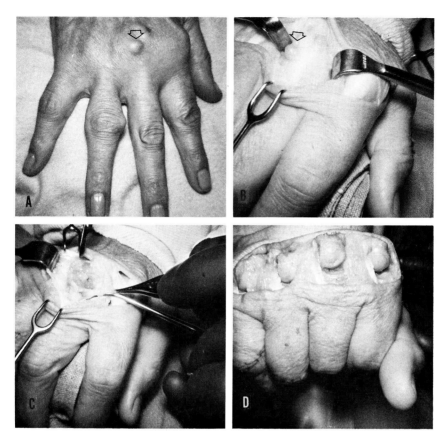

FIG. 8-16 Rheumatoid arthritis of the hand. A. Swelling of the synovial tissue is obvious in the proximal interphalangeal joint of the fourth finger, and a dorsal swelling protrudes from the metacarpal-phalangeal joint of the third finger (arrow). B. Surgical view showing the synovium (arrow) protruding through the extensor hood on the ulnar side. C. The extensor hood opened to show synovial hyperplasia in the joint. D. Exposure of the metacarpal heads to show the destruction of the articular surface by the proliferating synovium.

their great strength may also produce stretching of the accessory collateral ligaments attached to the volar plate that will cause further deformity of the hand. With ulnar deviation of the common extensor tendon and drifting into the valley between the metacarpal heads, further loss of extension occurs and in some cases the extensor will act as a flexor of the metacarpal-phalangeal joint. Because of this imbalance, the intrinsic muscles will tend to cause further subluxation of the metacarpal-phalangeal joint and to increase the ulnar drift. Contracture of the first volar

interosseous, third and fourth dorsal interosseous, and the abductor digiti quinti also will contribute to further ulnar deviation of the hand (Fig. 8-21).

The synovial disease of rheumatoid arthritis can also involve the flexor tendon sheaths, as well as the extensor tendons on the dorsum of the hand and beneath the dorsal retinaculum of the wrist. Severe proliferative synovitis can lead to destruction of the tendons with rupture and loss of function.

The proximal interphalangeal joint is frequently involved by rheumatoid disease producing characteristic deform-

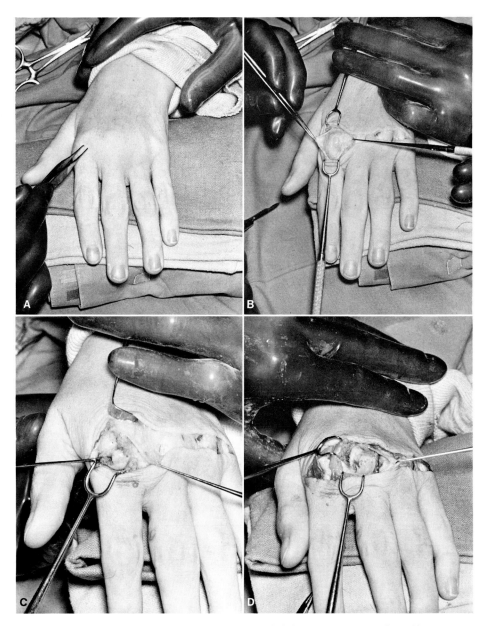

FIG. 8-17 Rheumatoid arthritis of the hand. A. Minimal deformities seen on clinical examination. B. Surgical view of the metacarpal-phalangeal joint of the index finger showing swelling of the synovium. C. Exposure of the metacarpal head to show destruction and erosion. D. Exposure of the metacarpal head of the third finger to show the destruction. Erosions were seen in the roentgenogram.

ities. Early in the course of the disease of the proximal interphalangeal joint the synovial component plays the greatest role. There is proliferation of the synovial lining of the joint with stretching and disruption of the dorsal capsule beneath the common extensor slip. A characteristic of rheumatoid arthritis is the spindle-shaped appearance of the swelling of the synovial tissue that leads to loss of flexion and extension at the proximal interphalangeal joint. Pro-

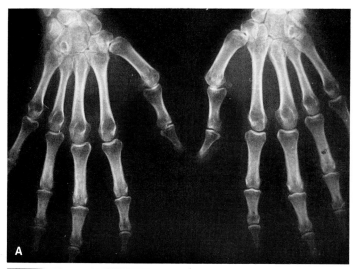

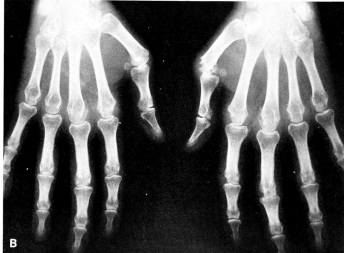

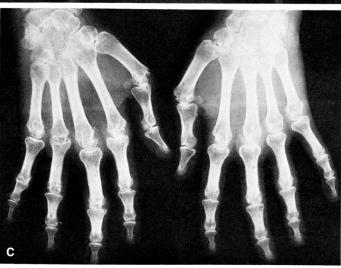

FIG. 8-18 Roentgenograms showing progressive destruction of the hand from rheumatoid arthritis. The patient was 26 years old when first examined. A. Early subluxation of the thumbs with reasonable joint spaces in the metacarpalphalangeal joints. B. One year later. Erosions and punched-out lesions in the metacarpal of the thumbs with beginning subluxations. The radial ulnar joint of the wrist is also severely involved, and there is narrowing of the metacarpalphalangeal joints. C. Two years later. Destructive lesions involving the metacarpal heads, as well as the proximal interphalangeal joints and thumbs, are seen. Severe destruction is noted in the region of the radial-ulnar joint.

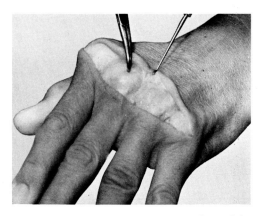

FIG. 8-19 Surgical view showing stretching of the transverse fibers of the hood that produces the ulnar drift of the extensor tendon.

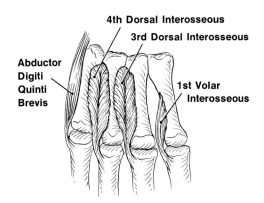

FIG. 8-21 The intrinsic muscles which contribute to ulnar drift.

longed synovitis frequently produces destruction of the articular cartilage with permanent loss of function of the proximal interphalangeal joint.

Rheumatoid arthritis in the thumb will start out as a synovitis involving the metacarpal-phalangeal joint with grad-

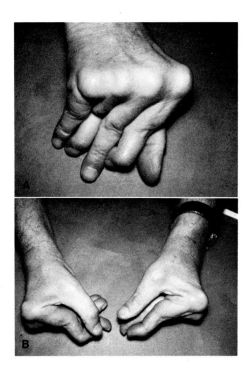

FIG. 8-20 Severe swan-neck deformity. A. Dorsal view. B. Lateral view. Note dislocation of meta-carpal-phalangeal joints.

ual subluxation of the joint. As the disease process continues, the extensor pollicis longus tendon and the adductor expansion are displaced toward the ulnar side. The interphalangeal joint may be spared or can be fixed in hyperextension due to contracture of the extensor mechanism (Fig. 8-22). If the joint itself is severely involved with a synovial process resulting in destruction, permanent dislocation and instability can occur. If the head of the proximal phalanx protrudes into the soft tissue of the thumb, the digit will function poorly. A large bursa, or callus, can develop over the head of the proximal phalanx.

Characteristic of rheumatoid arthritis of the hand are the boutonnière deformity and the swan-neck deformity. The swan-neck deformity is also known as an intrinsic contracture. It is possible to have swan-neck deformities in several fingers and boutonnière deformities in several other fingers of the same hand (Fig. 8-23).

Boutonnière Deformity. Active synovitis within the proximal interphalangeal joint leads to the development of the boutonnière deformity (Fig. 8-24). The synovial proliferation gradually destroys the capsule and invades the central slip of the extensor tendon. This synovial tissue can lead to weakening and rupture of the central slip. A

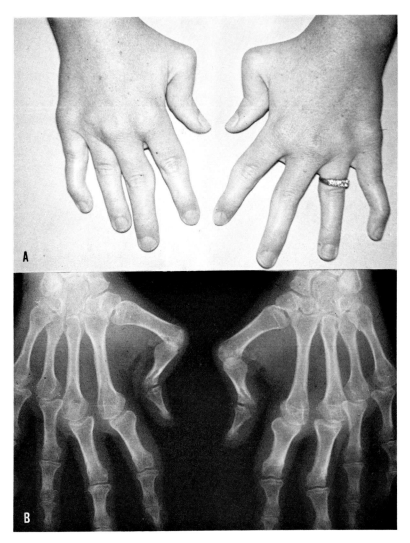

FIG. 8-22 Rheumatoid arthritis in the thumb. A. Photograph of a severe boutonnière deformity from dislocation of the metacarpal-phalangeal joint and the interphalangeal joint. This patient also had advanced intrinsic contractures of the fingers. B. The roentgenogram revealing the changes in the thumb.

gradual flexion deformity develops as the central slip of the extensor tendon and the lateral fibers of the hood are stretched so that there is volar displacement of the lateral bands below the axis of the proximal interphalangeal joint (Fig. 8-25). Since at this stage the lateral bands will act as a flexor of the proximal interphalangeal joint rather than as an extensor, the distal phalanx will become hyperextended. As the process continues, the proximal joint erodes through the central tendon, producing a fixed deformity, and the head of the proximal phalanx protrudes beneath the skin with dislocation of the joint. The distal interphalangeal joint gradually becomes hyperextended with subluxation or dislocation of the distal phalanx on the dorsum of the middle phalanx. Weakening of the extensor mechanism produces a hole in the center through which the proximal interphalangeal joint protrudes. The term *boutonnière* is derived

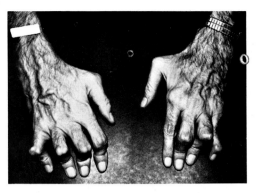

FIG. 8-23 Combination of swan-neck and boutonnière deformities. The patient's right hand has severe fixed boutonnière deformities. On the left hand there is an intrinsic contracture of the index finger with the lateral bands displaced over the dorsum of the finger. Severe boutonnière deformities are seen on the third and fourth fingers, and a swan-neck deformity on the fifth finger. Dislocation of the metacarpal-phalangeal joint of the thumb is also noted.

from the resemblance to a buttonhole. In long-standing disease, the joints become stiff and fixed in the deformed position.

Intrinsic Contracture—Swan-neck Deformity. Swan-neck deformity is believed to be a result of contracture of the intrinsic muscles of the hand which produces hyperextension at the proximal interphalangeal joint. As the hyperextension becomes more severe, the profundus tendon is stretched over a longer distance so that flexion of the distal phalanx occurs. The appearance of the finger from the side tends to resemble a swan's neck, hence the name of the deformity (Fig. 8-26). It is believed that the intrinsic contracture is usually due to persistent spasm of the intrinsic muscles when the metacarpal-phalangeal joints are inflamed.

In the early stages swan-neck deformity produces hyperextension but still allows complete flexion of the proximal interphalangeal joint (Fig. 8-27). As the contracture progresses, however, it tends to become permanent, and flexion of the proximal interphalangeal joint is gradually lost (Fig. 8-28). This can be masked somewhat by the ulnar drift of the fingers and the subluxation at the metacarpal-phalangeal joint. As the patient attempts to forcibly flex the fingers, there is more and more stress on the metacarpal-phalangeal joint with gradual dislocation toward the volar side. This deformity can severely limit the grasp of the hand and prevent the normal ability to pinch.

At times a swan-neck deformity can occur in the thumb, but it is not as common as the boutonnière deformity.

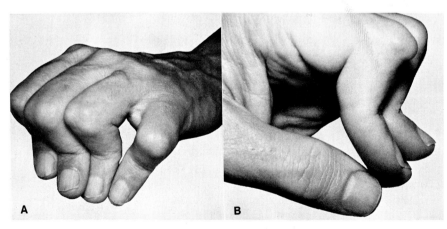

FIG. 8-24 The boutonnière deformity on hand of a 43-year-old man. A. Dorsal view. B. Lateral view showing the complete dislocation of the proximal interphalangeal joint and hyperextension of the distal interphalangeal joint.

RHEUMATOID FINGER DEFORMITY

Type: Boutonniere (Button Hole)

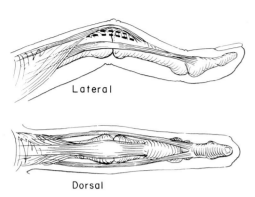

Lateral

Dorsal

FIG. 8-25 Lateral and dorsal views of the boutonnière deformity. The lateral bands are displaced volarward and pass beneath the axis of the proximal interphalangeal joint, flexing it.

Usually it is associated with disease involving the carpal-metacarpal joints with subluxation of this joint or complete dislocation. As the patient loses the ability to abduct the metacarpal of the thumb, attempts to gain further abduction will produce gradual hyperextension of the metacarpal-phalangeal joint.

Severe loss of function occurs with this type of deformity (Fig. 8-29).

The usual test for determining whether an intrinsic contracture is present is to place the finger in its normal position at the metacarpal-phalangeal joint and extend this joint to 180°, maintaining the proximal phalanx parallel to the metacarpal. The proximal interphalangeal joint is then flexed by the examiner and it should normally exceed 90° of flexion. As the intrinsic contracture becomes more severe, less and less flexion is possible at the proximal interphalangeal joint.

Conservative Treatment

The early or conservative treatment of rheumatoid arthritis of the hand, in general, has consisted of either bracing to try to prevent deformity when possible and maintain a position of function or physical therapy to try to relieve the patient's symptoms during the acute stage and maintain motion.

Since rheumatoid arthritis is a systemic disease with involvement of the

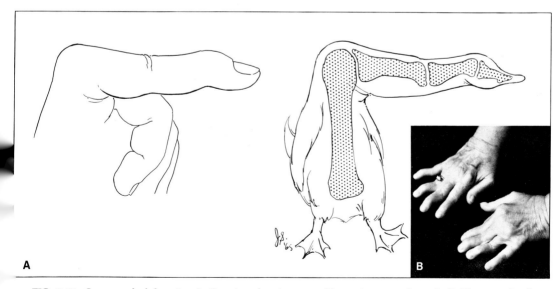

A   B

FIG. 8-26 Swan-neck deformity. A. Drawing showing resemblance to a swan's neck. B. Photograph of patient's hands.

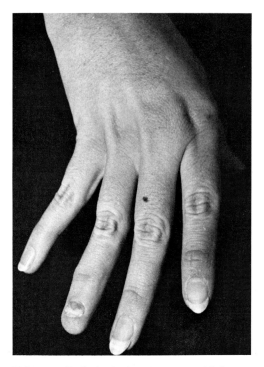

FIG. 8-27 Early intrinsic contracture with hyper-extension of the proximal interphalangeal joints. This patient illustrates ulnar drift with displacement of the lateral bands over the dorsum of the proximal interphalangeal joints.

synovial tissues, early care is mainly supportive for the patient. The disease process will continue despite various modes of therapy because the exact etiology is not known and there is not a definitive medical treatment.

In the past it was felt that bracing could prevent deformities of the hand. At the present state of knowledge, it is apparent that bracing will not prevent deformity. The disease process will continue with destruction of the joints despite immobilization in a position of function. When there is progressive functional loss of the hand and simple methods of treatment do not succeed, it is now generally believed that operative treatment may be indicated for the control of the deformities.

Treatment of the synovitis is paramount in preventing the progression of the disease and destruction of the joints in the hand. The local injection of steroids into the metacarpal or proximal interphalangeal joints can at times bring immediate relief of the synovitis in these joints. Local injection can be utilized to try and control the patient's symptoms, especially when there is a contraindication to surgical procedures.

Studies have been conducted with nitrogen mustard and thiotcpa. Flatt has recommended thiotepa injections into the joints to control the local synovitis. Brooks has also recommended the use of thiotepa which is a much safer drug than the nitrogen mustards and has reported that better results can be obtained if repeated injections are given within a short period of time. Repeated injections

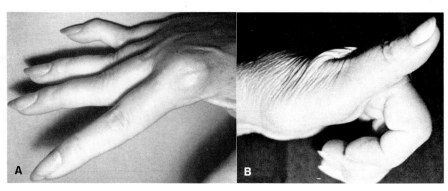

FIG. 8-28 Hyperextension deformities of the proximal interphalangeal joint. A. Full flexion is prevented. B. The fingers will not reach the palm of the hand.

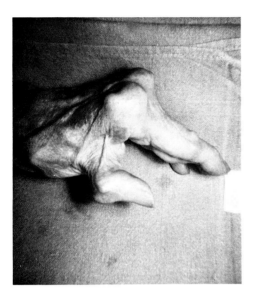

FIG. 8-29 A severe swan-neck deformity of the thumb with hyperextension at the metacarpal-phalangeal joint, dislocation at the carpal-metacarpal joint, and a fixed deformity of the distal interphalangeal joint.

of thiotepa, one week apart, for three injections in series, have given much better results than a single injection alone. The drug is supplied in 15 mg ampules, which are diluted with 2 or 3 cc sterile water injected into the ampule, to make a solution containing either 7.5 mg or 5 mg per cc. A small No. 25 or 26 needle is inserted into the involved joint and 1 percent lidocaine (Xylocaine) is injected on the dorsal aspect of the joint. If the needle is within the joint, the joint can be filled to distension with the Xylocaine. The needle is left in place and then approximately 0.5 cc thiotepa is injected into the joint, and the needle is removed. The joint should be massaged to disperse the fluid uniformly throughout the joint.

In some cases, relief from the synovial distention can be obtained for up to 6 months. The series of injections can then be repeated if necessary.

Exercises can also be utilized to strengthen the intrinsic muscles on the radial side of the finger. Atrophy of the first dorsal interosseous is seen very early in rheumatoid disease of the hand. The patient should be taught to exercise the finger toward the radial side and to work each finger separately to develop the intrinsic muscle on the radial side. Exercises should be attempted also to fully extend each one of the joints at the metacarpal-phalangeal and proximal interphalangeal joints.

Paraffin baths may bring considerable relief for some patients. This type of therapy can often be conducted by the patient at home after simple instructions. The value of the paraffin bath is that it is a simple and efficient method of applying a fairly high degree of surface heating to the hand. Ordinary commercial paraffin to which has been added a little mineral oil melts around 130° Farenheit. The skin temperature in a paraffin bath after the formation of a protective glove is around 116° Farenheit. The patient is advised to obtain a double boiler or any two large containers so that the hand is easily placed in the paraffin. The lower part of the boiler is filled with hot water, and the upper part contains the paraffin oil. The boiler is heated until the paraffin is melted, and then the boiler should be removed from the hot plate or stove. Before dipping the hands into the melted paraffin, the patient should check the temperature to prevent burning. The hand is quickly dipped into the paraffin and lifted out so that only a thin coat of paraffin congeals on the skin. The dipping is repeated from six to twelve times or until a thick glove has been formed, at which time the hand is then wrapped in a towel for 20 or 30 minutes. At the end of this time, the glove can be easily peeled off and put back in the boiler for use again.

The usual mixtures are as follows: 3 pounds of paraffin to a 1/2 pint of mineral oil or 13 pounds of paraffin to 1 quart of mineral oil.

The Metacarpal-Phalangeal Joint

One of the earliest changes that occurs in the hand afflicted with rheumatoid arthritis is swelling of the metacarpal-phalangeal joints. This has been even more frequent than involvement of the proximal interphalangeal joints.

The synovial lining of the metacarpal-phalangeal joint becomes severely inflamed and swollen, producing a persistent synovitis with stretching of all of the supporting structures about the joint. It is during this early stage of synovitis that prophylactic surgery can be considered. If conservative measures fail and the disease cannot be controlled, a synovectomy may be of value in preventing further destruction. Once the deformity of ulnar drift begins to develop, conservative management has failed, and the deformity usually cannot be corrected by bracing, drug therapy, or local injections (Fig. 8-30).

The indications for surgery on the metacarpal-phalangeal joints of the hand of a patient with rheumatoid arthritis are as follows:

1. Persistent swelling of the metacarpal-phalangeal joints despite good medical therapy and local conservative care (Fig. 8-31).
2. Roentgenographic evidence of early bone destruction or loss of the joint space.
3. The presence of ulnar drift of the fingers without subluxation of the metacarpal-phalangeal joints.

The major contraindication for early surgery and synovectomy of the metacarpal-phalangeal joints is subluxation of the metacarpal-phalangeal joint. If the joint is slightly subluxed or dislocated, a synovectomy will not be adequate. It is at this stage that surgery should be deferred. Subluxation, therefore, is a contraindication to early surgery. It is better to allow the patient to continue using the hand until the function is compromised, at which time an arthroplasty can be considered.

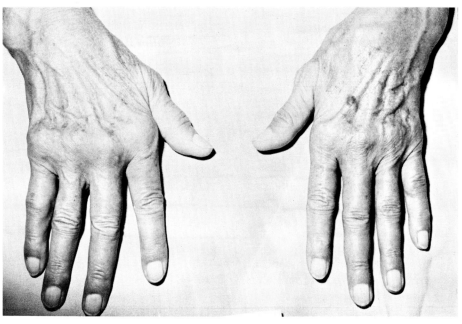

FIG. 8-30 Synovitis of the metacarpal-phalangeal joints. There is beginning ulnar drift of both hands. Synovectomy can be of value if subluxation has not occurred.

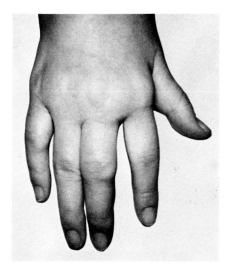

FIG. 8-31 An indication for early synovectomy —persistent swelling of the metacarpal-phalangeal joints that does not respond to good medical therapy.

A synovectomy can be considered in a patient with a subluxed joint to relieve the pain in the hand, but the deformity will recur because of further subluxation taking place with the passage of time. If the patient is aware that the deformity will recur, a synovectomy can be utilized to control symptoms in this type of patient.

Palpation and roentgenograms are two ways to determine whether subluxation exists in the hand. Clinical palpation of the metacarpal-phalangeal joint by manually pushing the proximal phalanx up and down against the metacarpal head will demonstrate whether the proximal phalanx can be subluxed. If there is grating and a tendency for the phalanx to slip volarward, one can be sure that subluxation does exist.

Roentgenograms also are of value in determining the status of these joints (Fig. 8-32). Some surgeons feel that roentgenograms should be taken with the hand elevated and away from the x-ray film to reveal the true deformity (Fig. 8-33). The anteroposterior and oblique views will often demonstrate subluxa-

tion in the metacarpal-phalangeal joint, and this evidence will aid in the final judgement as to what procedures should be performed or whether surgery is indicated. At the time of surgery, the joint changes are often much worse than the clinical signs and radiologic findings. The roentgenograms are of value in determining the extent of early changes in the metacarpal-phalangeal joints.

If the joint is badly subluxed and will not reduce easily at the time of the operation, the joint will resume its position of deformity and the patient and surgeon will be dissatisfied with the result. The most common cause of failure of surgery in rheumatoid arthritis of the hand is the improper selection of the operation to be performed on the metacarpal-phalangeal joints. If the deformity is not corrected passively at the time of surgery and there is a tendency for the deformity to recur at the end of the operation, one can expect a recurrence of the deformity in a short time postoperatively.

Frequently, the disease is more advanced in the index and middle fingers which often can be dislocated, whereas the ring finger and fifth finger are much less involved. In such a situation, an arthroplasty may be performed on the index and middle fingers and a synovectomy on the fourth and fifth fingers.

Synovectomy

At one time there was a great deal of enthusiasm about synovectomy for the metacarpal-phalangeal and other finger joints, but this has tapered to a more realistic approach to what can be accomplished. Careful selection of the patient for synovectomy is important in order to obtain good results. As was pointed out earlier, it is extremely important to be sure that subluxation of the joints has not occurred because the re-

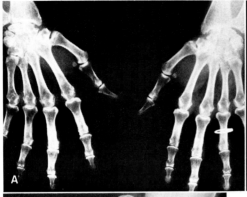
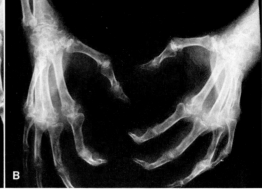
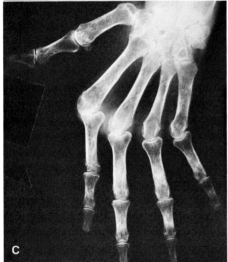

FIG. 8-32 Roentgenograms to determine whether subluxation has occurred in the metacarpal-phalangeal joints. A. This patient has advanced disease of the joints with loss of joint space and erosions of the metacarpal head. B. The oblique view in a patient with advanced disease reveals erosions of the metacarpal heads and subluxation of the phalanx. C. A dorsal view of the metacarpal-phalangeal joints reveals advanced rheumatoid disease with subluxation of the phalanx.

sult then will not be as satisfactory as desired. The patient will have a good deal of relief of pain, but there will be subluxation postoperatively, and a prominence at the metacarpal-phalangeal joint of the metacarpal head can resemble the previous synovitis, although it will not be as prominent as preoperatively. It is important that the patient be advised of stiffness following surgery and of the necessity for early motion to regain the function that he had preoperatively. Proper motivation, preoperative instruction, and postoperative care are of value in obtaining a good result.

Patients with fulminating synovitis of all of their joints that cannot be con-trolled by medical therapy should be approached with caution. These patients often have recurrences of their disease soon after surgery and are difficult to manage. This is not to say that surgery cannot be performed in a joint that is extremely active with rheumatoid arthritis. It is only in the fulminating type of the disease throughout the body that one should be cautious. Ellison, Kelly, and Flatt feel that patients with a history of progressive, severe systemic illness or in an active stage of disease at the time of surgical evaluation are much less likely to obtain a good result from synovectomy than other patients.

The aim of surgery is to remove the diseased synovium to obtain relief of

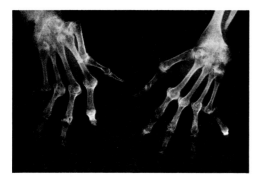

FIG. 8-33 Roentgenogram taken with the hand elevated from the x-ray plate to reveal the true deformity present.

pain and to try to prevent the development of other deformities. Recurrent disease will occur in some of the patients following surgery at varying intervals of time. Although this does happen and there is a recurrence of the disease, the patient may have relief from pain and arrest of joint destruction for long periods (Fig. 8-34).

Synovectomy of the metacarpal-phalangeal joints can be combined with other procedures such as synovectomy of the proximal interphalangeal joints, arthrodesis of any of the joints or thumb, or arthroplasty of some of the fingers.

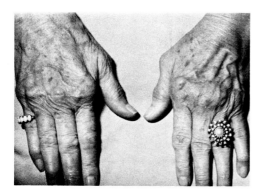

FIG. 8-34 Hands of patient 14 years after a synovectomy of the metacarpal-phalangeal joints of the right hand. The right hand is free of pain and synovitis, although some subluxation is visible. The left hand reveals evidence of some synovitis with subluxation. Ulnar drift has not recurred in the right hand.

Operative Technique. Synovectomy of the metacarpal-phalangeal joints is performed under tourniquet control with the arm placed on a hand operating table. The surgeon and his assistant should be seated for comfort and for ease of performing the operation. The hand is positioned on several folded towels, and a dorsal transverse skin incision is made over the metacarpal-phalangeal joints from the radial side of the index finger to the ulnar side of the fifth finger. The skin incision should be made carefully to preserve the dorsal veins in order to prevent postoperative edema of the hand (Fig. 8-35). The best way to do this is to proceed slowly through the skin. Then the surgeon and his assistant, each using a skin hook in one hand, the assistant's hook opposite the surgeon's hook, should lift the skin and carefully divide it to expose the extensor hood and the veins. In this way the important structures can be protected from inadvertently cutting them with the skin incision.

The skin flap should be turned back to give adequate exposure of all of the metacarpal-phalangeal joints at one time and should be handled carefully, especially in patients with paper-thin skin who have had steroid therapy. Starting on the index finger after exposing the ex-

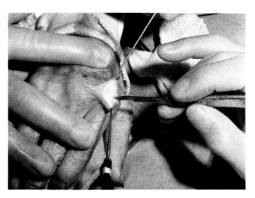

FIG. 8-35 The skin incision made transversely over the metacarpal-phalangeal joints.

tensor hood, the surgeon should place a small skin hook on the proximal and distal skin flap and a blunt retractor on the radial and ulnar side of the extensor hood for exposure. An incision is made through the extensor hood on the radial side parallel to the common extensor tendon (Fig. 8-36). There it is carefully dissected free from the capsule to which it may be quite adherent. The synovial tissue can bulge through the capsule and erode into the extensor tendon in very active disease. The best way to separate the two layers from each other is to start distally over the phalanx because the capsule ends at the base of the phalanx and the extensor hood continues on into the finger and may be easily isolated from it. The extensor hood is carefully turned back, and then the blunt retrac-

tors are used to protect it when excising the capsule and synovium. The collateral ligaments should be protected because they are necessary for stability of the joint. The articular cartilage should look normal and the fingers should not sublux at this stage of the operation.

The finger is flexed, and the area beneath the collateral ligaments along the side of the metacarpal head should be carefully cleaned of synovium. This can be done with dental tools or a small rongeur to scrape away the synovial tissue. It is difficult to remove all of the synovial tissue, especially from the volar aspect of the joint. However, most of the synovial destruction will be present on the dorsal side of the joint because the volar capsule has less synovial tissue.

In a similar manner, the synovium is

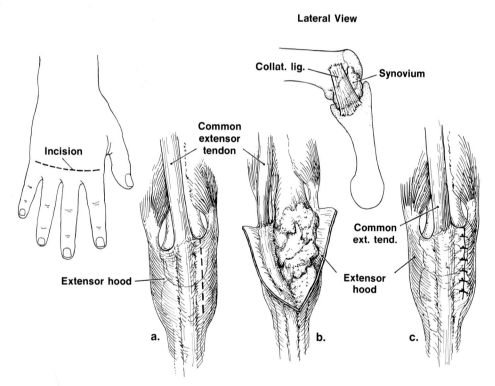

FIG. 8-36 Synovectomy of the metacarpal-phalangeal joints. a. A transverse skin incision is made over the joints. Another incision is made on the radial side of the hood parallel to the common extensor tendon. b. The extensor hood is retracted out of the way to expose the joint. c. The extensor tendon is then repositioned over the top of the joint by plicating the radial side.

excised from the metacarpal-phalangeal joints of the third, fourth, and fifth fingers. If there is any tendency to ulnar drift, the abductor digiti quinti tendon may be divided at its insertion into the base of the fifth proximal phalanx (Fig. 8-21). The fingers are then placed in the corrected position or in slight radial deviation, the extensor hood is plicated on the radial side with 4-0 white silk sutures, and the excess hood is over-lapped and sutured to the ulnar portion of the extensor hood. This should re-place the extensor tendon over the top of the metacarpal-phalangeal joint. It is im-portant to repair the hood distally where it joins the oblique fibers of the extensor hood to prevent ulnar drift and to aid in the radial pull of the intrinsic muscle.

At one time it was recommended that the indicis proprius tendon be trans-planted beneath the common extensor tendon to the first dorsal interosseous tendon to provide a dynamic correcting force (Fig. 8-37). This is not recom-mended because one often finds loss of full extension of the index finger if the transplant is placed too far volarward or at times the indicis propius can act as a flexor if it is placed below the axis of the metacarpal-phalangeal joint. It is better to suture the common extensor tendon

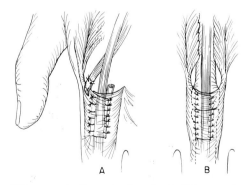

FIG. 8-37 A. Transplanting the indicis proprius under the common extensor to the radial side of the hood. B. Repair of the common extensor tendon over the metacarpal-phalangeal joint by plicating the radial side of the extensor hood.

more toward the radial side when plicat-ing the hood than to transplant the ind-icis proprius tendon.

It has also been suggested in the past that the fifth metacarpal-phalangeal joint be arthrodesed to prevent recurrent drift of the fingers. This is not recommended because it does not prevent drift of the other fingers either over or under the fused finger.

The extensor digiti quinti tendon, which is located on the ulnar side of the extensor hood, can be removed from the hood and passed under the common extensor tendon to the radial side of the hood where it may be sutured to provide a correcting force. Usually there are a number of extensor tendons to the fifth finger and the extensor digiti quinti, which is the most ulnarward tendon, can easily be transferred without interfering with the extensor power of the fifth finger.

The incision is closed subcutaneously with 3-0 plain catgut interrupted sutures, and the skin is sutured with 5-0 nylon. The fingers are placed in the corrected position, and a bulky compression fluff dressing is applied in the palm of the hand. No dressings are placed between the individual fingers to prevent ulnar drift. The hand is wrapped with a soft bandage, carefully keeping it in a cor-rected position, with the wrist in a posi-tion of function and then two 3-inch wide plaster splints, five splints in thick-ness, are placed on the volar and ulnar aspects of the hand and wrist to main-tain the position obtained at surgery and to prevent recurrent ulnar drift. The tourniquet is released at this stage. It is important to inspect the position of the fingers carefully at the close of the oper-ation and to hold the fingers in a cor-rected position while the dressing is applied. Many of the failures of correc-tion occur at this stage because of poor positioning of the fingers. It is extremely important the night of surgery to split the dressing on the radial side of the hand between the thumb and the index finger, cutting the bandage down to the skin from the fingers to above the wrist to relieve the pressure and pain. Pain and swelling are increased if the bandages are not split the night of the operation. The bandage can be loosely approximated with adhesive tape to keep it from falling off. The ulnar and volar splints will maintain the position of the hand, and it is surprising how much less pain the patients have following this operation. Elevation and ice packs also help considerably. Usually by the following morning patients will be comfortable, and there will be minimal swelling of the hand.

The proximal interphalangeal joints and distal joints are left free, and early motion is encouraged both actively and passively on the first postoperative day to maintain good function and to prevent further swelling of these joints. It is wise to advise the patient to exercise the elbow and shoulder as well to prevent postoperative loss of motion.

About the second postoperative day, the dressing can be completely changed and reapplied, leaving more of the finger joints free, but protecting the meta-carpal-phalangeal joints. At the time of this dressing change, the hand should be carefully positioned to prevent any ulnar drift. After the dressing change, the patient may be discharged the following day, and further postoperative care given in the office.

The dressing is removed on the tenth to the fourteenth postoperative day, and if the incision is healed, the sutures may be removed. A protective ulnar plaster splint is worn at night for 6 weeks to prevent ulnar drift. The night splint is made by folding five strips of plaster, 3 inches by 15 inches, and placing them on a thickness of soft padding which is then pulled into a tube of 3-inch stockinette to act as a covering. This is then bandaged with a 2-inch Ace bandage to the ulnar side of the hand from the fifth finger at the proximal interphalangeal joint to the midforearm. The bandage and splint should not be placed too tight, and the patient should be cautioned to avoid pressure over the ulnar head which can become painful and prevent the wearing of the night splint.

When patients have more advanced rheumatoid disease and an ulnar drift deformity that is resistent to correction, further operative procedures may be necessary to correct this ulnar drift. After the synovectomy, the first volar, third dorsal, and fourth dorsal interossei are divided at their tendinous insertions into the ulnar side of the proximal phalanx and the extensor hood. The best way to do this is to grasp the ulnar side of the extensor hood with a single hook and pull it up while deviating the finger radially. The intrinsic will come into view. A small hemostat can be passed through the hood beneath the intrinsic tendon, pulling it upward, and then the tendon can be divided with a sharp knife. Directly beneath the tendon is the neurovascular bundle which should be protected during this portion of the procedure. Release of the intrinsic tendon on the ulnar side will often relax the finger, and it will correct spontaneously.

The extensor digiti quinti, which is located on the ulnar side of the hand, is removed from the extensor hood, tracing it as far distally as possible without destroying the hood, and then is passed beneath the common extensor to prevent kinking. A small incision is made on the radial side of the hood so that the extensor digiti quinti tendon can be pushed through this hole and sutured back upon itself on the radial side. This will then act as a spontaneous correcting force for ulnar drift of the fifth finger. This procedure combined with tenotomy of the abductor digiti quinti tends to correct ulnar drift of the fifth finger.

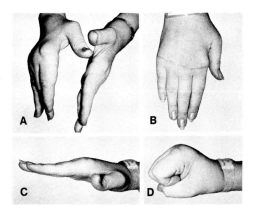

FIG. 8-38 Synovectomy on rheumatoid hand of 21-year-old woman to relieve pain. A. Preoperative photograph shows ulnar drift and loss of extension. B. Six months after the operation the patient had complete relief of pain with correction of the ulnar drift. C. The extension was improved. D. Flexion was excellent. (From Marmor, L.: Surgical treatment of the rheumatoid hand. Proc. Roy. Soc. Med., 58:567, 1965.)

Results. Early operation on the rheumatoid hand has given dramatic relief of pain and increased strength. If the synovectomy is done early enough, return of function is reasonably rapid, and the normal anatomic relationships can often be preserved (Fig. 8-38).

Vainio reported 84 percent good results from synovectomy of the metacarpal-phalangeal joints when erosions were absent or minimal. If severe erosions were present, the results fell to 45 percent. Ellison, Kelly, and Flatt in their survey of 67 patients with synovectomies of 390 joints found that 43.2 percent of the patients had either excellent or good results with a length of follow-up from 3 months to 10 years and a mean for all patients of 4.5 years. Aptekar and Duff found a recurrence rate of 36 percent in their series of 25 hands and 16 patients. Their patients were not in the early stages and had evidence of advanced disease in the metacarpal-phalangeal joints. Although 36 percent had a local recurrence, over 60 percent had good or excellent results, with an average follow-up time of 7.1 years from the date of operation (Fig. 8-39).

Bäckdahl-Myrin H-Graft

The H-graft was designed to provide a solid post in the center of the hand to prevent recurrent ulnar drift. The proximal phalanges of the third and fourth fingers are fixed together by a bony dowel graft, and a syndactyly of the fingers is performed (Fig. 8-40). Only a small number of cases have been reported so far so that this procedure must await further evaluation. The procedure is used mainly to stabilize the center of the hand and must be combined with a synovectomy or arthroplasty of the metacarpal-phalangeal joints if further destruction is to be prevented and the deformity of the hand corrected.

Resection Arthroplasty

At the present time, most of the patients that are seen by the orthopaedic surgeon have far advanced disease of the metacarpal-phalangeal joints with involvement of the entire hand (Fig. 8-41). Patients who are seen late in the course of the disease already have extensive destruction and dislocation of the joints. The most common deformity seen is ulnar drift of the fingers with volar subluxation or dislocation of the proximal phalanx. The ability to restore function to these unstable, dislocated joints with soft tissue contractures still is one of the most challenging problems in reconstructive surgery of the hand (Fig. 8-32; 8-33). This type of hand will not respond to synovectomy alone and requires an arthroplasty with resection of the metacarpal head to restore function. Unless the soft tissues are released by shortening the bone, the phalanx cannot easily be reduced and the deformity will recur postoperatively.

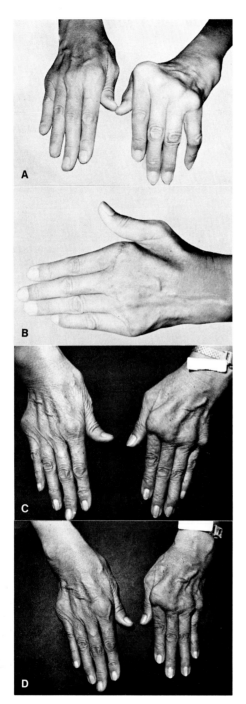

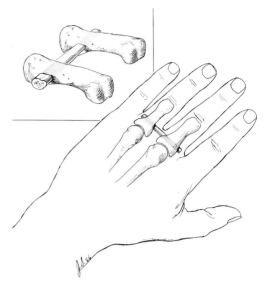

FIG. 8-40 The Bäckdahl-Myrin H-graft. A bone graft is inserted through the proximal phalanges of the third and fourth fingers.

It is believed that the pathologic changes in the metacarpal-phalangeal joints are due to the synovial disease which weakens and stretches the collateral ligaments of the joint so that it loses stability. The accessory collateral ligament also undergoes stretching which relaxes the volar plate. The pull of the flexor tendon upon the volar plate adds additional stress to the accessory collateral ligament and allows the volar plate to sublux toward the flexor side. The transverse fibers of the extensor

FIG. 8-39 Results of synovectomy. A. The patient had advancing ulnar drift with synovitis due to rheumatoid arthritis. B. Six months postoperatively the hand maintained its correction. There was no evidence of subluxation, and the ulnar drift had been corrected. C. Patient's left hand 11 years after surgery shows some evidence of subluxation. The patient is free of pain and still able to use the hand without difficulty. D. The left hand 14 years after synovectomy.

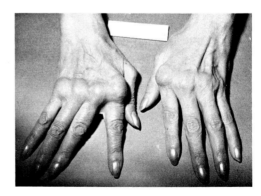

FIG. 8-41 Hands with far-advanced disease of the metacarpal-phalangeal joints.

hood are stretched by the synovial swelling, and gradually there is a dislocation of the common extensor toward the ulnar side. Further use of the extensor tendon will increase the ulnar drift and result in a progressive deformity.

Basically arthroplasty of the metacarpal-phalangeal joint should accomplish three things: (1) remove the synovial tissue, (2) correct the deforming muscular forces about the joint, and (3) restore stability to the joint. A number of operative procedures are available for achieving these goals, and several of the resection and implant techniques will be described. The resection arthroplasty has been used for over a decade and has given satisfactory results in a large number of patients with good finger joints (Fig. 8-42). However, one of the problems has been recurrent subluxation of the metacarpal-phalangeal joint. The failure

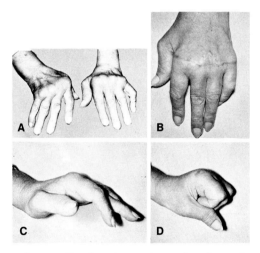

FIG. 8-42 Results of resection arthroplasty. A. Preoperative photograph showing severe painful deformities from rheumatoid arthritis. B. One year following arthroplasty, the patient had excellent function and cosmetic improvement. C. Extension of the fingers was good, except for the index finger because of a transfer of the indicis proprius too far toward the volar side. D. Grasp of the fingers was excellent. (From Marmor, L.: Surgical treatment for arthritic deformities of the hands. Clin. Orthop., 39:191, 1965.)

of the simple resection arthroplasty will not preclude the use of one of the various implant techniques that have been developed in recent years.

Marmor Technique. The operative procedure for resection arthroplasty is performed under tourniquet control, and a transverse skin incision similar to that in a synovectomy is made over the metacarpal-phalangeal joints (Fig. 8-35). Because of the thin skin of patients with advanced rheumatoid arthritis, it is important to be careful not to damage the extensor hoods by the initial incision. The skin flaps are carefully turned back for exposure. The index finger is corrected first.

An incision is made on the radial side of the extensor hood, and the hood is carefully separated from the capsule (Fig. 8-43). It is important to preserve the hood because it will be needed in repairing the ulnar drift. The hood may be extremely thin and the synovium may have perforated it in several places (Fig. 8-16B). If this occurs, it is safer to take some of the capsule with the hood to preserve the thickness of the hood. Otherwise, there will be nothing left with which to repair the ulnar drift. The hood is carefully retracted out of the way, using blunt retractors to protect it, and the capsule and synovium are excised from the joint. The collateral ligaments are divided at their attachment to the metacarpal head and removed.

The metacarpal head is removed with a rongeur piecemeal to avoid crushing the neck of the metacarpal. Enough bone must be removed to allow easy reduction of the phalanx. At this stage the finger is flexed 90°, and the proximal phalangeal base will become visible in the operative field. The volar plate is carefully stripped from the base of the phalanx being careful to protect the flexor tendon (Fig. 8-44). By releasing the volar plate distally and the ulnar attachments of the intrinsic muscle, the phalanx is released

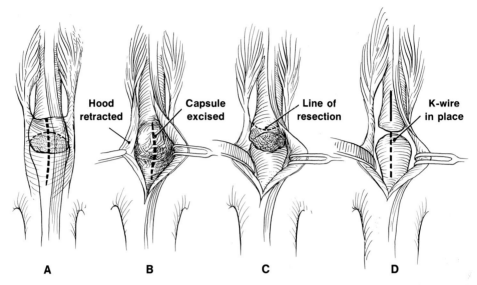

FIG. 8-43 Arthroplasty—Marmor technique. A. The extensor hood is opened on the radial side parallel to the common extensor tendon. B. The extensor hood is retracted out of the way to expose the capsule. C. The capsule, synovium, and collateral ligaments are excised. D. The phalanx is reduced and fixed with a Kirschner wire.

from the volar pull of the flexor tendons. If an adequate release has been obtained, the phalanx will have no soft tissue restrictions and can easily be placed on top of the neck of the metacarpal. The remaining metacarpal head or neck can be smoothed with a rasp or a rotary cup reamer and a power tool. This will usually reshape the head, giving a very nice smooth surface that will gradually be covered with fibrocartilage.

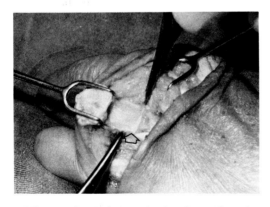

FIG. 8-44 Surgical view of arthroplasty. The volar plate has been cut to release the pull of the flexor tendon on the proximal phalanx (arrow).

The index finger at this stage of the operation usually can be easily placed in a corrected or overcorrected position without any tendency for it to drift back to the ulnar position. If ulnar drift is present or it is difficult to hold the finger easily in a corrected position, the contracted intrinsic muscle on the ulnar side of the finger must be released. The four muscles involved are the first volar, third dorsal, fourth dorsal interossei, and the abductor digiti quinti. These muscles are exposed between the metacarpal heads and divided at their musculotendinous junction. The neurovascular bundle should be protected in the depths of the exposure. Straub suggests transferring the tendon to the radial side of the hood of the opposite finger so that the intrinsic tendon may act as a correcting force. Generally these intrinsics are extremely contracted and fibrotic and do not always function as desired. However, this step can be carried out if the surgeon is so inclined.

When the procedure has been completed on all four fingers, the index finger is placed in the corrected position, and with the joint slightly distracted and slightly overcorrected a few degrees toward the radial side, the 0.045-inch Kirschner wire is drilled from the metacarpal neck into the phalanx with the finger flexed approximately 25° (Fig. 8-45). The wire will maintain the correct position as well as distraction of the joint. All four fingers are corrected in a similar manner, but the middle finger is placed directly against the index finger when the wire fixation is carried out. There should be no spaces between the fingers as the procedure is carried out; otherwise ulnar drift will be present in each finger.

The surgeon should hold the proximal phalanx between his index finger and thumb, with the index finger on the dorsal surface of the proximal phalanx and the thumb on the volar surface. If the surgeon holds the proximal phalanx on its lateral surface, his finger displaces the middle phalanx of the patient toward the ulnar side. If the remainder of the fingers are then positioned in an incorrect manner, ulnar drift will be present across the entire hand.

The Kirschner wires may be either cut off subcutaneously or brought out through the proximal skin flap. The common extensor tendons are then dissected proximally, freeing all transverse bands, to prevent an ulnar pull on the adjacent tendon. The tendons are then placed on the radial side of the wires to aid in a more radial pull while they are healing. If necessary, the extensor digiti quinti may be transferred to the radial side of the hood of the fifth finger to provide a dynamic correcting force. The subcutaneous tissue is closed with 3-0 plain catgut suture, and the skin with 5-0 nylon.

A bulky dressing is placed in the palm of the hand, using fluffs to maintain the proper position of the fingers and to act as a compression dressing. The hand is wrapped carefully with a bias stockinette or similar type of stretch dressing, and a volar and an ulnar molded splint are incorporated in the dressing, leaving the fingers free to start early motion on the first postoperative day (Fig. 8-46). The tourniquet is then released, the hand is elevated, and ice bags are placed on it for 24 hours. The dressing should be split the night of surgery between the index finger and the thumb up to the forearm

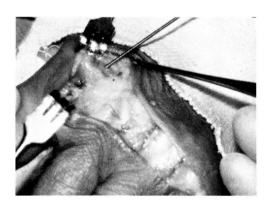

FIG. 8-45 Surgical view of arthroplasty. A Kirschner wire is drilled across the joint.

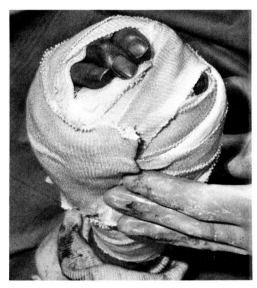

FIG. 8-46 Stockinette enclosing bulky dressing and volar and ulnar splint.

to relieve the swelling and reduce the patient's postoperative pain. On the second or third postoperative day, when the swelling has receded, the hand should be redressed to prevent any drift. No dressing should be placed between the fingers, as this will contribute to ulnar drift. The patient is usually discharged on the fifth postoperative day or whenever comfortable.

Between the tenth and fourteenth postoperative days, the patient is seen as an outpatient, and under local anesthesia the wires are removed so that early motion may be started. Early removal has allowed better motion without the recurrence of ulnar drift. If the wires are left in place for 3 to 4 weeks, the joints may remain stiff because of the scar tissue contracture. An ulnar plaster night splint is worn for 6 weeks to prevent drifting of the fingers.

Results. The results of resection arthroplasty have remained reasonably good over the years. Recurrent drift has not been a problem, but subluxation of the metacarpal-phalangeal joint does occur with the passage of time (Fig. 8-47).

Fowler Technique. The Fowler arthroplasty is performed through the transverse dorsal approach. The capsule and synovium are excised through an ulnar incision in the hood, and the common extensor tendon is dissected out of the hood, and the head of the metacarpal is reshaped into a point. If the base of the phalanx has several large osteophytes, they should be trimmed. The phalanx should be reduced, and a tenodesis of the common extensor tendon to the dorsal surface of the phalanx is an important part of this arthroplasty. A bony gutter is made in the phalanx on the dorsal surface, and a drill hole is made at each end to accept a 4-0 braided wire suture (Fig. 8-48). The hood is repaired to the common extensor by looping the stretched radial side of the hood under the extensor tendon and back on itself to form a sling. A Kirschner wire is used for 3 weeks to maintain the fingers in a corrected position.

Vainio Technique. This arthroplasty is performed through a transverse incision made over the metacarpalphalangeal joint. The common extensor

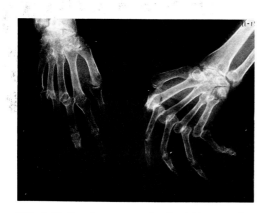

FIG. 8-47 Roentgenogram of patient 10 years after resection arthroplasty of the right hand. The third and fourth metacarpal-phalangeal joints are dislocated, but the patient continues to have painless use of the hand and no evidence of ulnar drift. The left hand, which was not operated upon, has deformities and ulnar drift.

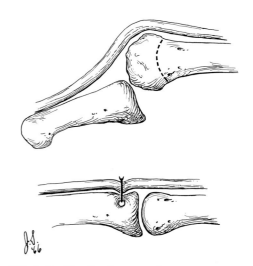

FIG. 8-48 The Fowler procedure to prevent or correct subluxation of the metacarpal-phalangeal joint. The metacarpal head is excised (top) and the extensor tendon is sutured to the phalanx (below).

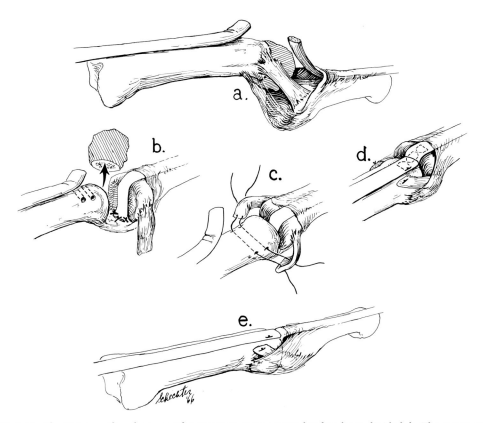

FIG. 8-49 The Vainio arthroplasty. a. The common extensor tendon has been divided. b. The metacarpal head is excised, leaving the collateral ligaments attached to the phalanx, and the common extensor is sutured into the volar plate over the base of the phalanx. c. The collateral ligaments are repaired to the remaining metacarpal for stability. d. The common extensor tendon is sutured to the extensor tendon remaining on the top of the base of the proximal phalanx. e. The final repair.

tendons are dissected out of each extensor hood, and the hood is turned back out of the way (Fig. 8-49). The metacarpal head is resected distal to the attachment of the collateral ligaments to allow good joint motion. A thorough synovectomy of the joint is performed at this stage, and then the extensor tendon is cut proximal to the joint, and the distal end of the extensor tendon is sutured over the phalanx to the volar plate. This tends to shorten the extensor tendon and provide an interposition substance or spacer between the ends of the metacarpal and the phalanx. The proximal end of the extensor tendon is resutured to the extensor at the dorsal edge of the proximal phalanx. The two sides of the

extensor hood are sutured back to the common extensor tendon, and the incision is closed. The dressing and the volar splint on the proximal interphalangeal joints are applied to the forearm with the metacarpal-phalangeal joints in complete extension.

Tupper Technique. A transverse skin incision is made over the metacarpal-phalangeal joints. The skin flaps are mobilized to expose the extensor hoods. The transverse fibers on the ulnar side of the extensor hood are released to each finger, and the abductor digiti quinti is divided at its insertion into the proximal phalanx of the fifth finger. The fifth finger is done first. An incision is made on the radial side of the extensor tendon, and the tendon is retracted out of the way with the hood. Synovium is dissected off the top of the metacarpal head, the joint is opened, and then the radial collateral ligament is released from the metacarpal neck at its proximal end. The ulnar collateral ligament is divided, and a synovectomy is carried out. The metacarpal head is then resected to expose the joint. The volar plate is incised transversely at the junction of its fibrocartilaginous and membranous portions. This is usually found at the level of the original metacarpal neck. This transverse incision through the volar plate at this level will expose the profundus tendon. The exposure is further developed laterally, and then the flexor retinaculum is released from the volar plate distally to its phalangeal attachment. A lateral incision is made longitudinally in the volar plate along the retinacular attachments, revealing the lumbrical muscle on the radial side. The proximal end of the volar plate is gradually reflected up into the joint on its distal attachment. The proximal end of the volar plate is sutured to the dorsal lip of the metacarpal stump, providing a thick interposition membrane completely blocking any bone-to-bone contact. Tupper feels that this elevates the proximal phalanx and reestablishes a strong anchorage of the volar plate to the metacarpal. Attachment of the volar plate to the metacarpal stump can be aided at times by drilling small holes with a Kirschner wire for passage of sutures.

An important step is the reattachment of the radial collateral ligament which should be shortened and reattached to the metacarpal stump. The precise point of insertion is important, and this should be on the dorsal-radial aspect of the metacarpal stump. When properly placed, the ligament will cause some radial deviation and mild supination of the digit. The ulnar collateral ligament need not be repaired. At the completion of this part of the surgical procedure, the fingers should be stable and have no tendency to recurrent drift. It is also suggested that the radial collateral ligament should be sutured with the joint in 45° of flexion to prevent the development of an extension contracture. The radial hood is then shortened to correct the ulnar drift of the extensor tendons. Kirschner wires have not been used postoperatively for fixation. A volar splint with a gutter along the ulnar side of the fifth finger is used for 2 or 3 weeks. Then motion is started using a movable splint.

Implant Arthroplasty

Various implants have been tried for replacement of the metacarpal-phalangeal joint in an attempt to stabilize the joint and improve the function of the hand. Kettelkamp, Alexander, and Dolan tried to restore the articular surface of the metacarpal head by transplantation of an osteochondral graft, but this procedure did not result in a better range of flexion than that from a simple excision of the metacarpal head. A metal prosthesis was developed by Brannon and improved by Flatt, but metal in general has been unsatisfactory in the arthritic hand because of bone absorption and osteoporosis. The stem of the implant tends to migrate through the bone, resulting in loss of stability and often in infection and breakdown of the incision. The development of synthetic materials that can be tolerated by the human body led to the use of plastic implants by Swanson and other investigators.

Silastic, a unique material belonging to the silicone family, has given the orthopaedic surgeon a flexible rubber-like substance that is easily molded into various shapes. The medical grade silicone is extremely inert, but if contaminated by foreign materials, it can produce a foreign body reaction. Some of the silicone implants for the hand have been encapsulated (Calnan-Nicolle) or impregnated with Dacron (Niebauer-Cutter). The same conditions that indicate a resection arthroplasty are indications for an implant arthroplasty.

Swanson Technique. Under tourniquet control, a dorsal transverse skin incision is made over the metacarpal heads. The dorsal veins are protected as in a routine resection arthroplasty, and the extensor hoods are carefully exposed. The index finger is repaired first. An incision is made on the radial side of the hood parallel to the common extensor tendon (Fig. 8-50). The hood is carefully turned back to expose the capsule of the joint. The capsule is excised with the collateral ligaments and synovial

tissue. The metacarpal head is removed down to the neck with a ronguer or power tool. Enough bone should be removed to allow for easy reduction of the phalanx and also room enough for the Silastic Swanson prosthesis to be inserted.

It is important to look at the oblique roentgenogram of the hand to determine whether the proximal phalanx has been eroded on its dorsal surface from rubbing against the underside of the metacarpal head. If this is so, it may be necessary to cut a portion of the proximal part of the phalanx away to give a broad, flat surface for support of the stem of the Swanson prosthesis. Therefore, less metacarpal head should be removed (Fig. 8-51). The finger is then flexed 90°, and the volar plate is carefully dissected off the base of the

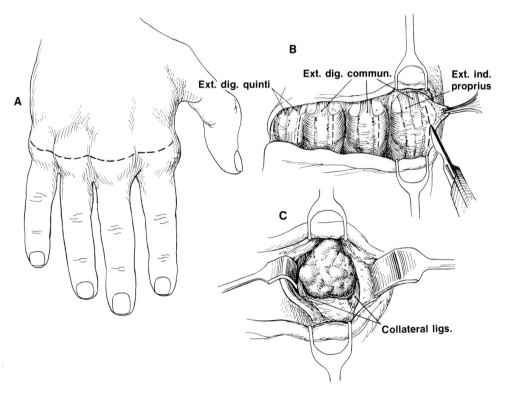

FIG. 8-50 The Swanson implant arthroplasty. A. Transverse incision is made over the metacarpal-phalangeal joints. B. The extensor hood is opened on the radial side parallel to the common extensor tendon. C. The collateral ligaments are exposed and excised from the metacarpal head.

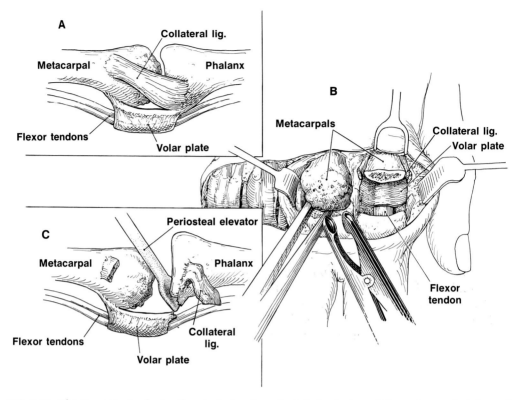

FIG. 8-51 The Swanson implant arthroplasty (continued). A. Lateral view of the metacarpal-phalangeal joint revealing the collateral ligament, volar plate, and flexor tendons. B. The metacarpal head is excised along with the collateral ligaments on the index finger. The volar plate has already been divided to expose the flexor tendon. The middle metacarpal head is ready for removal with a rongeur. C. The volar plate is dissected free from the base of the phalanx to allow the flexor tendon to drop away and prevent postoperative subluxation.

phalanx to expose the flexor tendon and release the phalanx from the flexor tendon and the attachments of the intrinsics. If the ulnar intrinsic tendon is tight, it should be released in its tendinous portion. The tendon of the abductor digiti quinti is also divided to the fifth finger.

A broach is passed up the medullary canal of the metacarpal as far as possible without using force (Fig. 8-52). Then a power tool is used to cut a hole in the base of the phalanx into the medullary canal. The broach is inserted into the phalanx a shorter distance than into the metacarpal. Special burs are available for use with the power tools in cutting out the medullary canal. In a patient

with subluxation of the proximal phalanx or dislocation, the metacarpal head will erode away the dorsal surface of the phalanx, and some must be removed for proper insertion of the prosthesis. Enlarging the canal allows for easy seating of the trial prosthesis.

The proper size of trial implant is selected, and the stem of the implant is fitted into the metacarpal and the opposite end is pushed into the phalanx. The largest sized implant that will fit the canal should be selected. This procedure is then carried out for all of the remaining digits to be operated upon (Fig. 8-53). The fourth metacarpal often has a small medullary canal, and it has to be prepared carefully to avoid splitting the shaft. Frequently a larger sized Silastic prosthesis can be inserted in the fifth finger than in the fourth. If there is impingement of the implant in extension, it is advisable to remove a small amount of bone and release the soft tissue to prevent this. Once all the implants are in place, the finger should stay in a corrected position without effort. The ulnar side of the extensor hood should be released, if tight, to allow the extensor tendon to come up over the top of the implant, centering it over the metacarpal-phalangeal joint (Fig. 8-54). The extensor hood is plicated on the radial side, overlapping the excess, using 4-0

white silk sutures. The skin incision is closed with interrupted 5-0 nylon sutures, and Swanson inserts two small drains of silicone rubber to prevent a hematoma. A large bulky dressing is applied to the hand, a narrow plaster splint is applied to the palmar side, and the tourniquet is released. The wound is inspected on the second day if drains are used, and they are removed. Swanson tends to use a dynamic brace on the third to fifth postoperative days. In our experience, a bulky dressing has been left in place for 10 to 14 days, at which time the hand bandage is removed and exercise is started.

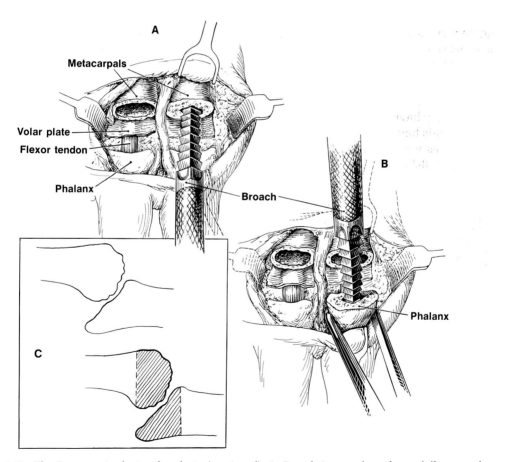

FIG. 8-52 The Swanson implant arthroplasty (continued). A. Broach is passed up the medullary canal. B. After drilling a hole in the base of the phalanx, the surgeon passes the broach into the proximal phalanx. C. The shaded area reveals the amount of eroded area to be removed for reduction and proper insertion of the Swanson prosthesis.

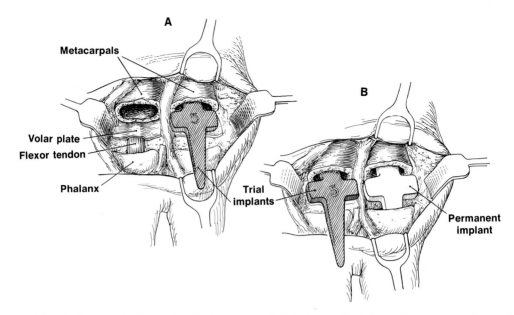

FIG. 8-53 The Swanson implant arthroplasty (continued). A. Trial prosthesis is inserted into the metacarpal to determine a proper fit. B. The permanent implant has been placed in the index finger, and the trial component is being inserted into the middle finger.

The results of the Swanson Silastic arthroplasty have remained good to date. The patients have been satisfied with the cosmetic as well as functional improvement (Fig. 8-55). Recurrence of the de-

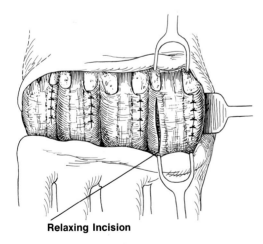

FIG. 8-54 The Swanson implant arthroplasty (continued). The common extensor tendons are sutured to lie over the top of the metacarpal-phalangeal joint. If the ulnar side is contracted, a relaxing incision should be made to allow centering of the extensor tendon.

formities has been seen with the Silastic arthroplasty and tearing of the prosthesis has occurred (Fig. 8-56). The development of a stronger Silastic material should prevent some of these problems as well as the surgical technique of flattening the base of the proximal phalanx and smoothing off any rough edges that could tear the prosthesis.

Niebauer-Cutter Technique. The Niebauer-Cutter prosthesis differs from the Swanson prosthesis in that it contains an outer layer of Dacron mesh. The purpose of the Dacron mesh is to allow bone and fibrous tissue to infiltrate into it, providing stability of the prosthesis.

The operative procedure is performed through either a transverse incision over the metacarpal-phalangeal joints or a longitudinal incision over each metacarpal-phalangeal joint. The operation is performed under tourniquet control, and every effort is made to spare the dorsal veins. The joint is approached through an incision which runs parallel to the extensor tendon on the ulnar side

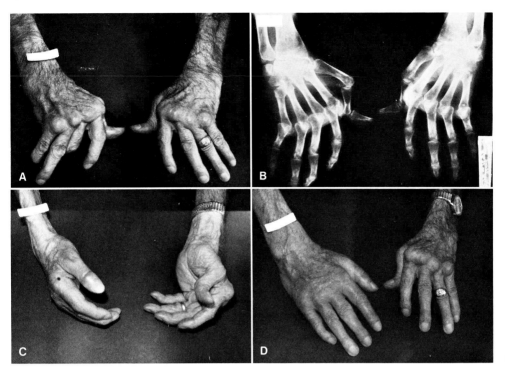

FIG. 8-55 Results of Swanson implant arthroplasty. A. Preoperative photograph showing severe deformities in both hands. B. Roentgenogram showing dislocation of the metacarpal-phalangeal joints, boutonnière deformity of the thumb, and involvement of both wrists. C. Postoperative photograph after Swanson arthroplasty and arthrodesis of the metacarpal-phalangeal and proximal interphalangeal joint of the thumb. D. Dorsal view showing improvement in appearance and increased function of right hand. The patient is free of pain.

of the hood, releasing the hood so that it may be retracted to the radial side of the joint. The joint is exposed by incising the capsule longitudinally and then transecting the metacarpal origin of the collateral ligaments.

The metacarpal heads are resected at approximately the level of the origin of the collateral ligaments. A sufficient amount of bone should be resected to allow easy reduction of the dislocated phalanx. It is recommended that approximately ³/₈-inch clearance should be present when the finger is reduced to aid in easy insertion of the prosthesis and to avoid tension. The resection of the metacarpal head is performed perpendicular to the anteroposterior plane of the bone, but it is angulated toward the radial side of the hand in the lateral plane. A syn-

ovectomy should then be performed with a rongeur.

If the base of the phalanx is not perpendicular, it should be resected to give a flat base for insertion of the prosthesis. A power reamer or special sizing broach should be used to open the metacarpal and phalangeal medullary canals. If the special Niebauer broaches are used, the prosthesis will correspond to the size of the broach that is used. It is preferred that the prosthesis not fit tightly in the intramedullary canal. The sizes of prostheses most commonly used in the metacarpal-phalangeal joints are numbers 3, 4, and 5. The hand should correct easily after the insertion of the prostheses, and every attempt should be made to re-establish the extensor mechanism with the extensor tendon over the

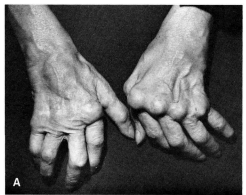

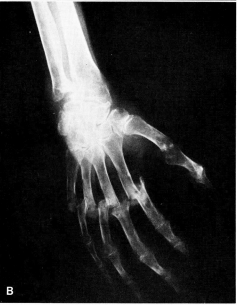

FIG. 8-56 A. Photograph of patient's hands 6 months after Swanson arthroplasty. Dislocations of the metacarpal-phalangeal joints have recurred in the right hand. B. Roentgenogram. The Swanson prosthesis has torn in all four fingers. A new Swanson prosthesis of stronger Silastic should avoid this complication.

dorsum of the joint. After the repair has been carried out, the tourniquet is released, and a bulky dressing is applied to the hand with immobilization splints. Immobilization for this technique is recommended for 3 to 4 weeks; and then exercises are instituted with a precaution not to place ulnar deviating forces on the fingers for several weeks.

Calnan-Nicolle Technique. The Calnan-Nicolle encapsulated finger joint is an intramedullary prosthesis with an integral hinge (Fig. 8-57) made of polypropylene. The capsule is made of Silastic, and there are 2.5 mm perforations to allow filling with interstitial fluid. There are seven different sizes of encapsulated finger joints, the larger four being intended for metacarpal-phalangeal joint replacement.

Under tourniquet control, the metacarpal-phalangeal joints are exposed through separate longitudinal skin incisions avoiding the dorsal veins. The extensor hood is incised along the radial aspect of the common extensor tendon. The capsule is opened, and the metacarpal head is removed along with 3 to 4 mm of the proximal phalanx. Release of soft tissue is vitally important where marked ulnar drift and volar contracture exist. A set of reamers corresponding to the sizes of the finger joints has been developed to open the medullary canal. After the proper size has been selected, the implant is inserted by flexion and traction on the finger. The extensor tendon is then relocated over the top of the finger and imbricated on the radial side. A dressing with a volar pressure splint is applied for 3 weeks. After 3 weeks, active exercises are started to regain motion.

The prostheses can also be inserted into the proximal interphalangeal joint.

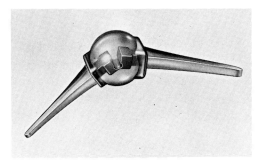

FIG. 8-57 The Calnan-Nicholle encapsulated finger joint.

There have been some reports of failure of the prosthesis; and further follow-up is indicated.

Postoperative Physical Therapy. The basic exercise program for most patients will not vary too much, regardless of the procedure performed. It is important in most hand patients to encourage them to exercise the elbow and shoulder and to be sure to put the arm above the head at least once a day. Patients tend to keep the arm at the side for fear of injuring the hand and often will develop stiffness in the shoulder or elbow joint that can be prevented much easier than trying to correct it later. Upon discharge from the hospital, the patient is generally instructed to elevate the hand at rest to prevent swelling of the fingers and to exercise the finger joints as much as possible to prevent stiffness.

At the end of 2 weeks when the hand is removed from the immobilization splints and dressing, the patient is advised to wear a night splint for 6 weeks that runs along the ulnar border of the hand and is wrapped on with an elastic bandage. To prevent ulnar drift of the bandage, the patient is instructed to avoid wrapping the bandage beyond the scar over the index finger. The night splint should extend on the ulnar border of the hand beyond the metacarpal-phalangeal joint to prevent ulnar drift. This splint is generally made by taking five thicknesses of 3 by 15-inch plaster splints, folding them over, and coating them with a layer of soft cast padding. This is then pulled into a 3-inch stockinette tube and molded as a splint to the ulnar border of the hand and wrapped loosely with an Ace bandage. Be careful to pad very well over the ulnar head which can become uncomfortable if the padding is not adequate.

The patient is instructed to soak the hand 10 minutes, twice a day, and to exercise each finger while using a sponge in the water. The fingers should also be exercised into extension and flexion individually and assisted by either the patient's other hand or the therapist to gain further passive motion. To build up the intrinsic musculature, the patient is instructed to place the hand flat on a smooth tabletop that has been dusted with talcum powder. Keeping the hand flat, the patient should exercise all fingers toward the radial side (thumb) and should try to bring the fifth finger alongside the fourth. Crazy putty, soft sponge, or a soft rubber ball for continuous exercise of the finger joints is also valuable if used carefully to prevent ulnar positioning of the fingers. It should be stressed that the hand should not be painful at the end of the exercise period. Better results are obtained from several brief exercise periods daily rather than from one long session. Encouragement by the therapist or surgeon will stimulate the patient to perform better.

The scar may be massaged with cocoa butter or lanolin ointment daily to free the skin and to aid in the healing process. Some patients feel that vitamin E oil is beneficial for massage of scars. Paraffin baths and hydrotherapy can be added to the routine when the incision is well healed.

The patient should be instructed not to lift anything heavy with the hand during the postoperative recovery period. The hand can be used for light activities such as eating, shaving, and putting on makeup. When the hand is at rest, the patient should put it in a position so that gravity will work against the ulnar drift and tend to maintain the correction.

If patients are gaining motion slowly, it is possible when the wound is healed to utilize a Bunnell knucklebender splint to gain flexion and a reverse knuckle-bender to gain extension. The splint should be worn for 5- or 10-minute periods several times each day to prevent undue pressure from the brace on the incision and postoperative edema.

For some patients, it is possible to use small aluminum splints on the proximal interphalangeal joints to transfer the force of the flexor tendons to the metacarpal-phalangeal joint and aid in gaining better flexion post-surgery. The splints should be removed several times a day to prevent stiffness of the proximal interphalangeal joints. A return of extension may be slower in patients having an excisional arthroplasty, and full extension may never be possible. Better extension has been gained with the Silastic implants, and the return of function has been quicker.

The majority of patients will benefit from a general exercise program planned to gain or maintain full range of motion of all joints. These exercise periods should be limited to less than 15 minutes a day so as not to overtire the patient.

The best program of therapy can be accomplished by setting up a group therapy clinic where the patients work together under the supervision of a trained therapist. It is surprising how this helps the morale of the patients. Since the patients are usually seen once a week in the clinic, the program is basically a home program. The patient's relatives should be encouraged to take an active interest in the exercise routine.

Arthrodesis

In the past, some doctors have recommended arthrodesis of the metacarpal-phalangeal joints in a position of function as a method of correcting rheumatoid destruction. Unfortunately, rheumatoid arthritis is a progressive disease, and if the metacarpal-phalangeal joints are fused, it is possible that there will be loss of motion in the proximal-interphalangeal joints that will lead to a rigid, stiff hand with loss of total function. Although pain relief and permanent correction of the ulnar drift can be ob-

tained by fusion, the procedure is not recommended for use in the rheumatoid hand (Fig. 8-58).

Some authors have recommended that the metacarpal-phalangeal joint of the fifth finger be fused to prevent drifting of the other fingers. Arthrodesis has not been satisfactory, since the fingers can drift over or below the fused fifth finger and still produce deformities.

The Proximal Interphalangeal Joint

The proximal finger joint may become involved in rheumatoid arthritis (Fig. 8-59). Synovitis with swelling of the proximal interphalangeal joints can develop, and the synovial tissue will tend to stretch the capsule dissecting proximally because of the attachment of the central slip of the extensor tendon to the base of the middle phalanx (Fig. 8-4). The synovium can gradually stretch the central slip and the attaching fibers of the lateral bands, leading to a loss of extension and a flexion deformity of the joint. The synovium may erode into the

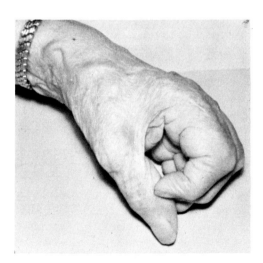

FIG. 8-58 Arthrodeses of the metacarpal-phalangeal joints placing them in a position of function. Although the pain and deformities were corrected, the patient was unhappy with the result because of stiffness and deformities in her distal finger joints that limited the use of her hand.

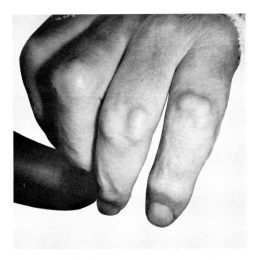

FIG. 8-59 Swelling of the proximal interphalangeal finger joints from synovial proliferation in rheumatoid arthritis.

articular surface of the joint to cause deformities and destroy the articular cartilage. Far-advanced disease will result finally in a boutonnière deformity that is difficult to correct. The proximal interphalangeal joint can also be influenced by disease of the metacarpal-phalangeal joint. It is a well-known fact that in joint disease, the muscles passing the joint will often go into spasm and become involved when there is disease within the joint. This holds true for the intrinsic muscles which pass the metacarpal-phalangeal joint to insert into the base of the proximal phalanx and the extensor hood. Persistent spasm of the intrinsic muscles often leads to subluxation and dislocation of the metacarpal-phalangeal joints. The shortened intrinsic tendons will produce an intrinsic contracture leading to the common swan-neck deformity of rheumatoid arthritis.

Conservative Treatment

The early conservative treatment of the proximal interphalangeal joint is directed toward controlling the synovitis and attempting to prevent the development of deformities. Local injections into the proximal interphalangeal joints can be considered. It is surprising how well the synovitis can be controlled in some patients and how long they will have relief of the synovial swelling after injections of steroids or thiotepa. If the synovitis cannot be controlled, serious thought should be given to surgical intervention to prevent the development of fixed deformities. Once a severe boutonnière deformity has developed, it is extremely difficult to correct and may require fusion of the joint.

Synovectomy

The indications for surgery in the proximal interphalangeal joint are persistent synovitis that cannot be controlled conservatively. If the patient continues to have swelling of the joints, it is advisable to consider early synovectomy to prevent the severe destruction and deformities that can occur. If the roentgenograms show beginning erosions of the edges of the joint, as well as loss of the joint space, synovectomy should be undertaken without delay. The patient must be cautioned that early motion is essential and they they will have to exercise to regain their flexion and extension. They must also be cautioned that some loss of motion can occur with this procedure. It is extremely important not to use prolonged immobilization after operating on the proximal interphalangeal joints to avoid stiffness.

Operative Technique. A proximal interphalangeal joint is approached through a transverse incision over the joint itself. The skin incision should be made carefully not to divide the extensor hood, and there are several blood vessels that should be cauterized on approaching the dorsal surface of the hood. The extensor hood and central slip are exposed, and the joint may be approached by incising between the central tendon and the lateral band or by lifting the lateral edge of the hood, exposing the capsule and the synovium (Fig. 8-60). The synovium should be thoroughly excised, using a rongeur and small instruments such as dental tools to get into tiny crevices. The edges of the joint can be scraped to remove all evidence of synovial tissue from the articular margins. It is possible to work from both sides of the hood, medial and lateral (Fig. 8-60B). If the extensor hood has been opened, it can be repaired with several interrupted 4-0 white silk sutures, but if the lateral band has just been lifted up, it can be dropped back into place and will generally remain in the proper position. If it tends to ride up, several 3-0 chromic sutures tacked into the soft tissue will hold it in place.

All of the proximal interphalangeal joints can be operated on at the same time, and the synovectomy can even be combined with a synovectomy of the metacarpal-phalangeal joints, or any other combination of procedures, as long as the total operating time is less than 2 hours. The rapidity of doing this surgery will depend upon the experience of the surgeon, and he should take into consideration the length of time for all of the procedures.

Postoperatively, motion of the fingers should be started as soon as possible to maintain function and prevent stiffness. As soon as the sutures have been removed, hydrotherapy and the use of crazy putty should be encouraged.

Synovectomy of the proximal interphalangeal joints has given good results in a number of patients (Fig. 8-61). Because it is difficult to remove all of the synovial tissue, a recurrence is possible, and this should be explained to the patient preoperatively.

Lipscomb Technique. Lipscomb has

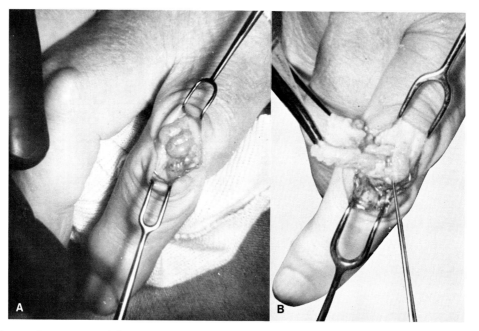

FIG. 8-60 Synovectomy of the proximal interphalangeal joint. A. The synovial tissue can be seen protruding through the extensor mechanism. B. The extensor mechanism is retracted to remove the synovium. A hook may be used to pull the lateral band out of the way, and the synovial tissue is excised.

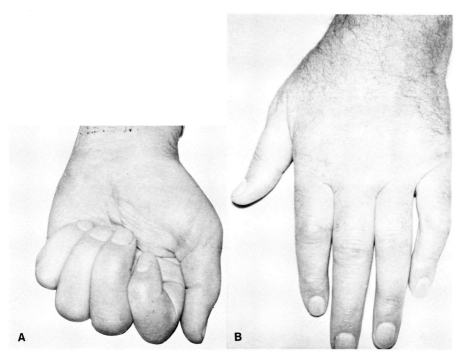

FIG. 8-61 Twelve months after synovectomy of the metacarpal-phalangeal joints and proximal interphalangeal joints. A. There is no evidence of swelling in the hand. B. The patient has an excellent range of motion in the proximal interphalangeal joints.

described a technique for doing a synovectomy of the finger joints that allows excellent visualization of the joints with simplicity of technique.

A lateral incision 1-$\frac{1}{2}$ inches long is made in a longitudinal direction between the dorsal and volar skin creases, and the skin flaps are carefully elevated. The lateral band of the extensor mechanism is retracted upward, and the capsule and collateral ligament are sectioned transversely at the level of the joint. The area of the volar plate is carefully detached distally to about the midline of the finger. Care must be exercised not to damage the extensor mechanism, or a postoperative deformity will develop. All of the visible synovium is removed, and exposure is increased by dislocating the finger joint and using the intact collateral ligament on the opposite side as a hinge. The margins of the articular surface should be curetted to remove any excess synovium and to prevent pannus formation.

Following removal of the synovium, a thin Kirschner wire is inserted diagonally across the joint with the finger flexed 20° to 30°. The ends of the collateral ligament are repaired with mattress sutures of 4-0 chromic catgut. Lipscomb also suggested placing 1 or 2 drops of hydrocortisone solution into the joint prior to closure of the wound.

Postoperatively, a bulky dressing is used with a plaster-of-Paris splint to hold the hand and wrist in a position of function. This is usually left in place for 10 or 12 days, after which the sutures and Kirschner wires are removed.

Reconstruction of Boutonnière Deformity

In the early stage of the boutonnière deformity which can be corrected passively or in which the flexion deformity can be corrected preoperatively by physical therapy or dynamic splinting, soft tissue surgery can be considered. The results of this type of surgery are poor, however, and the patient should be cautioned in regard to this fact. If a flexion contracture of the joint is present, it is difficult to reconstruct the deformity by soft tissue repair.

A number of procedures are available for reconstruction of the boutonnière deformity. Fowler has recommended division of the attachment of the lateral bands to the distal phalanx. This tenotomy releases the pull of the intrinsics on all of the finger joints and allows flexion of the distal joint (Fig. 8-62). The extensor hood is released and slides proximally, producing better extension of the proximal interphalangeal joint. This procedure has not been extremely satisfactory, and in the advanced stage when there is no active extension of the proximal interphalangeal joint and the finger is flexed to 90° with a severe hyperextension deformity of the distal phalanx, arthrodesis is the best procedure. The Littler and Eaton and the Heywood techniques have been more satisfactory and will be described in more detail.

Littler and Eaton Technique. In the

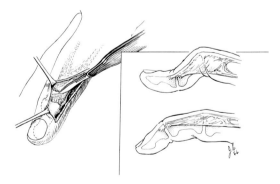

FIG. 8-62 The Fowler procedure for the treatment of a boutonnière deformity. The distal attachment of the extensor mechanism is released to produce a mallet finger and correct the hyperextension to the distal phalanx.

Littler and Eaton technique for the correction of a boutonnière deformity, a dorsal incision is made over the finger joint, and the lateral bands are identified. The lumbrical tendon and the radial retinacular ligament are dissected from the main portion of the radial lateral band. On the ulnar side, the lateral band is separated from the oblique retinacular ligament, maintaining the attachments of the ligament. The lateral bands are then folded dorsally to the midline of the finger where they are sutured with the proximal joint in full extension, thereby reinforcing the weakened central slip. For 2 weeks following operation, the proximal joint is maintained in full extension by a thin, transarticular Kirschner wire. If there is evidence of an active synovitis within the joint, the synovial tissue should be removed prior to closure of the skin incision and repair of the extensor mechanism.

Heywood Technique. A soft tissue technique for the boutonnière deformity has also been suggested by Heywood. An incision is made over the dorsum of the middle and proximal phalanges, using a lazy-Z incision. The skin and subcutaneous tissue are lifted up in one sheet, exposing the extensor mechanism. The central slip, which has been stretched by the disease process, is incised transversely approximately 4 mm proximal to the proximal interphalangeal joint. The central slip is dissected proximally for about 2 cm and lifted free. The distal portion is carefully preserved and elevated to allow a synovectomy of the joint if there is active synovium present (Fig. 8-63).

The lateral bands are freed from the volar retinacular fibers and brought dorsally together with their delicate transverse connecting fibers. The ulnar lateral band is cut distally from its insertion into the conjoined tendon attaching to the distal phalanx and anastomosed end to the side of the radial lateral band.

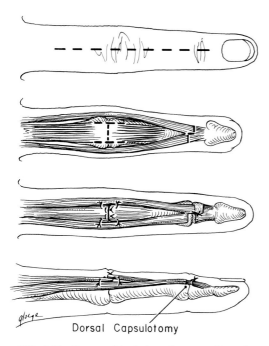

Dorsal Capsulotomy

FIG. 8-63 Heywood technique for correction of a boutonnière deformity. The finger is approached through a dorsal incision. The extensor slip that has been stretched out is divided, and a synovectomy can be carried out in the proximal interphalangeal joint. The lateral bands are brought upward and sutured to central slip to reinforce it.

This junction is made centrally just distal to the joint line.

The central slip is now pulled distally and overlapped to its distal attachment to the base of the middle phalanx. The joint is then fixed with a thin Kirschner wire at 10° to 15° of flexion. An aluminum lightweight splint can be used to maintain the distal phalanx in slight flexion. Postoperatively, the wire is removed along with the sutures on approximately the tenth to the twelfth day, and motion is started.

Lateral Band Suture

Operative Technique. Suture of the lateral band is performed through a lateral incision extending from the distal one third of the middle phalanx through the proximal one third of the proximal

phalanx. The dorsal skin flap is mobilized along with the soft tissue and blood vessels and can be retracted well over the side of the finger, exposing the entire extensor mechanism over the proximal interphalangeal joint. The lateral bands are mobilized so that they cross the top of the proximal interphalangeal joint (Fig. 8-64). The adjacent borders of the tendon are freshened with a knife, and then they are sutured to each other distally with interrupted 4-0 white silk sutures. The central slip may also be incorporated in the sutures to strengthen the attenuated fibers. The joint should be immobilized in extension for approximately 10 days to allow healing together of the tendons.

The same approach can be used in the technique of crossing over the lateral bands. The bands are divided over the middle phalanx and then crossed over the top of the joint and sutured to each other, as well as to the distal stump.

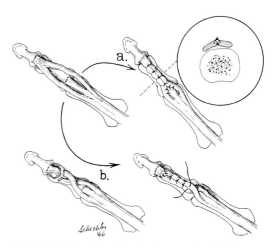

FIG. 8-64 Lateral band suture to correct a boutonnière deformity. One long extensor tendon is made by mobilizing the lateral bands and suturing them together distal to the proximal interphalangeal joint and then suturing the central tendon to the combined lateral bands (a). An alternate method for correction of a mild boutonnière deformity is to divide the lateral bands and cross them over the top of the proximal interphalangeal joint (b).

Arthrodesis

Arthrodesis is of value when the joint is badly destroyed and is in a severely flexed position or is ankylosed (Fig. 8-65).

Operative Technique. The joint may be approached in several ways: through a straight longitudinal incision, an S-shaped dorsal incision, or a lateral incision centered over the joint. The last incision is the most cosmetic of the three since it will lie between the fingers (Fig. 8-66).

The central slip and lateral bands are exposed; the central tendon is split and removed from the base of the middle phalanx if still attached. The collateral ligaments are divided along the proximal phalangeal head, and the joint is opened widely. The head is carefully debrided of remaining articular cartilage. A blunt point or dowel is made out of the cancellous bone. An awl or small curette is drilled manually into the base of the phalanx through the articular surface. Then gradually larger-sized curettes are used until a satisfactory fit of the proximal phalanx into the middle can be obtained. The two are then compressed together in about 30° of flexion and an 0.045-inch Kirschner wire is drilled across the joint from the proximal end and cut off subcutaneously. Only one wire is used to prevent distraction, and

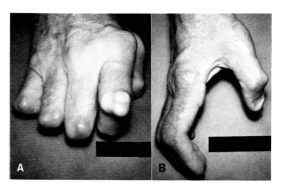

FIG. 8-66 A. Preoperative photograph of severe fixed deformities of the proximal interphalangeal joints. B. Photograph after arthrodesis using the lateral approach. Improvement in function and cosmetic appearance was gained.

rotation has not been a problem. Fixation in 45° of flexion seems to give a better grasp in the palm, but 30° seems to give a more acceptable result from a functional and cosmetic aspect. This method of arthrodesis has worked extremely well, and nonunion has not been a problem. The extensor hood is closed with several interrupted sutures (Fig. 8-67).

The hand is immobilized, including only the fingers that were involved in the arthrodesis. This plaster immobilization is removed early to prevent stiffness in the other joints. At about 2 weeks a small aluminum splint immobilizing only the finger joint is used, and warm soaks are instituted. The finger is protected for 6 weeks after which, if there is evidence of fusion on roentgenograms, full use is allowed. The Kirschner wire may be removed with the area locally anesthetized if it produces symptoms.

Correction of Intrinsic Contracture (Swan-neck Deformity)

Soft tissue surgical procedures can often correct the swan-neck deformity as long as the proximal interphalangeal joint is reasonably normal. It is important to determine by roentgenograms of

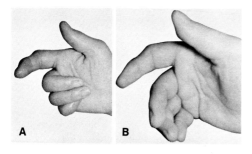

FIG. 8-65 Results of arthrodesis. A. Preoperative view shows the proximal interphalangeal joints fixed into the palm of the hand. B. A postoperative view of fingers fused in a position of function.

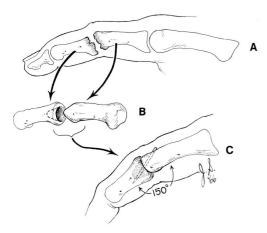

FIG. 8-67 Arthrodesis of the proximal inter-phalangeal joint. A. Destruction of the joint sur-face. B. Head of proximal phalanx shaped to fit into depression at base of middle phalanx. C. Joint compressed together and fixed with a Kirschner wire.

the hand the status of the joints. If there is extensive articular destruction and the deformity is firmly established, an in-trinsic soft tissue release will not correct the problem. In far-advanced cases arthrodesis may be necessary to fix the joint in a position of function or do an arthroplasty to replace the joint with a prosthesis if the tendon structures are still normal.

Bunnell described the first surgical treatment for correction of the swan-neck deformity. He stripped the interos-seous muscle from the shaft of the metacarpal and allowed it to slide dis-tally to lengthen the contracture. This approach to the problem, however, has not been too satisfactory and has been discarded by most surgeons.

In the past Littler has suggested that excising the oblique fibers of the exten-sor hood would release the contracture. This procedure has been of value in only the early stages of intrinsic contracture, and there is a tendency for the contrac-ture to recur.

Littler Release. The Littler release is intended for the patient with mild swan-neck deformities who has increasing

tightness of the intrinsic muscles. The finger may be approached through a midlateral incision exposing the oblique fibers on the ulnar side (Fig. 8-68). It is recommended that the fibers be released on the ulnar side only to prevent weak-ness of the radial structures which could contribute to further ulnar drift. The triangular section of the oblique fibers of the extensor hood is resected, leaving the central slip intact and cutting the lateral band. The transverse fibers of the hood are left intact to initiate flexion of the metacarpal-phalangeal joint and to hold the extensor tendon in its proper posi-tion over the metacarpal-phalangeal joint. It is not necessary to remove the ulnar side of the fifth finger because the intrinsic muscle inserts into the phalanx rather than into the hood.

The test for an adequate intrinsic

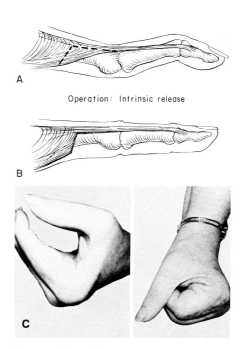

FIG. 8-68 The Littler release for intrinsic contrac-ture of the finger. A. The dotted line indicates the portion of the oblique fibers to be excised. B. The transverse fibers should be left intact. C. The pa-tient with severe intrinsic contractures of the fingers had improved function of the hand follow-ing intrinsic release.

release at the time of surgery is to maintain the metacarpal-phalangeal joint at 180° and to flex the proximal interphalangeal joint at least 90°. If this is not possible, it is necessary to resect more fibers of the hood. The incisions are closed, and the finger is placed in a position of function. Early flexion should be instituted under the direction of a therapist or the surgeon. Full extension of the joint should be avoided for at least 2 weeks and only flexion movements allowed.

Littler Tenodesis. Most soft tissue procedures have been developed in an attempt to produce a tenodesis across the proximal interphalangeal joint to prevent hyperextension and the recurrence of the swan-neck deformity. Littler has described a method of tenodesis using either a slip of the flexor sublimis tendon in the finger or one of the lateral bands.

The lateral band method is utilized quite frequently, and there are several minor variations possible. The finger may be approached through a lateral incision, with the dorsal flap being turned back to get complete exposure of the extensor mechanism or through a Z-type incision over the extensor surface of the finger (Fig. 8-69). The lateral band on the ulnar side can be carefully dissected out from the extensor hood and traced proximally and then distally to its insertion on the base of the distal phalanx to remove it from the oblique fibers. The slip of tendon is then carefully passed beneath Landsmeer's ligament below the axis of the proximal interphalangeal joint and sutured carefully into the flexor tendon sheath in the region of the proximal phalanx with the finger flexed approximately 20° to 30° at the proximal interphalangeal joint. This produces a check-rein effect, preventing hyperextension and the recurrence of the deformity. The opposite lateral band is left intact to maintain function of the distal phalanx (Fig. 8-71).

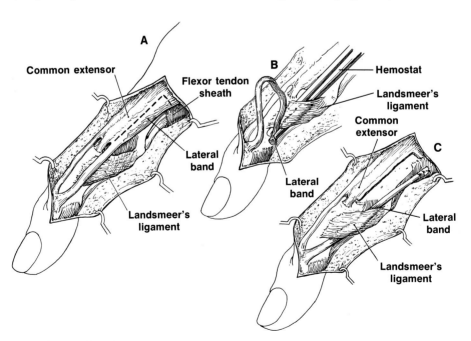

FIG. 8-69 Littler tenodesis for intrinsic contracture. A. The dotted line indicates the section of the lateral band to be dissected. B. The lateral band is dissected free from the central slip. C. The slip of the lateral band is passed beneath Landsmeer's ligament and sutured into the flexor tendon sheath.

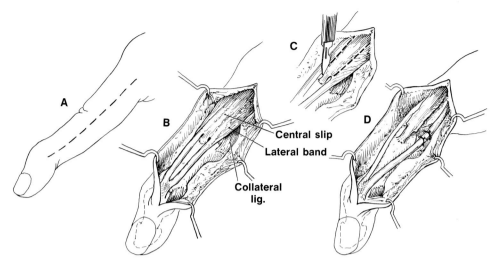

FIG. 8-71 Modification of the Littler tenodesis. A. Lateral approach to the finger is used. B. The collateral ligament is visualized along with the central slip. C. The lateral bands are dissected free from the central slip. D. With the finger flexed at the proximal interphalangeal joint, the lateral band is sutured into the collateral ligament below the axis of the proximal interphalangeal joint.

In a modification of this technique the lateral band is sutured into the collateral ligament at the proximal interphalangeal joint on the ulnar side. The fibers are cut obliquely, leaving the deep fibers intact, and then sewn over the lateral band to give a check-rein effect (Fig. 8-70).

It is possible to take one slip of the flexor sublimis tendon and suture it into the middle phalanx through a drill hole in the bone. Swanson uses pull-out button technique and makes a trough in the cortical bone on the volar aspect. The tendon then will adhere to the bone, producing a tenodesis effect on the proximal interphalangeal joint that will prevent hyperextension.

Mallet Finger

A synovitis may also occur in the distal finger joint or in the interphalangeal joint of the thumb. The synovitis can proliferate up through the capsule of the joint, leading to destruction of the attachment of the extensor tendon to the distal phalanx. This will result in the development of a mallet finger or loss of extension at the distal interphalangeal joint. If a deformity is severe, arthrodesis is probably the best method of treating this problem.

Arthrodesis

Arthrodesis of the distal interphalangeal joint is best performed by making a small tunnel in the base of the distal phalanx with a rongeur and curettes and rounding off the head of the middle phalanx. The two can be fitted together reasonably well and a Kirschner wire, 0.045 inches in diameter, can be drilled down the medullary shaft and out beneath the nail of the finger. The finger is then placed in the corrected position, and the wire is then drilled from the distal end, retrograde, into the middle phalanx with the finger in slight flexion of 10°. The wire is cut off subcutaneously in pulp of the finger so that it can be removed easily under local anesthesia in approximately 6 weeks. An aluminum splint can be used postoperatively for protection for about 3

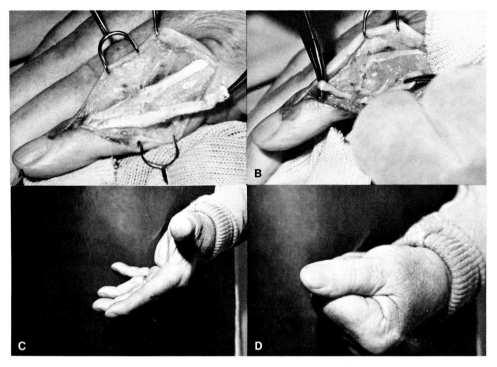

FIG. 8-70 Littler technique for correcting intrinsic contracture. A. The lateral band has been dissected free from the central slip. B. The lateral band has been passed beneath Landsmeer's ligament. C. Extension is improved postoperatively in a patient who had severe limitation. D. Full flexion is possible.

weeks, and if the patient allows the finger nail to grow out, it protects the area surrounding the pin from becoming irritated with use of the hand.

Carpal-Metacarpal Joint of the Thumb

The thumb differs from the remainder of the fingers because it has the greatest range of motion at the carpal-metacarpal joint and has only two phalanges rather than three. The hypermobile metacarpal-carpal joint is dependent on its collateral ligaments for stability. The tendon of the abductor pollicis longus attaches to the radial side of the base of the first metacarpal, and the tendon of the extensor pollicis brevis gives some fibers to the extensor hood and also inserts into the base of the proximal phalanx (Fig. 8-72). Because of

its attachment to the extensor hood, it may assist in extending the metacarpal-phalangeal joint, as well as the interphalangeal joint. The extensor pollicis longus passes on the ulnar side of the thumb to insert into the base of the distal phalanx. The long extensor can extend the metacarpal-phalangeal joint and the interphalangeal joint, as well as adduct the thumb into the plane of the palm of the hand. The adductor pollicis brings the thumb toward the palm and inserts into the ulnar side of the base of the proximal phalanx of the thumb (Fig. 8-73). The adductor has two heads, the oblique and the transversus.

Three basic types of deformities are seen in rheumatoid arthritis of the thumb:

1. A boutonnière type of deformity which involves primarily the metacarpal-phalangeal joint.

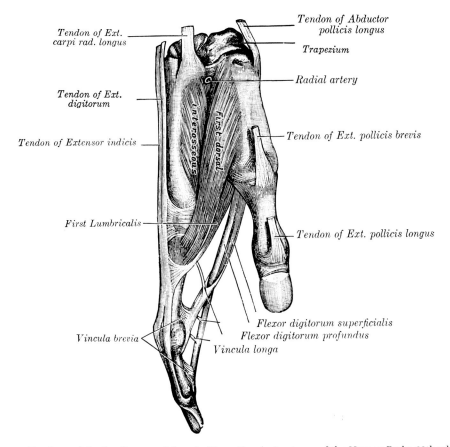

FIG. 8-72 Tendons of the forefinger and thumb. (From Gray's Anatomy of the Human Body, 29th ed. C. M. Goss, editor. Philadelphia, Lea & Febiger, 1973.)

2. The swan-neck deformity which primarily involves the carpal-metacarpal joint.

3. Pain, stiffness, or instability of the carpal-metacarpal, metacarpal-phalangeal, and interphalangeal joints.

The carpal-metacarpal joint is a saddle type of joint that is important in opposition, flexion, extension, abduction, and rotation of the thumb. Although the disease process in general affects more than one joint of the thumb at a time, occasionally the major involvement may be in the carpal-metacarpal joint (Fig. 8-74). Altered function at the carpal-metacarpal joint will lead to secondary changes in the distal joints. The synovial disease will destroy the integrity of the joint, allowing subluxation or dislocation of the metacarpal on the trapezium. This usually is not painful late in the disease and in the subluxed thumb, the examiner can feel the metacarpal sliding up and out of the joint, but the patient has reasonably good function with hypermobility of the thumb. Restricted motion with pain tends to adduct the thumb, limiting the web space considerably. Repeated attempts by the patient to hold large objects produces a hyperextension deformity at the metacarpal-phalangeal joint. Gradually this hyperextension deformity becomes fixed, and flexion of the proximal phalanx on the metacarpal gradually is lost, resulting in a swan-neck deformity of the thumb (Fig. 8-75).

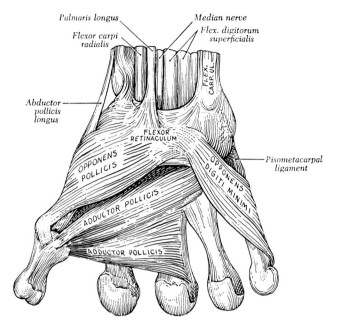

FIG. 8-73 The muscles of the thumb. (From Gray's Anatomy of the Human Body, 29th ed. C. M. Goss, editor. Philadelphia, Lea & Febiger, 1973.)

Arthrodesis of the carpal-metacarpal joint in rheumatoid arthritis is not advised because of the disability which is usually present in the other joints of the thumb and the loss of motion that results from arthrodesis.

At times the carpal-metacarpal joint may have spontaneously fused, and if the thumb is adducted or in a poor position, resection of the trapezium is

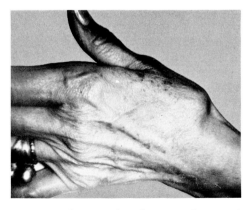

FIG. 8-74 Rheumatoid arthritis in the carpal-metacarpal joint. Note the subluxation and dislocation of the base of the thumb.

indicated to produce an arthroplasty. The insertion of a Silastic prosthesis can be considered in this type of deformity. If the adductor muscle is contracted, stripping the attachment of the adductor to the thumb or releasing it from the third metacarpal is of value to improve the grasp of the thumb and to improve web space.

In the swan-neck deformity with collapse of the metacarpal-phalangeal joint and subluxation of the carpal-metacarpal joint, the treatment of choice is generally to replace the trapezium with a Silastic prosthesis and fuse the metacarpal-phalangeal joint of the thumb in a position of function of about 20° to 25° of flexion. If there is a full range of motion in the metacarpal-phalangeal joint, it is not necessary to consider arthrodesis. It is only indicated when there is a loss of flexion at the metacarpal-phalangeal joint of the thumb. If the interphalangeal joint is dislocated or destroyed, arthrodesis can be combined with this procedure.

A severe boutonnière deformity is

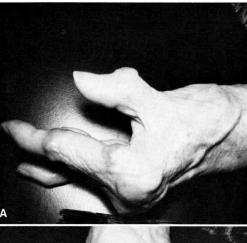

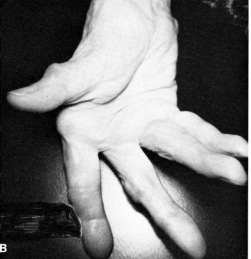

FIG. 8-75 Swan-neck deformity related to subluxation of the carpal-metacarpal joint of the thumb. A. Lateral view. B. Volar view.

usually accompanied by dislocation of the metacarpal-phalangeal joint and a hyperextension dislocation at the interphalangeal joint. Arthrodesis of both joints will produce a functioning thumb (Fig. 8-76).

Arthroplasty, Excisional Type

Excisional arthroplasty is a well-recognized procedure for regaining motion and restoring function of the joints of the body. Excisional arthroplasty can be considered in the treatment of rheumatoid arthritis of the carpal-metacarpal joint when there is ankylosis, limited function, or severe pain.

Operative Technique. An incision is made along the radial border of the metacarpal-carpal joint paralleling the extensor pollicis brevis tendon. The superficial sensory branch of the radial nerve passes on the dorsal side of the incision, and care must be taken not to injure the nerve during the approach or closure. The capsule of the joint is carefully opened longitudinally, and an attempt is made to preserve as much of the attachment as possible for closure after the excision of the trapezium. The dorsal surface of the trapezium is exposed, and in the proximal area the branch of the radial artery, should be protected from injury. It is possible to remove the bone in one large piece, but it is generally easier to excise it piecemeal, using a rongeur. It may even be necessary to free the base of the first metacarpal from the radial side of the second metacarpal, since occasionally the two may be fused together by the disease process. The flexor carpi radialis tendon should be carefully preserved in the depth of the wound beneath the undersurface of the trapezium. The trapezium is a large bone, and one is often confused by its size and tends to take less bone than is indicated. The articular surface of the navicular, as well as the side of the second metacarpal and the trapezoid bone, should be visible. After removal of the trapezium, the area can be filled either with Gelfoam or a portion of tendon as recommended by Froimson. The capsule is repaired, and the thumb is dressed in abduction and opposition for approximately 3 weeks to maintain the proper position and allow for scar tissue to form and preserve the position of the base of the thumb.

The thumb can be released if fixed in the palm because of soft tissue contracture. A dorsal incision is made along the

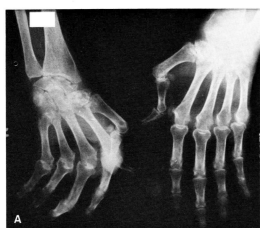

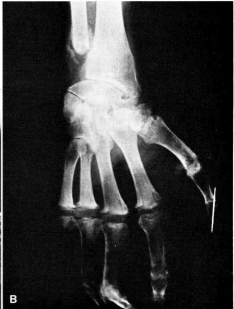

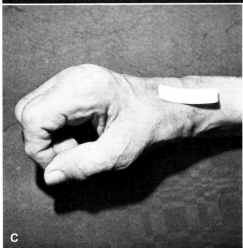

FIG. 8-76 Arthrodesis for boutonnière deformity of the thumb. A. Roentgenogram before surgery reveals collapse of the metacarpal-phalangeal joint and the interphalangeal joint. B. Roentgenogram after arthrodesis and a Swanson arthroplasty of the metacarpal-phalangeal joints 2, 3, 4, and 5 reveals the solid arthrodesis of the metacarpal-phalangeal joint of the thumb, as well as of the interphalangeal joint. The Kirschner wire is still in place in the interphalangeal joint. The Swanson prostheses are visible in the metacarpal-phalangeal joints. C. Photograph reveals the cosmetic appearance of the thumb, as well as the stability and excellent pinch obtained with arthrodesis of the metacarpal-phalangeal and the interphalangeal joints.

shaft of the first metacarpal from the base of the shaft to the metacarpal-phalangeal joint as suggested by Flatt. This can be connected with a Z-plasty skin incision (Fig. 8-77). The first dorsal interosseous muscle is stripped from the shaft of the first metacarpal to gain motion. The tendon of the adductor is located next and released from its insertion on the metacarpal of the thumb. The neurovascular bundle lies on the palmar side of the tendon and should be pro-

tected. The flaps of the skin are rotated to complete the Z-plasty, and the thumb is dressed in full opposition and abduction to open the web space. As soon as the wound is healed, stretching exercises should be instituted to increase the web space.

Implant Arthroplasty

The implant technique as described by Swanson utilizes the Silastic trape-

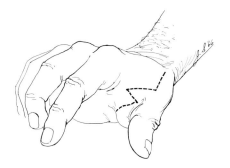

FIG. 8-77 A Z-plasty of the skin with release of the adductor tendon to increase the web space of the thumb.

zium prosthesis. A similar approach is made as for an excisional arthroplasty.

Operative Technique. After removal of the trapezium, the base of the thumb is flattened, and any osteophytes and sclerotic bone are removed. The surface should be smooth to prevent any sharp spicules from damaging the Silastic prosthesis. The medullary canal is then drilled with a power tool to open the canal prior to the use of a reamer or curette. Five sizes of Silastic implants are available, and the trial sizes should be inserted to find one that will adequately fill the defect left by the trapezium. The trial is inserted and tested to see if the thumb is reasonably stable. One of the problems encountered with this type of procedure is that there is a tendency for subluxation of the prosthesis outward from the navicular, producing a deformity and prominence. It is important to preserve as much of the capsule as possible for repair, and if necessary, it can be reinforced with the surrounding tissue, including the abductor pollicis longus tendon.

A modification suggested by Swanson uses the flexor carpi radialis tendon. The tendon is passed dorsally and radially around the metacarpal rather than through the shaft. The distal insertion of the flexor carpi radialis is left attached to the base of the second metacarpal, and a half of the tendon is split

and retracted distally and passed around the abductor pollicis longus tendon and through a rent in the capsule and then sutured over the dorsum of the capsule to reinforce the area and prevent subluxation of the trapezium. It is always advantageous to advise the patient preoperatively that there may be some subluxation of the base of the thumb and although there is a prominence, it generally will be painless and will not interfere with the function of the hand.

If there is a hyperextension or fixed deformity at the metacarpal-phalangeal joint, it should be fused prior to closure of the capsule to prevent disruption of the sutures and the repair at the carpalmetacarpal joint.

Metacarpal-Phalangeal Joint of the Thumb

The synovial swelling produced by rheumatoid arthritis in the metacarpalphalangeal joint will stretch the capsule and extensor hood and result in a flexion deformity that progresses to subluxation and finally dislocation (Fig. 8-78A). It is important in considering surgical procedures on the metacarpal-phalangeal joint of the thumb to inspect the carpalmetacarpal joint as well as the interphalangeal joint (Fig. 8-78B). If the interphalangeal joint is stable, it need not be included in surgical procedures on the metacarpal-phalangeal joint.

Arthrodesis

Early in the course of rheumatoid disease of the thumb, soft tissue repair has been suggested by some authors, and synovectomy can be carried out at the time of transfer of the intrinsics of the thumb to the short extensor attachment. Arthrodesis in general is the operation of choice in advanced disease of the metacarpal-phalangeal joint (Fig. 8-79).

Operative Technique. Under tourni-

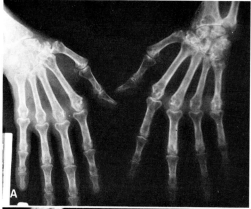

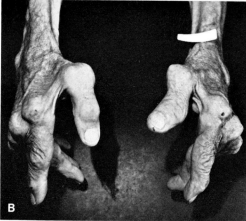

FIG. 8-78 Rheumatoid arthritis of the hand. A. Roentgenogram revealing erosions of the joints due to synovitis. Note the beginning subluxation and the punched-out lesions of the metacarpal-phalangeal joint of the thumb. B. Photograph showing dislocations of the metacarpal-phalangeal joints of the thumbs in an advanced stage of the disease.

quet control, a slightly curved incision is made over the metacarpal-phalangeal joint of the thumb. The extensor hood is exposed and opened on the radial side and retracted out of the way. The synovial tissue is excised along with the collateral ligaments to expose the metacarpal head (Fig. 8-80). The metacarpal head is shaped into a round ball with a rongeur or various finger reamers (Fig. 8-80A). The base of the proximal phalanx is reamed with a matching ball

reamer to develop a cup for acceptance of the rounded metacarpal head (Fig. 8-80B). The two are impacted together in approximately 10° of flexion at the metacarpal-phalangeal joint. A Kirschner wire 0.045 inches in diameter is drilled across from the metacarpal through the joint into the proximal phalanx (Fig. 8-80C). Generally one wire is adequate and prevents distraction of the joint surfaces and is better than using crossed wires. The wire is cut off subcutaneously, and the extensor mechanism is repaired with 4-0 silk sutures. A soft bulky dressing with a plaster splint may be utilized for about 10 days, and

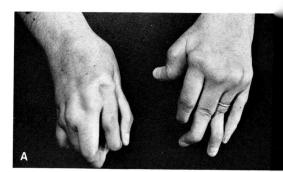

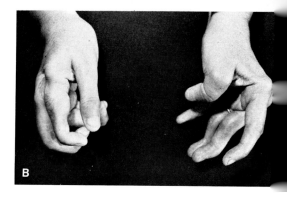

FIG. 8-79 The hands of a young woman with severe deformities. The right thumb shows a fixed hyperextension deformity at the metacarpal-phalangeal joint, subluxation of the carpal-metacarpal joint, and fixed flexion of the distal thumb joint. The left hand has a severe flexion deformity of the metacarpal-phalangeal joint and an unstable interphalangeal joint. A. Dorsal view. B. Lateral view.

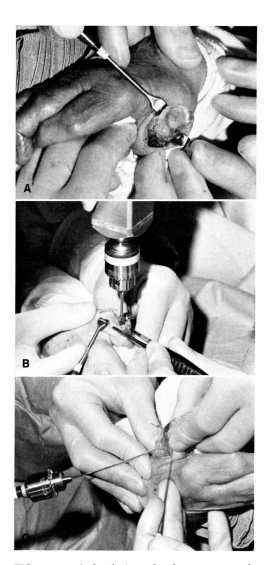

FIG. 8-80 Arthrodesis of the metacarpal-phalangeal joint of the thumb. A. The metacarpal head is rounded into a ball. B. Developing a depression in the base of the phalanx to form a socket for the rounded metacarpal head. C. Drilling a Kirschner wire across the joint to fix it in a position of function.

then an aluminum splint can be taped to the hand to prevent displacement of the operated area. Generally, within 6 weeks union has occurred, and the wire can then be removed under local anesthesia. Frequently the thumb may be fused at the time of reconstruction of the entire hand.

If a boutonnière deformity is present with hyperextension and complete dislocation of the interphalangeal joint (Fig. 8-81). Then it is suggested that an arthrodesis of the distal joint be carried out at the same time. This joint can be fused in 10° to 15° of flexion as required by the patient. The distal interphalangeal joint is fused generally through a separate transverse incision, and the long extensor tendon is detached from the base of the distal phalanx. The capsule and synovial tissue are excised along with the collateral ligaments and the head of the proximal phalanx is shaped into a small ball with a rongeur or with reamers of a power tool. The base of the phalanx is tunneled out with a curette or with a small ball reamer. The two are interdigitated together for a good snug fit. The joint is then taken apart, and the Kirschner wire is drilled retrograde out through the tunnel in the distal phalanx, under the nail, and through the pulp of the finger. After the two bones have been impacted together, the wire is drilled into the proximal phalanx for good stability. The wire is cut off beneath the nail and allowed to disappear under the skin. It should be left in place approximately 6 weeks and then removed. Occasionally two wires are necessary to maintain coaptation. The shortening incurred by the interdigitation of the bones tends to relax any intrinsic contracture and improve the function of the thumb.

Extensor Tendon Rupture

Rheumatoid arthritis of the extensor pollicis longus frequently results in rupture of the tendon and loss of extension of the distal phalanx of the thumb. The site of the disease process is near Lister's tubercle where a synovial proliferation will result in attrition and rupture of the tendon (Fig. 8-82). The rupture is generally painless and the patient will consult

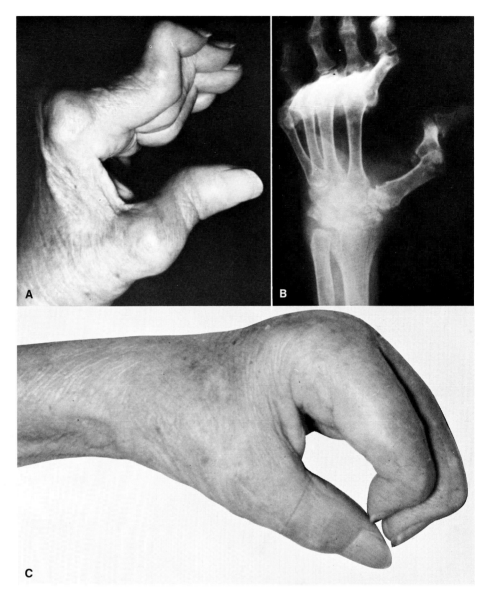

FIG. 8-81 Correction of boutonnière deformity of the thumb. A. Preoperative photograph showing flexion of the metacarpal-phalangeal joint and hyperextension of the interphalangeal joint. B. Roentgenogram revealing destruction of the thumb. C. Improvement of thumb in pinch after arthrodesis of the metacarpal-phalangeal and interphalangeal joints.

his physician because of a loss of extension of the thumb. Surgical repair generally consists of tendon transfer at the wrist. The indicis proprius can be utilized as a motor and sutured to the remaining distal portion of the extensor pollicis longus.

Flexor Tenosynovitis

Rheumatoid arthritis often produces a stenosing flexor tenosynovitis of the tendon sheaths of the hand or "trigger" finger that is frequently overlooked because of the long-standing complaints

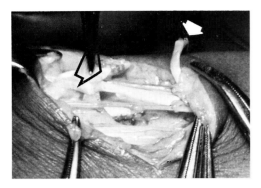

FIG. 8-82 Surgical view of rupture of the extensor tendon of the thumb (arrows).

of the arthritis patient. The process starts as a synovitis producing a thick boggy swelling involving both the tendon and its sheath. Scudamore reported the occurrence of tenosynovitis in 1827, and Necker in 1893 regarded "trigger fingers" as rheumatoid in origin. Heleveg in 1924 reported "snapping" tendons associated with rheumatoid disease, and Edstrom in Sweden noted that 42 percent of chronic rheumatoid patients showed involvement of the tendons in their hands. The most common location was in the flexor tendons. Howard in 1955 described an operation for the surgical treatment of rheumatoid tenosynovitis, and Jacobs, Hess, and Beswick in 1957 reported cases in which the earliest sign of rheumatoid disease was involvement of the synovium of the tendon sheaths. There are four basic types of involvement: (1) a rheumatoid nodule may occur in the tendon proximal to the sheath which will cause locking in flexion, (2) in less severe cases, there will be a snapping finger, (3) the nodule may be in the profundus tendon distal to the bifurcation of the sublimis and cause locking in extension, and (4) extensive involvement of the entire sheath may result in stiffness without snapping of the finger.

Pathologic changes in the synovial-lined tendon sheaths consist of a villus hypertrophy with an increase of the stroma, infiltration with lymphocytes, and hypertrophy of the lining cells. The synovium is heaped up in villus folds, infiltrates the flexor tendons, and gradually destroys them. Interference with the normal blood supply by the proliferating granulation tissue also contributes to the destruction of the tendon. Nodule formation within the flexor tendons in rheumatoid disease will produce a "locking" or "snapping" of the finger. The nodule frequently occurs on the profundus tendon and tends to catch at the bifurcation of the sublimis over the proximal phalanx.

The first clinically recognizable condition seen in early rheumatoid involvement of the hand is that of "snapping" or "triggering" of the finger. The patient will complain of pain in the finger, especially in the region of the proximal interphalangeal joint, rather than over the palmar crease and the finger may stick or catch when flexed into the palm, requiring the patient to extend the involved finger forcibly with the other hand. Slight pressure exerted by the examiner's finger over the distal palmar crease of the involved finger or fingers will produce pain, and the nodule can often be palpated as the patient forcibly flexes the finger. It is also important to palpate over the volar surface of the phalanx to rule out a nodule in the profundus tendon catching in the sublimis bifurcation. Thickening of the finger can be seen if there is a synovial proliferation in the digital sheath (Fig. 8-83).

The patient usually has a history of triggering of the fingers, but this disappears as the disease progresses. The tendons no longer slide through the narrow tunnel and tend to bind because of the synovial thickening about the flexor tendons (Fig. 8-84). The patient will complain of stiffness of the fingers, especially in the morning, and the inability to flex fully, although there is no pain. This syndrome can occur with or

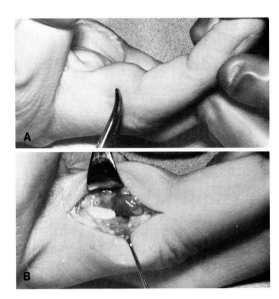

FIG. 8-83 Flexor tenosynovitis. A. Thickening of the finger as a result of synovial proliferation in the digital sheath. B. Operative procedure revealing the proliferating rheumatoid synovium covering the flexor tendon.

without finger-joint involvement. Whenever a patient with rheumatoid arthritis cannot flex his fingers actively and the proximal interphalangeal joint is not stiff or ankylosed, stenosing tenosynovitis of the flexor tendons should be suspected. Three things are pathognomonic of late stenosing tenosynovitis: the ability to move the joints of the finger passively

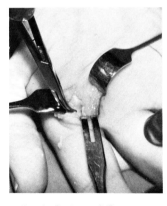

FIG. 8-84 Surgical view of flexor tenosynovitis. The clamp points to the flexor tendon sheath which is stretched and swollen by the synovial tissue.

through a good range of motion; the ability of the examiner to flex the finger into the palm further than the patient can actively do so; and the palpation of crepitus over the flexor sheath in the palm.

Conservative Treatment. If tenosynovitis is in an early stage and has not been present for many months, improvement can be obtained with the local injection of hydrocortisone and an anesthetic into the tendon sheath. The needle is inserted into the palm at the distal skin crease over the involved tendon sheath, and the injection is made distally. This injection is also utilized as a diagnostic test because, if the patient improves for a short while because of the antiinflammatory effect of the steroid, one can be certain that surgical release will provide a more permanent result. If relief of symptoms does not occur with an injection, a rheumatoid nodule should be suspected.

Tenosynovectomy

Operative Technique. The patient may be prepared for a tenosynovectomy by an axillary block. Under tourniquet control a 1-inch incision is made parallel to the tendon in the palm from the web space to the distal palmar crease between the metacarpal heads. In order to avoid pain from the scar, the incision should not be placed over the bony prominences of the metacarpal head or base of the phalanx. If this incision is properly placed between the tendons, it allows the flexor tendons of the second and third fingers to be released through one incision and those of the fourth and fifth fingers through another (Fig. 8-85). The thumb is released through a transverse incision in the proximal skin crease at the base of the proximal phalanx.

The operation must be done under tourniquet control to allow adequate

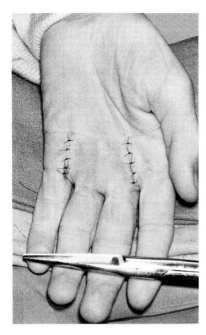

FIG. 8-85 Flexor tenosynovectomy. Two incisions, one between the metacarpal heads of 2 and 3 and another between those of 4 and 5, allow the flexor tendons of the four fingers to be released through two incisions, and the scar is not over the metacarpal head where it can be painful.

visualization of the digital nerves and vessels. The tendon sheath will be thickened and filled with synovial tissue (Fig. 8-82B). It should be completely split over the proximal phalanx. By lifting the flexor digitorum profundus and sublimis tendons from the sheath, the bifurcation of the sublimis can be visualized to reveal a nodule on the profundus tendon or a constriction of the sublimis tendon bifurcation.

If the sublimis is constricted, the opening may be easily enlarged by splitting the tendon proximally. The thickened sheath, as well as all the synovium, may be partially excised.

The patient is encouraged to use his fingers as much as possible postoperatively. The sutures should be left in place for 2 weeks.

If a more extensive procedure is necessary, a transverse skin incision parallel to the distal palmar crease will give adequate exposure. Patients who have synovial thickening in the sheath over the proximal and middle phalanges are best operated upon through a mid-lateral incision along the finger.

Results. Many patients have a dramatic return of function after flexor tenosynovectomies. A 21-year-old girl had a three-year history of rheumatoid arthritis with gradual loss of flexion of her fingers on both hands (Fig. 8-86). Examination revealed loss of active flexion, but passive motion was complete. Roentgenograms showed no evidence of joint involvement. At operation the tendon sheaths of the right hand were found to be thickened and filled with edematous granulation tissue. Surgical release of the flexor tendons made full flexion possible in the right hand and improved flexion in the left hand (Fig. 8-87).

Flexor Tendon Rupture

Prolonged involvement of the digital sheaths with invasion of the tendons gradually leads to rupture of the flexor tendons within the sheath between the middle phalanx and the distal palmar crease. Erosion and invasion of the tendon mass by proliferating synovium and granulation tissue tend to weaken the tendon. Avascular necrosis also occurs due to prolonged compression and interruption of the blood supply.

The patient usually has a history of rheumatoid tenosynovitis preceding the rupture of a flexor tendon. When the rupture occurs, it is in general not painful, but the patient may note some discomfort and the inability to use the involved finger. If only the sublimis tendon ruptures, the loss may go unnoticed by the patient. To determine the loss of the sublimis tendon the remaining fingers of the hand should be hyperextended with the profundus tendon fixed so that

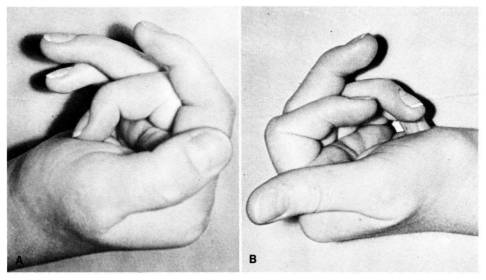

FIG. 8-86 Flexor tenosynovitis. A. Flexion of the fingers was limited in the right and left hands. B. Active motion in the left hand was equal to that seen in the illustration, but complete passive flexion of the fingers was possible.

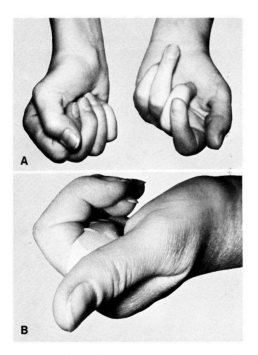

FIG. 8-87 After a flexor tenosynovectomy. A. The flexor tendons have been surgically released in the right hand, and full flexion is now possible. B. The left hand immediately after surgical release reveals the improvement of the flexion of the fingers.

flexion is impossible. Then the suspected finger is left free, and the patient attempts flexion. If the finger flexes at the proximal interphalangeal joint, the sublimis is intact (Fig. 8-88A). The profundus may be tested by stabilizing the proximal interphalangeal joint, leaving the distal joint free to flex (Fig. 8-88B). If the patient can forcefully flex the finger, the profundus tendon is intact.

Exploration of the ruptured tendon usually reveals that the ends are frayed and the tendon is covered by brownish synovial tissue because of old hemosiderin (Fig. 8-89A). When the profundus tendon ruptures, it will sometimes retract into the palm of the hand. The proximal end may wrap around the sublimis tendon and cause discomfort (Fig. 8-89B).

If the sublimis alone is ruptured, repair is not indicated, since the profundus will function quite well.

Tendon Graft

If both flexors rupture, the sheath should be cleaned out and a free tendon

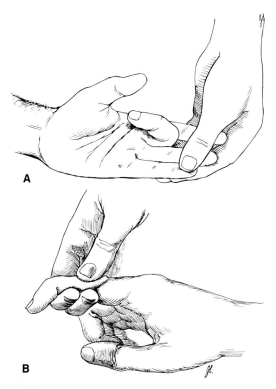

FIG. 8-88 Tests for rupture of the flexor tendons. A. The test for sublimis function in a finger. B. The test for profundus function in a finger.

graft inserted. The sublimis tendon should not be repaired, but only the profundus. The proximal portion of the sublimis may be utilized as a free graft if it is in good condition; otherwise the palmaris longus tendon should be selected.

Operative Technique. A skin incision is made in the palm of the hand under tourniquet control to expose the proximal portion of the digital tendon sheath, and another incision is made along the lateral aspect of the finger. The tendon sheath and all proliferating synovium should be excised, leaving the annular ligaments to prevent bowstringing of the graft. The sublimis tendon is removed, and a small slip of profundus is left attached to the distal phalanx. The remaining tendon is split longitudinally, and the distal phalanx is roughened at the attachment of the tendon. A pull-out wire is utilized with a button to attach the distal end of the graft, and the remaining profundus tendon is sutured about the distal graft. The graft is then

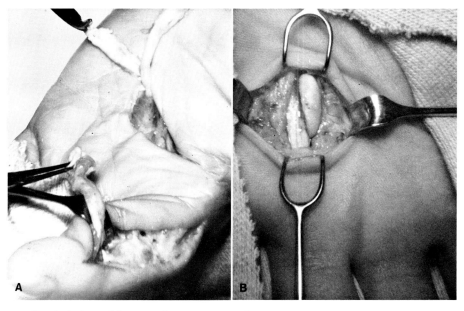

FIG. 8-89 Surgical views of flexor tendon ruptures. A. The proximal and distal ends of the ruptured tendon to the index finger are visible in the photograph. B. The ruptured profundus tendon has retracted into the palm of the hand, and the proximal end is wrapped around the sublimis tendon.

placed beneath the annular ligaments and brought into the palmar incision. The proximal profundus tendon is cut off in the palm, and the graft is sutured to the proximal profundus tendon. The correct tension is most difficult to determine, but it should flex the repaired finger slightly more than the other fingers with the wrist in the position of function.

The hand is immobilized with a plaster slab with the wrist and fingers flexed. Great care must be used because of the rheumatoid patient's tendency to stiffen rapidly. The plaster should be removed in two weeks and careful, controlled exercises of the fingers and wrist instituted.

Osteoarthritis

Osteoarthritis frequently results in deformities of the distal interphalangeal joints as well as of the proximal interphalangeal joints of the hand. Kellgren and Moore and Wardle have described a primary generalized osteoarthritis that occurs in middle-aged women and involves the hands. In 1961 Crain reported 23 patients with interphalangeal osteoarthritis. He described this disease as "a localized form of arthritis involving the finger joints, characterized by degenerative changes with intermittent inflammatory episodes leading eventually to deformities and ankylosis." The patients described by Crain were predominantly middle-aged women with disease confined to the cervical spine and the interphalangeal joints of the hand (Fig. 8-90).

Osteoarthritis of the hands tends to present two types of disease. One type of patient tends to have Heberden's nodes primarily and the other type the patient has an erosive disease of the proximal interphalangeal joints associated with Heberden's nodes, but with no clinical evidence of rheumatoid arthritis (Fig. 8-91). This type of erosive osteoarthritis is not rare and seems to represent an advanced form of type 1 with Heberden's nodes. Pathologic specimens taken from both types are identical in many respects.

Erosive osteoarthritis of the hand, which produces swelling and destructive changes, is frequently misdiagnosed as rheumatoid arthritis. The two diseases can be distinguished by clinical, laboratory, and roentgenographic characteristics. Erosive osteoarthritis can produce severe destruction in the finger joints but does not involve the larger joints nor does it produce systemic symptoms such as fever, weight loss, or anemia. In contrast to rheumatoid arthritis, erosive osteoarthritis of the hands characteristically affects the distal interphalangeal joint early and affects the proximal interphalangeal joint later in the disease (Fig. 8-92). It is not associated with the typical rheumatoid deformities of the hand, such as ulnar drift, swan-neck, or boutonnière deformities. The sedimentation rate is usually normal, and the latex fixation test is negative. Rheumatoid arthritis tends to produce osteoporosis in the hand when the disease is active, but osteoporosis is absent in erosive osteoarthritis.

Osteoarthritis in the hand can remain localized to the distal interphalangeal joint, or it may also involve the proximal interphalangeal joint. Occasionally the disease will start in the proximal interphalangeal joint rather than in the distal joints. Pain and swelling are characteristic of this disease, and the joints tend to enlarge with the formation of bony osteophytes (Fig. 8-93). In contrast to rheumatoid arthritis, however, there is no early morning gel phenomenon nor is there involvement of the metacarpalphalangeal joints. Roentgenograms re-

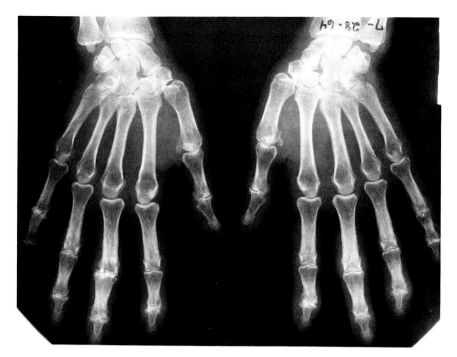

FIG. 8-90 Roentgenogram showing evidence of osteoarthritis in the proximal interphalangeal and the distal interphalangeal joints. Characteristically, the metacarpal-phalangeal and the carpal joints are normal.

veal destruction of the bone around the distal interphalangeal joint with little osteoporosis. Sclerosis of the articular surfaces and osteophytes are present early before the destructive phase starts (Fig. 8-93B, C). These can be associated with osteoarthritic changes in the carpal-metacarpal joint of the thumb.

Proximal Interphalangeal Joint

The patient with osteoarthritis with involvement of the proximal inter-phalangeal joint can be at one of two stages of the disease. In the early stage, the synovium has an invasive character and tends to erode the bone and con-tribute to the patient's symptoms. During this early stage, synovectomy may give reasonably good results and arrest the disease process. For the patient with a severely painful and unstable joint and radiologic evidence of complete destruc-tion, arthrodesis would be the operation of choice or arthroplasty with a Silastic

implant. In the past, the proximal inter-phalangeal joint of the toe has been grafted to replace the proximal inter-phalangeal joint of the hand. However, since the joint tends to go on to ankylosis or limited motion, the surgical procedure is not justified.

Synovectomy

The patient with erosive osteo-arthritis with a very active synovitis can be aided by synovectomy if the joint is reasonably stable and does not have advanced destruction.

Operative Technique. The operation is performed under tourniquet control, and a transverse incision is made over the proximal interphalangeal joint, ex-posing the extensor tendon. The joint may be approached from either the radial or ulnar side first by carefully incising along the edge of the lateral band and lifting the band upward. The synovial tissue tends to herniate up

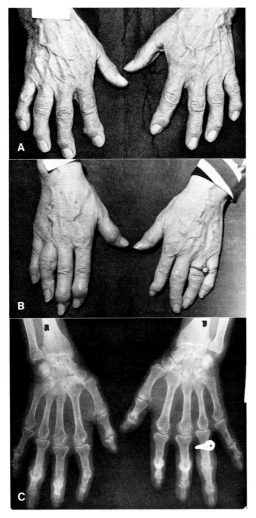

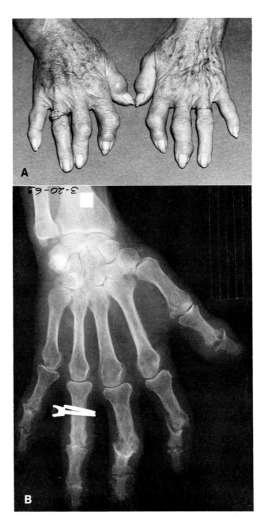

FIG. 8-91 Osteoarthritis of the hands with involvement of the distal interphalangeal joints. A. This patient has active disease with radial deviation and formation of Heberden's nodes. B. A patient with active swelling and involvement of the proximal interphalangeal joint of the fourth finger of the right hand and both distal joints of the thumb. C. Roentgenogram revealing destruction of the proximal interphalangeal joints. Note that there is no evidence of disease in the metacarpalphalangeal joints as would be common in rheumatoid arthritis.

FIG. 8-92 Erosive osteoarthritis of the hands. A. Photograph showing the characteristic swelling of the proximal interphalangeal joints. This type of swelling should not be confused with the spindletype swelling seen in early rheumatoid arthritis. The metacarpal-phalangeal joints show no evidence of the swelling usually seen in rheumatoid disease. B. Roentgenogram showing synovial invasion of the proximal interphalangeal joints and destruction of the joint surfaces. There are no evidences of the disease in the metacarpal-phalangeal joints.

under the central slip and forms a large sack that protrudes both laterally, medially, and superiorly. This sack can be excised from the joint along with the capsule, but the central slip must be

carefully preserved to the base of the middle phalanx. The best way to remove this tissue is to use a fine rongeur or small curettes and scrape the synovium along the edges of the articular margins.

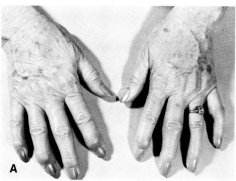

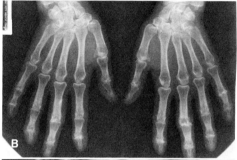

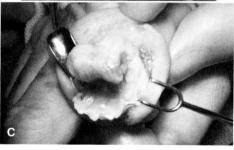

FIG. 8-93 Osteoarthritis of the hands. A. Photograph shows the painful swelling of the distal interphalangeal joints and involvement of the proximal interphalangeal joint of the third fingers. B. The roentgenogram reveals the characteristic changes of osteoarthritis. C. Surgical view reveals that the osteoarthritic joints are devoid of articular cartilage and have numerous ridges from constant rubbing of the bony surfaces. The synovial disease has subsided.

This approach can be carried out from both sides of the joint to allow removal of most of the synovial tissue. After removal of the synovial tissue, the extensor mechanism is allowed to fall back into place. The collateral ligaments have been preserved so that stability has not been compromised. The skin incision is closed, and a dressing applied. The patient is allowed to exercise the fingers as soon as he can comfortably do so postoperatively to regain as much motion as possible.

Arthroplasty

Arthrodesis was at one time the operation of choice in osteoarthritis of the proximal interphalangeal joints involved with severe disease and instability. However, the Silastic (Swanson) prosthesis has given good results in selected cases and certainly should be considered in those patients who desire to regain motion or maintain it (Fig. 8-94).

Operative Technique. The operation is performed under tourniquet control, and an incision is made along the ulnar side of the finger, midway between the dorsal and volar surface, toward the distal interphalangeal joint and also proximally toward the metacarpalphalangeal joint. The skin flap is lifted up and pulled toward the radial side, exposing the extensor mechanism. The lateral band is carefully dissected free from the surrounding ligamentous attachments to the soft tissue and pulled upward to the base of the middle phalanx where the central slip is attached. The collateral ligament on the ulnar side is then cut on the bias so that it may be easily repaired on closure. This will allow the joint to rock open, giving good exposure of the entire joint. The head of the proximal phalanx should be removed with a rongeur to facilitate the insertion of the Swanson prosthesis. It is important to have some form of power tool to be able to ream out the medullary cavity, which is quite hard and narrow, in the phalanx. The base of the middle phalanx is also drilled out to accept the Swanson trial prosthesis.

Various sizes of prostheses are tried to find the one that fits the best, since

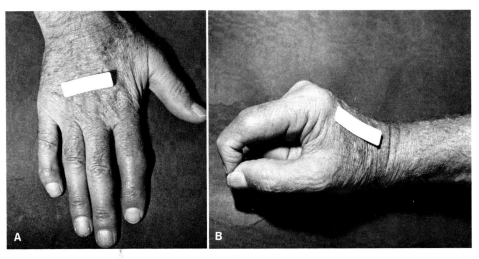

FIG. 8-94 Photographs of hand after Swanson arthroplasty for osteoarthritis involving the proximal interphalangeal joint of the index finger. A. Dorsal view. The index finger lacks 10° of full extension. There is a Heberden's node on the fifth finger. B. Lateral view. The patient has a good pinch and a limited range of motion in the proximal interphalangeal joint.

there is not much room to insert a prosthesis. If it fits well, then an adequate amount of bone has been removed. If it tends to buckle or is too tight, more bone should be removed until a good fit is obtained. The trial prosthesis is replaced with the permanent prosthesis. Then the collateral ligament is repaired with 4-0 silk sutures, and the extensor mechanism is allowed to drop back over the top of the finger. The skin is closed and a dressing applied. Generally, the finger will be quite stable. If there is any instability, an aluminum splint attached to the finger, with sponge rubber protecting the finger, will provide stability until healing has occurred. Leaving the radial collateral ligament tends to give excellent stability for pinching. With early motion, a fair degree of extension and flexion can be obtained without pain. If the arthroplasty were to fail, the finger still could be fused by adding a bone graft across the resected joint (Figs. 8-95; 8-96).

Arthrodesis

Arthrodesis has been the mainstay operation for destructive arthritis of the proximal interphalangeal joint. Arthrodesis can give a patient a strong, painless finger, but at the sacrifice of motion. If the finger is fused at approximately 30°, a cosmetic appearance as well as the best function can be obtained (Fig. 8-97). If more flexion is desired, the finger can be fused at 45°, but this is not cosmetically as acceptable to the patient.

Operative Technique. The operation of arthrodesis is performed under a tourniquet for hemostasis, and a midlateral incision is used, either on the radial or ulnar side. The skin flap is turned back, exposing the extensor mechanism (Fig. 8-98). Generally, the incisions are placed on the ulnar side of the finger, especially of the index finger, to prevent scarring which might cause discomfort on pinching.

If the distal interphalangeal joint, as well as the proximal, is to be fused, then one need not concern himself greatly with the extensor mechanism. If, however, only the proximal interphalangeal joint is to be fused, then the extensor mechanism must be preserved. The lateral band is carefully lifted up, and the central slip is dissected off the base of the middle phalanx and turned

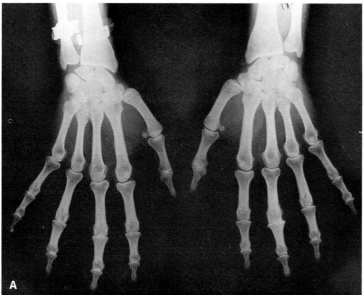

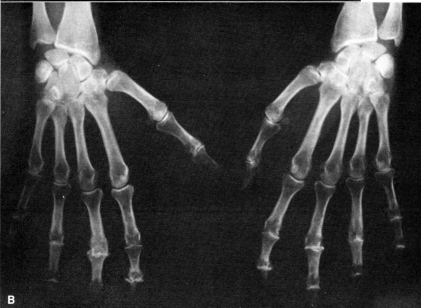

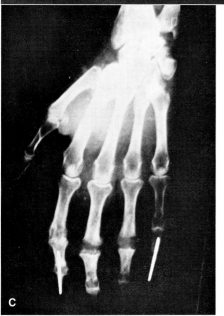

FIG. 8-95 Roentgenograms of hands with advanced osteoarthritis. A. Beginning stage. B. Ten years later. Advanced destruction of the finger joints is evident. C. After surgical correction of the distal interphalangeal joints of the left hand by Swanson arthroplasties of the third and fourth fingers and arthrodeses of the second and fifth fingers.

245

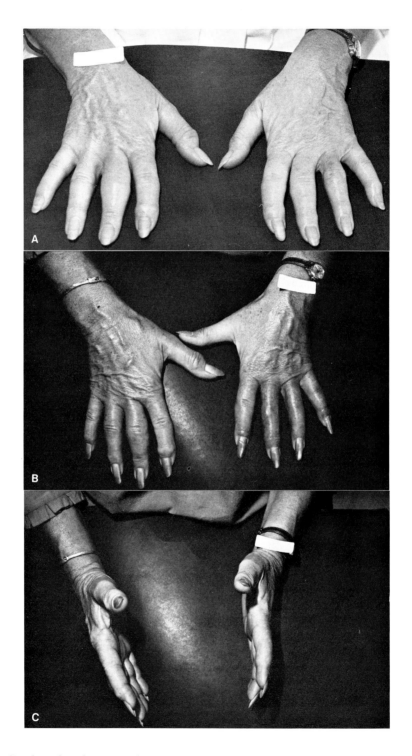

FIG. 8-96 (See legend on facing page.)

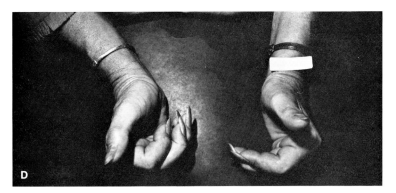

FIG. 8-96 Photographs of hands of patient with advanced osteoarthritis. A. Before surgical correction. Swelling indicates involvement of the proximal interphalangeal joints, Heberden's nodes are seen on some of the distal joints, and there is some deviation and instability. B. After surgical correction of the left hand by fusion of the distal interphalangeal joints of the second, and fifth fingers and a Swanson arthroplasty of the third and fourth fingers. C. Note cosmetic improvement in the left hand and patient's ability to open the hand without pain. A painful Heberden's node is on the index finger of the right hand. D. Flexion possible in the proximal interphalangeal joints of the left hand after operation.

toward the opposite side with the extensor mechanism. The collateral ligaments are divided, and the joint is rocked open like a book, giving excellent exposure. The proximal phalanx is rounded with a rongeur and polished with a small female reamer and a power tool. The base of the middle phalanx is drilled also with a power tool and a small bur to make an indentation for the proximal phalanx to fit into. If a good fit has been obtained, cancellous bone should be matching cancellous bone.

With the finger set about 30° of flexion and in neutral position, a Kirschner wire is drilled from the proximal phalanx across the joint into the middle phalanx for good fixation. The wire is cut off subcutaneously. The extensor mechanism is brought back over the top of the finger and dropped into place. The skin is closed, and a dressing is applied. The finger is usually splinted with an aluminum splint for 6 weeks to allow healing of the arthrodesis site. At 6 weeks, if a roentgenogram shows union, the Kirschner wire can be removed in the office under local anesthesia and with sterile technique. It is wise to have special Kirschner wire pliers or extractor

available, as it makes it much simpler to remove these wires when they are intrenched in the bone. The average wire is usually loose and can be removed with a straight clamp.

One of the problems arising in performing an arthrodesis in patients with severe erosive osteoarthritis is the loss of bone about the joint. In these problem cases, after removal of the synovium and reshaping of the joint surfaces to obtain as much bone contact as possible, a drill hole is made from the proximal phalanx into the middle phalanx, and a cortical bone peg is hammered across the joint along with a Kirschner wire. Bone chips are packed into the bony defects to aid in fusion. Immobilization should be maintained until there is radiologic evidence of solid union (Fig. 8-99).

Distal Interphalangeal Joint

Osteoarthritis can produce symptoms of pain and deformity in the distal interphalangeal joint. The earliest sign of osteoarthritis of this joint results from an active inflammatory condition of the synovium which produces a mucous cyst outpouching from the joint space (Fig.

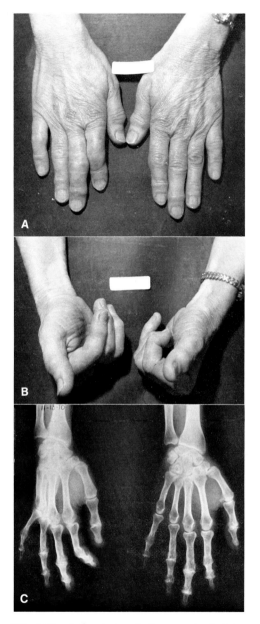

FIG. 8-97 Arthrodesis of the proximal interphalangeal joint of the index finger of the right hand. The patient, a secretary, complained of severe pain and limitation of the ability to pinch. A. Dorsal view. B. Flexion. The position of the index finger is approximately 45°. C. Roentgenogram reveals solid fusion of the index finger.

8-100A). Generally the cysts will persist for a long time and then gradually disappear, leaving a prominent osteophyte (Fig. 8-100B). Once the inflammatory

phase has subsided, the patient's pain will also disappear. These osteophytes are usually located beneath the collateral ligaments and cannot easily be removed for cosmetic reasons without destroying the ligaments.

Conservative Treatment

Mucous cysts that develop in osteoarthritis may often be treated with soaks in warm water, salicylates, or nonsteroidal anti-inflammatory drugs to relieve the inflammatory process. Puncture of the cyst with a sterile needle and the instillation of a drop of local steroid solution may also decrease the inflammatory process (Fig. 8-101). Excision of the cyst is not recommended, and if it is carried out, often a small skin graft may be required.

Arthrodesis

Osteoarthritis can produce grossly unstable distal interphalangeal joints that limit the function of the hand. If the joints are extremely painful, cosmetically unacceptable, or grossly unstable, arthrodesis can be considered (Fig. 8-102).

Operative Technique. Arthrodesis is carried out through a transverse incision in the distal skin crease over the interphalangeal joint. The extensor attachment is removed, and the collateral ligaments are divided (Fig. 8-103). The osteophytes are excised, and the head of the middle phalanx is shaped into a small dowel with a rongeur. A tunnel is made in the distal phalanx with an awl and a curette to accept the middle phalanx. In some cases it is not possible to make a ball-and-socket-type joint, and it may be necessary to shape the middle phalanx into a small rectangle and create a rectangular defect in the base of the distal phalanx.

A Kirschner wire is drilled retrograde

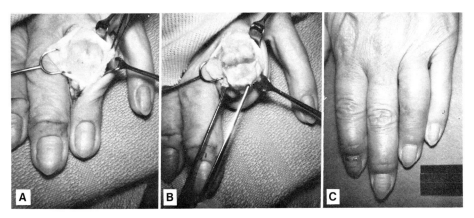

FIG. 8-98 Arthrodesis of the proximal interphalangeal joint. A. The extensor mechanism is turned back to expose the joint. Note the synovial hyperplasia. B. The collateral ligaments have been divided and the articular destruction and synovial changes in this joint can be noted. The other fingers reveal the cosmetically acceptable transverse incision in the distal interphalangeal joints for arthrodesis. C. The postoperative photograph reveals cosmetically acceptable hand with arthrodeses of the distal interphalangeal joints of the index and middle fingers and of the proximal interphalangeal joint of the fourth finger. The lateral approach to the fourth finger produces a scar that is not visible on the dorsum of the hand.

from the base of the distal phalanx out through the pulp of the finger beneath the nail. The pointed end is then drilled back across the distal interphalangeal joint which is forced together at about 170 to 180° of extension. Excellent fixation can be obtained with one wire in most cases. If instability is noted, two

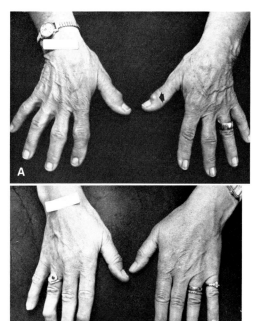

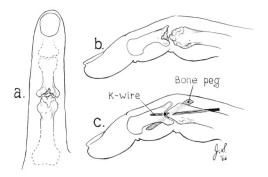

FIG. 8-99 Arthrodesis of the severely involved proximal interphalangeal joint. Dorsal view showing destruction of the proximal interphalangeal joint (a). The lateral view of the finger showing the destruction of the joint (b). Lateral view after reshaping the joint surfaces (c). A single Kirschner wire and a bone peg are nailed across the joint to fix it. (Marmor, L., and Peter, J.: Osteoarthritis of the hands. Clin. Orthop., 64:164, 1969.)

FIG. 8-100 Signs of osteoarthritis of the distal interphalangeal joints. A. The arrow indicates a mucous cyst on the left thumb. B. Heberden's nodes have developed on the index and fourth fingers of the right hand after subsidence of mucous cysts.

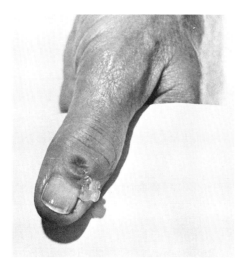

FIG. 8-101 A mucous cyst after aspiration with a large needle. Cystic fluid is exuding from the cyst.

wires may be used parallel to each other. The wire is cut off subcutaneously with a wire cutter pushed against the skin, and the end is tapped beneath the surface of the skin (Fig. 8-104). Small bone chips may be packed about the arthro-

desis site, and if possible, the extensor tendon may be repaired. The skin is closed with interrupted sutures, and a bulky dressing is applied. Generally this bulky dressing is removed in a few days after the operation, and the involved joint is splinted with a small aluminum splint to allow motion in the other joints of the hand and finger (Fig. 8-105). The Kirschner wire is usually left in place approximately 6 weeks to allow fusion to occur. It may then be removed under local anesthesia in the office. This method of fusion is satisfactory and produces a high rate of union. The use of crossed wires tends to distract the joint and may lead to nonunion which is not unusual at this distal interphalangeal joint with that type of technique.

After arthrodeses of the distal interphalangeal joints patients usually obtain relief from pain. Stability is regained and function is improved. Those who have lost the ability to pinch often regain that function (Fig. 8-106).

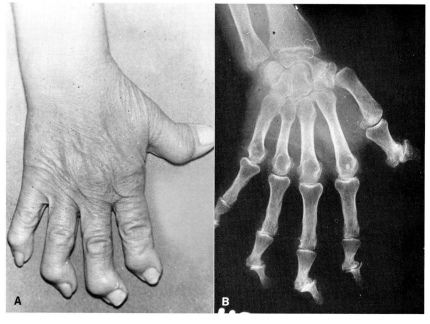

FIG. 8-102 Osteoarthritis of the distal interphalangeal joints. A. Photograph showing swelling and dislocation of the joints. The patient has lost the ability to pinch. B. Roentgenogram revealing instability of the joints.

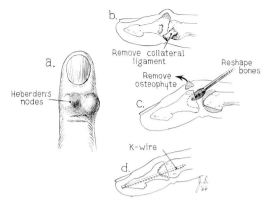

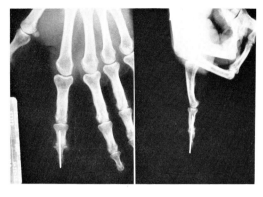

FIG. 8-103 Arthrodesis of the distal interphalangeal joint. a. Heberden's nodes are frequently seen in osteoarthritis as a bony spur on the distal interphalangeal joint. b. Arthrodesis is carried out by dividing the collateral ligaments. c. The osteophytes are removed, the head of the phalanx is reshaped, and the base of the phalanx is tunneled to accept the rounded head of the middle phalanx. The two are fitted together in the position of function, and a Kirschner wire is drilled retrograde across the joint space for fixation. (Marmor, L., and Peter, J.: Osteoarthritis of the hands. Clin. Orthop., 64:164, 1969.)

FIG. 8-104 Roentgenograms showing Kirschner wire in place after arthrodesis of the distal interphalangeal joint of the index finger. The ball-and-socket method was used. Dorsal view (left). Lateral view (right).

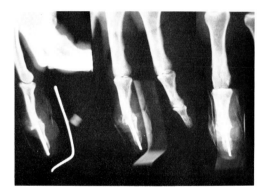

FIG. 8-105 Roentgenograms after placement of aluminum splint to immobilize the distal interphalangeal joint. Note that the proximal interphalangeal joint is left free for motion and that the splint is bent over the tip of the finger to protect the end of the wire, which is located subcutaneously.

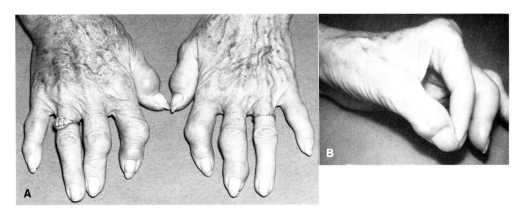

FIG. 8-106 Restoration of function after arthrodesis for severe erosive osteoarthritis of the hand. A. Preoperative view. B. Postoperative view showing ability to pinch.

Scleroderma

Scleroderma is a systemic disease of connective tissue which produces inflammatory changes in the skin with fibrosis and loss of the smooth muscle of internal organs. It is frequently a chronic, slowly progressive disease that can cause death by cardiac failure, hypertensive renal disease, intestinal absorption difficulty, or pulmonary complications.

In a majority of patients, the initial complaint is gradual thickening of the skin or else evidence of Raynaud's phenomenon. The patients will often have articular symptoms with a polyarthritis that could simulate rheumatoid disease. When the hands are involved, they can require orthopaedic management.

The exact cause of scleroderma is not known at the present time. However, specific changes in the skin produce edema, induration, and atrophy. Edema occurs early in the disease and lasts for several months, resulting in thickening and tightening of the skin. Raynaud's phenomenon appears to be related to paroxysmal spasms of the vascular system in the fingers and occurs in over 90 percent of the patients with systemic scleroderma.

The first manifestation of scleroderma is often seen in the fingers and wrists. As the disease progresses, there is increasing stiffness of the finger joints with loss of soft tissue in the hand. The proximal interphalangeal joints frequently become involved and severe flexion deformities can develop (Fig. 8-107). The skin over the proximal interphalangeal joint is thin, and ulceration is common. These ulcerated areas tend to heal slowly, and surgical wounds may also have delayed healing. In advanced cases, ulnar drift of the fingers can occur with stiffening and loss of function (Fig. 8-108). Involvement of the bone itself may occur with collapse and loss of

length of the fingers. Calcification in the soft tissue of the fingers can result in ulcerations that become extremely painful and extrude calcific material that prevents healing of the ulcer (Fig. 8-109).

Conservative Treatment

At the present time, there is no specific treatment for scleroderma. In some cases treating the skin with dimethyl sulfoxide has thinned the skin and returned it toward normal. In most cases, however, deformities gradually develop, producing severe flexion of the fingers and ulnar drift.

Surgical Treatment

The deformities can become severe and limit the function of the hand so that the patient may become helpless unless something is done surgically to correct the deformities. Surgical intervention is possible, and healing will generally occur, although in some patients it will be somewhat delayed. Patients with calcium deposits through the skin are difficult to treat. Although the material can be curetted out of the soft tissue and joint, the defect will leave little tissue to work with.

Arthrodesis or arthroplasty can be successfully carried out under either a general anesthesia or an axillary block. Careful handling of the thick skin is imperative to allow for closure. Frequently it is difficult to suture the skin. The patients should also be cautioned about the possibility of gangrene, a complication that also can occur in the disease without surgery because of the poor vascular supply to the fingers. Local ring blocks of the finger should be avoided.

Proximal Interphalangeal Joints

The treatment in general for the flexion deformities of the proximal interphalangeal joint is arthrodesis.

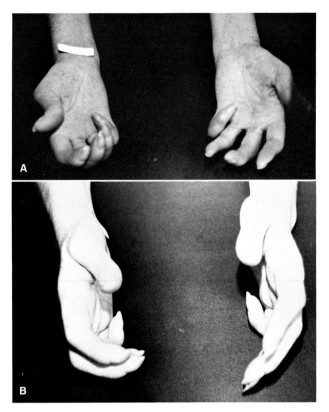

FIG. 8-107 Photographs of the hands of a patient with severe scleroderma resulting in involvement of the proximal interphalangeal and the distal interphalangeal joints. A. Volar view. Note that the fifth fingers are fixed in the palm of the hand. Characteristic deformities of the thumb have also occurred. B. Lateral view. The maximum extension with the fifth fingers fixed in the palm of the hand is illustrated.

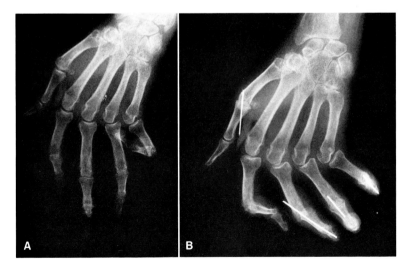

FIG. 8-108 Roentgenograms of left hand of patient with scleroderma. A. Before arthrodesis. Note the fixed deformity of the fifth finger and beginning ulnar drift. B. Six months later after reconstruction of the finger joints by fusion to improve their function. The ulnar drift has considerably increased.

253

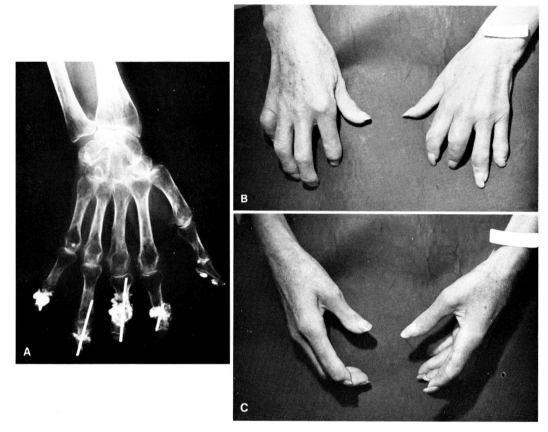

FIG. 8-109 Scleroderma. A. Roentgenogram shows severe calcium deposits in fingers and projection into the skin. B. Clinical photograph after arthrodesis of the proximal interphalangeal joints of the second and third fingers and the distal interphalangeal joints of the fourth and fifth fingers of the left hand. There is an ulceration on the left index finger. C. Improvement in function after correction of flexion deformities and unstable joints.

Operative Technique. The skin may be turned back by a transverse incision over the proximal interphalangeal joint or by a longitudinal incision running along the midlateral aspect of the finger and then turning the dorsal flap upwards. In some patients with severe ankylosis of the joint, it is possible to remove a dorsal wedge of the bony joint allowing the finger to come up into a better position of function. The fingers should be fused about 30° to 40° to allow a good pinch as well as a moderate grasp. In some patients, a tunnel may be made in the base of the middle phalanx, and the proximal phalangeal head may be reshaped to fit into it. This reshaping shortens the finger and allows easier skin closure. One Kirschner wire drilled across the joint generally will maintain fixation. The extensor mechanism is usually thin over the top of the proximal interphalangeal joint and in some patients is nonexistent. It is advisable to operate on the proximal interphalangeal joints first, as this procedure may improve the function of the hand without requiring surgery on the metacarpal-phalangeal joint.

Metacarpal-Phalangeal Joints

The metacarpal-phalangeal joints in scleroderma can become extremely stiff and fixed in a position of flexion with ulnar drift. The result is a poor hand for function. Arthroplasty can be carried out in scleroderma utilizing the Swanson Silastic prostheses (Fig. 8-110). The same procedure is carried out as is performed for rheumatoid arthritis.

Operative Technique. A dorsal skin incision is made over the metacarpal-phalangeal joints and the skin flap is turned back carefully. The skin is usually thick and brawny and hard to dissect from the extensor mechanism. Once exposure has been gained, the extensor mechanism is opened on the radial side, and the hood is turned back from the capsule and underlying tissue. The capsule, collateral ligaments, and metacarpal head should be excised from the joint, and then the volar plate is stripped from the base of the proximal phalanx. The medullary canal is reamed out with a power tool, and the base of the phalanx is opened into the medullary cavity for the broach to be inserted. After sizing the canals, the proper trial prostheses are inserted for a fit. In many cases it is necessary to release the ulnar intrinsics that are tight to gain further correction of the fingers. The hood is plicated on the radial side with 4-0 white silk, and the hand is treated postoperatively in the same manner as the rheumatoid hand.

Immobilization is carried out for approximately 12 days, and then motion is instituted in the metacarpal-phalangeal joints. It is imperative that healing be complete before hydrotherapy is started to prevent contamination of the Silastic prosthesis.

Thumb

The deformities from scleroderma of the thumb are similar to those for rheumatoid arthritis and severely limit the patient's ability to use the hand. In general, arthrodesis of the metacarpal-phalangeal and proximal interphalangeal joints can be carried out at the same time, if necessary, or the particular joint that is involved may be fused in a position of function. Arthrodesis is carried out exactly as performed for rheumatoid arthritis. If the carpal-metacarpal joint is involved, a Swanson arthroplasty can be performed to insert a Silastic trapezium.

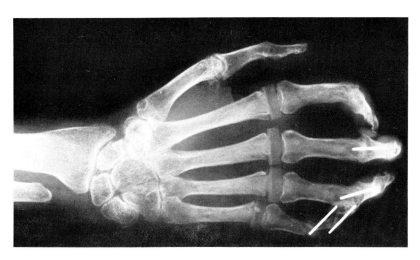

FIG. 8-110 Roentgenogram after arthroplasty on hand of a patient with severe scleroderma. The metacarpal-phalangeal joints have been replaced with Swanson prostheses to improve the range of motion. Arthrodesis of the distal finger joints has also been carried out to improve function. Excision of the ulnar head has relieved the pain. (See Figs. 8-107 and 8-108.)

Bibliography

Rheumatoid Arthritis

Adamson, J. E., Horton, C. E., and Crawford, H. H.: The surgical reconstruction of the rheumatoid hand. South. Med. J., *57*:928, 1964.

Aptekar, R. G., and Duff, J. F.: Metacarpophalangeal joint surgery in rheumatoid arthritis. Clin. Orthop., *83*:123, 1972.

Bäckdahl, M., and Myrin, S. O.: Ulnar deviation of the fingers in rheumatoid arthritis and its surgical correction: A new operative method Acta Chir. Scand. *122*:158, 1961.

Brand, P.: Personal communication.

Braun, R. M., and Chandler, J.: Quantitative results following implant arthroplasty of the proximal finger joints in the arthritic hand. Clin. Orthop., *83*:135, 1972.

Brewerton, D. A.: Hand deformities in rheumatoid disease. Ann. Rheum. Dis., *16*:183, 1957.

Brooks, A. L.: Personal communication.

Bunnell, S.: Surgery of the rheumatic hand. J. Bone Joint Surg., *35-A*:88, 1953.

Bunnell, S.: Surgery of the rheumatic hand. J. Bone Joint Surg., *37-A*:759, 1955.

Clayton, M. L.: Surgery of the thumb in rheumatoid arthritis. J. Bone Joint Surg., *44-A*:1376, 1962.

Cregon, J. C. F.: Indications for surgical intervention in rheumatoid arthritis of the wrist and hand. Ann. Rheum. Dis., *18*:29, 1959.

Curtis, R. A.: Treatment of ulnar deviation of the metacarpophalangeal joints in rheumatoid arthritis by shortening of the radial collateral ligaments. Rev. Chir. Orthop., *54*:335, 1968.

Ellison, M. R., Flatt, A. E., and Kelly, K. J.: Ulnar drift of the fingers in rheumatoid disease. J. Bone Joint Surg., *53-A*:1061, 1971.

Ellison, M. R., Kelly, K. J., and Flatt, A. E.: The results of surgical synovectomy of the digital joints in rheumatoid disease. J. Bone Joint Surg., *53-A*:1041, 1971.

Fearnley, G. R.: Ulnar deviation of the fingers. Ann. Rheum. Dis., *10*:126, 1951.

Flatt, A. E.: Restoration of rheumatoid finger joint function. J. Bone Joint Surg., *43-A*:733, 1961.

Flatt, A. E.: Intra-articular Thio-tepa in rheumatoid disease of the hands. Rheumatism, *18*:70, 1962.

Flatt, A. E.: Salvage of rheumatoid hand. Clin. Orthop., *23*:207, 1962.

Flatt, A. E.: Surgical rehabilitation of the rheumatoid hand. Ann. R. Coll. Surg. Engl., *31*:283, 1962.

Flatt, A. E.: The Care of the Rheumatoid Hand, St. Louis, C. V. Mosby Co., 1963.

Fowler, S. B., and Riordan, D. C.: Surgical treatment of rheumatoid deformities of the hand. J. Bone Joint Surg., *40-A*:1431, 1958.

Froimson, A. I.: Tendon arthroplasty of the trapeziometacarpal joint. Clin. Orthop., *70*:191, 1970.

Girzadas, D. V., and Clayton, M. L.: Limitations of the use of metallic prosthesis. Clin. Orthop., *67*:127, 1969.

Goldner, J. L., and Clippinger, F. W.: Excision of the greater multangular bone as an adjunct to mobilization of the thumb. J. Bone Joint Surg., *41-A*:609, 1959.

Goodwin, M. A.: Surgical correction of the deformed arthritis hand. Br. J. Surg., *44*:628, 1957.

Harris, C., Jr., and Rutledge, G. L., Jr.: The functional anatomy of the extensor mechanism of the finger. J. Bone Joint Surg., *54-A*:713, 1972.

Henderson, E. D., and Lipscomb, P. R.: Rehabilitation of the rheumatoid hand by surgical means. Arch. Phys. Med., *42*:58, 1961.

Henderson, E. D., and Lipscomb, P. R.: Surgical treatment of rheumatoid hand. J.A.M.A., *175*:431, 1961.

Heywood, A. W. B.: Correction of rheumatoid boutonnière deformity. J. Bone Joint Surg., *51-A*:1309, 1969.

Howard, L. D., Jr.: Surgical treatment of rheumatic tenosynovitis. Am. J. Surg., *89*:1163, 1955.

Inglis, A. E.: Rheumatoid arthritis in the hand. Am. J. Surg., *109*:368, 1965.

Inglis, A. E., et al.: Reconstruction of the metacarpophalangeal joint of the thumb in rheumatoid arthritis. J. Bone Joint Surg., *54-A*:704, 1972.

Jacobs, J. M., Hess, E. V., and Beswick, I. P.: Rheumatoid arthritis presenting as tenosynovitis. J. Bone Joint Surg., *39-B*:228, 1957.

Jonsson, E.: Rheumatological hand and finger symptoms. Ann. Rheum. Dis., *8*:72, 1949.

Kellgren, J. H., and Ball, J.: Tendon lesions in rheumatoid arthritis: A clinico-pathological study. Ann. Rheum. Dis., *9*:48, 1950.

Kelly, M.: The correction and prevention of deformity in rheumatoid arthritis. Canad. Med. Assoc. J., *81*:827, 1959.

Kestler, O. C.: Histopathology of the intrinsic muscles of the hand in rheumatoid arthritis. Ann. Rheum. Dis., *8*:42, 1949.

Kettelkamp, D. B., Alexander, H. H., and Dolan, J.: A comparison of experimental arthroplasty and metacarpal head replacement. J. Bone Joint Surg., *50-A*:1564, 1968.

Kuhns, J. G.: The preservation and recovery of hand function in rheumatoid arthritis. Bull. Rheum. Dis., *10*:199, 1959.

Laine, V. A. E., Sairamen, E., and Vainio, K.: Finger deformities caused by rheumatoid arthritis. J. Bone Joint Surg., *39-A*:527, 1957.

Landsmeer, J. M. F.: Anatomical and function investigations on the articulations of the human fingers. Acta Anat., *24*(Suppl.), 1955.

Leaming, D. B., Walder, D. N., and Braithwaite, F.: The treatment of hands, a survey of 10,688 patients. Br. J. Surg., *48*:247, 1960.

Lipscomb, P. R., Surgery of the arthritic hand. Proc. Staff Meet., Mayo Clinic, *40*:132, 1965.

Littler, J. W., and Cooley, S. G.: Restoration of the retinacular system in hyperextension deformity of the proximal interphalangeal joint. J. Bone Joint Surg., *47-A*:637, 1965.

Littler, J. W., and Eaton, R. G.: Redistribution of forces in the correction of the boutonnière deformity. J. Bone Joint Surg., *49-A*:1267, 1967.

Marmor, L.: Hand surgery in rheumatoid arthritis. Arthritis Rheum., *5*:419, 1962.

Marmor, L.: Rheumatoid flexor tenosynovitis. Clin. Orthop., *31*:97, 1963.

Marmor, L.: Surgical treatment for arthritic deformities of the hands. Clin. Orthop., *39*:171, 1965.

Marmor, L.: Surgical treatment of the rheumatoid hand. Proc. Ry. Soc. Med., *58*:567, 1965.

Marmor, L.: The role of hand surgery in rheumatoid arthritis. Surg. Gynecol. Obstet., *116*:335, 1963.

Marmor, L., and Upshaw, M. J.: Physical therapy in rheumatoid arthritis of the hand. J. Am. Phys. Ther. Assoc., *44*:729, 1964.

Martel, W.: The pattern of rheumatoid arthritis in the hand and wrist. Radiol. Clin. North Am., *2*:221, 1964.

Nalebuff, E. A., and Potter, T. A.: Rheumatoid involvement of tendon and tendon sheaths in the hand. Clin. Orthop., *59*:147, 1968.

Niebauer, J. J., and Landry, R. M.: Dacron-silicone prosthesis for the metacarpophalangeal and interphalangeal joints. Hand, *3*:55, 1971.

Niebauer, J. J., Shaw, J. L., and Doren, W. W.: The silicone-Dacron hinge prosthesis: design, evaluation, and application. J. Bone Joint Surg., *50-A*:634, 1968.

Pulkki, T.: Rheumatoid deformities of the hand. Acta Rheum. Scand., *7*:85, 1961.

Rose, D. L., and Wallace, L. I.: A remedial occupational therapy program for the residuals of rheumatoid arthritis of the hand. J.A.M.A., *148*:1408, 1952.

Scudamore, C.: A Treatise on the Nature and Cure of Rheumatism. London: Longmans, Rees, Orme, Brown & Green, 1827.

Smith, E. M., et al.: Role of the finger flexors in rheumatoid deformities of the metacarpo-phalangeal joints. Arthritis Rheum., *7*:467, 1964.

Smith-Peterson, M. N., Aufranc, O. E., and Larson, C. B.: Useful surgical procedures for rheumatoid arthritis involving joints of the upper extremity. Arch. Surg., *36*:764, 1943.

Stecher, R. M.: Ankylosis of the finger joints in rheumatoid arthritis. Ann. Rheum. Dis., *17*:365, 1958.

Steindler, A.: Arthritic deformities of the wrist and fingers. J. Bone Joint Surg., *33-A*:849, 1951.

Straub, L. R.: Surgery of the arthritic hand. Western J. Surg., *68*:5, 1960.

Straub, L. R.: Surgical rehabilitation of the hand and upper extremity in rheumatoid arthritis. Bull. Rheum. Dis., *12*:265, 1962.

Straub, L. R.: The etiology of finger deformities in the hand affected by rheumatoid arthritis. Bull. Hosp. Joint Dis., *21*:322, 1960.

Straub, L. R.: The rheumatoid hand. Clin. Orthop., *15*:127, 1959.

Swanson, A. B.: The need for early treatment of the rheumatoid hand. J. Mich. Med. Soc., *60*:348, 1961.

Swanson, A. B.: Silicone rubber implants for replacement of arthritic or destroyed joints in the hand. Surg. Clin. North Am., *48*:1113, 1968.

Urbaniak, J. R., McCollum, D. E., and Goldner, J. L.: Metacarpophalangeal and interphalangeal joint reconstruction. South Med. J., *63*:1281, 1970.

Vainio, K., and Julkunen, H.: Intra-articular nitrogen mustard treatment of rheumatoid arthritis. Acta Rheum. Scand., *6*:25, 1960.

Vainio, K., and Oka, M.: Ulnar deviation of the fingers. Ann. Rheum. Dis., *12*:122, 1953.

Vaughan-Jackson, O. J.: Rheumatoid hand deformities considered in the light of tendon inbalance. J. Bone Joint Surg., *44-B*:764, 1962.

proximal and distal articulations. J.A.M.A., *175*:1049, 1961.

Ghormley, R. K., and Bateman, J. G.: Pathology of rheumatoid diseases, synovial membrane in osteoarthritis. *In* Rheumatoid Diseases. Based on the Proceedings of the Seventh International Congress on Rheumatic Diseases. Philadelphia, W. B. Saunders, 1952.

Kellgren, J. H., and Moore, R.: Generalized osteoarthritis and Heberden's nodes. Br. Med. J., *1*:181, 1952.

Marmor, L., and Peter, J.: Osteoarthritis of the hands. Clin. Orthop., *64*:164, 1969.

Nichols, E. H., and Richardson, F. L.: Arthritis deformans. J. Med. Res., *2*:149, 1909.

Peter, J. B., Pearson, C. M., and Marmor, L.: Erosive osteoarthritis of the hands. Arthritis Rheum., *9*:365, 1966.

Stecher, R. M.: Heberden's nodes. A clinical description of osteo-arthritis of the finger joints. Ann. Rheum. Dis., *14*:1, 1955.

Stecher, R. M.: Osteoarthritis and old age. Geriatrics *16*:167, 1961.

Wardle, E. N.: Primary generalized chronic arthritis. Rheumatism, *9*:51, 1953.

Scleroderma

Entin, M. A.: Scleroderma hand: A reappraisal. Orthop. Clin. North Am., *4*:1031, 1073.

Lipscomb, T. R., Simons, G. W., and Winkelmann, R. K.: Surgery for sclerodactylia of the hand. J. Bone Joint Surg., *51-A*:1112, 1969.

Osteoarthritis

Collins, D. H.: The Pathology of Articular and Spinal Diseases. London, Edward Arnold and Co., 1949.

Crain, D. C.: Interphalangeal osteoarthritis characterized by painful, inflammatory episodes resulting in deformity of the

The surgical treatment of arthritis of the hip has dramatically changed in the past decade. Before the advent of joint implantation the patient with bilateral hip disease was an extensive reconstruction problem requiring years of physical therapy and the use of crutches. The new developments in surgical technique now make it possible to reconstruct the hips of patients and return them to function in several months. However, any form of hip reconstruction must be based on a logical approach to the patient's problems.

A careful analysis of the entire patient should be undertaken and proper staging of the surgery should be considered prior to embarking on a hip operation, because of the possible involvement of other joints necessary for ambulation such as the feet, ankles, and knees. If the patient has severe disease with multiple involvement of the joints of the knees, feet, and hips, it is advisable to evaluate the patient's motivation and to explain to the patient the problems involved in the reconstruction. Generally several operations are required, and the patient must have a great deal of courage and expend much effort to achieve a good result. In a young,

well-motivated patient with severe involvement, surgical reconstruction is certainly worth trying.

Aufranc has suggested five broad indications for reconstructive surgery of the hip:

1. Relief or diminishment of pain in the hip.
2. Restoration or improvement of function of the joint.
3. Correction of a deformity.
4. Establishment of stability in a subluxed or dislocated hip.
5. Prevention of unnecessary changes in the joint involved as well as secondary changes in the opposite hip or in the knee on the same or opposite side (Fig. 9-1).

Wiles has stated, "The methods available for the treatment of the painful hip are those applying to most orthopaedic problems, move it, keep it still, or cut it out." When pain is severe, conservative therapy may be of little value. However, it should be attempted to reassure the patient that every possible step has been taken to aid his recovery without resorting to operative intervention. When the symptoms are severe, then a choice of the operation must be

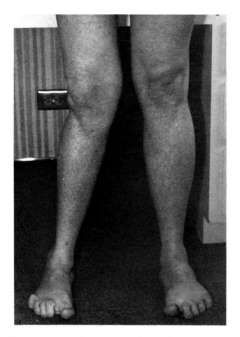

FIG. 9-1 Secondary changes in the knee joint from severe hip disease. This patient had a severe adduction contracture of the right hip which subsequently led to a valgus deformity of the right knee.

and this must be kept in mind. Problems of infection, loosening of the components, and thromboembolism are not to be taken lightly in the young patient. Arthrodesis, which at one time was the operation of choice in the young patient with unilateral arthritis, now must be carefully considered in light of our newer advances. Arthrodesis can be considered as a method of getting rid of pain, but one must consider also the status of the lower back and the knee on the same side. Although the patient may walk with only a slight limp, more energy will be expended in ambulation and stairs may be difficult because the patient must lead with the sound leg on each step. Some compensation must be made by the lumbar spine when the person sits in a chair, and the older patient may not be able to make the adjustment. In some series the rate of fusion failure requiring repeated operations may be as high as 40 percent.

made by the surgeon, and the choices must be explained to the patient. The development of the informed consent concept has made this mandatory in many parts of the United States.

The choice of the procedure depends upon the age and occupation of the patient, the range of movement of the hip, the condition of the spine and the knees, and the cooperation to be expected from the particular patient. It is extremely important to select the correct procedure for the individual patient. Although the total hip replacement has altered our thoughts considerably in our approach to surgery on the hip, Duthie has pointed out that it should in no way be the only operation considered. In the younger patient the cup arthroplasty and the displacement osteotomy may be of great value in preserving bony stock for future use. The total hip replacement is either a total success or a total failure,

Anatomy

The hip joint is essentially a ball-and-socket joint formed by the femoral head and the acetabulum. The articular cartilage on the femoral head is thicker at the center than at the periphery and covers the head except at the fovea capitis femoris where the ligamentum teres (ligamentum capitis) attaches (Fig. 9-2). The articular capsule is strong and thick and is reinforced anteriorly by the iliofemoral ligament. This ligament is of great strength and maintains the integrity of the joint anteriorly (Fig. 9-3). The synovial membrane is quite extensive in the hip joint and covers the margins of the femoral head, the neck within the joint, and then is reflected on the inner surface of the capsule and both surfaces

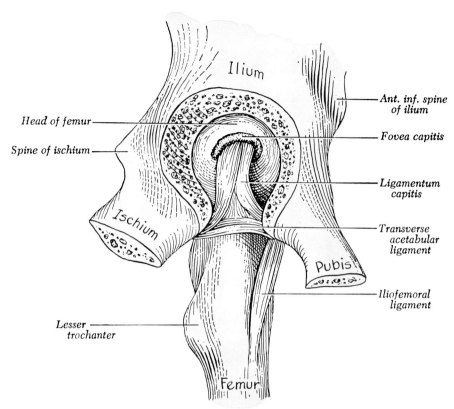

FIG. 9-2 Left hip joint viewed by removing the floor of the acetabulum to reveal the ligamentum capitis and the fovea capitis. (From Gray's Anatomy of the Human Body, 29th ed. C. M. Goss, editor, Philadelphia, Lea & Febiger, 1973.)

of the glenoid labrum, the ligamentum teres, and the fat pad in the depth of the acetabulum (Fig. 9-4).

The acetabulum has a horseshoe-shaped articular surface that is deepened by the fibrocartilaginous labrum. The position of the acetabulum has taken on considerable interest with the development of the total hip replacement. The cavity of the acetabulum faces obliquely forward, downward, and outward.

The angle formed by the femoral neck and shaft of the femur in the transverse plane is commonly referred to as the angle of anteversion. The average value for the angle of anteversion in the adult is approximately 12° with a wide range of normal. In patients with congenital dysplasia of the hip, anteversion may deviate widely from normal and

can present a problem in total hip replacement.

Numerous bursae about the hip are lined with a synovial membrane that can become affected by rheumatoid disease. The bursa overlying the trochanter is most frequently involved in rheumatoid disease, and a trochanteric bursitis with or without calcific deposit can be the cause of a good deal of discomfort.

The iliopsoas bursa is located between the iliopsoas muscle or tendon and the front of the hip joint. It is located just medial to the hip and extends from the region of the inguinal ligament to the level of the lesser trochanter. It can produce severe and excruciating pain when inflamed.

The hip moves through a remarkable range of motion because of the ball-and-

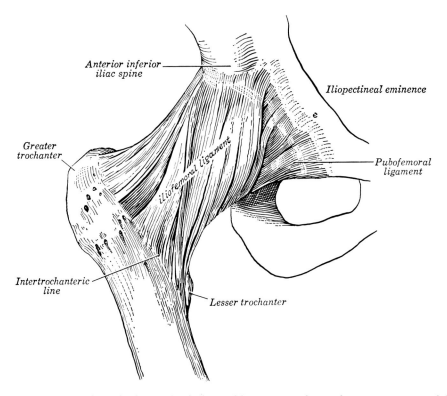

FIG. 9-3 Right hip joint from the front. The iliofemoral ligament reinforces the anterior aspect of the hip capsule. The vastus lateralis inserts along the intertrochanteric line. (From Gray's Anatomy of the Human Body, 29th ed. C. M. Goss, editor. Philadelphia, Lea & Febiger, 1973.)

socket type of joint that it is. The various muscles acting upon the hip joint tend to stabilize the hip as well as aid in locomotion of the body. Although it is felt that the gluteus medius is the main abductor of the hip joint. Charnley feels that a major abductor of the hip joint is the tensor fascia lata muscle which has a much better fulcrum for abducting the hip. This seems to be borne out in total hip replacement where avulsion of the greater trochanter has occurred with the gluteus medius muscle attached, and yet the patient has excellent abduction and stability. This also tends to correlate with the shoulder joint where the deltoid muscle acts as the main abductor and the short rotators are more for fixation and stabilization of the humeral head in the glenoid cavity.

Physical Examination

In order to perform an adequate examination of the hip joint, the patient must be suitably draped so that both lower extremities and pelvis can be visible to the surgeon.

Inspection

The patient is usually asked to stand, and the examiner should note whether the weight is borne on both legs or on one and whether there is an increase in the lumbar lordosis or a pelvic tilt. The patient should also be observed walking

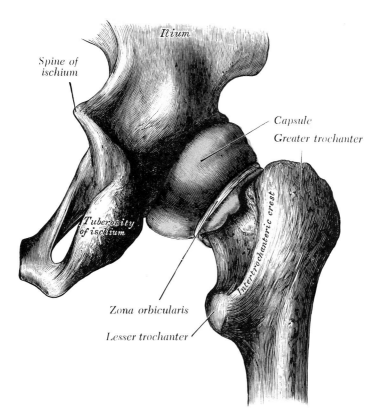

Spine of
ischium

Ilium

Capsule

Greater trochanter

Tuberosity
of ischium

Intertrochanteric crest

Zona orbicularis

Lesser trochanter

FIG. 9-4 Posterior aspect of the synovial tissue of the capsule of the hip joint (distended). (From Gray's Anatomy of the Human Body, 29th ed. C. M. Goss, editor. Philadelphia, Lea & Febiger, 1973.)

to determine if there is a limp or an abnormal gait pattern, and an attempt should be made to determine if the limp is due to a short leg or to pain. Any obvious deformity of the leg or pelvis should be noted. The Trendelenburg test can be carried out at this time. The patient should be asked to stand on one leg and raise the opposite leg off the floor. If the pelvis can be maintained on the raised side, the test is normal. If, however, the gluteus muscles are unable to hold the pelvis properly, a positive test is present.

Palpation

With the patient lying on the examining table, the hip joint can be palpated in an attempt to localize any areas of tenderness. Their location should be noted, either anterior or posterior, and special attention should be paid to both the anterior and the trochanteric areas of the hip joint. The trochanteric region can be palpated best with the patient lying on the opposite side with the legs crossed and with the trochanter area to be examined uppermost on the examining table. This position tends to expose the trochanter better, and more accurate palpation can be carried out.

Range of Motion

With the patient lying supine on the examining table, each hip should be put through a full range of passive motion, recording flexion, abduction, adduction, internal rotation, and external rotation.

The tests should also be carried out for hip flexion contracture by acutely flexing one hip, flattening the lumbar spine, and observing the position of the opposite hip which, if a contracture is present, will rise off the table.

Measurements

The length of the legs should also be measured with a tape measure to determine whether there is shortening of one leg or the other. The distance from the anterior superior spine to the medial malleolus should be measured and recorded for both legs. The spread of the legs is also measured by asking the patient to abduct both hips at the same time, and recording the distance between the medial malleoli.

Autotransfusion

Blood should be available for transfusion during major hip surgery. Autotransfusion is becoming more widespread for all surgery and has been used for many of our arthritis patients. This technique prevents transfusion reactions, as well as the development of hepatitis, a complication that has become more common with the use of stored blood and the purchase of blood from private blood banks.

A simple technique has been worked out, and most patients advised of the procedure are willing to cooperate. Approximately 3 weeks before the patient is to enter the hospital for the operation, the patient is seen as an outpatient by the clinical laboratories where his blood is typed and cross matched and one unit of blood is drawn. At five-day intervals, until three units of blood have been obtained, the patient is again seen as an outpatient, a hemoglobin and hematocrit are taken, and another unit of blood is drawn.

The patient is placed on iron therapy starting with the first unit of blood drawn to aid in the restoration of the blood volume. Generally upon admission to the hospital patients will have hemoglobins between 10 and 12 gm. We have had no problems drawing blood from patients, even from those in the 80-year-old category. If there is a history of heart trouble, 250 cc instead of 500 cc may be taken at more frequent intervals to obtain two or three units of blood. This blood is then transfused back during the operative procedure instead of using banked blood.

Postoperatively the hemoglobin can drop as low as 6.9 gm/100 cc with a hematocrit of 22, but in no case have we noted any major problems. Patients tolerate this low blood count without too much difficulty, although they may feel weak for the first 7 days after the operation. As long as the patient shows no evidence of air hunger or other symptoms of severe anemia, additional transfusions are not needed, but iron therapy, along with 1 mg folic acid, is continued daily. During the second week, the hemoglobin usually rises rapidly and prior to discharge will be up close to 10 gm. In our series there have been no problems with delayed wound healing or infection related to the low blood count.

Rheumatoid Arthritis

The hip joint is frequently involved in rheumatoid arthritis in association with disease of other joints of the lower limb.

Duthie and Harris, in a review of rheumatoid arthritis of the hip, found that in every case of hip involvement, there was also involvement of at least one other joint in the leg. The onset of the disease is insidious, and often the patient will not realize the gradual loss of function. The patient will usually note that some soreness develops in the hip after using it and tends to improve with rest. As the disease becomes more advanced, the patient begins to develop a limp. It is not unusual for patients with hip disease of this type to complain about pain in the knee, especially on the medial aspect, due to referral from the obturator nerve that supplies both the knee and the hip. Most often when the patient is seen with complaints in the hip joint, the disease has advanced considerably, and evidence of destruction and loss of the joint space will be seen in roentgenograms (Fig. 9-5). The major complaint of the patient at this time is severe pain and the inability to walk any distance at all.

Early in the disease process in the hip, the patient will develop a rheumatoid synovitis with pain and muscle spasm. If the pain and spasms persist, the range of motion in the joint will continue to decrease. Swelling of the joint will not be obvious because of the thickness of the capsule and the depth within the body. The pain may often be referred to the knee joint or front of the thigh. Roentgenograms at this stage of the disease may reveal a slight narrowing of the joint space, some early osteoporosis, and small erosive lesions of the subchondral bone (Fig. 9-6).

As the disease process continues, the roentgenograms will reveal even further narrowing of the joint space, evidence of cyst formation, and destruction of the femoral head (Fig. 9-7). Frequently in rheumatoid arthritis the femoral head will sink further into the acetabulum, producing a protrusio acetabuli (Fig. 9-8). Sometimes it is even worthwhile to take an anteroposterior view of the pelvis while the patient is standing to see if joint narrowing is present in the hip joint. This may be of value in the patient with severe symptoms but minimal evidence of narrowing on the routine roentgenogram with the patient supine.

Conservative Treatment

Little has been published in the past on the early treatment of the rheumatoid

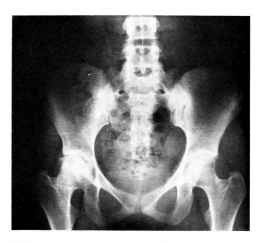

FIG. 9-6 A roentgenogram of the pelvis showing osteoporosis, small erosive lesions of the subchondral bone, and slight narrowing of the joint space that are characteristic of the early stage of rheumatoid arthritis.

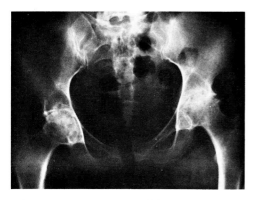

FIG. 9-5 A roentgenogram of the pelvis revealing advanced bilateral rheumatoid disease.

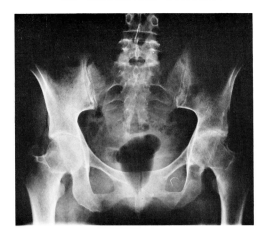

FIG. 9-7 A roentgenogram revealing changes of the left hip due to advanced rheumatoid arthritis. There are cyst formation, erosion of the femoral head, and early protrusion into the pelvis.

hip, since most patients are usually seen late in the disease when they are no longer able to ambulate or have severe pain. Usually the peripheral joints, which are involved early, occupy the attention of the patient and the physician.

The conservative treatment of the hip joint consists of local injection of corticosteroids into the joint, as well as the use of crutches or a cane to relieve the pressure of weight bearing. The local injection of corticosteroids can offer a great deal of relief to the patient with rheumatoid arthritis who is not a candidate for surgery or who is seen early in the progression of the disease.

Aspiration and injection of the hip joint can be performed with the patient supine. The patient's skin should be cleansed with an antiseptic solution similar to preparing for an operative procedure. The surgeon should wear sterile gloves and use sterile technique throughout. The left hand is used to palpate the anterior-superior iliac spine, with the index finger on the femoral artery and the middle finger on the pubic tubercle, to determine the landmarks for injection of the hip joint (Fig. 9-9). The thumb and the middle finger outline the inguinal ligament, and the index finger protects the femoral artery from insertion of the needle. The patient's skin is infiltrated with lidocaine (Xylocaine), approximately one inch below the inguinal ligament and lateral to the femoral artery and nerve. The Xylocaine is inserted down into the joint capsule with a #20 spinal needle until bone is felt with the needle. If there is any doubt concerning the position of the needle, an assistant should rotate the leg, and if the needle is in the correct position, the femoral neck will grate against it. If this maneuver is not carried out, one may strike the overhanging acetabular ridge and not inject the joint. One percent Xylocaine without adrenaline, approximately 5 cc, and a local corticosteroid preparation are injected into the joint. If

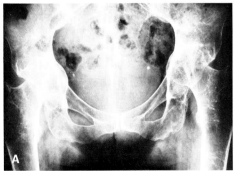
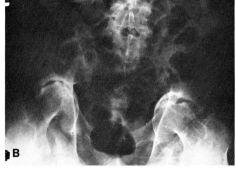

FIG. 9-8 Roentgenograms showing changes in advanced stages of rheumatoid arthritis. A. The femoral heads protrude into the acetabulum. B. Severe destruction can be seen in the hip joint.

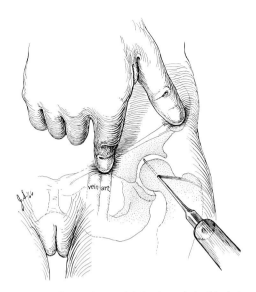

FIG. 9-9 Aspiration and injection of the hip joint through the anterior approach. The index finger is protecting the femoral artery as the needle is inserted into the capsule.

the joint has been successfully injected, the patient will experience dramatic relief upon getting up from the table and standing.

The patient should be cautioned that for the first 24 hours there may be pain in the hip joint but that this will gradually disappear and improvement can be expected. If there is no improvement within a few days, one can suspect that the joint was not entered with the needle and that the cortisone is outside the capsule. If symptoms recur rapidly and the roentgenograms show minimal joint narrowing with effusion, an early synovectomy of the hip is indicated to relieve the symptoms and try to prevent destruction of the joint.

When patients obtain dramatic relief lasting from 6 to 12 weeks, repeated injections can be given to avoid surgery and to allow the patient to function. Even in patients with radiologic evidence of advanced disease and joint narrowing, local injection can often give prolonged relief. The injection of 1 cc

Aristocort (triamcinolone) and 1 cc Aristospan (triamcinolone hexacetonide) in the same syringe with the Xylocaine has tended to give longer and better results than either one used independently. Patients whose symptoms are alleviated by the intra-articular injection should be instructed in exercises to put the hip through as complete a range of motion as possible daily and to strengthen the hip extensors and abductors, since there is a strong tendency to develop hip flexion and adduction contracture with rheumatoid disease.

Physical therapy can be combined with the exercise program, and the application of mild heat may bring comfort to the patient. Exercising in a swimming pool with heated water or hydrotherapy in a Hubbard tank is an excellent way of putting the hip through a good range of motion and building up strength. Gait training and the use of crutches when indicated will often be of great value to the patient during the acute phase and also before surgical intervention.

Surgical Treatment

The patient with rheumatoid arthritis and a severe hip problem often has a flexion contracture of both the hip and the knee (Fig. 9-10). When both contractures are severe, a problem exists as to what can be done for the knee, and possible solutions will be discussed in Chapter 10.

The total hip replacement has relegated many of the other operations to a lesser role in the management of the patient with rheumatoid arthritis. The results in properly selected patients have been spectacular to a degree not observed with any other form of hip reconstruction. Despite the spectacular success, a long list of complications must be taken into account when considering this form of surgical reconstruction.

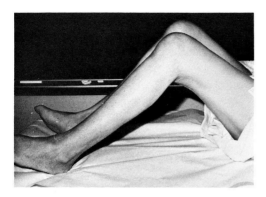

FIG. 9-10 Flexion contractures of the hips and knees.

Many surgeons utilize this one procedure for all hip disease regardless of the age of the patient, status of the bony stock, and involvement of the other joints in both lower limbs. The words of Charnley should not be forgotten in the rush to perform total hip replacement in the young person with unilateral hip disease. The long-term result of the total hip replacement in the young vigorous adult may be different from that in the elderly patient or the far-advanced rheumatoid arthritic who will put minimal stress on the new joint.

The selection of the operative procedure depends upon a number of factors, including age and the phase of the disease. At the present time procedures such as osteotomy, arthrodesis, and femoral head replacement are rarely of value in rheumatoid arthritis of the hip. The patient with early rheumatoid disease of the hip frequently is not seen by the orthopaedic surgeon. However, if a patient does have early symptoms with radiologic evidence of beginning erosions at the joint margin, the patient can be considered for a synovectomy. The patient with far-advanced disease with loss of the joint space and erosions of the articular surfaces can be considered for an arthroplasty. In the young patient with unilateral disease, the cup arthroplasty can still be considered a reasonable procedure, but a total hip replacement might be better for the patient with an early protrusio of the pelvic wall. In the middle-aged patient or the young adult with severe disease of both hips, a bilateral cup arthroplasty is a formidable procedure, and recovery is slow. For this type of patient the total hip replacement should be considered as the operation of choice.

Synovectomy

A synovectomy of the hip joint can be considered for the patient in the early stage of rheumatoid arthritis of the hip or for the young patient with juvenile rheumatoid arthritis when there is severe pain. spasm, and evidence of beginning destruction of the hip on roentgenograms. In the examination of this patient it is advisable to take a roentgenogram of the pelvis with the patient standing to determine whether the joint space is narrowed. Distension with joint fluid and synovial tissue may often simulate a good joint space in the patient who is lying on the x-ray table.

There are two schools of thought in performing a synovectomy for rheumatoid disease of the hip. One is to dislocate the hip to allow for better removal of the synovial tissue. This procedure carries the possibility of a complication due to the dislocation that may result in aseptic necrosis or changes in the femoral head. In general, the operation of choice would not include dislocation of the hip. Recent evidence seems to indicate that a total synovectomy is not necessary to achieve a reasonable result in rheumatoid arthritis. A satisfactory result can be achieved by removal of the synovial tissue around the articular surfaces without dislocation.

Operative Technique. The patient should be prepared and draped with the hip free. Either the anterior or the Watson-Jones approach can be utilized.

The Watson-Jones approach is recommended because it requires less extensive exposure. The incision can start near the anterior-superior spine and curve gently toward the trochanter (Fig. 9-11). The subcutaneous tissue is divided, exposing the tensor fascia lata, the gluteus medius, and minimus muscles. The interval between the tensor and the gluteus medius muscles is developed, and the tensor can be retracted medially to expose the anterior capsule of the hip joint. The capsule then is opened anteriorly and turned back, exposing the joint. Care should be exercised not to damage the articular surface of the femoral head. The synovial tissue should be removed from the margins around the femoral head and the neck of the femur. If the leg is manipulated, the various areas can be reached with a small rongeur. A small curette is also valuable

to scrape the synovial tissue from the areas of the articular margins. The capsule and wound should be closed in layers, and the patient can be placed in a balanced suspension sling for early exercise postoperatively. The patient should ambulate early, using crutches and partial weight bearing, and within two weeks full weight bearing can be allowed. The patient should be taught exercises to prevent the development of a flexion contracture postoperatively. Care should be exercised in positioning the patient in bed, and at some time during the day the bed should be flattened to stretch the hip into extension.

Arthroplasty

The cup arthroplasty has a definite place in the management of the patient with rheumatoid arthritis in the hip. The removal of the capsule and the synovium tends to arrest the destruction of the hip by the disease process. Unfortunately, the cup arthroplasty has been maligned by some surgeons because of the surgical techniques or the postoperative care. What many have called a cup arthroplasty in no way resembles the procedure that has been popularized by Smith-Petersen, Aufranc, Harris and others. The tendency often has been for the orthopaedic surgeon to read about a procedure and then decide to do it without any further instruction. Charnley has definitely established an important concept in hip surgery that the surgeon should know how to do the procedure and learn the techniques from someone who is skilled in the operation.

The cup arthroplasty at one time was quite difficult to perform because of the use of hand tools to develop an adequate acetabulum in sclerotic hard bone (Fig. 9-12). The development of new reamers and power tools has greatly simplified what was once a difficult procedure.

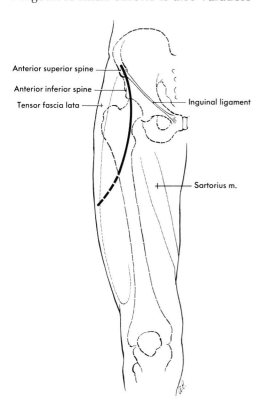

Anterior superior spine

Anterior inferior spine

Tensor fascia lata

Inguinal ligament

Sartorius m.

FIG. 9-11 The incision for a synovectomy of the hip.

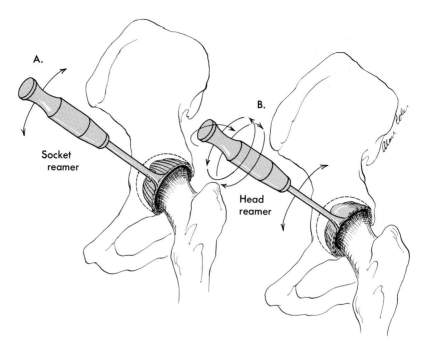

FIG. 9-12 Hand tools for cup arthroplasty. A. Socket reamer. B. Head reamer.

The major indication for a cup arthroplasty is unilateral hip disease (Fig. 9-13). Bilateral cup arthroplasties have been done, but the results are generally poor. The patient must have good bone in the femoral head before the surgeon considers a cup arthroplasty. If the head is fractured or aseptic necrosis is present, a cup arthroplasty would be contraindicated.

The value of the cup or mold arthroplasty is that it preserves the bony stock and does not prevent other procedures if failure does occur. It can be performed in the patient with a history of sepsis when other procedures such as total hip replacement may be contraindicated. A cup may be revised following an infection and the hip can be salvaged.

The patient must realize when considering a cup that it will require an investment of time and effort to achieve a good result. The hip must be protected from full weight bearing for a minimum of 6 months, and crutches may be required up to a year or longer. However,

the cup tends to improve with the passage of time, and long-term results up to 30 years have been reported (Fig. 9-14).

The results, however, are not as spectacular as those for the total hip replacement, but major complications are less and infection is not as severe a catastrophe. Revision of the cup because of pain is necessary in about 15 percent of the cases. The chances of pain relief in some series runs as high as 80 to 85 percent.

Two approaches, the anterior and lateral, are used most often for cup arthroplasty. The anterior approach will be described first because it leaves the lateral approach available for total hip replacement in the future if it should ever be necessary and does not require detachment of the greater trochanter. The lateral approach is recommended when shortening of the head-neck length is present or anticipated because the trochanter can be moved distally to increase the abductor power.

Anterior Approach. The patient is

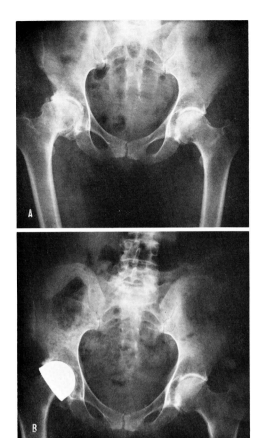

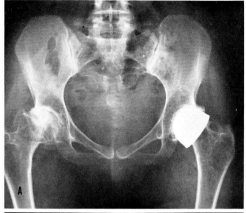

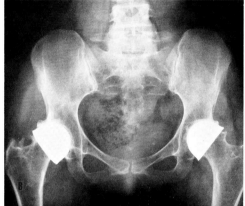

FIG. 9-13 Roentgenograms of young patient with unilateral hip disease. A. Preoperative view revealing changes in right hip 10 years after onset of rheumatoid arthritis. B. Postoperative view showing cup in place. The patient has an excellent range of motion and walks without support.

FIG. 9-14 Roentgenograms showing results of Smith-Peterson cup arthroplasty in a 36-year-old woman who had severe bilateral hip disease due to rheumatoid arthritis. A. Twelve years after the cup was placed in the left hip. The patient had a good range of motion but severe pain in the right hip. B. Sixteen years after placement of a cup in the right hip. The cup in the left hip had then been in place 28 years. The patient has no pain and walks without a cane.

placed supine on the operating table, and the intravenous needle is inserted into the arm opposite the hip to be operated upon so that the first assistant can stand next to the surgeon. The arm on the side of the hip surgery is usually folded across the chest out of the way. A folded sheet is placed beneath the buttock proximal to the hip joint to allow the hip to fall free of the sheet (Fig. 9-15). The hip is then prepared from the umbilicus to the knee and the entire circumference of the thigh. A plastic drape is applied to the umbilicus and perineum to remove them from the

operative area. Plastic drape is then placed over the anterior incision to protect the operative area from the skin edges. The leg must be draped free to allow for manipulation during dislocation of the hip.

The skin incision starts about one inch along the anterior iliac crest and continues over the anterior iliac spine distally for about 8 to 10 inches (Fig. 9-16). At the level of the anterior iliac spine several large veins and an artery

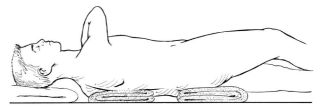

FIG. 9-15 Diagram showing the patient in position for a cup arthroplasty of the hip. A folded blanket is placed beneath the vertebral border from the scapula to the pelvis, and another blanket is under the buttock.

that pass transversely should be clamped and cauterized. The lateral femoral cutaneous nerve will be found slightly medial and distal to the iliac spine. If it cannot be preserved easily, it should be pulled distally and cut as proximally as possible with a sharp knife and allowed to retract. (It is wise to mention the fact to the patient preoperatively that anesthesia or a dead area will be present on the thigh.)

The interval between the tensor fascia lata muscle and sartorius is devel-

oped by finding the tendon of the rectus femoris distally where it has a shiny appearance like that of a fish belly (Fig. 9-16B). Tracing it proximally, one will develop the proper interval between the sartorius and the tensor fascia lata muscles.

The periosteum is stripped from the proximal one inch of the crest by sharp dissection with a knife and the tensor is stripped from the lateral wall of the ilium with a periosteal elevator. The area is immediately packed with a moist

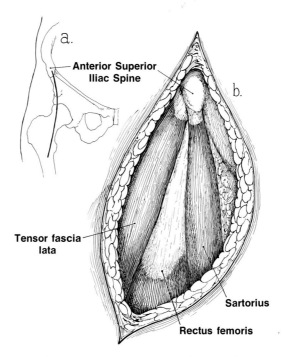

FIG. 9-16 Cup arthroplasty. a. The skin incision starts approximately 1 inch along the anterior iliac crest and then crosses over the anterior iliac spine distally for 8 to 10 inches. b. The rectus femoris muscle is visualized between the sartorius and the tensor fascia lata. (Courtesy of the Mira Company.)

laparotomy pad to prevent bleeding. In a similar manner the iliacus is swept from the inner wall and packed with a laparotomy pad for hemostasis.

The deep fascia over the rectus femoris muscle is carefully opened to expose the transverse circumflex vessels on its lateral side passing toward the tensor muscle (Fig. 9-17). It is best to ligate these vessels rather than cauterize them to prevent bleeding during the exposure of the hip joint. If this is done carefully, bleeding will be kept to a minimum.

The rectus femoris tendon is then traced proximally to its two heads, the reflected head to the acetabular rim and the direct head to the anterior inferior iliac spine. The reflected head is cut, and the direct head is removed, leaving a small portion for resuture of the rectus on closure of the incision. A large artery frequently encountered at this point near the anterior inferior spine should be watched for and cauterized to reduce blood loss.

The rectus femoris can then be mobilized distally and folded until the neurovascular pedicule is encountered on its medial aspect. This must be preserved to prevent paralysis of the muscle. The tendon of the rectus can be sutured to the skin with heavy silk 0 sutures distally to retract it out of the way. The capsule of the hip will now become visible. A blunt periosteal elevator can be used to expose the superior and inferior aspects of the capsule. If some fibers of the iliopsoas are present on the medial surface of the capsule, they are pushed out of the way. Abduction of the hip will facilitate the separation of the capsule from the gluteus tendon superiorly, and flexion adduction will aid in exposing the inferior aspect of the hip joint capsule.

The capsule is then opened anteriorly and should be removed entirely along

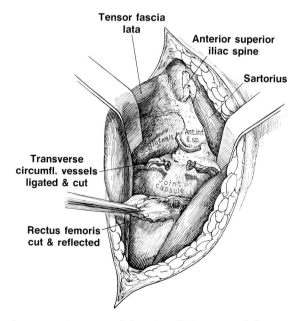

FIG. 9-17 Cup arthroplasty, anterior approach (continued). Exposure of the transverse circumflex vessels which have been ligated before cutting to prevent bleeding. The rectus femoris muscle has been cut from the anterior-inferior iliac spine and reflected distally to the neurovascular bundle attachment. (Courtesy of the Mira Company.)

the acetabular attachment, except for a small anterior portion which is left near its attachment at the intertrochanteric line or ridge. (The psoas tendon will be transferred here later.) In some patients the hip can be dislocated by external rotation and adduction of the leg, but too much force can fracture the femur.

If dislocation does not occur, the anterior ledge of the acetabulum and all its osteophytes should be removed from the inferior and superior aspects (Fig. 9-18). The psoas tendon may be removed at the lesser trochanter, and a suture of black silk placed through it to mark it and retract it out of the way. Careful retraction along the medial side will expose any further tight capsule on the inferior surface. Since the femoral nerve is beneath the medial retractor, one must be careful not to injure it by forceful retraction (Fig. 9-19).

The hip usually can be easily dislocated now by external rotation and adduction. A twisted gauze sponge may be placed around the femoral neck to aid in retracting the head laterally and upward out of the incision (Fig. 9-20).

At this stage the power tools and

Mira reamers are utilized. (The reamers are designed to cut slowly to prevent perforation of the acetabulum.) The femoral head is usually reamed first with the female reamers, starting with the larger sizes and working down to the smaller sizes (Fig. 9-21). To develop a valgus head, the reamer is placed on the femoral head from the superior aspect like a derby hat on a head. All osteophytes on the superior aspect of the neck should be removed with a rongeur to prevent them from forcing the cup into varus. It is not necessary to ream the head down completely to cancellous bone.

The male reamers are then placed into the acetabulum, starting with the smaller sizes and working up to the larger sizes (Fig. 9-22). The reamer should be inserted in a superior and posterior direction to develop a valgus position for the cup. If the bone is sclerotic, it will take a reasonable amount of reaming to develop a good cancellous acetabulum. Be careful not to injure the femoral head with the acetabular reamers. The assistant should keep the head pulled out of the way.

The femoral head should be reduced to fit in the new acetabulum. There must be room for the cup to fit without binding. If further reaming is necessary, remember the valgus position and always ream in valgus when deepening the acetabulum or narrowing the head. The reamer, however, can be rotated around the head and acetabulum to remove all rough surfaces.

Any style of concentric cup or mold may be used; however, we prefer the Laing cup because of its narrower neck or opening. This is an advantage against dislocation of the femoral head postoperatively. The proper size is selected by trying to fit the cup over the head in valgus position. The second or third size of the cup usually fits reasonably well. If the cup appears to fit, it can also be tested in the acetabulum. When the

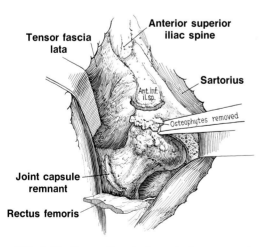

FIG. 9-18 Cup arthroplasty, anterior approach (continued). Removal of osteophytes around the acetabular margin to aid in dislocation of the hip. (Courtesy of the Mira Company.)

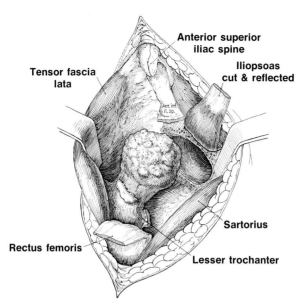

FIG. 9-19 Cup arthroplasty, anterior approach (continued). Retraction of the iliopsoas tendon from the lesser trochanter and dislocation of the femoral head. (Courtesy of the Mira Company.)

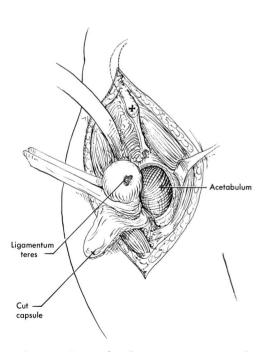

FIG. 9-20 Cup arthroplasty, anterior approach (continued). A twisted gauze sponge around the femoral neck aids in retracting the head laterally and upward out of the incision.

proper size has been selected, the cup can be forced to slip over the femoral head by using a femoral head prosthesis impactor or one's fist. Once the narrow portion of the cup opening slips over the head, it will fit loosely around the neck and the inner portion of the cup is large enough to fit loosely on the head without coming off easily. If the cup goes on too snugly, any prominences of the larger diameter of the head can be trimmed off to allow the cup to slip on easier. Any loose folds of capsule should be excised to prevent impingement by the cup. The cup should be easily placed in valgus (Fig. 9-23), and the hip should be reduced after irrigating the acetabulum well. A loose fit of the cup is desired, but as long as it moves easily with motion of the leg, the fit is adequate. The cup should be reduced well into the acetabulum, but a reasonable amount, say $\frac{3}{4}$ to 1 inch of cup, will remain out, depending upon the size of the cup and depth of the acetabulum. The cup should again be checked for a valgus position and manually pushed over the head into maximum valgus.

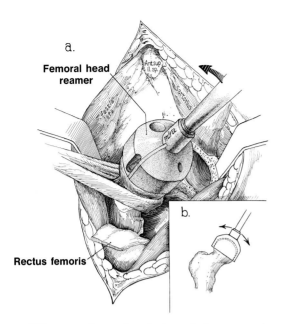

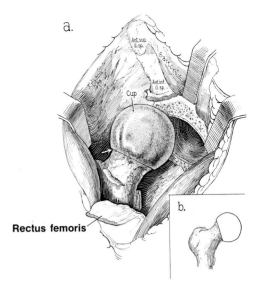

FIG. 9-21 Cup arthroplasty, anterior approach (continued). The female reamer is in place over the femoral head. Inset b. The reamer is used in a valgus position to develop a valgus head for placement of the cup. (Courtesy of the Mira Company.)

FIG. 9-23 Cup arthroplasty, anterior approach (continued). The cup should fit in valgus. Inset b. Varus positions generally produce a poor result. (Courtesy of the Mira Company.)

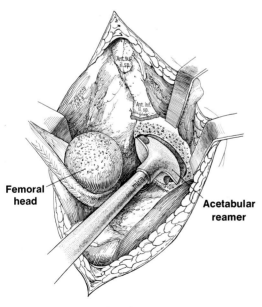

FIG. 9-22 Cup arthroplasty, anterior approach (continued). The male reamer has been inserted into the acetabulum in a superior and posterior direction to develop a valgus position of the cup. Note that the femoral head is being pulled out of the way. (Courtesy of the Mira Company.)

Then the iliopsoas tendon is brought over anteriorly by blunt dissection and sutured to the remaining anterior capsule on the femoral neck (Fig. 9-24). This procedure will aid in preventing dislocation of the cup and prevent the iliopsoas from being entrapped by the edge of the cup.

The rectus tendon is sutured to the anterior inferior iliac origin of its tendon (Fig. 9-25). After the deep fascia and the subcutaneous tissue and skin have been closed, a spica dressing of stockinette is wrapped from the foot up the leg and around the waist of the patient to give moderate compression of the incision.

The patient is then placed in a balanced suspension sling, with the leg in abduction and a folded bath towel under the trochanter, to prevent external rotation (Fig. 9-26).

Lateral Approach. An incision centered over the trochanter and about 10 inches in length is made along the lateral aspect of the hip (Fig. 9-27). The fascia lata is divided in the plane of the skin incision to expose the greater trochanter.

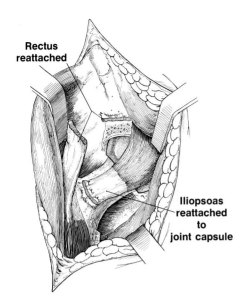

FIG. 9-24 Cup arthroplasty, anterior approach (continued). The iliopsoas tendon has been sutured to the remaining anterior capsule along the intertrochanteric line. The portion of the rectus tendon left for resuture is also visible. (Courtesy of the Mira Company.)

After exposure of the greater trochanter, the capsule of the hip joint is opened anteriorly (Fig. 9-28), and a heavy clamp is passed posteriorly over the superior aspect of the neck and behind the greater trochanter and brought through the posterior capsule. The end of the Gigli saw wire is grasped by the clamp and brought retrograde around the trochanter. The trochanter is removed by sawing parallel to the shaft of the femur toward the foot and then bringing the Gigli saw out laterally. A large portion of the trochanter should be excised to allow for replacing it postoperatively. The femur is dislocated by external rotation (Fig. 9-29). Hemostasis should be secured at this stage, as there is usually a reasonable amount of bleeding from the posterior aspect of the capsule and neck in this region.

At this stage the capsule can be completely excised, the hip can be dislocated, and, if necessary, the psoas tendon can be removed from the lesser trochanter for future transfer. The hip is

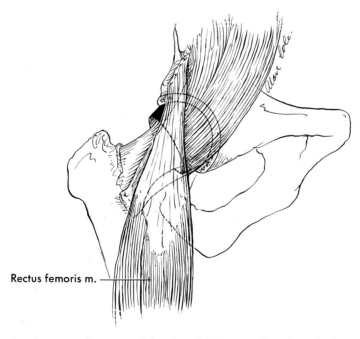

Rectus femoris m.

FIG. 9-25 Cup arthroplasty, anterior approach (continued). The rectus femoris tendon is sutured to its origin on the anterior inferior iliac spine.

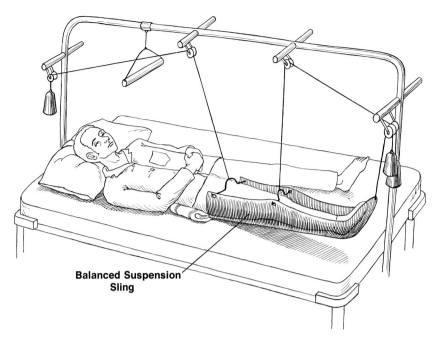

Balanced Suspension
Sling

FIG. 9-26 Cup arthroplasty, anterior approach (continued). The patient is placed in a balanced suspension sling with the leg in abduction and a folded bath towel beneath the trochanter to prevent external rotation. (Courtesy of the Mira Company.)

dislocated by adducting the femoral shaft and externally rotating the hip joint. Force is to be avoided because it may fracture the neck or shaft of the femur. All osteophytes should be removed from the anterior and lateral

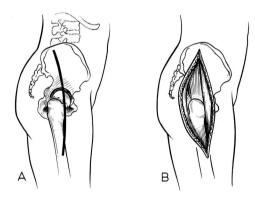

FIG. 9-27 Cup arthroplasty, lateral approach. A. An incision about 10 inches in length is centered over the trochanter. B. The facia lata is split in the plane of the skin incision to expose the greater trochanter. (Redrawn from Campbell's Operative Orthopaedics, 5th ed. H. H. Grenshaw, editor. St. Louis, C. V. Mosby, 1971.)

aspect of the acetabulum to permit easy dislocation. All tight structures should be divided, including the inferior portion of the hip joint capsule.

At this stage of the procedure the operation is then continued as illustrated in the anterior approach. Following the introduction of the cup into the hip joint, the iliopsoas muscle is transferred to a small remaining portion of the anterior part of the capsule, and the trochanter is brought down with some abduction of the leg to a snug fit distal to where it was previously removed and is wired into place (Fig. 9-30). The vastus lateralis is sutured over the wires to prevent the development of a painful bursa. A spica dressing of stockinette is wrapped around the leg as in the anterior approach, and the patient is placed in a balanced suspension sling with the leg in abduction.

Postoperative Care. The patient with arthritis should be started on early active and passive motion in order to regain as

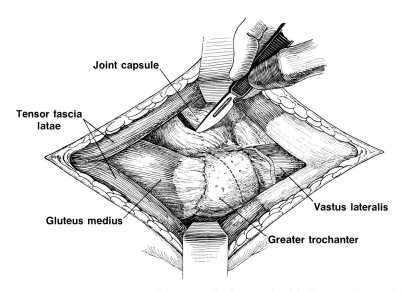

Joint capsule

Tensor fascia latae

Gluteus medius

Vastus lateralis

Greater trochanter

FIG. 9-28 Cup arthroplasty, lateral approach (continued). The capsule of the hip joint is opened. The broken line indicates where the greater trochanter is transected by a Gigli saw. (Courtesy of the Mira Company.)

much motion as possible before the scar tissue becomes mature and prevents stretching. Motion that is not obtained early usually cannot be regained at a later date. Therefore, exercises are started on the first postoperative day in the balance suspension sling. The patient is started on quadriceps-setting and knee extension exercises along with dorsiflexion of the foot. Other exercises to be encouraged are internal rotation of the hip and abduction as far as can be tolerated. By the second postoperative day the patient should be taught to lift the pelvis from the bed while extending the operated hip and flexing the opposite hip to hyperextend the lower back and hip joint, as this exercise is an aid in the prevention of a flexion contracture. It is extremely important to stress the fact

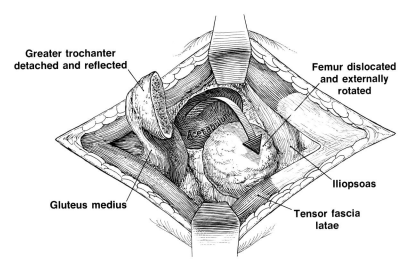

Greater trochanter detached and reflected

Femur dislocated and externally rotated

Acetabulum

Gluteus medius

Iliopsoas

Tensor fascia latae

FIG. 9-29 Cup arthroplasty, lateral approach (continued). The greater trochanter is detached and reflected up out of the way with the gluteus medius tendon still attached. (Courtesy of the Mira Company.)

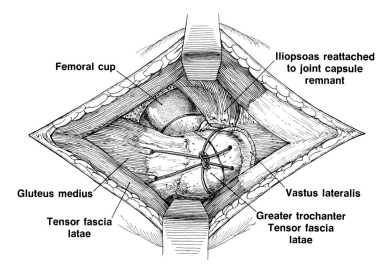

FIG. 9-30 Cup arthroplasty, lateral approach (continued). The trochanter is pulled distally to increase the length of the gluteus medius and is reattached with wires. The femoral cup is in place, and the iliopsoas has been reattached. (Courtesy of the Mira Company.)

that the patient should be straightened out completely flat in bed several times a day for a period of at least an hour to prevent a flexion contracture. The tendency is to adjust the bed so that the patient is half sitting with the knees in a flexed position because this position is comfortable.

A trapeze will help the patient to pull up in bed and to perform the hyperextension exercises. These should be performed several times a day to increase the patient's strength and also to develop the upper extremities.

Whenever possible, the patient should be taught crutch walking with partial weight bearing prior to the surgical procedure, as this is a great aid in ambulating the patient postoperatively. A skate board may be utilized to aid the patient in doing the abduction exercises.

Generally, around the third or fourth postoperative day, the patient may be removed from the balanced suspension for a half hour, three times a day, and by the end of the week, one hour three times a day. Longer periods should be avoided to prevent pressure on the heel. During the second postoperative week the patient is encouraged to continue an active exercise program to develop the control of the hip joint. After 2 weeks the sutures are removed, and the patient may be placed in the Hubbard tank to aid in gaining further motion and strength of the hip. With some patients a tilt board is utilized for a few days to prevent dizziness, and the patient is started on parallel bars or crutches immediately. By the end of the third week most patients will be walking with crutches and can be discharged. They should have a program of exercises similar to those done in the hospital. It is important to encourage minimal weight bearing of about 20 to 30 pounds to stimulate the calcification of the bone and prevent the development of hip flexion contractures from trying to walk on crutches with the leg flexed. Minimal weight bearing will also stimulate the healing of the joint, but too much weight will destroy the young regenerating surface. Full weight bearing should be restricted for a minimum of 6 months to allow regeneration of an articular surface and gradually allowed if it does not produce pain with crutches.

The patient with a hip arthroplasty must take care of his hip for the remainder of his life or until all symptoms disappear. Crutches or canes should be used for long-distance walking to protect the hip joint and to prevent recurrence of symptoms. As the symptoms disappear, the patient may be gradually switched to a cane, and when there is a negative Trendelenburg test the patient may begin to walk without support. It is important to prevent the patient from bearing weight too soon without support because he will develop a severe limp that may persist even when the hip is completely healed.

In a certain percentage of patients, revision of the cup may be necessary for persistent pain, or a total hip procedure may become a necessity. However, in general the patient can expect relief or diminishment of the pain in the hip joint to a reasonable level. Excessive activity can produce some pain and muscle aching about a hip joint, but with proper care and the use of support for long-distance walking, the patient may avoid these complications.

Complications. The usual complications of any surgery can follow a cup arthroplasty for arthritis of the hip. The most serious complication is infection. With proper care, however, the incidence of infection in cup arthroplasty of the hip is low and no greater than the average of any clean surgery in orthopaedics. If infection does occur, it can often be treated with appropriate antibiotics and frequently the cup may be left in situ. In severe cases the cup may have to be removed and the wound debrided. After proper and massive irrigation of the joint, a new cup may be inserted, and a loose closure may be carried out. Frequently, with antibiotic control, the cup may then be retained despite the previous infection.

Dislocation of the cup is extremely rare when the iliopsoas tendon has been transferred to the anterior portion of the capsule. The narrowed neck of the new concentric cups such as the Laing has prevented the head from rolling out of the cup, and dislocation from the acetabulum is quite rare. Transfer of the iliopsoas tendon also prevents it from occasionally catching on the rim of the cup and snapping, producing spasm and severe pain in the hip joint.

Occasionally the femoral head will collapse because of necrosis, severe rheumatoid cyst formation, or osteoporosis. The cup will tend to migrate distally down the neck as the head collapses (Fig. 9-31). In some cases, although the hip will be painful during the immediate collapse, the patient will gradually adjust to the new length and be quite comfortable. If severe destruction oc-

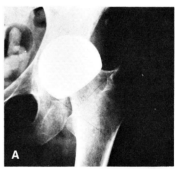

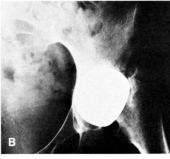

FIG. 9-31 Roentgenograms after cup arthroplasty. A. After the operation in August 1966 the cup is in excellent valgus position with a good length of neck. B. In February 1968 the head has collapsed and there has been shortening of the neck with impingement of the trochanter on the edge of the cup. Slight protrusion into the pelvis can also be noted.

curs, the neck may dislocate from the cup or the cup may drift into varus, and then total replacement of the hip joint should be considered (Fig. 9-32). It is unwise to place an intramedullary prosthesis such as an Austin Moore or a Thompson into a femoral neck when the acetabulum has been reamed for a cup because the prosthesis will migrate into the acetabulum. Total hip replacement is a much wiser choice in this situation.

Loss of motion can occur in a certain percentage of the patients, and this may limit the patient's ability to perform certain functions. However, if it is only unilateral, the loss of motion may be well tolerated if the pain is minimal. Early motion, however, tends to prevent a loss of motion in most rheumatoid and osteoarthritic patients. A gradual loss of motion can occur with the development of ectopic bone or myositis in the area about the hip joint. If the loss is severe, revision may be indicated.

Total Hip Replacement

The patient with rheumatoid arthritis of the hip has been a great problem for the orthopaedic surgeon because the overall results in the past have been unpredictable. The bone of the rheumatoid hip is much softer because of osteoporosis and steroid therapy. The results with the previously accepted surgical procedures such as the cup arthroplasty in rheumatoid arthritis tend to deteriorate with the passage of time. In Aufranc's review of 1,000 arthroplasties of the hip, 36 percent of the rheumatoid patients had a revision, and only 22 percent of the entire series had absolute pain relief. The results in patients with bilateral disease are even worse. The involvement of many of the joints in the lower extremity tends to rule out arthrodesis of the hip, and the use of a femoral head prosthesis tends to put additional stress upon the acetabulum and the shaft of the femur, resulting in migration of the prosthesis either into the acetabulum or down the shaft. In a number of our patients, as well as in patients in other series, it has been noted that the same type of absorption of the head and neck tends to take place with the passage of time after an arthroplasty, and the cup begins to settle with its edge resting at the base of the femoral neck in the region of the greater trochanter (Fig. 9-33). Migration of the cup into the pelvis has also been seen with the development

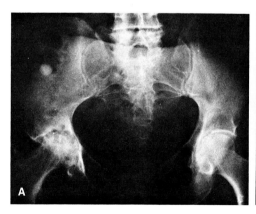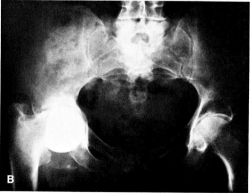

FIG. 9-32 Roentgenograms of patient with severe rheumatoid arthritis involving the right hip. A. Narrowing, destruction, and beginning protrusion of the joint are evident in the preoperative view. B. Roentgenogram taken 6 months later when the patient complained of pain revealed migration of the cup into varus and collapse of a portion of the head.

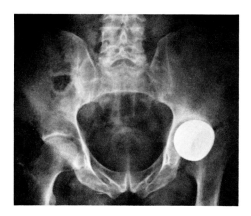

FIG. 9-33 Roentgenogram of patient who had a cup arthroplasty of the left hip. The femoral head has collapsed, and the cup is in a varus position. The patient's left leg was also shortened.

of a protrusio of the acetabulum (Fig. 9-34).

The total hip replacement has become a solution to the rheumatoid arthritic hip, but along with this solution can come a host of serious complications. The surgeon who is planning to do total hip replacement surgery must be thoroughly familiar with the operation and prepared to accept all the consequences associated with this major procedure.

The indications for total hip replacement in rheumatoid arthritis are as follows. If a Girdlestone pseudarthrosis would be an acceptable operation to the surgeon and the patient, total hip replacement can be considered (Fig. 9-35). One should always approach each individual case with the thought as to whether the patient would be better with some other procedure or the way he is as compared to the way he would be with a Girdlestone resection. When there is bilateral hip disease with extensive destruction of the femoral head and acetabulum, total hip replacement can be considered in the young adult because no other procedure is available to rehabilitate the patient to a reasonably normal life. The age limit has dropped considerably in the past 10 years, and it is no longer logical to limit the procedure to patients over a certain age. Each individual case must be considered on its own merits (Fig. 9-36). If revision is being considered because of failure of a cup arthroplasty, a replacement with a total hip is probably the procedure of choice.

A variety of total hip replacements are available to the surgeon at the present time. The two most popular techniques, the Charnley low friction arthroplasty and the Charnley-Müller total hip will be presented in detail because of their value in treating the patient with rheumatoid arthritis.

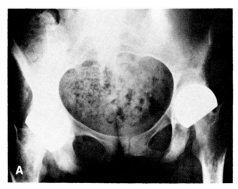
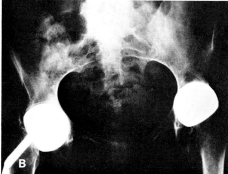

FIG. 9-34 Roentgenograms of patient who had bilateral cup arthroplasties for rheumatoid arthritis. A. Both cups were in a valgus position with a reasonable inner wall to the pelvis. B. Two years later the cups had migrated into the pelvic wall with the development of protrusion of the acetabulum. In the right hip the femoral neck, which had fractured, was treated by internal fixation.

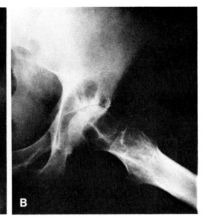

FIG. 9-35 Roentgenograms of patient with severe rheumatoid changes in the left hip. A. Note the massive cysts in the acetabulum and the femoral neck. B. Lateral view shows the large cysts in the femoral neck, head, and acetabulum.

The Ring total hip replacement, which is performed without cement fixation, is usually a poor choice for the patient with rheumatoid arthritis because of osteoporosis that will lead to the subsequent loosening of the prosthetic replacement. The introduction of methyl methacrylate for fixation of the total hip prosthesis has been of great value for the rheumatoid patient with osteoporosis and severe deformities (Fig. 9-37).

The McKee-Farrar procedure, although well accepted in many areas of the world, is gradually being used less

and less in the United States because of the metal-on-metal replacement. There is greater loosening of this prosthesis, as compared to the Charnley, which is one of its major disadvantages.

The Bechtol system is similar to the Charnley technique, except that the femoral head is slightly larger and the femoral component comes in a variety of neck lengths (Fig. 9-38).

Charnley Low Friction Arthroplasty

With the acceptance of total hip replacements throughout the world, there

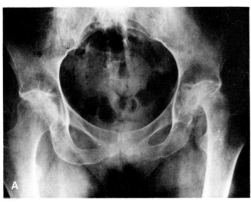
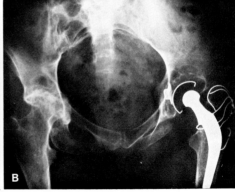

FIG. 9-36 Roentgenograms of patient who had complained of excruciating pain for 6 weeks. A. The left femoral head collapsed because of aseptic necrosis. B. View shortly after a total hip replacement when the patient experienced severe pain in the right hip. Comparison with the previous roentgenogram reveals the extensive rheumatoid changes in the right hip. The right femoral head rapidly collapsed.

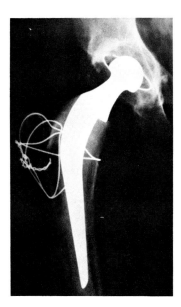

FIG. 9-37 Roentgenogram after total hip replacement fixed with methyl methacrylate in a patient with severe osteoporosis. Despite the osteoporosis, the patient has had no difficulty with migration or loosening of the prosthesis.

have been a number of modifications of the basic Charnley principles. However, Charnley's principles are still the foundation upon which the following technique will be presented. In certain areas of the operation where power tools can be utilized with safety, they will be presented as an alternate method of performing the operation. In the Charnley set there are a standard and a straight stem femoral component, and a heavy and an extra-heavy stem. The preparations for the surgical procedure can be instituted a week prior to the operation by allowing the patient to sterilize the skin by taking a shower with hexachlorophene (pHisoHex) before entering the hospital. Many of the patients are also started on buffered aspirin, 10 grains, four times a day, for the week prior to surgery and during the hospital admission in an attempt to reduce postoperative phlebitis. The patient is usually admitted to the hospital two days before the operation to allow for a medical evaluation and laboratory tests.

Although the preoperative orders may vary from surgeon to surgeon, the usual orders may consist of something similar to the following example.

Total Hip Replacement Preoperative Orders

1. Regular diet.
2. Shower or bath on admission day with hexachlorophene (pHisoHex).
3. Phospho-soda enema before shower or bath and antiseptic cleansing the night before surgery.
4. Sheepskin for bed and heel protector.
5. Balanced suspension sling set up on bed.
6. Shaving and antiseptic cleansing of the affected hip, pubic area, and the entire side of the body from nipple to toes and from midline anterior to midline posterior.
7. Sleeping medication of choice.
8. Pain medication of choice.
9. Stool softener.
10. Electrocardiogram.
11. Posteroanterior and lateral chest and anteroposterior pelvis roentgenograms.
12. Routine laboratory tests and chemistry panel, including erythrocyte sedimentation rate.
13. Typing and crossmatching of three units of whole blood.
14. Instruction by a physiotherapist in exercises and postoperative management of the hip.

Operative Technique. The patient is

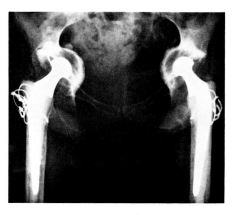

FIG. 9-38 Roentgenogram of a patient with protrusio of the acetabulum treated by bilateral Bechtol total hip replacements.

placed supine on the operating table with the pelvis level. The umbilicus, the perineum, and the anal area are excluded from the operative area by plastic drapes adherent to the skin. The entire leg is antiseptically prepared from the toes to the umbilicus, and the hip is draped so that the lateral aspect of the thigh, the greater trochanter, and the anterior-superior spine are visible to the surgeon. The skin area is covered with an adhesive plastic drape which tends to hold the drapes in place when the leg is manipulated. A Mayo stand cover is clipped to the opposite side of the table so that when the operative hip is dislocated, the foot can be placed inside the Mayo stand to prevent contamination.

The leg is flexed and adducted slightly to help accentuate the trochanter and to allow the fatty tissue of the thigh and buttock to fall away from the incision. The skin incision is made along the lateral aspect of the thigh, extending at least 3 inches proximal to the tip of the trochanter and approximately 6 inches below the trochanter (Fig. 9-39). Skin

towels are applied to the edges of the skin and coated with triple antibiotic solution. The fascia lata is exposed and opened with a knife and then slit upward with a heavy scissors, exposing the trochanter and its bursa. If the patient's leg has been flexed, the fibers of the tensor fascia lata muscle will not be encountered, as they will be carried forward away from the incision. It is important not to cut too deeply at this time or one will encounter the fibers of the gluteus medius muscle in the upper area of the incision and perhaps cut some of these inadvertently. If the fascia lata is too tight, a relaxing incision can be made with a transverse cut proximal to the trochanter. This is not often necessary. The large bow-shaped initial retractor is now inserted with the bow directed toward the patient's feet and the rake portions opposite the middle of the trochanter. The retractor should fit into the fascia lata and hold it open for the surgeon. The plane of this retractor should lie at a 45° angle to the floor and is controlled by the position of the

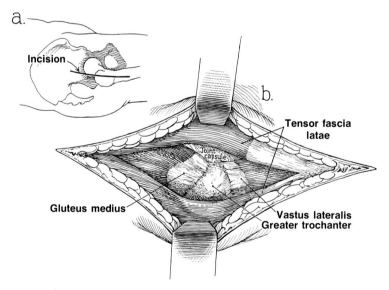

FIG. 9-39 Charnley low friction arthroplasty. a. Lateral incision is centered one third above the trochanter and two thirds below. b. After division of the facia lata, the gluteus medius, the greater trochanter, and the vastus lateralis become visible. The self-retaining retractor with the weight is inserted at this stage for better exposure. (Courtesy of the Mira Company.)

weight which hangs over the side of the table opposite the surgeon.

At this point in the procedure it is important to have the assistant place the leg flat on the table and externally rotate it to relax the muscles, allowing easier retraction of the gluteus medius. Then a Hibbs or Myerding retractor is used to scrape along the front of the hip capsule to expose its anterior aspect. A rake retractor can be used to retract the gluteus medius out of the way. This exposes the vastus lateralis muscle, which is detached from its origin on the anterior aspect of the neck and along the lateral aspect of the femur, utilizing the electric knife and cautery to decrease the blood loss. The intertrochanteric ridge can be palpated at the insertion of the capsule and the vastus lateralis muscle. The periosteal elevator is then used to strip the muscle distally from the shaft of the femur for approximately 1 inch. Hemostasis should be obtained at this time to prevent further blood loss.

The anterior capsule of the hip joint is opened over the neck of the femur for approximately 1 or 2 inches in a line parallel with its axis (Fig. 9-40). A Key elevator or Watson-Jones elevator may be inserted around the anterior and posterior aspect of the neck and gently levered outward to stretch the capsule and strong anterior ligaments. After carefully identifying the joint surfaces, a gallbladder clamp or other heavy clamp is inserted inside the capsule along the top of the femoral neck to the posterior aspect of the capsule, staying close to the bone, and the tip of the clamp is pushed through the posterior hip joint capsule, guided by the fingers of the surgeon's free hand. There is usually a thin point posteriorly where the clamp will pass through the capsule. The clamp should be opened with two hands to spread the tissues and enable the jaws of the clamp to be opened. A flat ribbon retractor can be inserted along the posterior aspect of the hip joint to expose the jaws of the gallbladder clamp and allow the assistant to see much better. The Gigli saw blade is inserted by the assistant into the clamp, and the saw blade is then pulled back around the femoral neck as the gallbladder clamp is removed. The handles of the Gigli saw are inserted into the loops, and the trochanter is removed by sawing toward the patient's feet, making sure that the wire passes posterior to the projection of the trochanter and parallel to the shaft of the femur

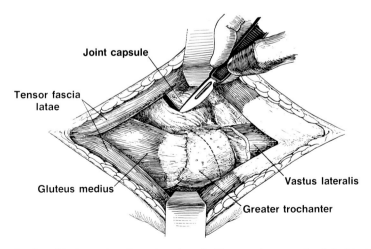

FIG. 9-40 Charnley low friction arthroplasty (continued). The anterior capsule of the hip joint is opened. The broken line reveals the site of detachment of the greater trochanter. (Courtesy of the Mira Company.)

(Fig. 9-41A). It is important to be sure the saw blade is completely around the trochanter and not around one of the superior prominences because it is necessary to remove a large piece of the bone to facilitate closure and to secure fixation of the trochanter later. Just before the trochanter is removed, the saw should be directed laterally to remove the complete trochanter. The trochanter should be pulled upward, out of the way, with a bone hook, and the leg is internally rotated to aid in clamping several large vessels that usually bleed at this point. After hemostasis has been secured, if the trochanter cannot be easily retracted, the external rotators may be divided at their insertion into the trochanter. The gallbladder forceps is passed behind the insertion of the external rotators into the trochanter to cut them at their insertion into the bone. The superior capsule should not be excised from the trochanter or the acetabulum margins as in a cup arthroplasty.

In some cases, it will not be possible to pass the gallbladder clamp around the neck of the femur because of previous trauma or surgery with adhesions. If difficulty is encountered at this stage, it is better to use a broad osteotome and remove the trochanter by starting distally parallel to the shaft of the neck and turning the trochanter upward with the gluteus medius tendon. Care should be exercised not to split into the neck but also to remove a large enough portion of the trochanter for later fixation.

The capsule may be divided transversely along the anterior-posterior aspects to aid in dislocation of the hip. Any large osteophytes should be removed to facilitate dislocation of the head of the femur. The leg is adducted across the opposite leg, and gentle external rotation is applied. A bone hook can be inserted along the neck of the femur to aid in dislocation. Force should not be excessive or fracture of the neck and shaft can

occur. When difficulty is encountered in dislocation, it is much safer and wiser to divide the femoral neck with a Gigli saw or osteotome and remove the head separately from the acetabulum. This is especially true in a protrusio of the acetabulum. *Preserve as much neck as possible,* as any excess can be removed later when it is decided what length of neck is required for stability.

If the hip can be dislocated easily without dividing the head, the trial prosthesis can then be placed over the head and neck to determine the proper neck length required and the angle at which to cut the neck of the femur. The trial prosthesis is superimposed over the femur so that the prosthesis head is close to the top of the femoral head (Fig. 9-41B). The femoral head can then be removed by a power saw, Gigli saw, or osteotome. If an osteotome is used, one must be careful not to split the posterior neck. Exposure at this stage may be limited because of adhesions to the neck of the femur, especially along the posterior aspect. Careful dissection close to the bone with a heavy scissors will release any scar and allow the femoral neck to move out of the way, giving better exposure of the acetabulum. The self-retaining east-west horizontal retractor is inserted between the stump of the femoral neck and the detached greater trochanter. If the bone is quite soft because of rheumatoid arthritis or osteoporosis, it is wiser to place the prongs of the self-retaining retractor against the calcar of the femur to prevent fracture or collapse of the neck. As the retractor is inserted, the leg should be adducted to aid in opening the retractor to gain exposure.

The acetabulum is then cleaned of synovium and fibrous tissue. Any anterior osteophytes on the acetabulum may be removed at this stage with a rongeur. It is important to see the superior aspect of the acetabulum to aid in determining

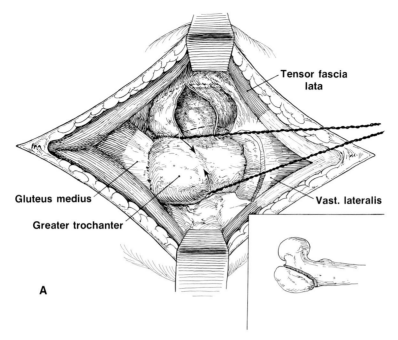

FIG. 9-41A Charnley low friction arthroplasty (continued). The Gigli saw is positioned to remove the greater trochanter by cutting parallel to the shaft of the femur (inset) to try to remove as large a piece as possible.

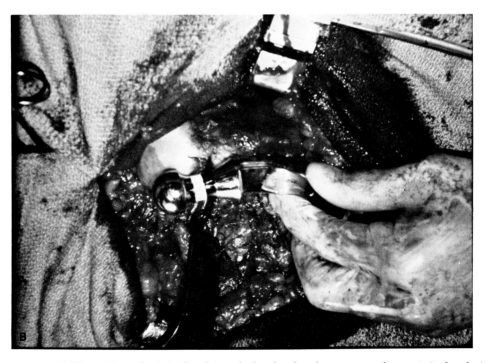

Fig. 9-41B A trial femoral prosthesis is placed over the head and neck to measure the exact site for placing the saw for removal of the head to preserve as long a neck as possible.

the depth of the prosthetic socket to be used.

At this stage, the surgeon should have determined from the preoperative roentgenogram whether a center hole is to be drilled into the acetabulum (Fig. 9-42). To prevent fracture of the entire inner wall of the acetabulum, a center or pilot hole should not be made if the roentgenogram reveals a thin or narrow medial wall. If the wall is relatively thick or normal, a pilot or center hole can be drilled. The anterior-superior spines should be marked with a large instrument placed across the spines to give a plane of reference. It is important to be sure that the pelvis is level and that the patient is not rotated because of the dislocation of the hip and placement of the leg across the table into the Mayo stand cover. The centering drill with the centering guide is inserted into the acetabulum and generally drilled at a 30° to 45° angle (Fig. 9-43). If the surgeon wishes to move the acetabulum upward, the 45° angle is used. If the acetabulum is to be moved

distally, a center hole is drilled at less than a 30° angle. The centering device is removed, and the drill is inserted through the inner table of the pelvis.

The depth of the pelvis can then be measured through this hole by either the surgeon's finger or a small hemostat inserted to the inner table of the pelvis. The projection of the deepening reamer is then engaged in the pilot hole, and four or five turns are made to clean the inner wall of the acetabulum, but no attempt is made to deepen it considerably at this stage. The instruments are used at an angle of 20° to 30° with the axis of the anterior-superior spine. The acetabulum should be measured at this time with the socket gauge to determine whether a small or a standard socket is to be utilized.

The expanding reamer is then inserted, and if a small socket is to be used, the reamer is not expanded fully. The Charnley expanded reamer is then used to cut away the cortical bone. Following this, the deepening reamer may be used

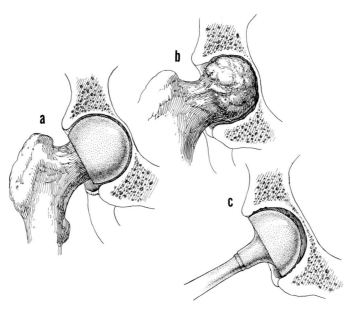

FIG. 9-42 Charnley low friction arthroplasty (continued). Contraindications for a center hole: a. cup arthroplasty with a thin medial wall; b. protrusion with a thin center wall; c. acetabulum roughened by reamers. (Courtesy of the Mira Company.)

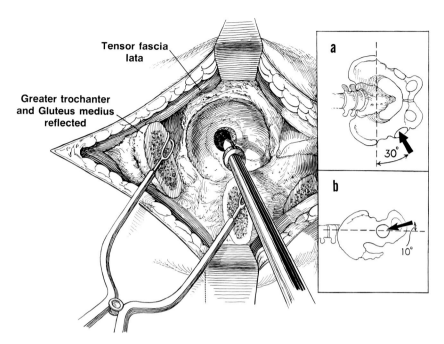

FIG. 9-43 Charnley low friction arthroplasty (continued). A drill with a centering guide is inserted into the acetabulum. Inset a. The drill is inserted at a 30° angle to the anterior superior spines. Inset b. The drill is also angled 10° posteriorly. (Courtesy of the Mira Company).

again to deepen the medial wall of the acetabulum until 6 to 8 mm of bone are present in the thinnest area of the acetabulum which is usually toward the patient's feet. As an alternate method, it is possible to use a slow-turning power tool with a hip reamer to perform the same procedure that the Charnley expanding reamer does by hand (Fig. 9-44). This method can be utilized especially in patients with a thin medial wall where a centering hole cannot be made for the Charnley reamers. Frequently the superior aspect of the acetabulum is not thoroughly cleaned with the Charnley reamer, and there may be some cortical bone remaining. Various grooving types of reamers can be used with power tools to score or groove the inner wall of the acetabulum to secure fixation of the cement (Fig. 9-45).

A one-half inch hole is drilled in the superior aspect of the acetabulum for fixation of the cement. In the Charnley low friction arthroplasty, further holes are not necessary in the inferior aspect of the acetabulum. Some surgeons, however, will drill holes into the ischium and pubis, but one must be careful not to penetrate the acetabular wall because cement may protrude into the posterior aspect of the pelvis and irritate the sciatic nerve.

At this stage, the associate surgeon or the nurse can begin preparation of the cement to be used in fixing the acetabular component. The cement is mixed until it is no longer sticky (approximately 4 minutes).

If the high posterior wall Charnley socket is used, the right or left marker on the socket has to match the socket holder right or left to prevent improper insertion. The prosthetic socket is clipped into the socket guide with the metal marker in the socket aligned with the handle of the guide. The iliac crest again should be carefully lined up to aid in

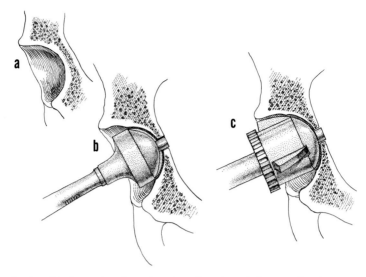

FIG. 9-44 Charnley low friction arthroplasty (continued). a. Acetabulum can be deepened to accept a total hip socket. b. A power deepening reamer can be used. c. An expanding reamer is also available for use with the power tools. Note that further penetration is not possible because the blades do not reach the inner wall. (Courtesy of the Mira Company.)

positioning the socket. The long-handled curette can be placed along the axis of the pelvis over the anterior-superior spines as a landmark. The acetabulum is irrigated, and a laparotomy pad is inserted to keep it dry while the surgeon changes his outer gloves. The laparotomy pad is removed, and the cement restrictor is inserted into the center hole at this stage.

Then the surgeon holds the cement until it begins to wrinkle on its surface. It is shaped into a ball or cup and carefully inserted into the acetabulum, avoiding contact with blood as much as possible. The cement should be pushed into the acetabulum and up into the superior fixation hole with a finger or the socket gauge. The polyethylene socket is now pressed into the cement and tilted forward toward the end of the table so that its edge is in contact with bone, and then the socket is pushed into the acetabulum until the shaft of the socket holder is parallel to the anterior iliac spine. The handle of the socket holder is kept parallel to the trunk of the patient or

rotated downward a few degrees to prevent retroversion of the socket.

The pusher is held against the socket holder while the excess cement is removed with a curette. The excess should be removed with care to prevent pulling the cement from behind the socket or changing the position of the socket holder. As the cement begins to harden, the pusher may be struck several sharp blows with the hammer to force the cement into the cancellous bone. Then the pusher is placed against the superior aspect of the socket to hold it in place and prevent movement of the socket, while the socket holder is carefully detached. The pusher is placed into the center of the socket and held, compressing the cement until it has hardened. When the cement has hardened, any excess cement, especially in the anterior region of the socket, should be removed with a rongeur to prevent dislocation of the hip. All large osteophytes and any thick scar tissue should be removed from around the edges of the acetabulum to prevent postoperative dislocation. All of

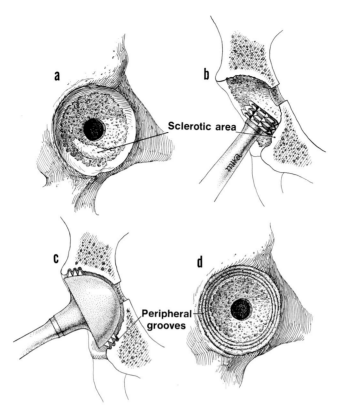

FIG. 9-45 Charnley low friction arthroplasty (continued). a. Small sclerotic areas may be left in the acetabulum after reaming. b. A small grooving reamer allows removal of these sclerotic areas for cement fixation. c. A grooving reamer can also be used to score the periphery of the acetabulum for better cement fixation. d. The scoring or grooves that can be placed around the periphery of the acetabulum. (Courtesy of the Mira Company).

the self-retaining retractors except the initial one are removed, and the wound is thoroughly irrigated with antibiotic solution.

The leg is now adducted further across the opposite leg with the tibia vertical off the table in the Mayo stand cover. The tapered reamer is inserted carefully into the neck and down the femoral shaft so as not to penetrate the cortex. This instrument tends to reveal the normal axis of the medullary cavity of the femur and tends to prevent piercing the lateral wall of the femoral shaft with the broaches. The first femoral broach is inserted down the medullary cavity of the femur with the "Tommy" bar parallel to the shaft of the tibia to prevent anteversion or retroversion of the prosthesis. The guide on the first broach should be parallel to the femur and directed toward the patella. The second broach, which is more curved, is now inserted to its full length, and then the trial femoral component of the prosthesis is inserted so that it fits easily. *All cancellous bone in the neck along the calcar should be removed to give strong bone for support of the cement.*

The trial reduction is carried out at this stage to test the stability of the hip. If the hip cannot easily be reduced and is extremely tight and cannot be brought down, the femoral neck should be shortened a few millimeters at a time until a reduction can be carried out. A snug fit that is not too loose and cannot be easily distracted from the socket gives the most security postoperatively. The hip should be flexed 90°, and internal rotation of 45° and external rotation of 45° should be carried out with the assistant carefully watching the position of the femoral head in the acetabulum. If the hip dislocates, one should look for an osteophyte on the femoral neck or the acetabular area or thick scar tissue from the capsule. Dislocation can also occur if the acetabular component has not been placed in the proper position. This should not have occurred if proper positioning of the socket holder has been carried out at the previous stage. Adduction and abduction should be carried out with the leg flat on the table and internal and external rotation to determine again the stability when the patient is lying flat.

The trochanter can be pulled down at this stage to determine where it will fit against the shaft of the femur. The male trochanteric reamer is then applied to the cut surface of the trochanter, and the undersurface is rounded to fit against the shaft of the femur. The female reamer is used on the shaft of the femur on its lateral surface where the trochanter will come to rest.

The hip is dislocated, and the trial femoral component is removed. The next step is to insert the wires for holding the trochanter. Two holes are drilled in the lateral femoral shaft 1 inch below the site determined for the reattachment of the trochanter. A stainless steel #16 wire is passed up through the neck through each hole and brought out through the cancellous bone where the trochanter has been removed. A transverse hole is drilled through the lesser trochanter, and a wire is passed through this hole and around the neck. The trial prosthesis is again inserted to be sure that it does not bind on the wires in the medullary cavity.

The leg is adducted, and the medul-

lary canal is suctioned while the surgeon changes his outer gloves. The nurse or associate surgeon mixes the cement, and then the surgeon rolls it into a sausage shape and inserts it into the femoral shaft after it has begun to show wrinkles on its surface. The surgeon forces the cement down the shaft with the slow, steady pressure of the index finger. It may take 20 to 30 pushes to insert the cement. There are various cement guns available which may supersede this manual procedure. A plastic tube may be inserted down the medullary cavity to remove the air and blood as the cement is inserted, but this is not always necessary because some air and blood will exit through the wire holes in the shaft of the femur.

The femoral prosthesis is slowly pushed down the shaft into the cement, and the prosthesis is pushed into valgus to allow cement to collect along the calcar region and along the lateral border of the femoral stem. It is very important to avoid anteversion or retroversion of the prosthesis at this time. The holder is carefully removed to avoid scratching the head, and the femoral head pusher is applied over the femoral head. The excess cement is removed from around the neck, and as the cement hardens the pusher is tapped several times with a mallet to force the cement into the cancellous bone.

The hip is then reduced carefully so as not to scratch the femoral head, and the reduction again may be tested for stability by flexing the hip 90° and internally and externally rotating it. If the cup and femoral component have been correctly inserted, dislocation should be no problem at this stage.

The trochanter is replaced by grasping it with a special holder. A hole is drilled anteriorly and posteriorly through the bone of the trochanter, and the transverse wires are passed up through these holes. The wire is then passed through the gluteus medius tendon proximal to the trochanter, and the two vertical wires are passed through the separate holes in the gluteus tendon. The vertical wires are grasped to pull the trochanter down to the prepared area on the shaft, and the transverse wires are tightened with a Harris wire tightener or a Kirschner traction bow. The transverse wire is twisted for about 1 inch and then cut off. A hole is drilled in the trochanter, and the end of the wire is inserted and impacted into the trochanter. The vertical wires are twisted in a similar manner and are impacted into the bone of the trochanter to avoid any sharp points. The leg is placed in a neutral position, and the vastus lateralis is sutured over the wires. If the vastus is sutured with the leg in abduction, the sutures may pull out when the leg is placed in a neutral position postoperatively. Suction tubes are inserted anteriorly and posteriorly into the hip joint and are brought out through the anterior thigh. The fascia lata should be carefully closed with nonabsorbable sutures, and then the subcutaneous tissue and skin should be closed in layers.

Postoperative Care. An abduction pillow is placed between the patient's legs for 4 days after the operation, and the patient is turned every 4 hours, or else placed in a balanced suspension sling. The balanced suspension sling is preferred over the pillow, especially for patients who have severe rheumatoid arthritis. Patients are much more comfortable because the sling allows them to get onto a bedpan much easier by lifting the leg and also tends to remove the pressure on the heel. The patient can exercise the leg in the sling and thus stimulate venous return. The usual postoperative orders consist of the following:

Total Hip Replacement Postoperative Orders

1. Vital signs q 15 min. until stable, then q 30 min. for 4 hr. and then q 4 hr.
2. Fluid and diet as tolerated.
3. Bed rest; do not turn.
4. Foot of patient's bed elevated 4 inches—Trendelenburg position.
5. Intake and output.
6. Closed suction drainage. Chart drainage from suction tubes every 4 hours.
7. Leg in balanced suspension in abduction.
8. Enema or laxative of choice in the evening.
9. Portable anteroposterior roentgenogram of hip, large film 14 x 17, in the recovery room.
10. Hematocrit and hemoglobin in the morning for 3 days.
11. Pain medication.
12. Medication for nausea.
13. Sleeping medication.
14. Stool softener.
15. $\frac{1}{6}$ Molar sodium lactate 1000 ml I.V. at 100 ml per hr.
16. Follow with 5 percent dextrose in water at 100 ml per hour to keep I.V. open.

The suction tubes are removed after 48 hours when the drainage has ceased. The intravenous fluid is generally stopped on the first postoperative day if the patient is able to take fluids by mouth. Catherization and indwelling catheters are avoided as much as possible to prevent genitourinary infection. Postoperative antibiotics have not been utilized, but there are two schools of thought, and the use of antibiotics must be determined by the individual surgeon. The decision to use anticoagulants also varies from surgeon to surgeon. In general, anticoagulants have been avoided because of the higher incidence of complications with their use. The incidence of phlebitis and pulmonary emboli in most series is much less in the rheumatoid arthritic patient. Whether this is due to the large doses of aspirin or some other factors is not known. However, aspirin can be given postoperatively as a possible anticoagulant in these patients.

The patient is allowed to stand on the fourth postoperative day, and if there is no evidence of dizziness on the fifth day, he may begin ambulating with the aid of a walker or crutches, putting partial weight on the operative leg. When patients have a feeling of lightheadedness, the legs may be wrapped with Ace bandages or thromboembolic stockings may be worn pre- and postoperatively to aid in the venous return. On the seventh day, the patient is allowed to go to the bathroom, an elevated commode being used to prevent severe flexion of the hip. Care must be exercised in toilet training because this is where most of the dislocations occur. The sutures are left in approximately 12 to 14 days, and the patients are usually discharged in 2 to 3 weeks. Prior to discharge a roentgenogram of the hip is obtained for further evaluation, and the patient is seen 6 weeks postoperatively when a recheck roentgenogram is obtained to determine whether the trochanter has united or not. If there has been no displacement, the patient is encouraged to put full weight on the hip and gradually discard the crutches or walker and use a cane until he is perfectly stable.

Complications. The late results of low friction arthroplasty of the hip reveal that after 9 years complete success is seen in approximately 92 percent of the patients. Charnley has stated that the four factors responsible for failure of the low friction arthroplasty are (1) infection, (2) loosening of the implant, (3) postoperative death, and (4) unexplained pain.

Infection. The most serious complication resulting in failure of the total hip replacement has been infection. Three types of infection are generally seen with total hip replacement: (1) early superficial infection occurring in the incision, (2) early deep infection developing in the wound, and (3) late infection occurring years after the operation. The incidence of infection tends to vary with the series reported. Reports have indicated infection rates as high as 15 percent in some series.

The use of clean air rooms and "space" suits has been reported to decrease the number of infections in some of the series. There is a considerable amount of debate as to whether this type of operating room and apparel is necessary. There is no doubt that the space-type suit tends to prevent contamination from the operating room personnel falling into the incision. Charnley himself has reduced his operative infection rate from 8.9 percent to less than 1 percent by using his clean air chamber. Other types of prevention, however, are available. Topical antibiotic irrigation of the wound with 50,000 units bacitracin, 5 gm neomycin, and 50 mg polymyxin dissolved in 500 cc normal saline solution has been used in many operating rooms. Suction drainage, double gloves, and rapid operating have all tended to reduce the number of infections. It should be noted that there is a much higher incidence of infection in patients who have had previous surgery, especially if a failed metallic device is present from the previous operation.

At the time of surgery cultures should be taken from the area where the failed metal device was located, and a specimen of the bursal tissue should be removed for biopsy. If a positive culture is obtained antibiotic therapy is indicated, even though there is only a small growth of organisms. The choice of drug will be determined by the sensitivity and the type of organism that was obtained. In general, intravenous antibiotics for 2 weeks should be given followed by oral antibiotics for 2 months. Although this is drastic therapy, every effort should be made to prevent a low-grade infection about a total hip prosthesis. It is even felt that routine antibiotics could be considered in patients who have failed metallic devices because of the high incidence of chronic infection about these devices.

Salvage of an infected total hip replacement may be possible in certain cases. Obtaining a culture of the organism, early wound drainage, and proper antibiotic selection can salvage a certain number of patients. The insertion of suction tube and irrigation drainage as suggested by Compere has been utilized in some patients with successful retention of the prosthesis and healing of the wound. A number of patients have had no recurrence of infection when the total hip replacement was removed and a new prosthesis was implanted within 6 to 8 weeks if the wound had healed. Each patient should be carefully evaluated because of the magnitude of the surgical procedure and the possible recurrence of infection. Buchholz has replaced infected total hips and incorporated antibiotics into the cement as an additional aid in controlling the infection.

When a deep infection does occur, it generally produces persistent pain that should alert the surgeon to the possibility of infection. Radiologic evidence of bone changes and thickening of the cortex with sclerosis is another indication of infection deep in the wound.

If the infection cannot be controlled by appropriate means and drainage continues, the entire prosthesis and cement must be removed. Generally the hip is converted to a Girdlestone arthroplasty and attempts at salvage or replacement can be considered in the future.

A number of infections have occurred many years postoperatively following septicemia. Chronic infections that require surgery—for instance, an infected gall bladder—can be a source of septicemia with subsequent infection of the total hip implant. Patients should be cautioned to notify their physicians or dentists that whenever a possible infected area is to be operated upon prophylactic antibiotics should be given. This is extremely important to prevent infection of the implant.

Mechanical Loosening. Mechanical loosening can occur due to infection, but in the absence of infection the incidence of loosening is quite small with the Charnley low friction arthroplasty. Either component can loosen because of incorrect cementing technique at the time of the operation or failure of the cement to adhere to the bone. The acetabular component can become loose by intrusion into the pelvis with fracture of the supporting bone about the cement bond (Fig. 9-46). This can occur more frequently in the patient with a protrusio of the acetabulum, and one must be extremely wary of the patient with a large failed cup arthroplasty. Deep reaming of the acetabulum is not recommended because of this problem. A large cup protruding into the acetabulum leaves very little inner support and bony attachment to the ischium and pubis. This is a potential area of stress fracture, and fractures have been reported in patients who have had total hip replacement. Charnley has also noted that in all of his mechanical loosenings, roentgenographic evidence was visible by the fourth postoperative year.

Stainless steel mesh can be used to line the inner wall with cement as reinforcement (Fig. 9-47). A layer of cement should be spread over the inner wall of the acetabulum. The mesh is placed over the cement, and another layer of cement is spread over the mesh before insertion of the socket.

Dislocations. It has been suggested by several authors that the small size of the Charnley total hip replacement (22 mm) would lead to dislocation of the prosthesis much more frequently than a large-sized femoral head (Fig. 9-48). However, proper operative technique in a large series of patients has demonstrated that dislocation is not a major problem with the Charnley prosthesis. The correct orientation of the prosthetic socket and the femoral component tends to prevent this. Reattachment of the greater trochanter distally also tends to increase

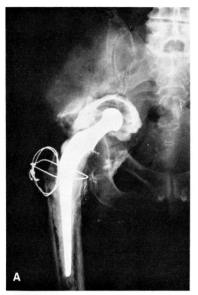

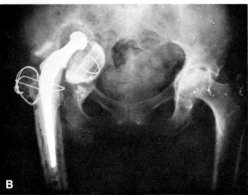

FIG. 9-46 Roentgenograms showing complications after Charnley low friction arthroplasty. A. The acetabular component can become loose and protrude into the pelvis when the inner wall is extremely thin and the cement breaks loose from the inferior aspect of the acetabulum. B. The components have dislocated, and the femoral head has eroded into the pelvic wall.

the tension, preventing dislocation. Removal of all osteophytes and scar tissue which could be a source of dislocation tends to prevent this complication. Proper education of the patient who has an excellent range of flexion within the first week postoperatively is important to prevent dislocation. The patient must be cautioned about flexing beyond 90°, especially in internal and external rota-

tion. Dislocation is much more common in the rheumatoid patient with poor tissue and weak musculature about the hip. If dislocation occurs in a rheumatoid patient, reduction can often be achieved by gradual pull on the leg by the surgeon over a period of time or by traction overnight. In some cases, reduction under anesthesia can be performed very easily, and then the patient may be placed in a balanced suspension for 1 to 2 weeks. The patient should again be cautioned about avoiding motions that precipitated the dislocation. Spica cast treatment is not generally recommended in the patient with severe rheumatoid arthritis.

Late dislocation can occur but is extremely rare (Fig. 9-49). Charnley has reported three late dislocations in patients who have had no previous trouble. One occurred 5 years after the surgery, one 8 years after the surgery, and the other 9 years following operation.

Trochanteric Problems. Many surgeons do not like to remove the greater trochanter in performing a total hip replacement because of the problems associated with removal of the trochanter. However, the advantages gained by removing the trochanter far exceed any of the problems encountered by its removal. The exposure is much better, and the ability to properly align the components is worth the additional surgery. In some rheumatoid patients, avulsion of the trochanter can occur because of osteoporosis or breakage of the wire, but in the long-term follow-up this has been of no consequence in the result obtained (Fig. 9-50). Occasionally the patients will complain of crepitation over the broken wires in the region of the trochanter and tenderness when lying on that side at night; however, this again has not been a great problem and occurs in a small percentage of patients. Removal of the wires in patients who have had difficulty has given complete relief.

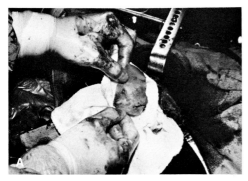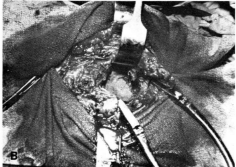

FIG. 9-47 Surgical views of repair of weak inner wall during a Charnley low friction arthroplasty. A. Stainless steel mesh used to reinforce the inner wall when a protrusio is present. B. The inner wall of the acetabulum lined with stainless steel mesh.

Thrombophlebitis. Thrombophlebitis occurs in a higher percentage of hip patients undergoing surgery and must be considered in all total hip replacements. The incidence again varies with the series under investigation by various authors, but the surgeon must be aware of this complication. Dextran and other anticoagulants were used in one series reported, but it is believed that the complications of these medications outweigh their prophylactic value. If a definite case of thrombophlebitis exists in the deep veins of the lower extremity or pelvis, one should seriously consider anticoagulant therapy postoperatively, the major concern being the development of a pulmonary embolus with a fatal outcome. Thromboembolic stockings may be used as a precaution. The stocking should be placed on the unoperative leg during the surgical procedures, as phlebitis can occur during the operation.

Fractures. Fracture of the shaft of the femur can occur on dislocating the hip

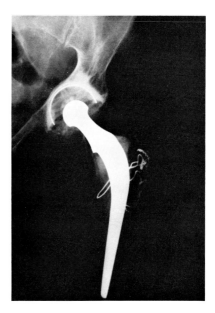

FIG. 9-49 Roentgenogram of a hip one year after dislocation of total hip replacement corrected by a closed reduction. Small fragments of cement are visible in the acetabulum, but these have caused no problems, and the patient is asymptomatic. Because of the patient's age and absence of symptoms no further surgery is contemplated.

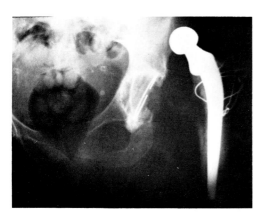

FIG. 9-48 Dislocation of a large-sized femoral head in a total hip replacement.

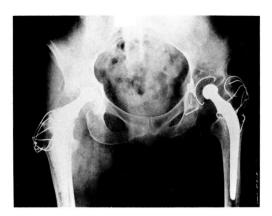

FIG. 9-50 Roentgenogram showing an avulsion of the greater trochanter 5 years after a total hip replacement on the left side. Although the wires have broken, there is no instability.

while performing the operation. If there is any difficulty in dislocation, it is always advisable to consider an osteotomy through the femoral neck and removing the head from the acetabulum without placing stress on the shaft of the femur. This is especially important in patients with a protrusio or with severe osteoporosis of the extremity. If fracture occurs, a long stem prosthesis is available to gain stability at the fracture site.

Urinary Retention. Urinary retention is a definite problem in the older age patient undergoing total hip replacement. In any elderly male with prostatic problems, it is always advisable to have the prostatic obstruction taken care of prior to considering total hip replacement. If catheterization or the use of an indwelling catheter can be avoided after total hip replacement, many genitourinary infections can be prevented. It is thought that some of the postoperative total hip infections may actually occur from septicemia involving the bacteria in the genitourinary tract. It was surprising that a large number of elderly women also have urinary retention postoperatively. Atony of the bladder is quite common in the elderly female and leads to urinary retention. Patients often are not aware of this, and the surgeon

must keep this in mind when treating older women. A clean-catch urine culture should be obtained preoperatively as a precaution against silent urinary infection.

Miscellaneous. Several other types of problems are seen occasionally in total hip replacement such as wound hematoma which should be evacuated and drained early with closure of the wound, transient peroneal nerve palsy from using Buck's traction postoperatively, paralytic ileus, pulmonary infection, coronary thrombosis, and sciatic nerve palsy. Wear of the acetabular component has not been a factor as yet. Charnley's latest report for patients with low friction arthroplasties reveals that the average wear is 1.2 mm in 10 years. However, 14 percent of the patients, or 10 out of 72, revealed wear up to 4 mm in 10 years, averaging 0.3 mm per year. Since there was no obvious connection between the weight of the patient and the physical activity, Charnley has concluded wear may be due to a difference in the quality of the high density polyethylene.

Resorption of the femoral calcar has been reported by Charnley and was noted to be present 5 years following the operation but did not materially increase thereafter. The exact significance of this at the present time is not known. No symptoms have been related to this change in the calcar.

It has become apparent in the past two years that fatigue fracture of the metal stem of the femoral prosthesis can occur. Charnley has reported 16 failures in 8,500 implants. The average age of the patient was 58 years with the oldest being 76 and the youngest 32. The commonest interval following surgery for fracture to occur was between $3\frac{1}{2}$ and 4 years. Twelve of the 13 typical stress fractures of the femoral component occurred in men and only one in a female patient. The average weight of these patients was 181 pounds, with a range from 144 to 224 pounds. The valgus position of the prosthesis is important in reducing the stresses on the femoral component, and it is important also to carefully curette the cancellous bone in the region of the calcar femoris. The weak spot in the femoral component is in the middle third section, especially in heavy male patients.

Because of fatigue fracture, the thickness of the stem has been increased in the Charnley prosthesis. An extra-heavy stem and a heavy stem are now available for insertion in male patients who weigh 181 pounds or more. It is not difficult to insert these extra-heavy components, but occasionally reaming of the canal is necessary in patients with a narrow canal.

Charnley-Müller Total Hip

The Charnley-Müller total hip replacement differs from the Charnley prosthesis in that the femoral head is 32 mm in diameter and the stem is curved more to allow easier insertion without removal of the trochanter (Fig. 9-51). It is available in a number of neck lengths. The acetabular socket is made of high density polyethylene similar to the material used for the Charnley socket.

Many surgeons prefer this technique because it allows an easy approach to the hip joint without removal of the trochanter, and a variety of neck lengths permits restoration of the abductor lever arm and also leg length. It is believed that the larger femoral head decreases the risk of dislocation, but this is open to question. The same preoperative precautions and orders are used as in the Charnley low friction arthroplasty.

Operative Technique. The patient is placed in a supine position on the operating table with a small roll under the buttock. The anterolateral incision is made using the Watson-Jones approach. The incision is placed approximately 1 inch distal and lateral to the anterior superior iliac spine and curves distally and laterally over the greater trochanter (Fig. 9-52). The skin and subcutaneous tissue are opened, and skin towels moistened with antibiotic solution are applied. The interval between the gluteus medius and the tensor fascia lata muscle is developed. This interval is not always easy to define and is best approached by working proximally from the distal area of the vastus lateralis. The

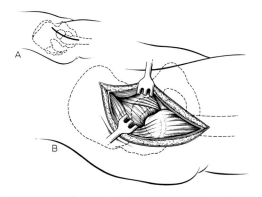

FIG. 9-52 The Charnley-Müller total hip replacement. A. The anterolateral incision. B. Exposure of the capsule of the hip joint. The gluteus medius muscle is pulled distally, and the tensor fascia lata is pulled anteriorly. (Redrawn from Campbell's Operative Orthopaedics, 5th ed. H. H. Grenshaw, editor. St. Louis, C. V. Mosby, 1971.)

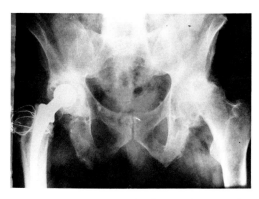

FIG. 9-51 Roentgenogram after implantion of a Charnley-Müller prosthesis. Compare the 32 mm-head with that of the Charnley prosthesis in Fig. 9-50.

gluteus medius is retracted with a Hohman retractor placed behind the neck and in front of the greater trochanter, and a second retractor is placed along the medial side of the neck directed toward the lesser trochanter. The fat over the articular capsule is scraped off with a periosteal elevator, and a third retractor is placed over the superior aspect of the acetabulum, exposing the capsule. The capsulectomy is performed, removing as much of the anterior medial and lateral capsule as possible. The femoral neck is divided at a 45° angle to the long axis of the neck and with 5° of anteversion approximately 1 inch proximal to the lesser trochanter. A corkscrew is inserted into the cut surface of the femoral head, and the head is removed from the acetabulum.

At this stage the posterior portion of the capsule is also removed. A Hohman retractor is inserted beneath the posterior rim of the acetabulum to aid in exposure and depressing the femur posteriorly. Charnley instruments can be utilized in preparing the acetabulum. The centering ring and drill is placed into the acetabulum at a 45° angle with the long axis of the body and in 10° of anteversion. The depth of the inner wall of the pelvis can be measured, and then the Charnley penetrating reamer is used to displace the socket inward. It should be pointed out that a center hole is not inserted if the inner wall of the pelvis is extremely thin. A Charnley expanding reamer is used to enlarge the acetabulum if necessary to 50 mm in diameter. Special reamers developed by Müller can be utilized to make the diameter of the acetabulum either 44 mm or 50 mm. The trial acetabular socket is inserted to determine the fit; then the various cement holes are made in the superior and inferior aspects of the acetabulum. The area is thoroughly dried, and the cement is mixed by the assistant surgeon or nurse. At this time the pillow is removed

by the circulating nurse from beneath the hip, and when the cement has reached the proper consistency, the cement restrictor is placed in the centering hole and the cement is forced into the acetabulum. The socket is inserted at a 45° angle to the long axis of the body, and at 10° of anteversion. Excess cement should be removed and the socket held firmly in place until the cement has hardened.

The femur is now prepared for the femoral prosthesis. It may be necessary to release a small area of the abductor gluteus minimus and medius from their insertion on the trochanter. The leg should be adducted and externally rotated, and at this stage if there are contractures of the external rotators, they should be released. A long pointed Hohman retractor is placed beneath the greater trochanter to lift the proximal femur up out of the wound to allow easy insertion of the rasp into the shaft of the femur. The rasp is introduced by hand to prevent penetration of the shaft of the femur. A mallet may be necessary in patients with hard bone. In preparing the shaft, the femoral component should be placed at about 0° to 5° of anteversion. A trial reduction should be carried out, and a femoral component with the proper length of neck should be selected to maintain the normal abductor tension. The tension should be reasonably moderate, and the hip should not dislocate through a normal range of motion. If dislocation occurs, it may be necessary to select a prosthesis with a longer neck and also to be sure there are no osteophytes or thick scar tissue posteriorly. At this stage another batch of cement is prepared and packed into the femoral shaft, and then the femoral prosthesis is forced down the shaft in the proper position with a slight amount of valgus. Following hardening of the cement, any excess cement should be removed, and then the prosthesis is reduced into the acetabulum. A range of motion test should be carried out to be sure dislocation will not occur. Suction tubes are placed into the hip joint and brought out through the anterior thigh, and the wound is closed in layers. The patient is treated postoperatively in the same manner as after the Charnley low friction arthroplasty.

Complications. The complications of the Charnley-Müller technique are quite similar to those from the Charnley low friction arthroplasty. Additional complications that can occur during the procedure are perforation of the femoral artery and vein by the Hohman retractor if it is incorrectly inserted on the medial aspect of the hip joint. It is also possible to injure the femoral nerve with the medial retractor. Fracture of the greater trochanter and perforation of the shaft with the rasp can occur because of inadequate exposure. The early postoperative complications are quite similar to those seen with any of the total hip replacements.

Girdlestone Resection

Although the Girdlestone technique has been advised for the treatment of severe disease of the hip, it has never

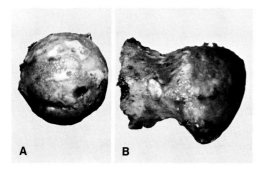

FIG. 9-53 Two views of the gross specimen of a femoral head removed at the time of a Girdlestone resection from a patient with severe rheumatoid arthritis. Because of the rheumatoid pannus the surface has been destroyed and no articular cartilage remains.

been widely accepted except as a salvage procedure or as a last resort in a patient who has an infected joint (Fig. 9-53). The major advantage of this procedure is the relief of pain in the majority of the patients. The patient will retain a wide range of motion, and in patients who have had serious infection of the joint, it allows for healing of the wound as well as a reasonable amount of stability from the scar tissue. The disadvantages are the loss of leg length and a marked limp. In some patients, however, a surprisingly good hip joint can still be obtained with this type of resection.

The surgeon who is going to undertake a Girdlestone resection on a patient must be aware of the results with this type of operation. A very positive outlook with reasonable explanation to the patient of what can be expected is extremely important in regard to the postoperative result. If the patient is cooperative, has good musculature and is willing to work, a reasonably stable hip can be developed.

Operative Technique. The operation is designed to create a pseudarthrosis, and an adequate amount of bone must be removed to prevent bony contact between the femoral neck and the acetabulum. The anterior iliofemoral or the Watson-Jones approach will give adequate exposure. If areas of the head or neck are still present, they should be resected down to the intertrochanteric line, and all diseased tissue should be excised if infection is present. The shaping of the femoral surface should be carried out with the leg in a neutral position and should run along the base of the neck (Fig. 9-54).

The acetabular margin should be smooth, and any osteophytes or ledges should be removed. After the area has been thoroughly prepared, the hip should be telescoped up and down to be sure that there is no bony spur that could abut against the acetabulum. It has been

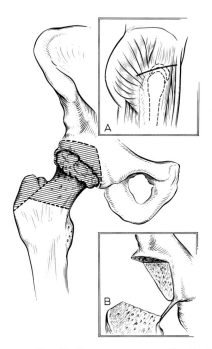

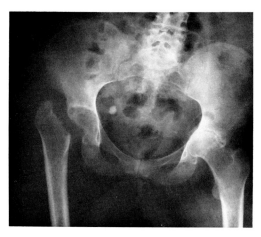

FIG. 9-55 Roentgenogram after a Girdlestone resection for rheumatoid arthritis of the hip. The patient's pain was relieved and there was an excellent range of motion, but ambulation was limited.

FIG. 9-54 The Girdlestone resection. The shaded area of bone should be removed at the time of resection. A. The transverse skin incision. B. After removal of the bone and reshaping of the femoral surface. (Redrawn from Campbell's Operative Orthopaedics, 5th ed. H. H. Grenshaw, editor. St. Louis, C. V. Mosby, 1971.)

recommended in some cases to move the iliopsoas muscle from the lesser trochanter to the anterior aspect of the hip in the region of the intertrochanteric line. All dense scars should be excised from the area, and two $\frac{1}{4}$-inch silicone perforated tubes should be inserted into the dead space in the anterior and posterior aspects of the hip. It is also recommended that the tubes be overlapped or in close approximation to prevent plugging with blood clots and debris. One tube is used for irrigation, and the other for suction to remove the irrigation fluid. The suction irrigation system can be started before the wound is closed to prevent plugging of the tubes and should be continued until all dead space has been obliterated.

Postoperative Management. Isometric exercises should be begun as soon as the patient is able to perform the exercises. Skeletal traction has been recommended for 4 weeks postoperatively to maintain length and prevent loss of the space between the femur and the acetabulum. Postoperatively, the patient should be advised to lie flat in bed for 4 weeks to avoid a flexion contracture of the hip. Abduction and adduction exercises can be performed with the aid of a skateboard. Patients are allowed up after the fourth week and begin walking with crutches, with partial weight bearing. Because of the shortening of the leg, a raised heel is often necessary along with a sole to provide approximately 1-$\frac{1}{2}$ inches of length. The patient will continue to improve years after the operation. With proper care and good musculature a reasonably satisfactory hip can be obtained free of pain and with good motion (Fig. 9-55).

Osteoarthritis

Osteoarthritis of the hip joint has become a major source of pain in the older patient since man assumed the upright position. Patients who have worked all

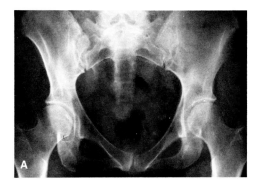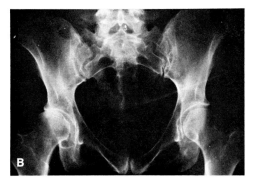

FIG. 9-56 Roentgenograms showing development of primary osteoarthritis. A. In June 1971 the hip joints appeared normal, and there was no evidence of disease. B. By October 1972 advanced osteoarthritis had developed in the right hip, with loss of the joint space and increasing pain.

of their lives and are ready to retire and enjoy life suddenly become disabled with increasing pain and the inability to walk. Any condition producing incongruity in the hip joint tends to increase the wear and tear of the joint and accelerate the development of osteoarthritis.

Basically two types of osteoarthritis tend to develop in patients. *Primary* osteoarthritis occurs with no evidence of preexisting disease (Fig. 9-56). *Secondary* osteoarthritis occurs following Legg-Perthes disease, congenital dysplasia of the hip, slipped femoral epiphysis, and trauma (Fig. 9-57). Key and Ford stated that mechanically unsound hips will develop osteoarthritis if the patient lives long enough. Tuberculosis, infection, any vascular necrosis, collagen diseases, sickle cell anemia, and other diseases can lead to secondary osteoarthritis.

Murray in a review of radiographs of patients with primary osteoarthritis of the hip noted some change in the femoral head tilt in approximately 40 percent of the cases. It has been proposed that perhaps minor anatomic changes in the proximal femur can produce osteoarthritis, and that, in fact, primary osteoarthritis may be secondary to them.

Osteoarthritis (malum coxae senilis) usually produces symptoms in patients over the age of fifty. There is a much higher incidence in the male, and it is usually unilateral in approximately two thirds of the cases.

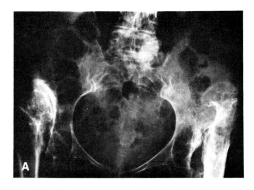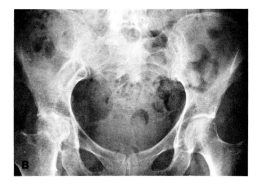

FIG. 9-57 Roentgenograms showing development of secondary osteoarthritis. A. This patient has bilateral congenital dislocations of the hip with secondary osteoarthritis of the right hip. B. This patient suffered a subcapital fracture of the right hip with the development of osteoarthritis and loss of the articular cartilage and joint space (traumatic arthritis).

The onset of the disease process is usually insidious, with the patient developing occasional discomfort and pain in the groin, buttock, or thigh. Occasionally symptoms will be referred to the knee with no complaints referable to the hip, and only a careful physical examination of the patient can rule out knee disease. The patient will complain of pain and limping which are generally relieved by rest. Symptoms may be present for years before the patient seeks care from the orthopaedic surgeon. When patients are seen by the orthopaedic surgeon, limitation of hip motion may be present, along with the development of a flexion contracture.

Radiographs can be extremely valuable in the evaluation of the patient with osteoarthritis of the hip. In many cases, an anteroposterior roentgenogram of the pelvis is sufficient to reveal the disease process. In other cases, views should be obtained in internal rotation, neutral, abduction, and adduction. These are especially important if an osteotomy is to be considered.

In evaluating the roentgenogram, there are two types of primary osteoarthritis that can be noted on the x-ray film. Pearson and Riddell noted that 85 percent of the patients with primary osteoarthritis had a superior-lateral type of involvement with narrowing of the joint space (Fig. 9-58A). This has also been our experience. In a smaller group of patients there is evidence of medial displacement of the femoral head into the acetabulum with loss of rotation (Fig. 9-58B). Exostoses are quite common, especially along the inferior medial aspect of the femoral head (Fig. 9-59A). Osteophytes also develop about the acetabulum with loss of the joint space and eburnation and sclerosis of the femoral head (Fig. 9-59B). Cystic formation in the acetabulum and femoral head usually occurs with advanced degenerative arthritis of the hip (Fig. 9-60).

It is important to realize that changes observed in roentgenograms cannot always be correlated with clinical symptoms. Patients with far-advanced disease may have minimal symptoms, except for loss of motion or flexion contractures with shortening of the involved extremity. It is important, also, to realize that for patients with minimal radiologic findings but with maximum symptoms, roentgenograms repeated within several months can be valuable because rapidly advancing destruction of the joint will become much more obvious on the subsequent films. Cases that progress rapidly may be associated with pathologic fractures in the femoral head (Fig. 9-61).

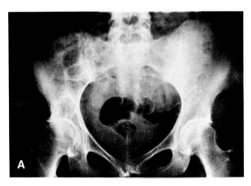 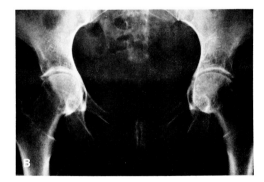

FIG. 9-58 Roentgenograms of the hips of patients with primary osteoarthritis. A. The superior-lateral type of involvement with narrowing of the joint space. B. Medial displacement of the femoral head into the acetabulum with loss of rotation.

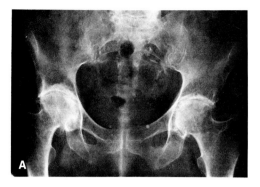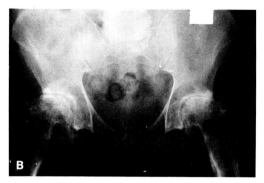

FIG. 9-59 Roentgenograms of patients with primary osteoarthritis. A. Exostoses appear along the inferior medial aspect of the femoral head. B. There are osteophytes in the region of the acetabulum, loss of joint space, eburnation, and sclerosis of the femoral head.

Osteoarthritis is believed to be a mechanical situation created by stresses on the weight-bearing cartilage and bone during standing or walking. The smaller the area exposed, the greater the stress. During the stance phase of walking, the body weight is balanced over the hip joint and is supported by the pull of the abductor muscles. All of the muscles about the hip contribute to the intra-articular pressure, especially if the hip is painful and the muscles are in spasm. Any change in the distribution of forces about the hip joint produces an alteration of the condensed bone in the acetabular roof. It is believed these abnormal stresses occur because of loss of articular cartilage, an incongruous joint, or a joint with a small acetabulum only partly covering the head and therefore increasing the stress on the smaller weight-bearing surface of the femoral head.

Knodt and others believe that the femoral head becomes altered in shape and gradually changes into two zones which are different in function and structure. The first zone, which is somewhat funnel-shaped in the central area, carries the major weight-bearing stress. Areas of sclerosis and cyst formation occur. Microscopically there are cellular areas with increased vascular activity. The second zone tends to surround the central one and expands into available space where the joint is not subjective to pressure or weight transmission. In these areas, microscopically there is fatty marrow with no sclerosis or necrosis.

Conservative Treatment

There has been an explosive change in the treatment of the patient with osteoarthritis of the hip over the past 10 years. Despite these rapid advances in the treatment of osteoarthritis of the hip surgically, one should not lose sight of the magnitude of the problem. Whenever possible, the patient should be

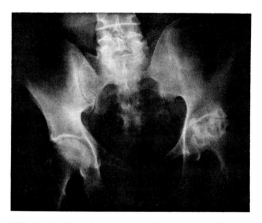

FIG. 9-60 Roentgenogram of patient with advanced degenerative arthritis of the hip. Cysts have formed in the acetabulum and the femoral head.

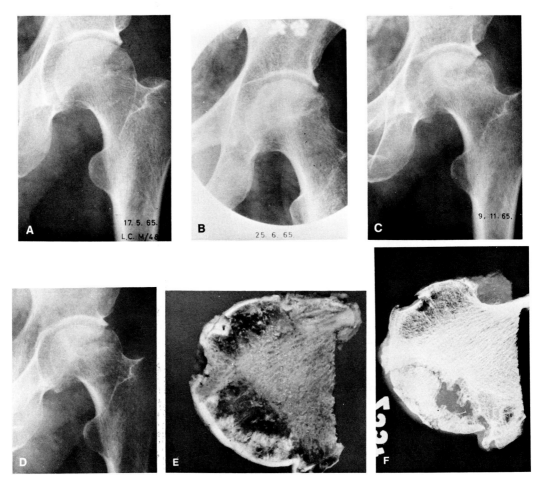

FIG. 9-61 Series of roentgenograms showing development of osteoarthritis of the hip. A. Early osteoarthritis of the femoral head. B. One month later. Beginning irregularity of the femoral head can be seen. C. Five months after B. A pathologic fracture is occurring through the superior aspect of the femoral head. D. Three months after C. The fragment is avascular and the change in the femoral head is very obvious. E. Cross section of the femoral head removed at surgery. F. A roentgenogram through the head reveals the fracture. (Courtesy of Department Orthopaedics, University of Hong Kong).

treated conservatively during the early phase of the disease. The majority of patients tend to be in the older age group and have numerous medical problems. In some instances they have tolerated their hip disease for a decade with minimal complaints until the last few years of the disease process. Therefore, during the early acute episode the patient with aches and pains and some limitation of motion due to osteoarthritis of the hip, conservative therapy should be considered.

The conservative management of osteoarthritis of the hip differs from that for rheumatoid arthritis because a great deal of improvement can be obtained by resting the hip joint during the early phase of the disease. The use of a cane as a support for the hip in walking is of great value in relieving the mechanical stress upon the hip joint. Crutches can also be of great value during this phase. Salicylate therapy and the use of anti-inflammatory drugs other than steroids may greatly alleviate the patient's discomfort. Many times the acute phase will subside, and the patient will be extremely comfortable. The orthopaedic surgeon can inject local steroids into the hip joint. These injections can give prolonged relief, especially in patients with an acute inflammatory episode related to osteoarthritis. The elderly patient who is a bad surgical risk may often be carried along with local steroid injections at 6- to 8-week intervals free of symptoms and able to continue daily activities.

Patients should be instructed in exercises to aid in putting the hip through a full range of motion and also to prevent flexion contractures. Physical therapy and hydrotherapy can also be used along with the exercise program to aid in strengthening the hip and obtaining a good range of motion.

Surgical Treatment

The operative treatment of the osteoarthritic hip differs somewhat from the treatment of the patient with rheumatoid arthritis of the hip. More procedures are available. The surgeon has the opportunity to consider more conservative procedures than the total hip replacement.

Pauwels believes that the key to successful treatment of osteoarthritis of the hip is to eliminate the abnormal stresses, and that the osteoarthritic hip has a remarkable regenerative power regardless of the stage of the disease or the age of the patient. This view is not shared by all surgeons interested in arthritis.

The results obtained with an osteotomy do not equal the results that could be obtained with a total hip replacement. If a displacement osteotomy is considered, one should always keep in mind that if a future total hip replacement is necessary, the distortion of the femoral neck and shaft may prevent the insertion of the prosthesis. Osteotomy certainly can be considered in the younger patient with early osteoarthritis.

The arthroplasty developed by Charnley and by McKee-Farrar has had phenomenal success in giving a painless, movable hip. However, the surgeon must be cautioned about the skill required in performing this operation and the numerous complications that can occur, some of which may be catastrophic. The cup arthroplasty is still a good operation in the young patient with osteoarthritis where an attempt is made to preserve bony stock. The advantages and disadvantages have been discussed in the section on rheumatoid arthritis. The skin arthroplasty which has been reported by Kallio has also given a reasonable number of satisfactory results. However, it has never been popular throughout the world.

The stem prosthesis of the Austin-Moore and Thompson type became extremely popular in the early 1960s, and thousands of these have been inserted. Although the procedure is reasonably easy to do, its long-term results have been poor, and a large number have eventually failed with the passage of time. It is an excellent prosthesis for the elderly patient with a fractured hip that has a good acetabulum, but protrusion into the pelvis can occur in a certain percentage of the cases.

The failed femoral replacement can be salvaged by the total hip operation, but removing the Austin-Moore prosthesis becomes a difficult problem in the osteoporotic patient with a protrusio of the pelvis. It is much easier to remove the Thompson head which does not have the holes in the stem for bone ingrowth. The cementing in of the stem prosthesis has become somewhat popular in the management of the fractured hip.

For the elderly patient or the middle-aged patient who has severe osteoarthritis of the hip and must earn a living, the total hip replacement should be considered. The patient with bilateral hip disease does not respond well to bilateral cup arthroplasty, nor will he do well with stiff hips. The rapid recovery after the total hip replacement has revolutionized the management of patients with severe and bilateral hip disease. The work of Charnley has now shown that the high-density polyethylene sockets wear little over 10 years and the age limit of the patients selected for the operation has been consistently dropping down, depending upon the severity of the hip problem.

The final selection of the operative procedure to be performed depends upon the age of the patient, the skill of the surgeon, and the individual problems presented by that particular patient.

Voss Hanging Hip Operation

The hanging hip operation was developed by Voss in an attempt to reduce the articular pressure. This operation was popular for a while but has few proponents at the present time. It consists of a tenotomy of the fascia lata, release of the greater trochanter, adductor tenotomy, and tenotomy of the rectus femoris.

Various reports in the literature state that pain is decreased in walking in the majority of the cases but no increase in mobility is obtained. Failure can be anticipated when the articular pressure is concentrated at the corner of the acetabulum as in a subluxated femoral head. This operation was originally recommended for the elderly patient because it required a minimum amount of surgery.

Operative Technique. The leg is adducted and internally rotated if possible. The patient may be positioned on the unaffected side in order to approach the trochanter. An 8 cm incision is made along the lateral aspect of the thigh. The fascia lata is split for 10 cm below the trochanter and then cut across trans-

versely. The trochanter is exposed and cut with an osteotome to displace it upward. The leg is then abducted, and the adductor tenotomy is performed. The rectus femoris is severed at its origin on the anterior inferior iliac spine. Some surgeons also recommend cutting the iliopsoas muscle.

Postoperative Care. Postoperatively, the patient is started on active motion, and in some cases hip traction of 5 to 10 pounds is utilized for 3 weeks. The patient is then allowed on crutches without weight-bearing.

Osteotomy

Osteotomy is a popular operation in various parts of the world, and a number of large series of cases have been accumulated. The mechanism for relief of pain by an osteotomy is still unknown. Many authors believe that adduction or displacement is not important and that division of the bone is the important thing. Studies by Trueta have called attention to the increased vascularity of the femoral head in osteoarthritis. Some think that the osteotomy actually decreases the blood supply to the femoral head, relieving the symptoms of osteoarthritis.

Osteotomy is indicated for patients who have pain in the hip and a deformity related to primary osteoarthritis. Generally, the ideal candidate for this type of procedure must have primary osteoarthritis with severe pain, especially at night, and still have 60° of hip flexion or more. The roentgenogram should reveal a reasonable preservation of the joint space with a round femoral head that is not subluxed.

Pauwels believes that there is necessity to consider either a varus or valgus osteotomy, depending upon the results of roentgenograms in adduction and abduction, to see which osteotomy would give the best fit of the femoral head in the acetabulum. In general, it appears not to be too important whether an abduction, adduction, or rotation osteotomy is performed (Fig. 9-62).

Adams and Spence have found that age has no bearing on the results obtained. As a rule, the operation is contraindicated for patients with osteoarthritis secondary to other disease, rheumatoid arthritis, and avascular necrosis.

At the present time, osteotomy usually is combined with some form of internal fixation. A compression-type device used by Müller is quite popular.

Operative Technique. The operative procedure can be carried out on a normal operating room table or on a table with orthopaedic traction. The latter allows more accurate positioning of the hip. A lateral approach to the trochanter is made approximately 6 inches in length, starting about the level of the greater trochanter and extending down the lateral aspect of the thigh. The fascia lata is divided, and the base of the trochanter is exposed. The vastus lateralis is detached from the oblique line of the trochanter and retracted out of the way to expose the lesser trochanter. The osteotomy generally starts at the base of the greater trochanter and is angled toward the upper aspect of the lesser trochanter. It is advisable to insert guide wires along the line of the osteotomy and also for the line of the blade plate. This will allow accurate placement of the osteotomy and the blade plate which can be checked by roentgenograms during the operative procedure.

The osteotomy line runs at approximately 10° to 20° of angulation with the shaft of the femur, and this line is outlined with drill holes. The blade of the compression plate is then inserted so that it will lie parallel to the osteotomy line and stay inside the femoral neck. The blade should be short enough so that it will not strike the medial femoral calcar and break through it. Once the blade is inserted, the osteotomy is completed with an osteotome or a power tool. The medial femoral cortex, which is quite fixed, should be divided first, and then the posterior cortex is divided to prevent splintering of the inferior femoral neck. Once the osteotomy has been completed, the femoral shaft can be displaced inward easily, and the compression plate blade is driven in snugly against the shaft of the femur. The osteotomy site is compressed tightly by the compression technique, and the plate is screwed to the side of the femur. The fascia lata is then repaired, and the

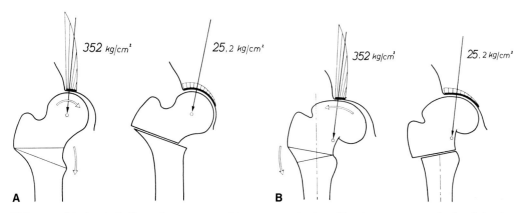

FIG. 9-62 Mechanical effect of osteotomy of joint stress. A. An adduction osteotomy. B. An abduction osteotomy.

wound is closed in layers. Suction tubes can be used postoperatively to reduce the pain and the hematoma formation.

Postoperative immobilization is not required because of the firm fixation of the compression plate. Postoperative exercises are instituted gradually. The patient is allowed to ambulate with crutches bearing partial weight until solid union has occurred in 3 to 6 months.

Stem Type Prostheses

The insertion of the Austin-Moore or Thompson stem type of prosthesis is an operation that replaces the femoral head but does not repair the acetabular surface. The procedure therefore can be classified as a hemiarthroplasty (Fig. 9-63). A number of excellent hemiarthroplasties have been performed for hip disease. The stem type of prosthesis can be used when the femoral head is

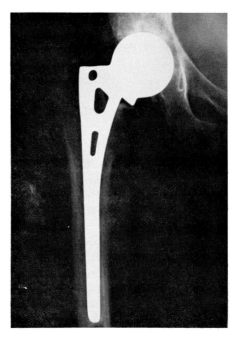

FIG. 9-64 Roentgenogram of patient who had an Austin-Moore replacement for osteoarthritis of the hip 5 years earlier. The acetabulum shows no evidence of articular cartilage at this time, and the patient is experiencing increasing discomfort in the hip joint. The prosthesis also appears to be loose in the shaft of the femur, and there is some evidence of sclerosis about the lower end of the prosthesis where a radiolucent line is seen adjacent to the stem.

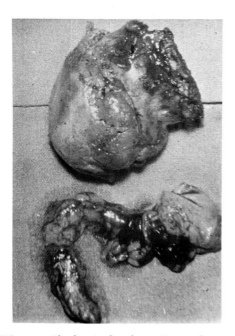

FIG. 9-63 The hemiarthroplasty. Severe destruction of the articular surface can be seen on this femoral head which has been removed for an Austin-Moore prosthesis.

affected by osteoarthritis if there is a reasonable acetabulum. It is not indicated following cup arthroplasty where the acetabulum has been previously reamed, as there is a high incidence of protrusio in this type of patient. There has been a tendency in the past to use the Austin-Moore prosthesis because it seemed to give the best results (Fig. 9-64). However, it is not advisable to cement a Moore prosthesis into place, as it becomes extremely difficult to remove. The Thompson prosthesis is easier to remove if total hip replacement becomes indicated in the future.

Operative Technique. Several approaches have been used for the insertion of the stem prosthesis. The anterior

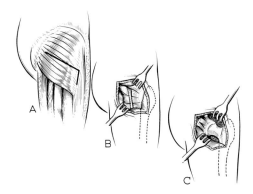

FIG. 9-65 Austin-Moore procedure. A. The posterolateral approach or "southern exposure." B. Separation of the fibers of the gluteus medius muscle to expose the sciatic nerve and the external rotators. C. Retraction of the sciatic nerve and division of the external rotators and capsule for exposure of the hip joint. (Redrawn from Campbell's Operative Orthopaedics, 5th ed. H. H. Grenshaw, editor. St. Louis, C. V. Mosby, 1971.)

approach is much more difficult than the "southern exposure" of Moore. The patient is placed on the unaffected side, and the thigh is flexed approximately 45° (Fig. 9-65). The incision is started low on the buttock, about 2 inches distal to and toward the outer side of the posterior inferior spine of the ilium. It runs downward and outward just beneath the greater trochanter and extends along the outer side of the thigh for approximately 4 inches below the trochanter. The fascia lata just below the greater trochanter is opened, and this incision is continued upward to divide the aponeurotic fibers of the gluteus maximus. The lower fibers of the muscle are spread upward, taking care to avoid the superior gluteal vessels, which are located about $1\frac{1}{2}$ inches above the lower border of the muscle body. The thigh is now flexed to a right angle of 90°, and the gluteus muscle upper fibers are retracted out of the way. The sciatic nerve lies fully exposed in the lower part of the incision. It should be carefully retracted medially. Over the lower portion of the capsule of the hip joint there is a layer of fatty tissue which

should be removed, and the insertions of the short external rotators, the gemelli, and the obturator internus tendon are divided. This will expose the posterior capsule of the hip joint. In some patients, it is necessary to release the insertion of the piriformis or the upper portion of the insertion of the quadratus femoris. The capsule of the joint is then opened parallel to the femoral neck up to the acetabular margin. The distal end of the capsule is also released from its attachment to give better exposure of the posterior portion of the neck. The lesser trochanter can now be visualized and is an important landmark. Dislocation of the femoral head should be carried out by flexing the thigh to a full right angle and adducting and internally rotating the leg (Fig. 9-66). Excessive force should be avoided to prevent fracture of the shaft in dislocating the femoral head. The neck of the femur should be cut across with a saw or power tool, $\frac{1}{2}$ to $\frac{3}{4}$ of an inch above the lesser trochanter. The cut should be made in the proper plane so that the prosthesis will fit well. The rasp should be used to ream the medullary canal.

The prosthesis is then driven down the shaft into place after selecting the proper size of femoral head. This can be done by measuring with a caliper the size of the femoral head removed and replacing it with a proper fit. The quadriceps muscle can be relaxed by extending the knee joint before applying traction to replace the femoral head. The prosthesis is carefully guided into place by manipulating the extremity from the position of internal rotation into neutral and a more anatomic position. The muscles and tissue will fall back into place, and only a few sutures will be required to close the wound.

Postoperative Management. Postoperatively the patient lies in bed with the limb extended and externally rotated to prevent dislocation. The patient may

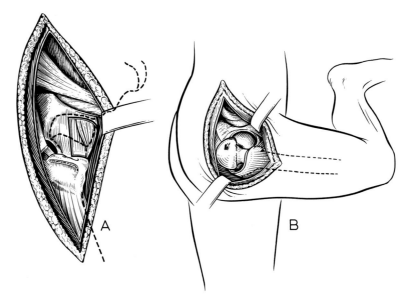

FIG. 9-66 Austin-Moore procedure (continued). The hip is adducted and internally rotated to dislocate the femoral head from the acetabulum. (Redrawn from Campbell's Operative Orthopaedics, 5th ed. H. H. Grenshaw, editor. St. Louis, C. V. Mosby, 1971.)

be out of bed in a few days and up on crutches with partial or full weight bearing, depending upon progress.

Cup Arthroplasty

The cup arthroplasty can be a valuable tool for treating patients with primary or secondary osteoarthritis of the hip (Fig. 9-67). However, when used for patients with bilateral hip disease, especially in the older-aged group, it should be considered second to the total hip replacement. It is especially valuable in the younger patient in an attempt to preserve bony stock (Fig. 9-68). The surgical technique and postoperative management are exactly the same as for the rheumatoid patient (page 269).

Total Hip Replacement

The indications for the total hip replacement in the treatment of osteoarthritis of the hip have changed with the passage of time and experience gained by various surgeons. The wear has been much less than anticipated and the results are holding up well even after 10 years. Candidates for the operation are generally patients over the age of fifty who have severe painful hip disease or a short life expectancy. Even patients below the age of fifty have been considered for reconstruction of their hips

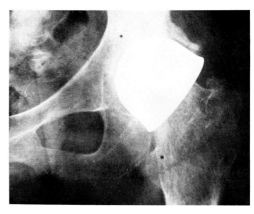

FIG. 9-67 Roentgenogram 17 years after a Smith-Peterson cup arthroplasty. The patient still walks well without pain, although she has limited motion. Bone growth is obvious along the acetabular margin and along the top of the cup; however, the head and neck length have been maintained.

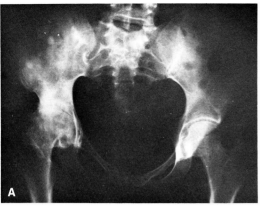 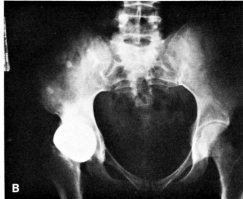

FIG. 9-68 Roentgenograms of the hip of a young patient who developed osteoarthritis after a septic hip. A. Preoperative view showing narrowing of the joint space. B. Two years after a cup arthroplasty to preserve the bone. The patient manages very well and is extremely active, although at times she requires Indocin to relieve her symptoms. At the time of surgery the cultures were negative.

when they have severe bilateral hip disease. Patients who have had destruction of the femoral head and neck for which the only procedure once available was a Girdlestone replacement may also be candidates for total hip replacement (Fig. 9-69). Recent infection, however, has been an absolute contraindication to total hip replacement.

The operative technique is the same as that described for rheumatoid arthritis (page 284).

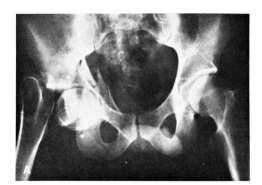 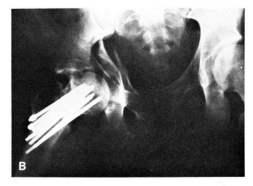

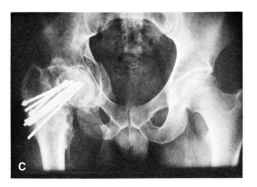

FIG. 9-69 Roentgenograms of the hips of a 25-year-old man who was injured in a motorcycle accident. A. Fractures of the acetabulum and femoral neck can be seen in the right hip joint. B. An open reduction was carried out with multiple pin fixation of the femoral neck fracture. Dislocation of the head centrally is noted in the postoperative film. C. A follow-up study revealed nonunion of the femoral neck. The patient had limited motion and severe pain in the hip joint. Arthrodesis was contraindicated because of severe injuries that made the knee joint unstable. A total hip replacement was carried out, and the patient is doing well one year postoperatively.

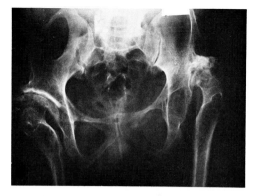

Congenital Problems. Patients with congenital dysplasia of the hip present a special problem in reconstruction with the total hip replacement. These patients generally have had multiple surgical procedures that have distorted the normal anatomy (Fig. 9-70). The osteotomies about the hip tend to result in loss of the normal neck shaft angle which can occasionally be a problem in the insertion of the stem of the femoral portion of the total hip replacement. Since congenital hip patients tend to have marked anteversion, this must also be taken into

FIG. 9-70 Roentgenogram of a patient who has had an osteotomy and shelf procedure of both hips because of congenital deformities. Note the large defect in the pelvis from a prior bone graft and the valgus deformity.

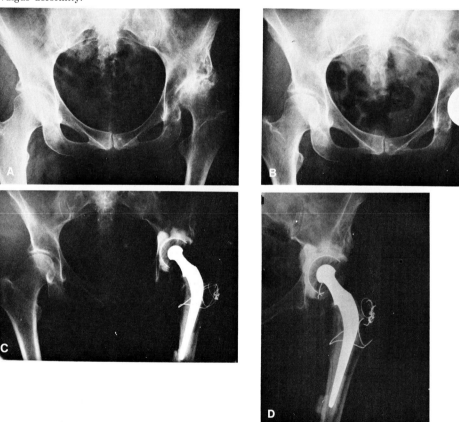

FIG. 9-71 Roentgenograms of patient who had a congenital subluxation of the left hip as a child and had a shelf procedure performed. A. Severe osteoarthritis is present, but there is adequate bony stock in the superior aspect of the acetabulum. B. The patient's postoperative course was good for several years after a cup arthroplasty. C. The cup was removed because of the recurrence of pain, and a total hip replacement was carried out. Note the protrusion of the cement at the base of the stem of the prosthesis. D. One year later the patient developed symptoms related to the wire breakage. The wires were removed, and the patient has been asymptomatic for 3 years after the total hip replacement.

consideration when the femoral component is inserted. It is important to insert the Charnley femoral component in a neutral position to prevent postoperative dislocation. The angle of anteversion of the congenital hip must be disregarded, and the femoral shaft must be reshaped in a neutral position without anteversion or retroversion.

Patients who have had a previous shelf procedure frequently have adequate bony stock in the region of the acetabulum to allow for insertion of the cup portion of the total hip replacement (Fig. 9-71). The shelf procedure thickens the superior aspect of the acetabulum and provides good bony support for the plastic socket (Fig. 9-72).

It is important to have the various sizes of small and extra-small acetabular cups to be sure that an adequate fit can be obtained in a congenital dysplasia of the hip. It may not always be possible to insert the acetabular component in the old true acetabulum. However, the most important factor is to have satisfactory bone coverage of the acetabular component.

Patients who have had previous osteotomies as children may still have retained internal fixation that can present a severe problem in removal of the old metal plates. Screws will tend to break, and various reaming tools should be available for their removal.

The patient with congenital coxa vara also presents a similar type of deformity with distortion of the femoral portion of the hip. The patient may have an extremely short femoral neck, and a prosthetic component with a longer neck may be required to insure stability postoperatively (Fig. 9-73). Usually the medullary canal will have to be reamed with a power tool because of the narrow canal in these congenital femurs.

Traumatic Arthritis. Patients with traumatic arthritis also present a special situation in total hip replacement. Frac-

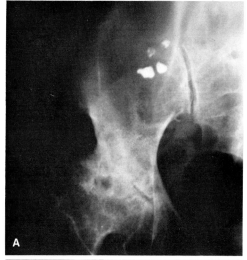

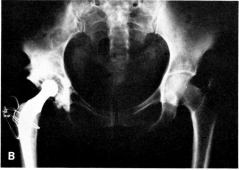

FIG. 9-72 Roentgenograms of patient who had a shelf procedure for a congenital hip. A. The preoperative view reveals severe disease of the hip joint but an adequate bony shelf for the the acetabular socket. B. The postoperative view shows excellent fixation of the cup after a total hip replacement.

tures of the hip joint can severely disrupt the normal anatomy and prior surgery can increase the risk of infection as well as prolong the operative procedure because of distortion of the anatomy or buried internal fixation devices. The blood loss in these patients is frequently increased over the average case because of the scar tissue. The aged patient who has had a fracture with internal fixation may go on to aseptic necrosis or nonunion. The acetabular cartilage is often severely involved and hemiarthroplasty does not give the same results as seen in fresh fractures. A loose internal fixation

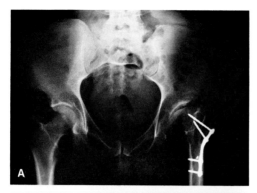

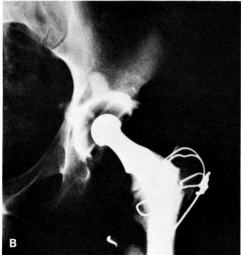

FIG. **9-73** Roentgenograms of a patient with congenital coxa vara. A. Preoperative view showing internal fixation done 30 years earlier. B. Postoperative view after a total hip replacement. Adequate fixation of the socket was obtained. Cement is noted protruding from the shaft of the femur, and a small piece of screw is visible in the soft tissue. As much bone as possible was saved to preserve the neck length.

device may be easy to remove, but when devices for treatment of the fracture are not of the usual type, severe problems can be encountered. The use of the Z-nail allows bony ingrowth through the holes in the nail that will make this type of device difficult to remove. It is advisable to have a similar nail available so that it can be hammered down over the preexisting nail to allow for easy removal and cutting of the bony ingrowth from the nail itself (Fig. 9-74).

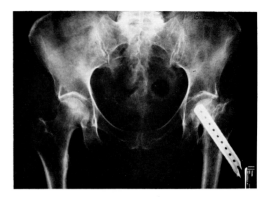

FIG. **9-74** Roentgenogram of patient whose hip has been fixed with a Z-nail. Another Z-nail is driven down over the existing nail to aid in removal of the device.

Severely comminuted fractures involving the hip may also constitute a difficult problem (Fig. 9-75). The medullary canal of the upper femur may be distorted by fracture callus preventing the entrance of the rasp down the medullary canal. It is advisable to have a power tool with a rotary rasp to open the medullary canal. This is the easiest way to allow for insertion of the femoral component.

Loss of the Femoral Neck and Head. Patients with destruction of the femoral head and neck resulting in a Girdlestone-type hip have severe shortening of the extremity and a very unstable gait. The problem of 1 to 2 inches of shortening can be overcome by the total hip replacement. Preoperative skeletal traction in long-standing cases has generally resulted in no improvement in stretching of the scar tissue or the roentgenogram appearance. Some telescoping may be present and can be determined from the radiologic examination by push-pull films. Generally the release of scar tissue must be carried out at the time of the operative procedure. The crucial point in the procedure is to be sure that there is adequate bony stock in the region of the acetabulum for secure fixation of the acetabular component. The acetabulum

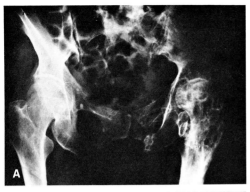

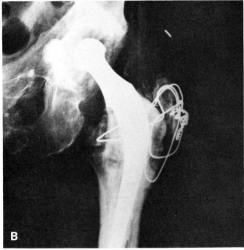

FIG. 9-75 Total hip replacement for patient with comminuted fractures. A. Preoperative roentgenogram revealing multiple fractures of the pelvis, the proximal femur, and the hip joint. B. Postoperative view of the prosthesis in place. Note that there is a nonunion of the trochanter, but this is asymptomatic. The result has been excellent.

is generally filled with extremely thick scar tissue, and dissection has to be carried out carefully to determine the appropriate site of the previous acetabulum. Once the scar tissue has been freed from its bony attachments in the acetabulum, the socket will gradually develop nicely. It would be advisable prior to cementing in the socket to determine how far distally the femur can be pulled for insertion of the trial femoral prosthesis. If it cannot be inserted and reduced, it may be necessary either to shorten the femoral neck or to advance

the acetabulum superiorly. This should be determined before final cementing of any of the components (Fig. 9-76).

Failed Cup Arthroplasty. Patients with a failed cup arthroplasty present a special problem in the reconstruction of the hip. The cup tends to weaken the inner wall of the acetabulum and frequently results in a loss of bony substance (Fig. 9-77). The extremely thin smooth inner wall allows for poor fixation of the cement, especially at the area of the ischium and pubis. These patients also have a higher incidence of loosening of the acetabular component. Cement holes should be drilled up into the superior aspect of the acetabulum and, if possible, a hole into the region of the ischium. An extremely thin inner wall can be reinforced with a stainless steel wire mesh, which comes fabricated in sheets that can be cut into various sizes to line the inner wall or in a cup shape. It is advisable to put a layer of cement in first after cleaning out the acetabulum of all soft tissue and forcing the cement up into the drill holes that have been placed in the acetabulum at the superior aspect and in the inferior aspect. The screen should be cut out to allow the cement to pass into these holes. The reinforced wire screen tends to increase the strength of the acetabulum and may prevent breaking of the inner wall with loosening of the component (Fig. 9-78).

Failed Hemiarthroplasty. A common cause of failure of a hemiarthroplasty is a poor acetabulum with no articular cartilage (Fig. 9-79). The failed hemiarthroplasty also increases the problems of total hip replacement. The Austin-Moore type of prosthesis is extremely difficult to remove at times because of the bony ingrowth. A thin-bladed osteotome can be used to slide down along the shaft of · the prosthesis to cut the bony growth into the holes of the Austin-Moore prosthesis. Care must be exercised in dislocating these prostheses to prevent shat-

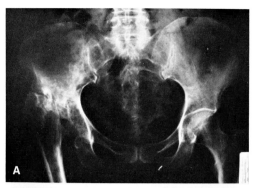

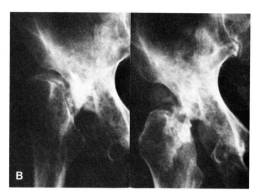

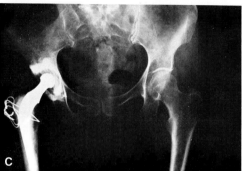

FIG. 9-76 Roentgenograms of hip of patient who had a Girdlestone resection and then a total hip replacement because of loss of the femoral neck and head. A. The patient had destruction of the hip joint which at first was suspected to be due to infection. Exploration and debridement of the joint revealed no evidence of active infection. B. The push-pull films reveal some telescoping of the femur. C. One year later, after total hip replacement.

Fused Hip. The major candidates for replacement of a fused hip are patients who are having increased low back pain or whose hip is fused in a bad position. A fused hip tends to increase the stresses on the lumbar spine and on the opposite hip. Loss of motion and increased pain in the only movable hip can produce severe disability in walking and sitting (Fig. 9-80). Hips that have been fused surgically or spontaneously by nature can be

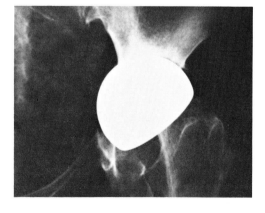

tering the femur and producing spiral fractures. All of the scar tissue should be dissected, and any bony overgrowth should be removed with an osteotome from the area of the acetabulum to allow for easy dislocation. Once the prosthesis has been dislocated and removed, the total hip replacement can be carried out in a routine fashion.

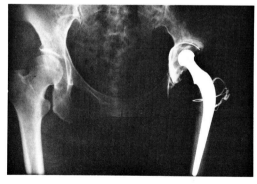

FIG. 9-77 Roentgenograms of patient with a failed cup arthroplasty, showing protrusion of the cup through the inner wall of the acetabulum.

FIG. 9-78 Roentgenogram after a total hip replacement for a failed cup arthroplasty because of a weak inner wall. A layer of wire mesh has been inserted between the cement and the defect in the medial wall.

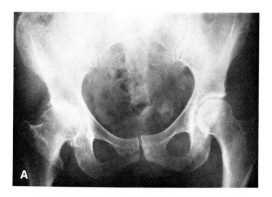

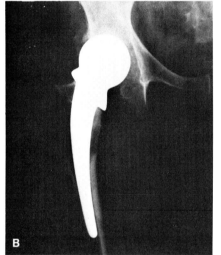

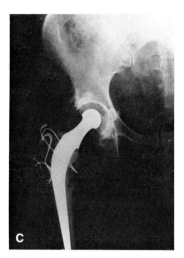

FIG. 9-79 Roentgenograms of total hip replacement for a failed hemiarthroplasty in a 74-year-old woman with severe pain from osteoarthritis in the right hip. A. Preoperative view. B. After insertion of a Thompson prosthesis. The patient continued to have increasing pain in the hip because of the poor acetabulum with no evidence of articular cartilage. C. After removal of the Thompson prosthesis and a total hip replacement.

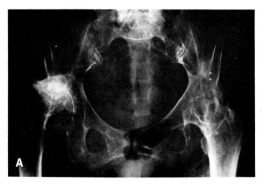

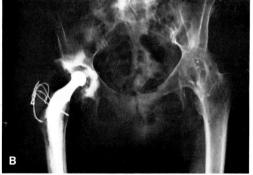

FIG. 9-80 Roentgenograms of total hip replacement in a 74-year-old patient with a fused hip on the opposite side. A. Preoperative view showing extensive osteoarthritis involvement of the right hip. The patient had severe pain in the low back and loss of motion. B. Postoperative view. The wires broke and avulsed a portion of the trochanter because the stiff left hip put undue stress on the right hip when the patient attempted to get up and walk. However, the result was not compromised, and the patient continues to do well.

replaced with the total hip. It is surprising that even though the hip may have been fused for 43 years, the musculature will develop and produce a reasonably sound movable hip. Patients with fused hips, however, recover much slower than those with the ordinary total hip replacement and tend to have increased pain postoperatively because of stretching of the muscles and movement in musculature that has been immobilized for many years. When hips have been fused in severe flexed positions, it is advisable not to attempt leg lengthening because of the possible injury to the femoral or sciatic nerve. This is especially true in patients who have had fused hips since early childhood.

Nonunion of the Trochanter. The trochanter is removed in many cases for better exposure in doing a total hip replacement through the lateral approach. Although other techniques are available, the one chosen is dependent upon the surgeon and the type of problem comfronting him. Wire breakage has been a problem in some cases and may require removal of the wire postoperatively.

Nonunion has not been a serious problem as far as function of the hip with total hip replacement was concerned. Late union of the trochanter can occur, and reattachment is not indicated in most cases (Fig. 9-81).

Arthrodesis

Arthrodesis of the hip can be considered in patients with septic hips, tuberculosis, poliomyelitis with a flail hip, and Charcot's joint. Arthrodesis may also be used for unilateral osteoarthritis when the patient requires a strong, painless hip. In evaluating the patient, it is important to realize the high incidence of pseudarthrosis in many cases. The difficulties in a patient with a hip fusion have been described earlier in this chapter.

Operative Technique. The operative technique varies considerably among orthopaedic surgeons, and various combinations of intra-articular and extra-articular arthrodeses have been described. The general approach is an anterior Smith-Peterson approach. The

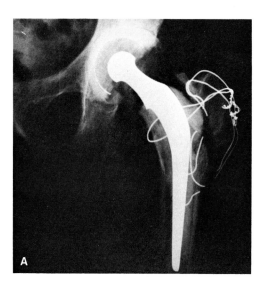
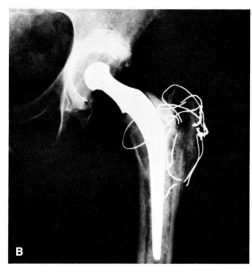

FIG. 9-81 Roentgenograms after a total hip replacement. A. Postoperative view showing nonunion of the trochanter and breakage of the wires. B. One year later. The trochanter has united spontaneously, and excellent bony union is present.

articular cartilage is removed from the femoral head and the acetabulum with various gouges. A bone graft or flap can be turned down from the anterior ilium into the neck of the femur for additional bone contact. The ideal position for fusion is flexion of 30° with 5° to 10° of external rotation and 5° of abduction. If the skin incision has been brought down laterally, the trochanteric area of the femur and shaft can be also exposed through this incision. Some form of internal fixation may be used, either a large Smith-Peterson nail or another variety of hip fusion nail. A graft may also be removed from the ilium and impacted across the joint from the pelvis to the femur. In most cases a 1 ½ hip spica cast is applied. It has been our policy to bivalve the posterior aspect of the leg of the cast behind the knee down to the toes to allow this to be removed and the knee flexed and extended in the cast. Knee motion will be regained earlier than when the leg is immobilized in a cast for a long period of time.

Bibliography

Rheumatoid Arthritis

Aufranc, O. E.: The adaptability of Vitallium mold arthroplasty to difficult hip problems. Clin. Orthop., 66:31, 1969.

Aufranc, O. E.: Constructive hip surgery with mold arthroplasty. Am. Acad. Orthop. Surgeons, Lect., 11:163, 1954.

Aufranc, O. E.: Constructive Surgery of the Hip. St. Louis, C. V. Mosby, 1962.

Aufranc, O. E.: The surgical treatment of the hip in rheumatoid arthritis. Am. J. Orthop., 3:102, 1961.

Aufranc, O. E., and Sweet, E. B.: Study of patients with hip arthroplasty. J.A.M.A., 170:507, 1959.

Blount, W. P.: Blade-plate internal fixation for high femoral osteotomy. J. Bone Joint Surg., 25:319, 1943.

Charnley, J.: The long-term results of low friction arthroplasty of the hip performed as a primary intervention. J. Bone Joint Surg., 54-B:61, 1972.

Charnley, J.: Postoperative infection after total hip replacement with special reference to air contamination in the operating room. Clin. Orthop., 87:167, 1972.

Charnley, J.: Total hip replacement by low friction arthroplasty. Clin. Orthop., 72:7, 1970.

Clayton, M. L.: Care of the rheumatoid hip. Clin. Orthop., 90:70, 1973.

Colonna, P. C.: A new type of reconstruction operation for old ununited fracture of the neck of the femur. J. Bone Joint Surg., 17:110, 1935.

Colonna, P. C.: The trochanteric operation for ununited fractures of the upper end of the femur. J. Bone Joint Surg., 42-B:5, 1960.

Conaty, J. P.: Surgery of the hip and knee in patients with rheumatoid arthritis. J. Bone Joint Surg., 55-A:301, 1973.

Coventry, M. B., Polley, H. F., and Weiner, A. D.: Rheumatoid synovial cyst of the hip. J. Bone Joint Surg., 41-A:721, 1959.

Dupont, J. A., and Charnley, J.: Low friction arthroplasty of the hip for the failures of previous operations. J. Bone Joint Surg., 54-B:77, 1972.

Duthie, R. B., and Harris, C. M.: A radiographic and clinical survey of the hips in sero-positive rheumatoid arthritis. Acta Orthop. Scand., 401:346, 1969.

Johnston, R. C., and Larson, C. B.: Biomechanics of cup arthroplasty. Clin. Orthop., 66:56, 1969.

Kennedy, W. R., et. al.: Massive articular osteolysis in rheumatoid arthritis, treated by total hip replacement. Case report and review of the literature. Clin. Orthop., 90:161, 1973.

Law, W. A.: Post-operative study of Vitallium mold arthroplasty of the hip joint. J. Bone Joint Surg., 30-B:76, 1948.

Marmor, L., and Fishbein, M.: Cup arthroplasty reamers. A new design concept. Clin. Orthop., *85*:148, 1972.

McKee, G. K., and Watson-Farrar, J.: Replacement of arthritic hips by the McKee-Farrar prosthesis. J. Bone Joint Surg., *48-B*:245, 1966.

Milch, H.: The resection angulation operation for arthritis of the hip. Geriatrics, *5*:280, 1950.

Milch, H.: Surgery of Arthritis, Baltimore, the Williams & Wilkins Co., 1964, pp. 166–168.

Müller, M. E.: Total hip prostheses. Clin. Orthop., *72*:46, 1970.

Schwartzman, J. R.: Arthroplasty of the hip in rheumatoid arthritis. J. Bone Joint Surg., *41-A*:705, 1959.

Schwartzman, J. R.: Reconstruction of the hip in rheumatoid arthritis. J. Bone Joint Surg., *49-A*:398, 1967.

Shorbe, H. B., and Blaschke, J. A.: Flanged acetabular cup replacement prosthesis in patients with rheumatoid arthritis. Clin. Orthop., *36*:66, 1964.

Wilde, A. H., et. al.: Reankylosis of the hip joint in ankylosing spondylitis after total hip replacement. Arthritis Rheum., *15*:493, 1972.

Osteoarthritis

Appel, H., et. al.: Effect of osteotomy on pain in idiopathic osteoarthritis of the hip. Acta Orthop. Scand., *44*:710, 1973.

Aufranc, O. E.: Constructive hip surgery with the Vitallium mold. A report on one thousand cases of arthroplasty of the hip over a fifteen year period. J. Bone Joint Surg., *39-A*:227, 1957.

Aufranc, O. E.: Constructive Surgery of the Hip. St. Louis, C. V. Mosby, 1962.

Blount, W. P.: Don't throw away the cane. J. Bone Joint Surg., *38-A*:695, 1956.

Blount, W. P.: Osteotomy in the treatment of osteoarthritis of the hip. J. Bone Joint Surg., *46-A*:1297, 1964.

Charnley, J., et. al.: The nine and ten year results of the low friction arthroplasty of the hip. Clin. Orthop., *95*:9, 1973.

Coventry, M. B., et. al.: Hip arthroplasties, 2,012 total: A study of post-operative course and early complications. J. Bone Joint Surg., *56-A*:273, 1974.

Eiles, S. P.: The surgery of the osteoarthritic hip. Br. J. Surg., *193*:488, 1958.

Ferguson, A. B., Jr.: The pathological changes in degenerative arthritis of the hip and treatment by rotational osteotomy. J. Bone Joint Surg., *46-A*:1337, 1964.

Goldie, I. F., et. al.: Long-term follow-up of intertrochanteric osteotomy in osteoarthritis in the hip joint. Clin. Orthop., *93*:265, 1973.

Harris, W. H.: Surgical management of arthritis of the hip. Semin. Arthritis Rheum., *1*:35, 1971.

Heywood-Waddington, M. B.: Use of the Austin-Moore prosthesis for advanced osteoarthritis. J. Bone Joint Surg., *48-B*:236, 1966.

Kallio, K. E.: Arthroplastia cutanea. Acta Orthop. Scand., *26*:327, 1957.

Key, J. A., and Ford, L. T.: The treatment of degenerative arthritis of the hip. Geriatrics, *12*:399, 1957.

Knodt, H.: Osteo-arthritis of the hip joint. J. Bone Joint Surg., *46-A*:1326, 1964.

Kollberg, G., et al.: The Voss operation in osteoarthritis of the hip. Acta Orthop. Scand., *36*:82, 1965.

McElfresh, E. C., and Coventry, M. B.: Femoral and pelvic fractures after total hip arthroplasty. J. Bone Joint Surg., *56-A*:483, 1974.

McMurray, T. P.: Osteoarthritis of the hip. Br. J. Surg., *22*:716, 1935.

Moore, A. T.: The self-locking metal hip prosthesis. J. Bone Joint Surg., *39-A*:811, 1957.

Nissen, K. I.: The arrest of early primary osteoarthritis of the hip by osteotomy. Proc. R. Soc. Med., *56*:1051, 1963.

Pauwels, F.: New principles for surgical treatment of coxarthrosis. Verh. Dtsch. Orthop. Ges., 332, 1961.

Pearson, J. R., and Riddell, D. M.: Idiopathic osteo-arthritis of the hip. Ann. Rheumat. Dis., *21*:31, 1962.

Porter, D. S.: Moore's arthroplasty for primary osteoarthritis. Proc. R. Soc. Med., *59*:119, 1966.

Rangno, R. E.: The rationale of antibiotic prophylaxis in total hip replacement arthroplasty. Clin. Orthop., *96*:206, 1973.

Ring, P. A.: Total replacement of the hip joint. Clin. Orthop., *95*:34, 1973.

Robins, R. H. C., and Piggot, J.: McMurray osteotomy with a note on the "regeneration" of articular cartilage. J. Bone Joint Surg., *42-B*:480. 1960.

Salvati, E. A., et. al.: Long-term results of femoral head replacement. J. Bone Joint Surg., *55-A*:516, 1973.

Smith-Petersen, M. N.: A new supra-articular subperiosteal approach to the hip joint. Am. J. Orthop. Surg., *15*:592, 1917.

Trueta, J.: Studies on the etiopathology of osteoarthritis of the hip. Clin. Orthop., *31*:7, 1968.

Voss, C.: Die temporare Hangerhufte. Dtsch. Orthop. Ges., *23*:351, 1956.

The knee joint, which is extremely important in the function of the lower extremity, is frequently damaged by arthritis and trauma. The great advances made in orthopaedic surgery in the past decade in the treatment of hip disease have greatly increased the interest of the orthopaedic surgeon in the knee joint. Many of the basic operative procedures that are still of value in the treatment of arthritis of the knee will be described in this chapter. Since as many as 50 different types of total knee replacements have been described in the medical literature, no attempt will be made to describe all of them. A thorough discussion of the Marmor Modular Knee will be presented because of its conservative approach in the treatment of arthritic knee joints. However, it should not be construed that this is the only procedure available or recommended. Other types of joint replacements have also given excellent results.

Anatomy

The knee joint is a superficial joint and is the largest joint in the body. It is basically a hinge joint between the femur and tibia, but it does permit motions of flexion, extension, and rotation.

The knee joint can be considered to be composed of three separate joints: the patellofemoral joint, the medial femoral condyle with the tibial plateau, and the lateral femoral condyle with the lateral tibial plateau. Many animals actually have three distinct subdivisions of the knee with separate synovial cavities and ligaments. In man the arrangement of the collateral ligaments of the knee joint and the cruciate ligaments tends to form individual collateral ligaments for each compartment. The medial collateral ligament and the posterior cruciate ligaments form the collateral ligaments for the medial compartment, and the anterior cruciate and lateral collateral ligaments form the collateral ligaments for the lateral compartment.

The medial compartment, therefore, would consist of the medial femoral condyle, the medial tibial plateau, the medial collateral ligament, and the posterior cruciate ligament. The lateral compartment of the knee joint can be considered as a separate articulation consisting of the lateral femoral condyle, the lateral tibial plateau, the lateral collateral ligament, and the anterior cruciate ligament (Fig. 10-1).

When one observes the lower end of the femur, the femoral condyles are

Table 10-1. *Surgical Treatment of Rheumatoid Arthritis*

Stage	Clinical Picture	Roentgenograms	Operative Procedure
Early stage	Synovial effusion No fixed deformity	Osteoporosis Subchondral ero- sions	Synovectomy
Advanced stage	Loss of articular cartilage	Erosions, cysts Joint narrowing	Synovectomy and Marmor Modular Knee
Late stage	Severe joint destruction Varus or valgus deformity	Severe changes	Total knee replacement

separated anteriorly by the patellar surface. These condyles are not identical and are shaped differently. The lateral condyle is more prominent and broader in its anteroposterior and transverse diameters than the medial. The condyles are not parallel to each other but toe in superiorly (Fig. 10-2). At the patellar surface, the area between the two condyles on the superior aspect, the patella tends to articulate with the femur. It is well above the weight-bearing surface of the femoral condyle.

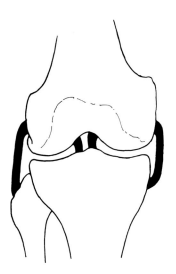

FIG. 10-1 Diagram of the knee. The cruciate ligaments act as collateral ligaments for the medial and lateral compartments.

During weight bearing most of the load is placed on the medial femoral condyle.

The patella is a flat, sesamoid bone which develops in the quadriceps tendon. It protects the front of the knee joint and improves the leverage of the quadriceps femoris muscle. It articulates with the patellar surface of the femoral condyles. In most people the contact between the two surfaces is not congruous.

The upper surface of the tibia contains two articulating surfaces: the medial and lateral tibial plateaus. Located between them is the intercondylar eminence or tibial spines. The articular surfaces of the tibia tend to slope toward the periphery in the anteroposterior view, and in the lateral view, the tibia tends to slope posteriorly.

The capsule of the knee joint is a thin, fibrous membrane that is reinforced by the fascia lata laterally and the tendinous expansion of the vastus muscle both medially and laterally (Fig. 10-3). The knee joint depends upon its ligaments for stability. Located on the medial side is a broad, flat medial collateral ligament that attaches from the medial epicondyle of the femur above to the medial plateau of the tibia and the body of the tibia below. This ligament has a deep and a superficial portion. The lateral collateral ligament is a strong, round band of fibers attached above to

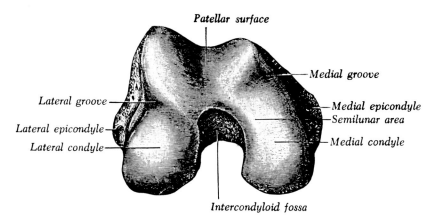

FIG. 10-2 Lower extremity of the right femur viewed from below. Note that the femoral condyles are not identical. (From Gray's Anatomy of the Human Body, 29th ed. C. M. Goss, editor. Philadelphia, Lea & Febiger, 1973.)

the lateral epicondyle and below to the side of the head of the fibula.

The cruciate ligaments are strong structures located in the intercondylar

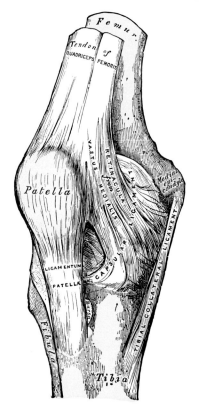

FIG. 10-3 Anterior view of the right knee joint. (From Gray's Anatomy of the Human Body, 29th ed. C. M. Goss, editor. Philadelphia, Lea & Febiger, 1973.)

region. The anterior cruciate ligament attaches to the depression located anteriorly on the intercondyloid eminence and passes upward, backward, and laterally to attach to the medial wall of the lateral condyle (Fig. 10-4). It acts as a collateral ligament for the lateral compartment. The posterior cruciate ligament is stronger and shorter than the anterior. It attaches to the back of the tibia and passes upward anteriorly and medially to attach to the lateral side of the medial condyle (Fig. 10-5). It acts as a collateral ligament for the medial compartment.

The menisci are located on the surface of the tibia. They are semicircular in appearance and are covered along their borders with synovial membranes (Fig. 10-6). The medial meniscus is larger and thinner than the lateral. The medial meniscus is attached to the coronary ligament of the medial collateral ligament, and the lateral meniscus is attached by the ligament of Wrisberg. These attachments tend to pull the menisci forward on extension and backward on flexion. It is believed that the menisci are actively involved in weight bearing because they cover most of the articular surface of the tibial plateau. They also function in carrying joint fluid up along the sides of the femoral condyle

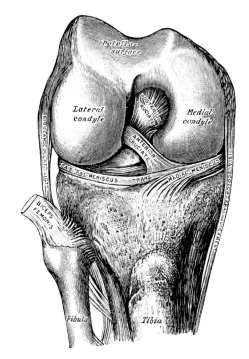

FIG. 10-4 The right knee joint, showing anterior ligaments. (From Gray's Anatomy of the Human Body, 29th ed. C. M. Goss, editor, Philadelphia, Lea & Febiger, 1973.)

and the tibial plateau. The lateral meniscus covers much more of the articular surface and is broader and more curved than the medial. The medial meniscus is thin anteriorly and has a broad posterior surface that covers much of the posterior aspect of the tibial plateau. The actual force applied to the joint surface on walking is approximately three times the body weight.

The articular cartilage, which is hyaline in nature, covers the articular surfaces of the femoral condyles, patella, and tibial plateaus. The average thickness of this cartilage is approximately 4 mm.

The synovial sac of the knee is the largest in the body and contains several large recesses such as the suprapatellar pouch which is interposed between the femur and the quadriceps tendon and extends upward for a varying distance from the articular surface of the femoral condyle (Fig. 10-7). It is separated from

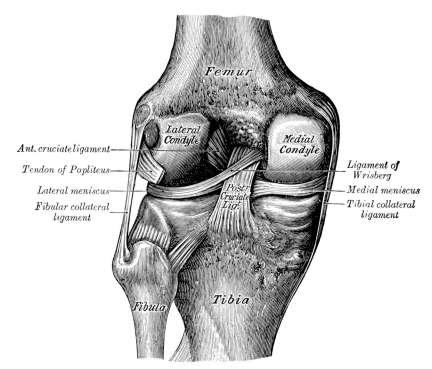

FIG. 10-5 Left knee joint, posterior aspect, showing posterior ligaments. (From Gray's Anatomy of the Human Body, 29th ed. C. M. Goss, editor. Philadelphia, Lea & Febiger, 1973.)

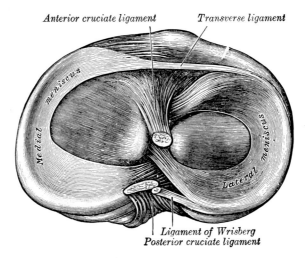

FIG. 10-6 Head of the right tibia seen from above, showing menisci and attachments of ligaments. (From Gray's Anatomy of the Human Body, 29th ed. C. M. Goss, editor. Philadelphia, Lea & Febiger, 1973.)

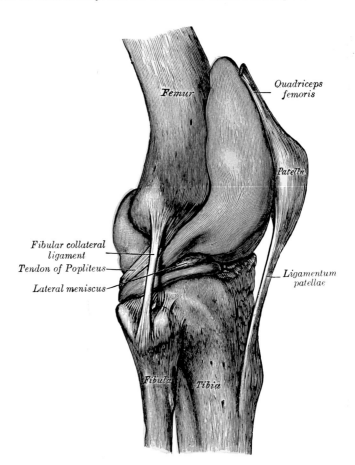

FIG. 10-7 Synovial membrane of capsule of right knee joint (distended). Lateral aspect. Note that the lateral meniscus is covered by the synovial tissue. (From Gray's Anatomy of the Human Body, 29th ed. C. M. Goss, editor. Philadelphia, Lea & Febiger, 1973.)

the patellar ligament by the infrapatellar fat pad. Several bursae located about the knee joint are of some importance. The anserine bursa is located on the medial surface of the tibia beneath the tendons of the sartorious, gracilis, and semitendinous muscles. It lies superficial to the insertion of the tibial collateral ligament. The prepatellar bursa is located superficial to the patella beneath the skin. When it is involved in trauma or rheumatoid disease, a large swelling is produced in the front of the knee joint.

The knee joint is controlled by the quadriceps femoris muscle and its subdivisions, the vastus lateralis, vastus medialis, vastus intermedius, and the rectus femoris. These muscles, which insert into a common tendon that contains the patella, produce extension of the knee joint when they are activated. It is believed that the vastus medialis is responsible for the last 10 degrees of full extension.

Flexion of the knee joint is produced by the action of the biceps femoris, semimembranosus and semitendinosus muscles. At times the gracilis, gastrocnemius, sartorius, plantaris, and popliteus muscles may also act as flexors.

Physical and Radiologic Examination

The patient should be suitably draped so that both lower extremities are available for examination.

Inspection

The patient's knees should be compared visually to see if there is any evidence of deformity, swelling, or malalignment. The patient should be asked to stand because when weight is born on the lower extremities, deformities such as genu varus or valgus become much more obvious. These deformities can often be overlooked when the patient is lying, relaxed, on the examining table. The patient should be observed walking to note whether there is a limp and also whether the knee joint tends to buckle in or outward due to a varus or valgus deformity when weight is borne on the joint. It is important to observe the popliteal space also because a large Baker's cyst or other mass can be easily overlooked. Any operative scars or discoloration about the knee joint should be recorded at this time.

Palpation

With the patient lying down on the examining table, the knee joint can be carefully palpated to determine any areas of tenderness or the presence of synovial effusion. Patients with varus deformities frequently have tenderness along the joint lines, which is located in most patients at the lower pole of the patella. The best procedure for detecting synovial effusion is for the examiner to place one hand over the superior aspect of the joint to press the fluid out of the suprapatellar pouch into the joint so that the fluid will collect beneath the patella. With the other hand, the patella may be tapped up and down against the femur, and the click will give an obvious sensation of fluid within the joint. When a swelling is present without any evidence of fluid, this is a sign of synovial thickness. Localized areas of heat can be detected by using the back of the hand in comparing the two knee joints as well as the surrounding tissues. The popliteal pulse should be palpated in the back of the knee and should be recorded in patients with pain in the leg. Vascular disease should not be overlooked in arthritis patients because of the high incidence of vasculitis and the advanced arteriosclerotic disease.

Range of Motion

The knee functions as a gliding hinge joint, and throughout its range of motion a combination of gliding, rotation, and flexion takes place. Range of motion should be measured in the knee joint both actively and passively. The average range of motion in a normal knee will start at 0° in full extension and pass through a range of approximately 135° of flexion. In some patients, hyperextension of 10° can be accepted as normal if it has been present all of their lives.

Ligament Stability

The ligaments should be tested about the knee joint. The knee should be abducted to test the medial collateral ligament and adducted to test the lateral collateral ligament. With the knee bent, to a right angle the cruciate ligament should also be tested for a drawer sign. Abnormal backward mobility of the tibia on the femur suggests rupture of the posterior cruciate ligament. Abnormal forward mobility of the tibia on the femur suggests rupture of the anterior cruciate ligament. Most patients with advanced rheumatoid disease will have some ligamentous laxity due to loss of the articular cartilage as well as involvement of the cruciate ligaments. The collateral ligaments are outside of the joint capsule and, therefore, are seldom involved in rheumatoid disease. Medial-lateral instability is usually due to bone loss within the joint rather than stretching of the ligament, except in traumatic arthritis when previous rupture of the collateral ligament may have occurred.

Roentgenograms

In addition to the clinical examination, the roentgenogram is extremely important in the evaluation of knee problems. Anteroposterior films obtained of the knee when the patient is lying down and standing should be compared to determine the loss of articular cartilage (Fig. 10-8). This loss is best

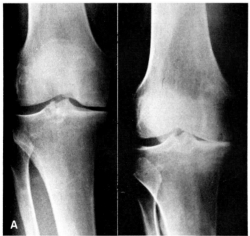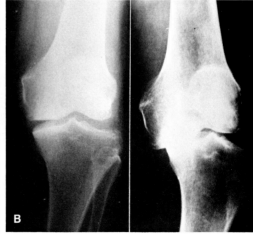

FIG. 10-8 Roentgenograms to evaluate joint space. A. The joint space appears reasonable in the nonstanding view (left), but the standing view (right) shows the narrowing of the medial compartment. B. The subluxation and destruction of the joint are obvious only in the standing view (right).

evaluated when weight is placed upon the joint because then the narrowing of the joint space becomes obvious. If the joint is filled with fluid or synovial tissue and the patient is lying down, the joint space may appear reasonable.

The lateral view of the knee is generally taken when the patient is lying down. Roentgenograms of the knee in full flexion and full extension are valuable in determining the preoperative range of motion and for comparing with the postoperative result. If necessary, an axial view of the patella or view through the intercondylar area also may be obtained for additional information.

Rheumatoid Arthritis

Rheumatoid arthritis frequently involves the knee joint where it often produces severe pain and disability. This joint may be involved early in the disease and frequently is the first joint to be affected in young women. Monoarticular arthritis in a young woman with chronic effusions should often alert the physician to the possibility of the onset of rheumatoid arthritis, especially when there is no history of trauma. Bilateral synovial involvement of the knees is often presumptive evidence of early rheumatoid arthritis.

The disease process may be insidious, or it may progress rapidly to destruction of the joint surfaces, with the development of flexion contractures and loss of motion (Fig. 10-9). The patient may be severely disabled and unable to walk. Most of the pathologic changes seen at various stages of rheumatoid arthritis in other joints occur in the knee. Since rheumatoid arthritis starts primarily as a synovial disease with extensive hypertrophy of the synovium within the joint, the enlargement of the synovium and joint effusion tend to distend the joint and stretch the capsule (Fig. 10-10).

It is believed that lysosomal enzymes can affect the articular cartilage and cause chondromalacia even before pannus forms (Fig. 10-11). Synovial tissue or pannus gradually grows over the articular surface to destroy the hyaline cartilage and then invades the cartilage along its subchondylar margin to undermine and destroy it (Fig. 10-12).

The anterior cruciate ligament, which is located within the synovial joint space, is frequently destroyed by synovial invasion in rheumatoid arthritis, but the posterior cruciate ligament and the collateral ligaments, which are outside the synovial layer, are seldom destroyed. The menisci, which are covered along their periphery by synovium, are frequently forced into the joint space by the proliferating synovium (Fig. 10-13). They often are trapped and ground down between the femoral condyle and the tibial plateau. Late in the disease process, the menisci are generally completely disintegrated so that no evidence of them can be found except around the peripheral margins of the joint.

If the synovitis cannot be controlled, the synovial tissue continues to destroy the joint. Most of the articular cartilage is lost, and there are adhesions and erosions throughout the surface of the joint (Fig. 10-14). This condition can lead to severe mechanical deformities with contractures of the knee joint, depression of the tibial plateau, and loss of function (Fig. 10-15).

Treatment

The basis for determining the treatment of the knee depends a great deal upon the pathologic condition within the

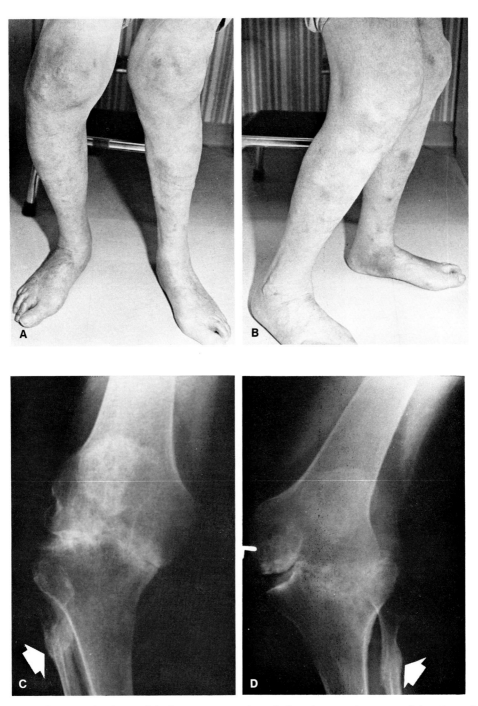

FIG. 10-9 Rheumatoid arthritis of the knee joints. A. The right knee has gone into varus deformity and the left knee into valgus deformity. B. The lateral view shows the flexion deformities of both knee joints. C. The roentgenogram of the right knee reveals loss of the tibial plateau, development of a varus deformity, and a stress fracture of the fibula (arrow). D. The roentgenogram of the left knee reveals severe valgus deformity, depression of the lateral condyle into the tibial plateau, and a stress fracture of the fibula (arrow).

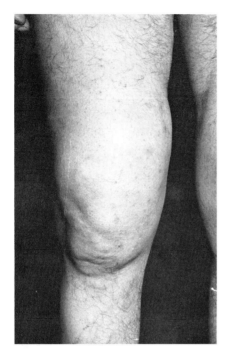

FIG. 10-10 Rheumatoid arthritis of the right knee joint. Swelling is a sign of synovial disease.

joint. As in rheumatoid arthritis in other joints, certain characteristics will be evident from the clinical and roentgenologic evaluations (Table 10-1).

In the *early stage* of the disease the patient will have an acute or chronic synovitis with an effusion in the joint and thickening of the synovial tissue. There is generally no fixed deformity, and a reasonably good range of motion is present. Within the joint itself, pannus will form early around the edges of a normal appearing articular cartilage. The roentgenogram at this stage may show some osteoporosis with very slight loss of bone at the subchondral area (Fig. 10-16). Small erosions may be present later in this early stage. There is generally no loss of joint space on the film obtained when the patient was standing. The treatment of choice at this time would be either conservative injections

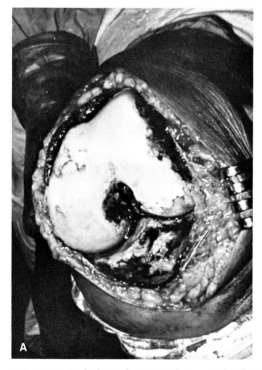

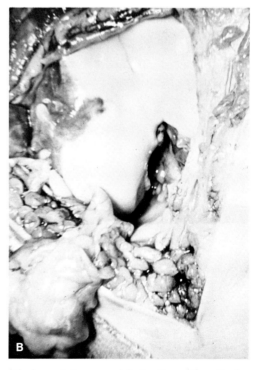

FIG. 10-11 Pathologic changes in rheumatoid arthritis of the knee. A. Lysosomal destruction of the articular cartilage. B. Beginning pannus formation on the medial femoral condyle.

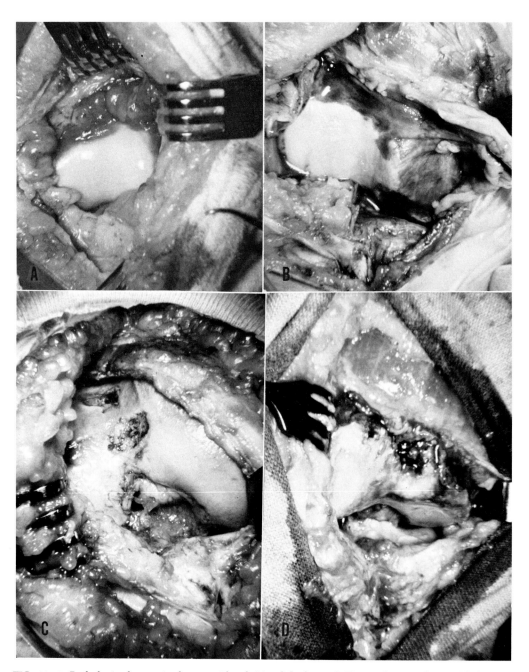

FIG. 10-12 Pathologic changes in rheumatoid arthritis of the knee. A. Encroachment of synovial tissue on subchondral margins of femoral condyle and destruction of articular surface along superior aspect of articular cartilage. B. Advanced pannus formation and destruction of large areas of the articular surface. C. Ulceration of articular cartilage and chondromalacia characteristic of advanced rheumatoid arthritis. D. Far-advanced destruction of femoral condyle and joint surfaces seen in late stage.

336

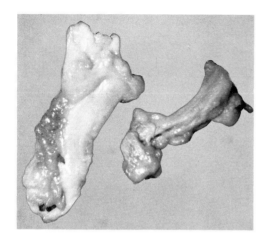

FIG. 10-13 Menisci removed from a patient's knee. Note the rheumatoid synovium around the periphery and changes in the articular margins.

of local steroids or synovectomy (Fig. 10-17).

In the *advanced stage* the joint will reveal loss of the normal appearance of the articular cartilage with thinning of its surface and synovial disease with villus formation. Pannus will be much further advanced with erosions into the edges of the articular margin extending out from the intercondylar notch and also from the medial and lateral femoral condylar areas. Subchondral erosion will be quite obvious along the tibial plateau area with undermining of the articular surface of the plateau (Fig. 10-18). The roentgenogram will reveal erosions in the subchondral area, cyst formation and joint narrowing (Fig. 10-18C).

Very early varus or valgus angulation may be noted at this stage of the disease, and one compartment may be much more affected than the other. This is important in predicting the postoperative result. If early varus or valgus angulation, with evidence of some narrowing of the joint space can be observed, one can predict that within 2 to 3 years further intervention may become necessary because of the deformity (Fig. 10-19). The treatment at this stage would consist of either synovectomy in a more

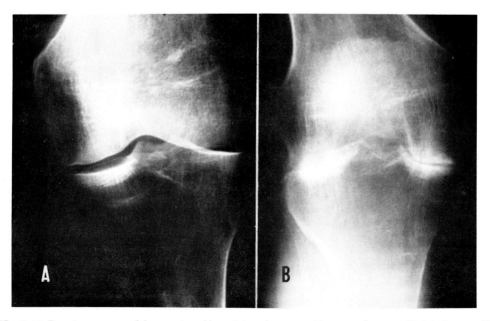

FIG. 10-14 Roentgenograms of destruction of knee joint when synovitis cannot be controlled. A. Reasonable joint space with active rheumatoid disease. B. Two years later. Almost no joint space after severe destruction of articular surfaces.

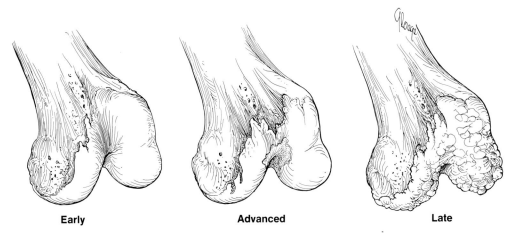

| Early | Advanced | Late |

FIG. 10-15 Pathologic changes at various stages of rheumatoid arthritis of the knee: early stage, involvement of periphery of joint; advanced stage, erosion of synovium from intercondylar area and around periphery of the articular surface and destruction of articular cartilage; late stage, destruction of entire joint surface.

conservative approach, or replacement of the articular surface by a tibial plateau prothesis or by a device like the Marmor Modular Knee. In selected cases of angular deformity with no evidence of active disease, however, one can still consider the osteotomy as an operation to salvage a knee when one does not wish to consider a total knee replacement (Fig. 10-20). The Geomedic, Polycentric, and other types of tracked knees should be reserved for more severe dis-

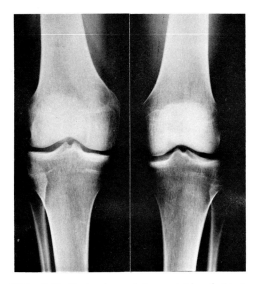

FIG. 10-16 Early stage of rheumatoid arthritis in the knee. Osteoporosis of the tibia of the left knee is evident in the roentgenogram, but there is no evidence of narrowing of joint space or destruction. The right knee is normal.

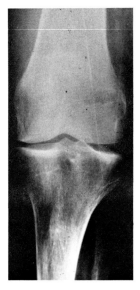

FIG. 10-17 Roentgenogram of knee joint of patient with the early stage rheumatoid arthritis. There is still a reasonably good joint space, and a synovectomy would be the procedure of choice.

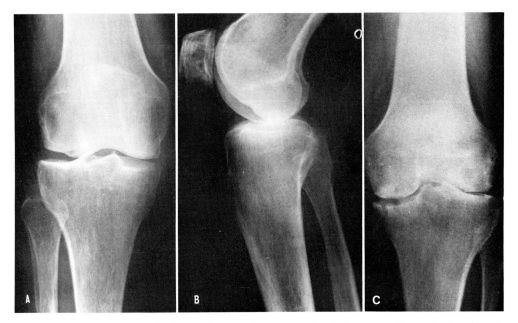

FIG. 10-18 Roentgenograms of advanced stage of rheumatoid arthritis in the knee. A. Anterior view revealing erosions in subchondral area, osteoporosis in the patella, and changes in the lateral compartment of the femoral condyle suggestive of articular destruction. B. Lateral view. C. Roentgenologic evidence of cystic formation, erosion of the articular surface, and narrowing of the joint space in a patient with advanced disease.

ease, as they require more bone removal.

In the *late stage* of the disease there is a severe loss of the joint surface with extensive destruction due to synovial tissue. No normal articular surface remains, and the menisci and possibly the

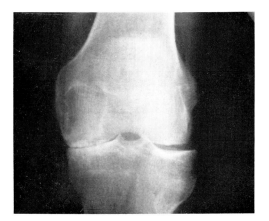

FIG. 10-19 Roentgenogram of knee revealing narrowing of one side of the joint and development of an angular deformity.

anterior cruciate ligament have been almost completely destroyed. The roentgenogram will reveal destruction of the joint with possibly a varus or valgus deformity due to loss of the tibial plateau and collapse of the bone structure (Fig. 10-21). At this stage a total knee replacement is indicated.

The early treatment of rheumatoid arthritis of the knee joint should be an attempt at medical control, if possible, including local injections of steroids into the knee joint. However, if injections and aspiration of the joint are required every few weeks to control the patient's symptoms, conservative therapy should be abandoned and surgical intervention should be considered.

In some patients repeated injections of thiotepa and prednisolone (Hydeltra-T.B.A.) may give remissions of up to one year. The usual technique is to inject, under sterile precautions, 1 to 2 cc

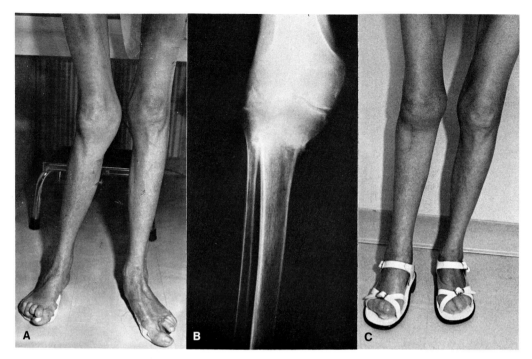

FIG. 10-20 Osteotomy to correct valgus deformity. A. Preoperative photograph. There was no evidence of active synovitis. B. Roentgenogram after osteotomy to realign the extremity. C. Photograph 3 years later. There is excellent alignment, and the patient can walk without discomfort.

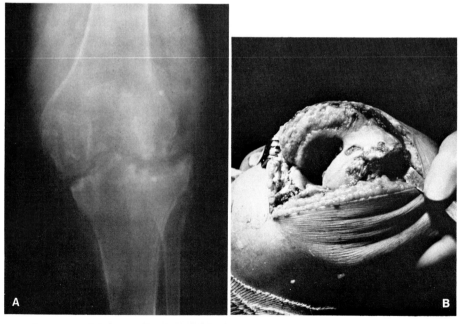

FIG. 10-21 Late stage of rheumatoid arthritis of the knee. A. The roentgenogram reveals severe destruction of the joint surface and collapse of the bony structure. B. Surgical view after synovectomy prior to total knee replacement reveals destruction of the femoral condyle and erosions in the lateral compartment.

thiotepa, approximately 7.5 to 15 mg, combined with 2 cc Hydeltra-T.B.A. into the joint at weekly intervals for 3 weeks.

Physical therapy may be of value in maintaining a full range of motion, as well as in preventing atrophy of the quadriceps muscles. Active exercises along with straight leg weight lifting can maintain an excellent function of the musculature about the knee joint. If muscle spasms and early flexion deformities are present, these are indications that conservative therapy may have to be discarded in favor of surgical intervention. The use of bivalved casts or wedging casts should be discouraged in favor of surgical intervention.

Synovectomy

The history of synovectomy is quite well known, and numerous papers have been written about the technique and the short-term results. In the early series that have been reported, many other conditions were lumped together with rheumatoid arthritis. These tended to obscure the final results and led to confusion when there was a comparison of the results obtained by different authors. In 1964, Aidem and Baker reported that excellent or good results were obtained from 23 out of 31 synovectomies performed for rheumatoid arthritis with an average follow-up of 4 years. Geens and his associates in 1969 in a small series of 23 patients found a definite correlation between the stage of the disease and the results obtainable by synovectomy of the knee. This also was my experience with 175 synovectomies reported in 1973.

The operation of radical synovectomy has been altered to improve the postoperative motion. It is well known by the orthopaedic surgeon that if the suprapatellar pouch is injured or removed surgically, knee motion is often lost. Therefore, in order to preserve motion, the synovium is thoroughly re-moved from the joint margins, except for the suprapatellar pouch. The removal of the synovium from the joint margins prevents articular destruction, but the remaining synovium in the suprapatellar pouch acts as a bursa for the quadriceps mechanism and prevents adhesions. In over 12 years of doing this in more than 300 patients, the remaining synovial tissue has not shown any evidence of growing back down into the joint or producing problems. The synovium regenerates, and the new synovium is not rheumatoid in nature. Its junction with the synovium in the suprapatellar pouch tends to prevent the rheumatoid synovium in the pouch from growing down over the condyles of the femur. Key and Wolcott have both demonstrated in animals that the synovium regenerates from granulation tissue within 3 weeks after a synovectomy. At the end of 2 months, the reformed joint lining was difficult to distinguish from normal synovium in their animal studies. Experience in reoperating on knee joints that have had prior synovectomies that are not involved in active rheumatoid disease or severe articular destruction has shown that the joints tend to have very benign thin synovial layers that are hard to distinguish from normal synovial tissue (Fig. 10-22).

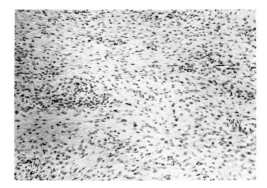

FIG. 10-22 Section of synovial tissue removed from patient at reoperation after a synovectomy ($\times$ 120). There is no evidence of active rheumatoid disease.

The patient with persistent pain that does not respond to good medical treatment within 6 months should be considered for surgical intervention by synovectomy. Evidence of progressive roentgenologic changes over a period of months again would substantiate the fact that early surgical intervention is indicated to prevent further destruction in the knee.

Flexion deformities of 10° to 15° with no evidence of bony block are not contraindications to synovectomy. Following removal of the diseased synovial tissue, the muscle spasm frequently disappears, and the knee flexion contracture will stretch out without any additional therapy. Preoperative traction or cast wedging is not indicated to correct this type of flexion deformity.

Operative Technique. The operation is performed under tourniquet control after expressing the blood from the leg with a Martin bandage. The operation was originally performed through a large median parapatellar incision, but it was found difficult to perform an adequate synovectomy on the lateral side and to gain exposure without injury to the quadriceps mechanism and the vastus medialis. Because of this, for the last 12 years I have used two incisions for all synovectomies and other knee operations that require access to both sides of the joint (Fig. 10-23). With this technique there have been no vascular complications to the skin flap as long as the edges of the incisions are kept separated at the upper and lower ends.

A median parapatellar incision is made one finger breadth medial to the edge of the patella and extends from the beginning lower edge of the vastus medialis to the tibial plateau, parallel to the patellar ligament. The medial expansion is opened, and it is not necessary to cut the vastus medialis, or at the most only 1 to 2 cm of its lower border, parallel to the rectus tendon. Often the

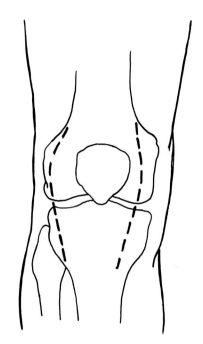

FIG. 10-23 Synovectomy of the knee joint. Diagram showing the locations of the two incisions.

synovial tissue will protrude from the joint on opening the expansion, and the synovial layer should be incised to expose the joint (Fig. 10-24). The synovial membrane can be separated from the medial expansion, and the patella can be retracted laterally to expose the infrapatellar fat pad (Fig. 10-24B). The infrapatellar fat pad should be excised to give better exposure of the joint while protecting the patellar ligament, as well as the medial expansion. The synovium is removed along the medial side of the patella from beneath the rectus tendon and the margin of the medial expansion.

At this stage, the attention is directed to the synovium along the superior aspect of the femoral condyle (Fig. 10-25). A knife is used to lift or scrape the synovial tissue along the medial superior aspect of the femoral condyle, and the synovial layer can be lifted up from the underlying areolar tissue. A scissors is slipped under the synovial layer and by spreading the scissors one can lift the

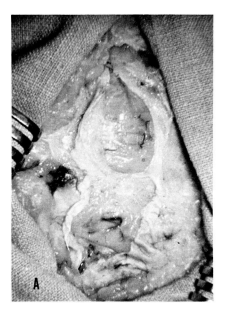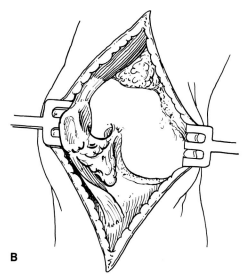

FIG. 10-24 Synovectomy of the knee joint (continued). A. Surgical view after medial expansion has been opened. Note the synovial tissue bulging from the joint. B. Drawing to show patella retracted laterally to expose the medial compartment and infrapatellar fat pad.

synovium up easily from the underlying tissue. It should be dissected upward for approximately 1 to 2 cm into the suprapatellar pouch but no further (Fig. 10-26). The synovium is then cut transversely away from the pouch toward the medial expansion (Fig. 10-26B), and all of the synovium is stripped off the femoral condyle on its superior aspect and then pulled distally with a rongeur, removing it in a thick layer but leaving the blood vessels intact on the areolar tissue. The area of the pouch left behind prevents adhesions of the quadriceps mechanism to the anterior aspect of the femur. The knee can be gradually flexed on the table by the assistant. This flexion exposes the medial wall of the femoral condyle so that the synovium can be pulled and removed with a rongeur. The subchondral edges of the articular margins should be curetted to remove all the vascular supply that could be contributing to the synovial hypertrophy. A retractor should be slipped under the medial collateral ligament with the knee flexed to allow

further exposure along the medial joint line and into the deep recesses of the posterior joint. If the medial meniscus is present, it should be excised carefully from the joint while the medial collateral ligament is protected.

Removing the meniscus allows access to the tibial plateau, and a more thorough synovectomy can be performed. Any protruding osteophytes should be removed from the femoral condyle and tibial plateau. With the knee flexed 90°, the intercondylar notch, which is usually filled with synovial tissue, is visible (Fig. 10-27). The synovium should be carefully removed from the cruciate ligaments and the inner sides of the femoral condyles (Fig. 10-27B).

After the medial compartment has been cleaned out, the knee is extended again, and a lateral parapatellar incision is made approximately two finger breadths lateral to the patella (Fig. 10-28). To protect the skin flap do not bring the ends of the incision toward the

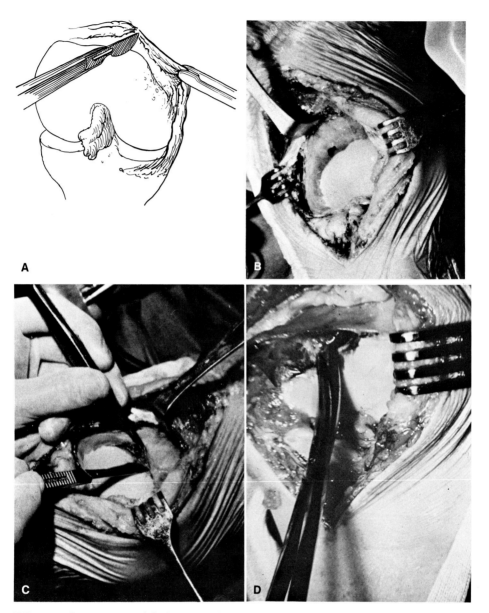

FIG. 10-25 Synovectomy of the knee joint (continued). A. Drawing showing freeing of the synovium along the superior aspect with a sharp knife. B. Clinical photograph of synovial tissue growing down over superior aspect of the femoral condyle, which has normal articular cartilage. C. Lifting the synovium from the superior aspect of the femoral condyle with a sharp knife. D. Scissors slipped under the synovial tissue and spread to lift it from the underlying areolar tissue.

medial incision. The thick fascia lata is opened, exposing the capsule and synovium. The joint is entered, and the patella is lifted upward with a retractor to expose the superior aspect of the lateral femoral condyle, and one can see where the synovium has been left behind from the medial incision. Starting here, one lifts up the synovial tissue and cuts across it laterally, leaving the suprapatellar pouch in place (Fig. 10-29). As one continues cutting laterally, one

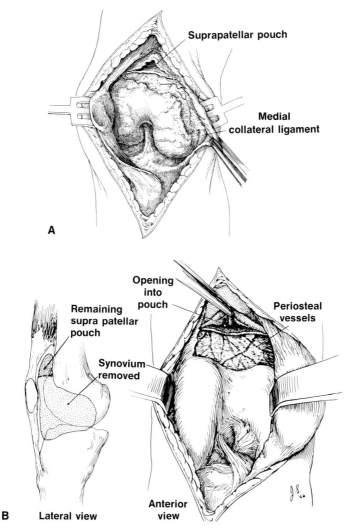

FIG. 10-26 Synovectomy of the knee joint (continued). A. Synovium dissected for about 1 inch toward the suprapatellar pouch and then swept down the medial side of the joint. B. Lateral and anterior views of area behind the suprapatellar pouch. The areolar blood vessels and the remaining pouch can be seen in the anterior view.

will see an area of fat that is the upper margin of the joint surface. The synovium can be stripped from the lateral wall of the femoral condyle, using a rongeur and gradually flexing the patient's knee. With the patient's knee flexed, the infrapatellar fat pad on the lateral side should be excised completely to give better exposure and to remove some of the diseased synovial tissue covering it. The lateral meniscus,

if present, should be detached anteriorly and then slipped into the intercondylar notch and removed. The popliteus tendon will be noted inserting into the lateral femoral condyle and should be protected.

The knee can be flexed 90°, and the collateral ligament should be lifted outward with a retractor to expose the posterior recess of the knee which contains synovial tissue. This tissue can be

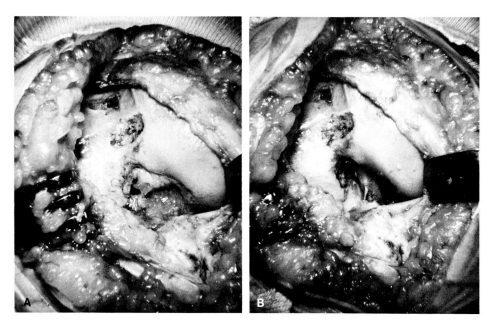

FIG. 10-27 Synovectomy of the knee joint (continued). A. Exposure of the intercondylar area through the medial incision. The cruciate ligaments are covered with synovial tissue. B. After debridement of the joint and intercondylar notch. The cruciate ligaments are visible.

removed with a small rongeur quite easily, and the edges of the articular margins should be curetted to remove all of the small vascular supply that feeds the synovial tissue. Any bony spurs should be removed from the condyle or tibial plateau with a rongeur. When the lateral compartment has been completed, the medial incision should be exposed with the patient's knee ex-

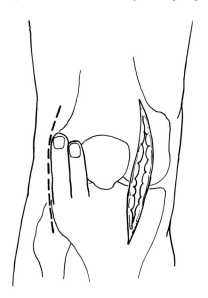

FIG. 10-28 Synovectomy of the knee joint (continued). The broken line indicates position for the lateral parapatellar incisions two finger breadths from the patella.

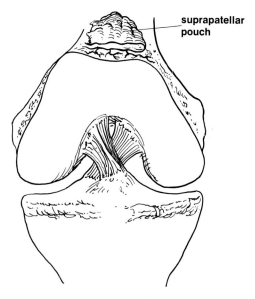

suprapatellar pouch

FIG. 10-29 Synovectomy of the knee joint (continued). The suprapatellar pouch left in place as a bursa.

tended, and the patella can be everted with a rake to reveal its surface (Fig. 10-30). All excess synovium and any osteophytes should be removed from its margin. It is advisable not to remove the patella at this time, no matter how bad the articular surface appears. Areas of chondromalacia may be seen but do not require treatment. A patellectomy can always be done in the future if symptoms warrant, but in my experience in operating on over 500 knees this has not been necessary, despite the appearance of the patella. (At this stage the surgeon would proceed to do a total knee replacement if it had been planned.)

The tourniquet may be released if a total knee replacement is not being inserted. I have done a large series of synovectomies in which the tourniquet was released at the end of the operation after a bulky dressing was applied, and I have also released the tourniquet and obtained hemostasis before closure. The latter procedure seems to be the one of choice and is recommended. Two small suction tubes are brought out through the suprapatellar pouch for post-operative drainage of the joint. The expansions are then repaired with either 0 chromic catgut or 0 silk sutures. The sutures are placed interrupted in the expansion to prevent breakage of a suture line with early motion. The knee may be flexed prior to closure of the subcutaneous tissue and skin to be sure that the suture line is secure, and it is wise to check that the suction tubes have not been sutured into the incision. The subcutaneous tissue is closed with 3-0 chromic sutures, and the skin is closed loosely with a 3-0 nylon continuous skin suture. We have found that 3-0 nylon tends to hold very well during early motion. Thinner sutures tend to break with the stress of early activity.

Postoperative Care. The leg is then placed in a large bulky Jones-type dressing using cotton batting or Dacron covered with bias stockinette (Fig. 10-31). This compressive dressing is left in place for 2 days, and the patient is started on immediate quadriceps muscle exercise and flexion within the confines of this dressing. At 2 days postoperatively the bulky dressing and the suction tubes are removed, and a small, lightweight dressing is applied. The patient is encouraged to exercise both actively and passively with the physical therapist and after the third day is allowed to sit on the edge of the bed to flex and extend the knee.

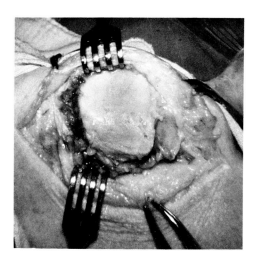

FIG. 10-30 Synovectomy of the knee joint (continued). Eversion of the patella with a rake to expose the articular surface. The osteophytes and synovial tissue around the periphery should be removed.

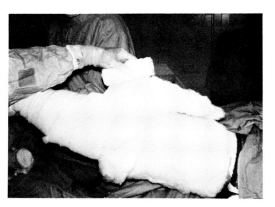

FIG. 10-31 Synovectomy of the knee joint (continued). Application of Jones-type dressing.

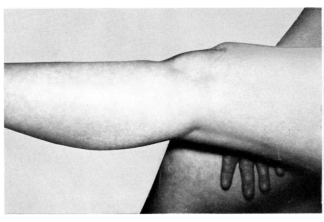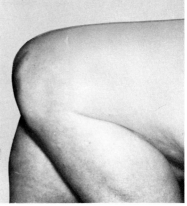

FIG. 10-32 Synovectomy of the knee joint (continued). Range of motion two years after operation on patient who had minimal joint destruction. The suprapatellar pouch was left in place.

Straight leg raising is included in the therapy routine, and if the quadriceps mechanism has not been damaged, it is surprising how quickly full extension is possible postoperatively. The patient is allowed full weight bearing on the knee on the fourth day. The patient is usually discharged from 7 to 14 days postoperatively, depending upon the home situation. If the incision is healed, the sutures may be removed by the twelfth to fourteenth day, and hydrotherapy may be started.

Results. The results of synovectomy of the knee correlate closely to the preoperative findings (Fig. 10-32). The major cause of failure of synovectomy occurred in patients with advanced destruction of the joint with loss of the articular cartilage that was observed on the preoperative roentgenogram and also noted at the surgical procedure (Fig. 10-33). These failures were all patients who were operated upon prior to the development of the total knee replacement. It is interesting, however, that the average patient in the group of failures due to articular changes did well for several years after synovectomy and had no symptoms. However, with the passage of time and use of the knee, symptoms gradually returned. These failures

were not actually recurrences of the disease following synovectomy but were the result of pain from the articular surface.

It is important also to point out that synovectomies were not successful in patients with evidence of an early varus or valgus deformity with unilateral narrowing of the joint space which could be

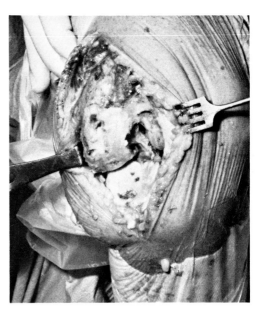

FIG. 10-33 Synovectomy of the knee joint (continued). Surgical view of advanced destruction of the joint and loss of articular cartilage.

confirmed by the roentgenogram (Fig. 10-34). It is also of interest that an excellent result can be obtained in the patients who have severe disease of the knee joint with evidences of advanced rheumatoid disease in roentgenograms (Fig. 10-35). Despite these changes, these patients have continued to do well with the passage of years (Fig. 10-36). The best results have been obtained in patients with a good joint surface with no evidence of articular destruction (Fig. 10-37). It is evident that the results of synovectomy are definitely related to the selection of the patient and the stage of the disease.

Patients with psoriatic arthritis also may develop severe chronic effusions due to synovitis. Synovectomy can be performed for treatment of the disease process (Fig. 10-38). Incisions through psoriatic lesions heal well.

Tibial Osteotomy

Rheumatoid patients can develop a varus or valgus deformity during the active stage of the disease. Occasionally the synovial disease will disappear, leaving the patient with a painful de-

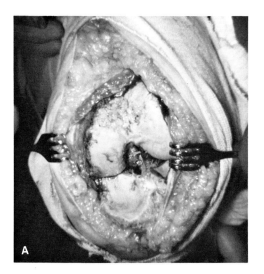

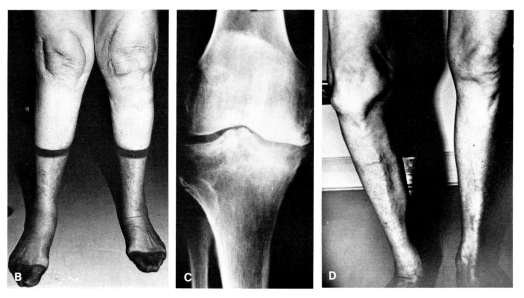

FIG. 10-34 Synovectomy of the knee joint (continued). Evidence of varus or valgus deformity is a cause of failure. A. Surgical view showing a depression in the tibial plateau and a grooved area in the tibia. B. Postoperative view 2 years later reveals valgus deformity. C. Roentgenogram of another patient with narrowing of the joint space on the medial side. D. Preoperative view showing the severe varus deformity requiring an osteotomy.

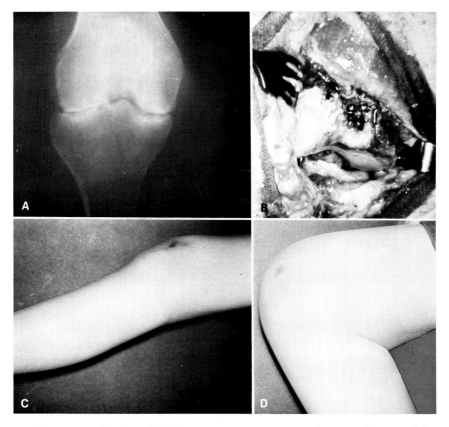

FIG. 10-35 Synovectomy (continued). A. Preoperative roentgenogram shows involvement of the joint. B. Surgical view shows destruction of femoral condyles and complete loss of articular cartilage. C and D. Ten years postoperatively the patient has excellent range of motion and is free of pain.

formity. These deformities can be associated with a flexion contracture of the knee, resulting in a poorly functioning joint. Often both knee joints may be diseased so that arthrodesis is not a very reasonable solution to the problem. Total knee replacement can be utilized, but when total knee replacement is not indicated or the surgeon is not familiar with the techniques, osteotomy can give satisfactory results in many cases. Osteotomy will correct the deformity, relieve the pain, and retain knee motion (Fig. 10-39). If failure does ensue, total knee replacement can always be carried out in the future.

Operative Technique—Low Tibial Osteotomy. The extremity is wrapped with a Martin bandage, and a tourniquet is inflated. A 3-inch skin incision is made from the tibial tubercle distally over the tibia in a vertical line (Figs. 10-40; 10-41). The subcutaneous tissue is divided down to the periosteum, which is incised in the same line as the incision. The periosteum is stripped from the tibia up to the insertion of the patellar ligament at the tibial tubercle to expose the flare of the base of the condyles and the tibial tubercle with the patellar ligament. The patellar ligament attachment to the tibia will be in the upper portion of the incision. On the medial side, sharp dissection with a knife is required to separate the fibers of the pes anserinus and a portion of the medial collateral ligament from the tibia.

Bennett retractors are inserted be-

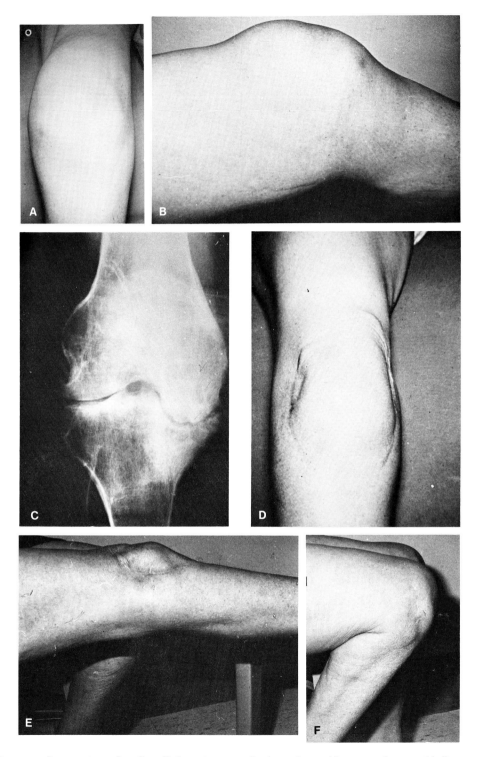

FIG. 10-36 Synovectomy (continued). Long-term results in patient with severe rheumatoid disease. A. Preoperative anterior view of swelling in knee. B. Preoperative lateral view. C. Preoperative roentgenogram showing destruction in the joint. D. Photograph 8 years after synovectomy. E and F. Range of motion without pain 8 years after synovectomy.

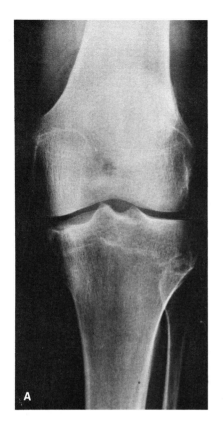

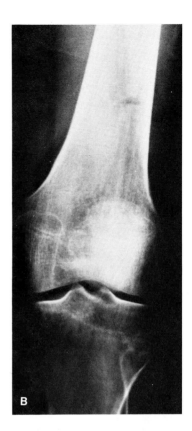

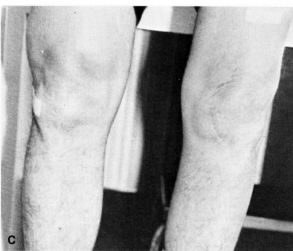

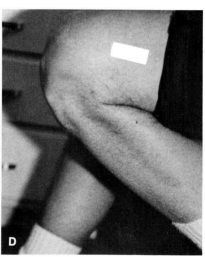

FIG. 10-37 Synovectomy of the knee joint (continued). Long-term results. A. Roentgenogram 10 years after operation on left knee reveals no evidence of loss of joint space when patient is standing. B. Roentgenogram 12 years later still reveals no evidence of narrowing of joint space. C. Photograph 13 years later. The patient has had no recurrence of pain or deformity in the left knee, but has effusion in the right knee. D. Flexion in the left knee is normal after 13 years.

FIG. 10-38 Synovectomy of the knee joint (continued). Psoriatic arthritis. A. Preoperative photograph shows effusion of the knee joint. The patient has had numerous aspirations. B. Preoperative roentgenogram reveals a reasonably normal joint despite the synovial disease. C. Surgical view reveals hyperplasia of the synovium. D. Surgical view also reveals changes in the articular cartilage. E. The lateral incision reveals a large pedunculated synovial mass (arrow). F and G. Postoperative photographs 8 years later showing no recurrence of disease process and an excellent range of flexion. The patient is free of pain. ⟶

352

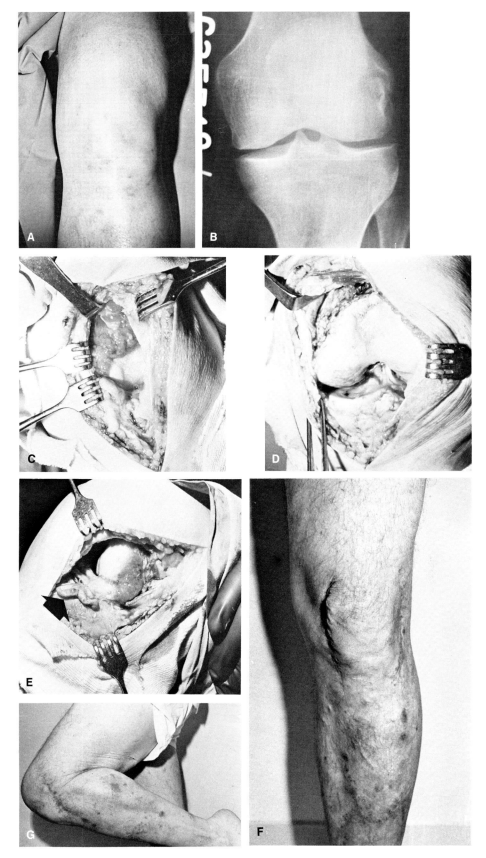

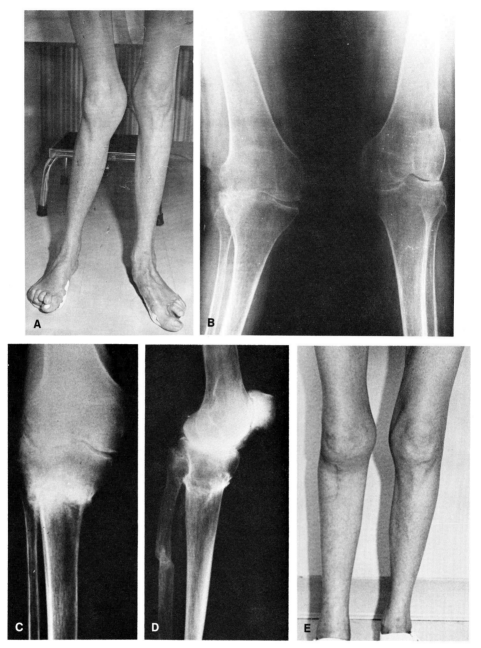

FIG. 10-39 Osteotomy of the knee. A. Preoperative photograph. The patient had advanced rheumatoid arthritis of the right knee with a severe valgus deformity but no active synovitis. B. Roentgenogram revealing rheumatoid changes in both joints. C. Roentgenogram after operation to correct alignment by impacting two fragments of proximal tibia together. D. Lateral view. E. Postoperative appearance of the leg.

hind the tibia, and holes are drilled transversely through the cancellous bone at the distal end of the tibial tubercle to mark the line for dividing the shaft of the tibia. The tibia is then divided with an osteotome (Figs. 10-40; 10-41). Care should be exercised to protect the posterior aspect of the tibia and to divide the entire cortex posteriorly. In patients with severe osteoporosis the tibia can be

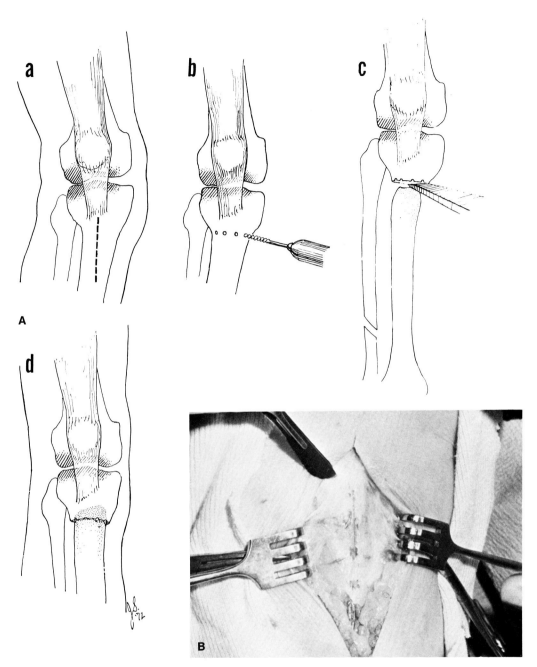

FIG. 10-40 Osteotomy of the knee. A. Technique for low tibial osteotomy adjacent to the tibial tubercle: skin incision(a); holes drilled(b); excision with osteotome(c); distal fragment impacted into the proximal(d). B. Surgical view of incision. The knife is pointing to the insertion of the patellar ligament on the tibial tubercle. (From Marmor, L: Salvage of the rheumatoid knee by osteotomy. J. West, Pacific Ortho Assoc., *11*:3, 1973.)

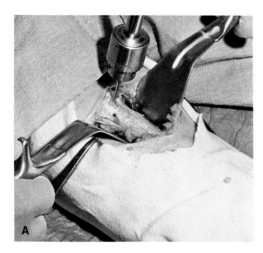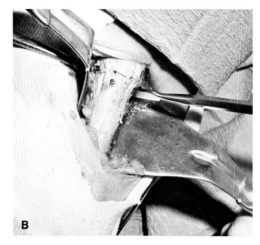

FIG. 10-41 Osteotomy of the knee (continued). A. Drilling holes across the tibia. Bennett retractors have been inserted behind the tibia. B. Cutting between the drill holes with an osteotome. The Bennett retractors protect the posterior aspect.

cracked manually, and the distal fragment can be impacted into the proximal fragment to correct the valgus or varus deformity, as well as the flexion deformity.

Next, a separate incision is made approximately two thirds down the fibula along the lateral side of the leg at the junction of the middle and lower third of the fibula where it is quite superficial. The fibula is exposed, and Bennett retractors are inserted behind it for protection. Holes are drilled through the fibula, perforating both cortices, and then the fibula is divided with an osteotome or a power tool. When correcting a varus deformity into valgus, it is wise to remove a small piece of the fibula (approximately 0.5 cm) to prevent impingement and loss of correction, which may produce distraction of the tibia and result in a delayed union or nonunion. In repairing the incision the deep fascia is closed to prevent a muscle hernia postoperative.

The medial incision over the proximal tibia is approached next. The distal shaft of the tibia is shaped with an osteotome and narrowed so that it will fit inside the medullary cavity of the proximal fragment. The two are impacted together in a corrected position (Fig. 10-42). Bone chips are turned down with a gouge, the chips are crossed over the osteotomy site, and the two fragments are firmly impacted.

The periosteum over the proximal tibia is resutured with 0 interrupted catgut sutures, the tourniquet is released at this stage, and hemostasis is secured. The subcutaneous tissue and the skin are closed.

It is generally advisable to slightly overcorrect the deformity. If the patient is in varus, it is wise to try to place the extremity in approximately 5° of valgus. If the patient is in valgus, it is wise to try to place the leg into slight varus. The patient should be advised of this possibility preoperatively so that there will be no confusion over the postoperative appearance. Unless overcorrection is obtained, the patient may continue to have symptoms because he may drop back on the diseased compartment during weight bearing.

After closure of the incisions, a long-leg cast is applied from the toes to the groin with the knee extended, to maintain the corrected position of the tibia.

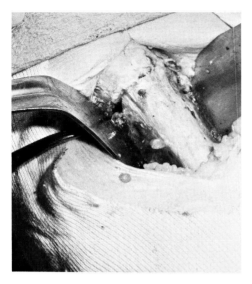

FIG. 10-42 Osteotomy of the knee (continued). Distal end of tibia reshaped and impacted into the proximal portion.

To allow for swelling it is advisable to split the cast by removing a 1 cm strip of plaster from the knee to the toes, across the anterior aspect of the cast. Cross hatches at 2-inch intervals can be made with the cast cutter to allow for easy spreading of the cast postoperatively.

Postoperative Care. When the swelling has receded, usually after 4 or 5 days, the cast is closed, and the patient is started on partial weight bearing with crutches. If the cast is loose at 10 to 14 days, it should be replaced to prevent motion at the osteotomy site. Full weight bearing is started after 2 weeks if symptoms have subsided and is encouraged until the cast is removed. At 6 weeks the cast may be replaced with a cast with a walking heel, and the patient continues to bear full weight on the leg for another 6 weeks. If union is evident, after 12 weeks clinically and roentgenologically, the plaster cast is removed. If there is any question about healing, it is safer to maintain the cast for another 6 weeks than to take if off too soon. After the cast has been removed, full weight bearing is allowed as tolerated. Support hose or an elastic bandage should be worn until all swelling has disappeared from the leg.

Results. Thirty-five osteotomies were performed from November 1964 through December 1971 for rheumatoid arthritis in a group of 30 patients with severe involvement of the knee joint. The average age of the patients was 52 years. Flexion contractures were present in 25 knees, and all but one was associated with a valgus or varus deformity. The average valgus deformity was 22°, with a range from 15 to 35°. The average varus deformity was 17°, with a range from 10 to 30°. The results were rated as excellent if the patient was able to walk without pain and had correction of the deformity. Patients who had mild pain, aching, or discomfort but who could do all of their daily activities were rated as having good results. Failures were patient who had pain, recurrence of the deformity, or the inability to walk. There were 25 excellent or good results in the 35 osteotomies performed (Fig. 10-43). There were 2 nonunions of the tibia and fibula in patients with advanced destruction of their knee joints. At the present time this type of patient would not be considered for osteotomy because of the severe involvement of both compartments of the knee.

One stress fracture of the distal tibia occurred one year after the osteotomy of a proximal tibia and fibula (Fig. 10-44).

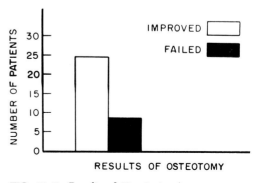

FIG. 10-43 Results of 35 osteotomies.

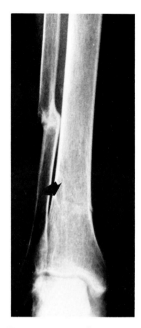

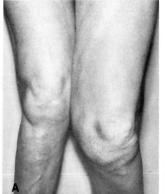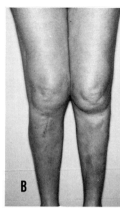

FIG. 10-45   Osteotomy to correct severe flexion-valgus deformities of both knees. The patient is a 42-year-old woman. A. Preoperative photograph. B. Photograph 2 years after correction of both knees.

FIG. 10-44   Roentgenogram showing stress fracture (arrow) of the tibia one year after an osteotomy.

In general, osteotomy of the tibia and fibula can be utilized for the treatment of rheumatoid deformities in patients with angular deformity without active synovitis within the joint (Fig. 10-45). The tibial osteotomy distal to the tibial tubercle allows correction of the osteotomy postoperatively by wedging of the cast. This is not possible if a high tibial osteotomy is carried out. The high tibial osteotomy (page 410), unless well performed, can result in recurrence of the deformity and extensive destruction of the articular surface of the joint if the osteotomy splits into the articular compartment (Fig. 10-46). The high tibial osteotomy has been used more often in the treatment of osteoarthritis.

Femoral Osteotomy

A supracondylar osteotomy can be utilized in the treatment of flexion contractures as well as varus or valgus deformities of the knee in rheumatoid arthritis. The closer the osteotomy is placed to the femoral condyle, the more cosmetic the result will be. In general, however, femoral osteotomy has many limitations and at the present time offers no advantage over the tibial osteotomy or total knee replacement in the rheumatoid patient. For the femoral osteotomy one must depend upon internal fixation of the femur. In the rheumatoid patient the bone is frequently osteoporotic so that fixation may be inadequate. Once the resection of bone has been carried out to correct the deformity and internal fixation is applied, further correction is impossible during the postoperative recovery period. It is easy to overcorrect or undercorrect in this type of osteotomy.

Patellectomy

Patellectomy is a procedure that is used seldom in the treatment of rheumatoid arthritis. In rheumatoid disease, there is practically no occasion when there is isolated patellofemoral disease without involvement of the articular surface of the remainder of the joint. Patellectomy should not be performed with other procedures such as synovectomy or total joint replacement because immobilization of the knee will result in stiffness postoperatively. In rare occasions, the patella may be a source of pain following total knee replacement, and

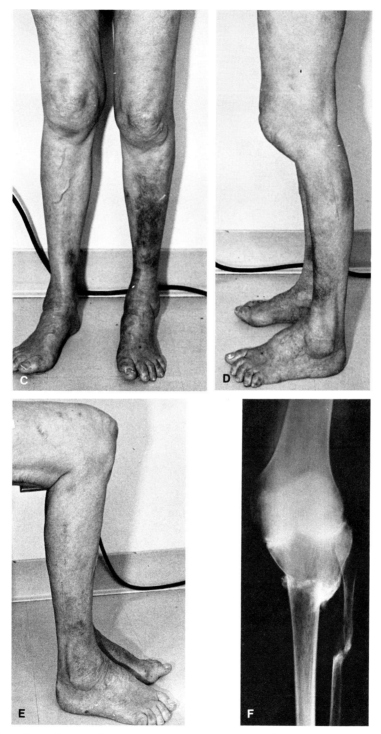

FIG. 10-45 (Cont'd.) Eight years later: C. Anterior view revealing maintenance of correction. D. Lateral view revealing offset of proximal tibia with distal tibia. E. Lateral view of both knees in flexion. F. Roentgenogram revealing impaction of the distal shaft into the proximal tibia. There is no joint space, but the patient is free of pain.

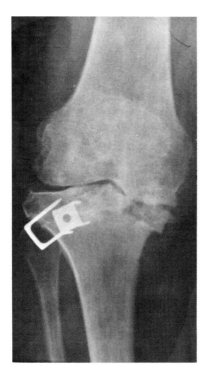

FIG. 10-46 Roentgenogram revealing fracture of the tibial plateau as a complication of a high tibial osteotomy.

symptoms will persist over a year. In such cases, a patellectomy may be indicated to relieve the patient's symptoms.

Operative Technique. A patellectomy is performed by flexing the knee 90° and then wrapping the leg with a Martin bandage and inflating the tourniquet. A transverse skin incision may be used over the patella, and then a vertical incision is made directly over the middle of the patella. By sharp dissection, the fibers of the patellar ligament and rectus tendon are peeled off the surface of the patella, leaving the tendon intact (Fig. 10-47). Gradually the joint is entered, and the patella is completely shelled out and removed. Since the longitudinal fibers of the ligament are still intact, the tendon can be repaired with No. 1 silk interrupted sutures. If a strong repair has been carried out, the knee can be flexed 90° and extended without any tension on the suture line. If the surgeon is satisfied,

then the wound is closed in layers. A compression dressing is applied, and the tourniquet is released. A cooperative patient will not need to be placed in a posterior splint if an adequate repair has been obtained. If there is any doubt in the surgeon's mind, the patient may be placed in a posterior molded splint or in a cylinder cast for 4 weeks.

Postoperative Care. Generally, a splint should be used during the immediate postoperative period to prevent damage on transfer from the operating room while the patient is anesthetized. Then if the repair is stable, the patient is cautioned against full flexion and is allowed to do quadriceps exercises and bend the knee to approximately 60°. Weight bearing is allowed with crutches or a walker within 3 to 4 days. This postoperative schedule allows rapid return of function and prevents atrophy, especially in the older arthritic patient.

Patellar Prosthesis

The patella in rheumatoid arthritis is frequently severely involved but is not

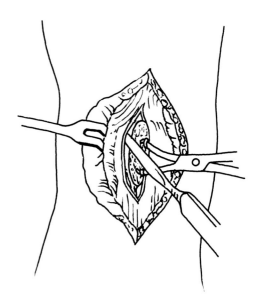

FIG. 10-47 Patellectomy of the knee—Boyd technique. Excising the patella from the quadriceps tendon.

usually a cause of symptoms. Hundreds of synovectomies have been performed upon patients with severe disease of the patella, and in few of these cases have patellar symptoms occurred postoperatively. However, devices have been developed for replacement of the patella. These may find more of a role in osteoarthritis than in rheumatoid arthritis. The patella in many cases of rheumatoid disease is quite eroded and thin, as well as osteoporotic, and it would be difficult to maintain a prosthetic device in opposition to its undersurface. During walking the forces on the patella are extreme, and the pull of the quadriceps muscle may tend to loosen most fixation devices. Patellar prostheses will be discussed in the section on osteoarthritis of the knee where they may have an occasional use.

Tibial Plateau

A number of prostheses have been developed for the replacement of the individual tibial plateau, both plateaus simultaneously, or the femoral condyles. McKeever and MacIntosh have both described prostheses for the tibial plateau which may be used separately for each plateau in contrast to the prosthesis for the entire tibial articular surface which was reported by Townley. These prostheses have been successful in the past and may still be valuable. They are a more conservative approach than unicompartment total knee replacement and may be used in place of this procedure for patients in the early stages of rheumatoid arthritis. In my experience, good results with the tibial plateau prostheses have been attained in less than 50 percent of the cases. There are still, however, a number of patients who are ambulatory because of the prosthesis and are able to work and carry on with their activities, despite some discomfort (Fig. 10-48). The prostheses available at the present time for the tibial plateau can be considered similar to those for

the femoral head hemiarthroplasty in arthritic patients. In many rheumatoid arthritic patients, the femoral condyles are severely diseased also, and the tibial plateau prosthesis cannot be used (Fig. 10-49). The tibial plateau prosthesis, however, will correct angular deformities that are not fixed deformities, and combined with the synovectomy in rheumatoid arthritis it can give reasonable results.

There are various types of tibial plateau prostheses. The McKeever prosthesis has a cruciate fin underneath it to anchor it into the tibia (Fig. 10-50). The MacIntosh is placed on a flat tibial bed after removal of the tibial plateau and is held in place by the capsule and collateral ligaments. The Marmor tibial plateau prosthesis is smaller in diameter than the patient's tibial plateau and can be inserted into the bone similar to inserting a filling in a tooth. The tibial plateau is designed with holes for ingrowth of bone into the metal for further fixation. Many years later subsequent exploration of some of the knees that have had these tibial plateau components has shown that they have become so firmly anchored in the bone that they have to be removed with an impactor.

Marmor Technique. The operation is performed under tourniquet control through medial and lateral parapatellar incisions. In rheumatoid arthritis patients with active disease, a synovectomy should be performed as described previously. After removal of all of the synovial tissue through the two incisions, the knee is flexed 90°, and the patella is retracted laterally. The tibial plateau is flattened with an osteotome to remove any ridges or irregularities from the arthritis.

The medial incision is used for the medial tibial plateau replacement. The tibial marking template is coated with methylene blue to outline the area to be removed (Fig. 10-51). If difficulty is en-

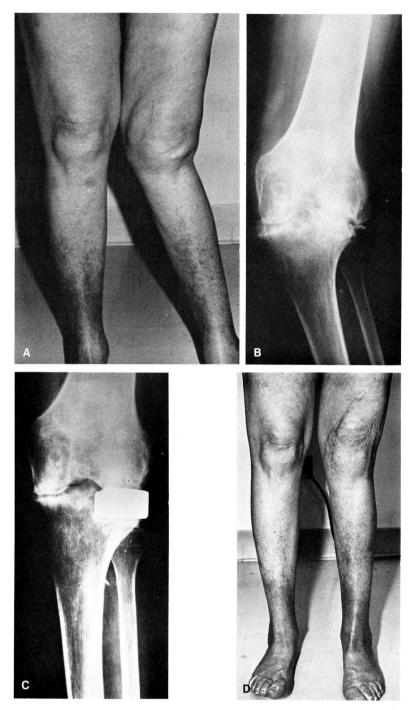

FIG. 10-48 Use of tibial plateau prosthesis and synovectomy to correct deformity from rheumatoid arthritis in left knee of 44-year-old woman. A. Preoperative view showing 50° valgus deformity. B. Preoperative roentgenogram revealing rheumatoid destruction of the joint. C. Postoperative roentgenogram one year after insertion of tibial plateau revealing correction of valgus deformity and old residual disease within joint. Six years after surgery: D. Anterior view showing correction of deformity.

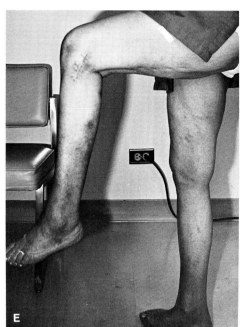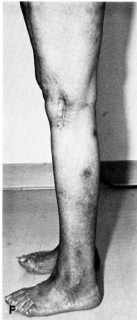

FIG. 10-48 (Cont'd.) E. Lateral view revealing flexion. F. Lateral view revealing full extension. The patient functions well without pain.

countered in placing the template, the knee should be fully flexed and approximately ¼ inch of bone can be removed from the posterior aspect of the femoral condyle with an osteotome. The template is coated with methylene blue dye and is positioned over the desired area on the tibial plateau, leaving several millimeters of posterior ledge for good fixation.

With a power tool such as the Hall air drill and a 5-mm bur, a trough is cut in the tibial plateau within the outlined area. The trough should be approximately 3 mm deep and should allow a good rim of remaining bone around its periphery (Fig. 10-52). The trial prosthesis should be inserted to check the dimensions. Since cement is not used in the Marmor technique to fix these devices, a tight fit is recommended. If cement (methyl methacrylate) is utilized, a tight fit is not necessary.

The prosthesis of the approximate thickness to restore the knee to a normal position is selected and impacted into the trough to restore the normal plateau height (Fig. 10-53). If the prosthesis tends to rock during flexion of the knee, the posterior portion of the tibia should be deepened to allow the femoral condyle to slide through easily. If the prosthesis is too tight, the joint will rock open. In replacing both plateaus during the same procedure, care should be taken to select the prosthesis of the proper thickness for each side. Suction drainage tubes are brought out through the suprapatellar pouch to prevent swelling and slow healing. The tourniquet is released, and hemostasis is secured. The quadriceps expansion should be repaired with 0 interrupted catgut or silk sutures and the subcutaneous tissue with 3-0 chromic sutures. The skin is closed with continuous 3-0 nylon sutures put in very loosely to prevent postoperative tension on the suture line.

Postoperative Care. A bulky compression dressing is used for 2 days postoperatively, at which time the suction tubes are removed and a small

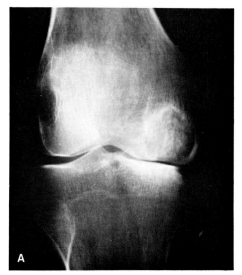

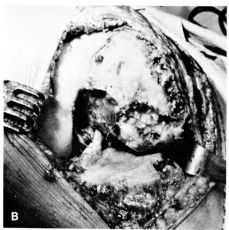

FIG. 10-49 Cystic lesion on weight-bearing surface of the medial femoral condyle. A. Roentgenogram. B. Surgical view revealing large defect.

dressing is applied. The patient is instructed to start early motion following surgery and is assisted with passive and active motion by the physical therapist on the day after the operation. Weight bearing with crutches generally is allowed after 5 days and is gradually increased until at the end of 6 weeks the knee is allowed to bear full weight.

Results. MacIntosh has previously reported that about 69 percent of his patients had good results, with relief of pain and improved function, and that the prostheses tended to last. Sbarbaro also reported in a lecture that for 45 rheumatoid arthritic patients 56 percent were in the excellent group and 29 percent were also improved. In my experience with 64 patients the good results were less than 50 percent in long-term follow-up. Many of these patients have required replacement of the tibial plateau with a total knee procedure. However, there are always exceptions, and several of the patients have had excellent results over 6 years (Fig. 10-54). In general, however, my impression is that the total knee replacement when there is bony destruction may be the procedure of choice for rheumatoid arthritis patients.

Total Knee Joint Replacement

The concept of a total joint replacement became a reality after the development of the total hip replacement by Charnley and McKee-Farrar. This was a dramatic event in the history of orthopaedic surgery. The spectacular results of hip replacement have withstood the test of time and have spurred interest in replacements for other joints in the body. The knee, being the most important joint in the lower extremity, has been a logical target for replacement for a long time.

The hinge knee device had its proponents for many years, but devices using the hinge principle have never been widely accepted by the orthopaedic surgeon because of the complications associated with them and the fact that the knee is not a hinge with a simple flexion-extension motion. The work of Gunston in developing a high density polyethylene and metal knee joint that could be cemented into place by methyl methacrylate opened the door to practical knee replacements.

From the Gunston design evolved the four-component tracked knee in which the femoral components drop into

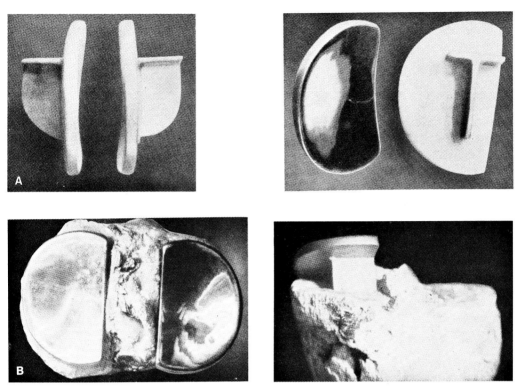

FIG. 10-50 McKeever tibial plateau prosthesis. A. Components. Note the cruciate fin underneath. B. The fin driven into the tibia to anchor the prosthesis.

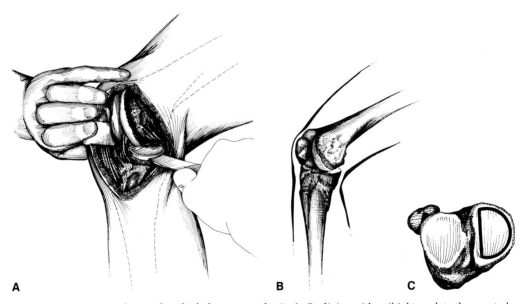

A   **B**   **C**

FIG. 10-51 Marmor technique for tibial plateau prosthesis. A. Outlining with a tibial template the area to be removed for insertion of the tibial plateau. B. Knee flexed 90° to remove ¼ inch of femoral condyle. C. Area outlined by tibial template. (Courtesy of Richards Manufacturing Co.)

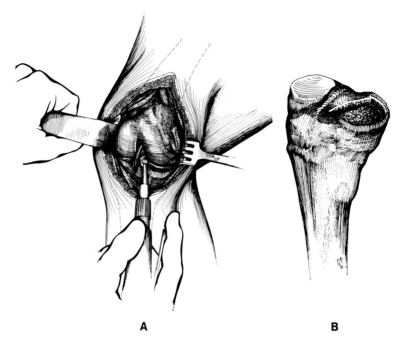

FIG. 10-52 Marmor technique for tibial plateau prosthesis (continued). A. Drilling trough with a power tool. B. The trough cut into the tibia. (Courtesy of Richards Manufacturing Co.)

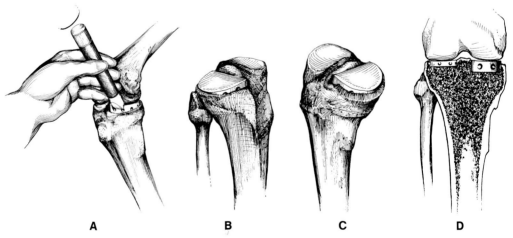

FIG. 10-53 Marmor technique for tibial plateau prosthesis (continued). A. Impaction of tibial plateau prosthesis into cancellous bone of the tibia. B. One plateau replaced in osteoarthritis. C. and D. Two plateaus replaced in rheumatoid arthritis, or osteoarthritis. (Courtesy of Richards Manufacturing Co.)

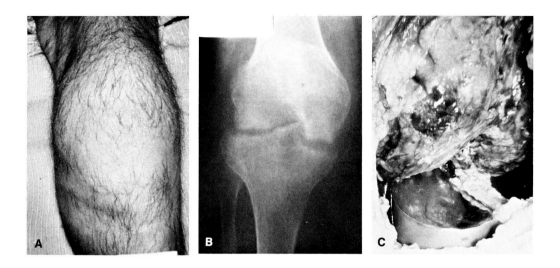

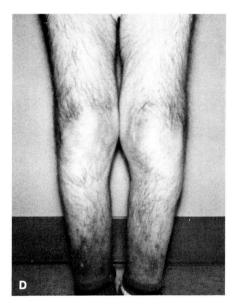

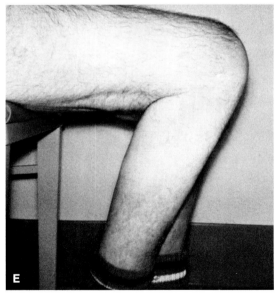

FIG. 10-54 Tibial plateau prosthesis in 54-year-old man with rheumatoid arthritis. A. Preoperative view showing swelling of the knee joint and atrophy of the quadriceps. B. Preoperative roentgenogram showing destruction of the joint. C. Surgical view showing destruction of the femoral condyles and tibial plateaus in place. Nine years after insertion of tibial prostheses in both knees: D. Anterior view showing extension. E. Lateral view revealing flexion possible. The patient has no pain and is able to work 8 hours a day.

grooves in the high-density polyethylene tibial component. Because of the difficulty of insertion of this device, the Geomedic prosthesis was developed. It is a two-part tracked knee device which replaces both femoral condyles and both tibial plateaus simultaneously. These knee replacements share the disadvantages of a complex insertion procedure. They require special cutting jigs to allow proper alignment of their femoral components and prevent normal rotation in the knee joint. This lack of rotation tends to increase the stress on the cement-bone bond and can lead to early failure of fixation. The complexity of the operative procedures, the restrictive rotation, and the loss of bony substance associated with these implants have tended to limit their popularity with many orthopaedic surgeons.

The experience gained with the metal tibial plateau prosthesis developed the idea of locking the tibial component into place by leaving a peripheral ledge of bone around the tibial plateau replacement (Fig. 10-55). Migration is less likely, and the bone tends to grow around the periphery of the plateau. In patients whose knee joints were explored many years later, the metal tibial plateaus were found to be well fixed in place without benefit of cement. The major cause of later difficulty with these prostheses was the loss of articular cartilage on the femoral condyle which was not replaced during the original operation. A component to replace only the femoral condyle also was not successful (Fig. 10-56).

The advent of the work performed by Charnley, McKee-Farrar, and Gunston and the newer materials led to the development of a modular concept for replacing the articular surface of the knee joint and leaving all of the ligaments and bony structure intact. The surgeon undertaking total joint replacement of the knee must realize the shortcomings of the lack of adequate follow-

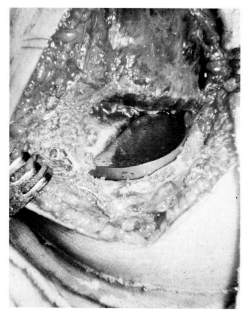

FIG. 10-55 Surgical view of the tibial plateau prosthesis locked into a trough cut in the tibia to prevent migration.

up, as well as the possibility of the future development of a better design. It is important, therefore, to be as conservative as possible and to leave as much bony stock behind as possible in case other surgical procedures become necessary or arthrodesis is required. We are standing at the threshold of an entire new era in knee replacement and what is present today should not be considered the ultimate solution.

The surgeon planning to undertake total knee replacement must consider taking proper precautions prior to embarking on such a procedure. As with the total hip, familiarity with the use of the instruments and the type of knee prosthesis to be inserted is paramount. The operation should be performed in a room that has been prepared for this type of implant surgery. Whether a laminar flow room is utilized or the room is kept sealed when in use to prevent contamination by opening and closing the doors is left to the judgment of the surgeon and the hospital infection committee. The use of "space" suits to shield the patient from the surgeons and nurse at the operating table may be more important than the laminar flow rooms. The helmet with the sterile face plate is of value because it prevents contamination when pieces of cement or bone fly out of the wound and strike the face mask.

The Marmor Modular Knee System

The Marmor Modular Knee system consisting of a femoral condyle of metal and a tibial plateau component of high-density polyethylene allows the surgeon to adapt the device to the patient rather than try to adapt a patient to the device. It is a conservative approach to replacement of the articular surface of the knee joint that will preserve as much bony stock as possible. Because there are no grooves in the plastic and a broad surface to the femoral component, full rotation of the knee is possible and stress on the cement-bone bond is prevented (Fig. 10-57). The varying heights of available tibial plateaus allow correction of varus or valgus deformities due to loss of bone. No complicated instruments are required for insertion of the components, and the various templates make it extremely easy to insert the components

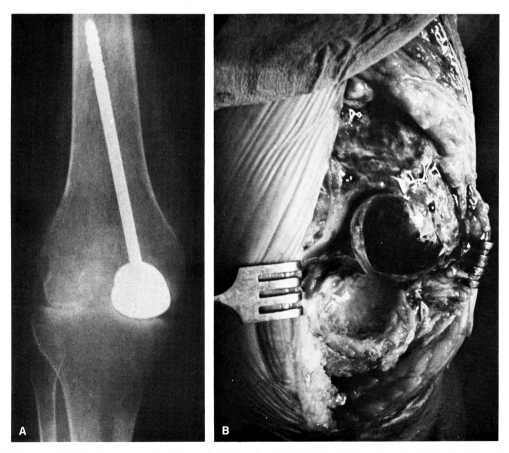

FIG. 10-56 A. Roentgenogram showing a metal stem prosthesis designed to replace the femoral surface. B. Surgical view at reoperation. Note the femoral component and the depression in the tibial plateau which resulted in pain and failure.

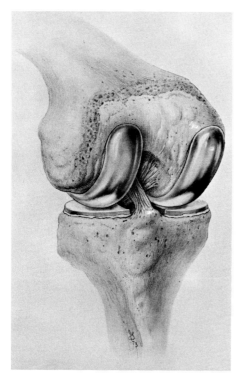

FIG. 10-57 The Marmor Modular Knee. It consists of a metal femoral condyle component and a polyethylene tibial plateau component with no grooves. (Courtesy Richards Manufacturing Company.)

into the knee (Fig. 10-58). The use of the trial prosthesis allows for adjustment of the various components to give maximum stability and correction of deformity. With the Marmor Modular Knee system it is possible to replace only what is necessary. Replacement of a single compartment is more common in osteoarthritis, however, and is extremely rare in rheumatoid arthritis because generally both compartments of the knee joint are involved.

The major indications for replacement of the joint surface in rheumatoid arthritis are to relieve pain, to correct joint stiffness, and to regain stability of the knee joint.

The major contraindications to replacement of a joint are infection, a previous surgical arthrodesis, or severe bone destruction with gross instability. The loss of a cruciate ligament or instability of a ligament due to bone destruction is not a contraindication to the use of the Marmor Modular knee, which replaces the bone destruction with the high-density polyethylene tibial plateau. The slack ligaments then become tight-

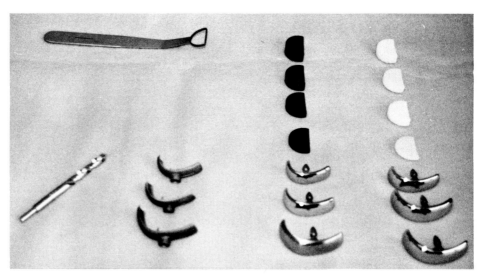

FIG. 10-58 Instruments and components for the Marmor Modular Knee: tibial template, black trial tibial components, white final tibial components, $\frac{3}{8}$-inch drill for use with femoral template, femoral trial and final components.

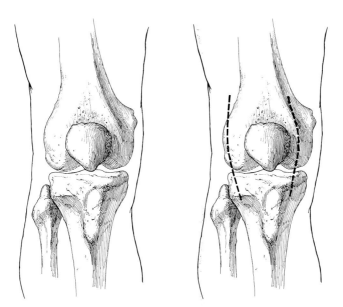

FIG. 10-59 Incisions for double compartment Marmor Modular Knee replacement. (Courtesy Richards Manufacturing Company.)

ened by the distraction of the joint space. Prior tibial osteotomy, severe flexion deformities, or varus and valgus deformities up to 40° also are not necessarily contraindications to replacement.

The patient with active rheumatoid arthritis will require a synovectomy combined with total knee replacement. The patient who has no evidence of active disease and whose main problem is articular destruction will not require a synovectomy at the time of total knee replacement.

Double Compartment Technique. The operation may be performed under tourniquet control, or in patients with vascular problems it can be performed without a tourniquet.

Two incisions are recommended for the Marmor Modular Knee replacement (Fig. 10-59). The medial parapatellar incision is made first approximately one finger breadth from the edge of the patella. It extends about one inch above it and one inch below it from the lower edge of the vastus medialis to the upper portion of the tibia. After the expansion

has been opened on the medial side in a patient with rheumatoid arthritis, the synovectomy is carried out as described on page 342. The second incision is a lateral parapatellar incision two finger breadths from the patella approximately the same length as the medial incision. To avoid necrosis of the skin it is important not to bring the skin incisions together. The dual incisions are similar to those described for synovectomy.

Following the synovectomy of both compartments, the medial incision is retracted with the knee flexed 90°, and the patella is pulled laterally with a blunt retractor which is slipped behind the lateral femoral condyle. Any remnants of the medial meniscus should be removed from the anterior surface of the joint in order to obtain better exposure. If there is a depression in the medial tibial plateau, the anterior ledge of the tibia is removed with an osteotome to flatten the tibial plateau.

With the knee flexed 90°, the posterior aspect of the femoral condyle faces against the tibial plateau and prevents the insertion of the tibial marking template. An osteotomy of the medial femoral condyle with a broad osteotome is carried out to remove approximately $\frac{1}{4}$ inch of the femoral condyle parallel to the tibial surface all the way through to the back of the joint (Fig. 10-60). The fragment can be levered out of the joint with an osteotome, or if the fragment is displaced posteriorly, a lamina spreader may be inserted into the intercondylar notch to lift the femoral condyle away from the tibial plateau to allow the fragment to be removed easily with a curette. If the posterior capsule cannot be seen easily, there is usually a retained portion of the posterior horn of the meniscus that should be excised. When this has been removed, a small clamp can easily be placed behind the posterior

tibial plateau against the capsule to indicate that there is no retained material. The tibial marked template is then placed on the medial tibial plateau, leaving a posterior margin of several millimeters. It is important to retain the posterior ledge if possible to aid in locking the tibial component in place. At times, some of the peripheral or anterior margins may be sacrificed without interfering with the postoperative result. If the tibial plateau appears to be too narrow, the surgeon should work toward the intercondylar eminence to gain width for the insertion of the tibial component, being careful not to sacrifice the insertion of the cruciate ligament if possible. In very small or young patients, it may be necessary to use a smaller tibial component, and then the inner

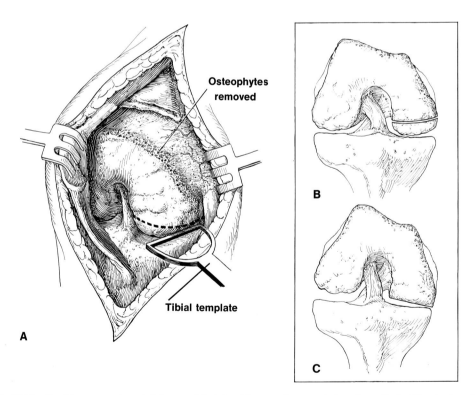

Osteophytes removed

Tibial template

A

B

C

FIG. 10-60 Double compartment Marmor Modular Knee replacement (continued). A. The broken line indicates the amount of bone to be removed to allow insertion of the tibial template. B. Diagram showing amount of femoral condyle to be removed. C. A diagram showing collapse of medial side to allow better exposure of the lateral compartment. (Courtesy Richards Manufacturing Company.)

aspect of the marking template should be used for measuring the amount of bone to be removed. In the patient in the advanced or late stage of arthritis, the femoral condyle will erode a large trough in the tibial plateau so that the smooth polished area of the plateau appears too small for the marking template. This depression on the tibia may be noted on the lateral roentgenogram preoperatively and should alert the surgeon to the problem. The anterior aspect of the tibia may have a large osteophyte and a bony prominence that can be removed with an osteotome to produce a broad, flat surface for the tibial component, and the tibial template will then fit (Fig. 10-61).

The upward protrusion of the anterior lip of the tibia as the tibial plateau erodes away is often the main cause of a persistent flexion contracture. Removal of the anterior ledge of the tibia will correct the flexion contracture and at the same time allow the knee to come up into almost full extension at the time of the operation (Fig. 10-62). Flexion deformities as great as 50° have been cor-

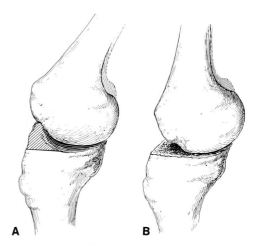

FIG. 10-62 Double compartment Marmor Modular Knee replacement (continued). A. Lateral view showing trough eroded in tibial plateau by femoral condyle. The shaded area is the anterior portion of the tibia which blocks full extension and produces the flexion deformity. B. Drawing after removal of the anterior lip of the tibia. (Courtesy Richards Manufacturing Company.)

rected in this manner with no difficulty at the time of surgery. In most cases the posterior structures have not been tight and do not cause persistent flexion contractures following this procedure.

When an adequate working surface has been developed on the tibial plateau, the tibial marking template is coated with methylene blue dye on its undersurface and is placed on the flattened tibial plateau where it will leave an outline for bone removal (Fig. 10-63). A 9- or 10-inch Pyrex sterile pie plate can be used to prevent bone dust and chips from flying up out of the wound when using the power tools (Fig. 10-64). The assistant surgeon should hold the knee flexed 90° and steady the lamina spreader to prevent it from falling out of the wound during bone removal. A high speed drill such as the Hall air drill (100,000 rpm) should be used to sculpture the bone (Fig. 10-65). If sharp burs are used, it is possible to avoid prolonged drilling time, as the bone will just melt away. The area should be cut out

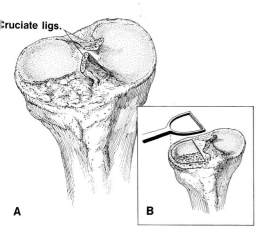

FIG. 10-61 Double compartment Marmor Modular Knee replacement (continued). A. A trough eroded in the posterior portion of the tibial plateau. B. The anterior portion removed so that the tibial marking template will fit. (Courtesy Richards Manufacturing Company.)

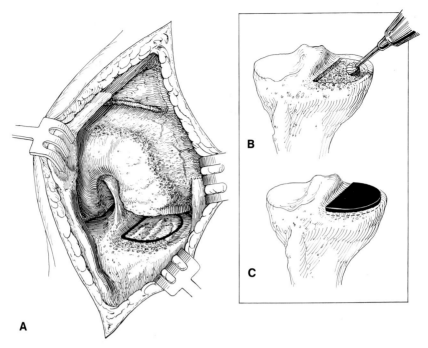

FIG. 10-63 Double compartment Marmor Modular Knee replacement (continued). A. Outline left by tibial template. B. Deepening the trough to about 5 mm with a high speed drill. C. Trial tibial component inserted to check dimensions of trough. (Courtesy Richards Manufacturing Company.)

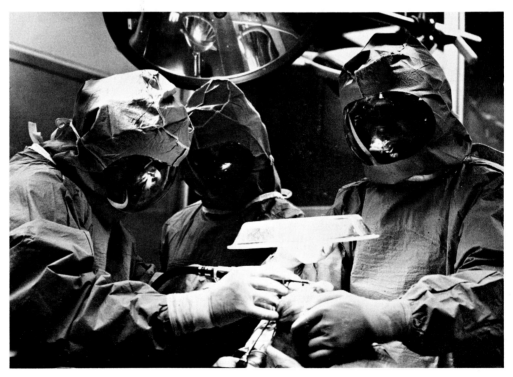

FIG. 10-64 Double compartment Marmor Modular Knee replacement (continued). The nurse is holding a Pyrex plate over the operating field. The members of the operative team are wearing "space" suits.

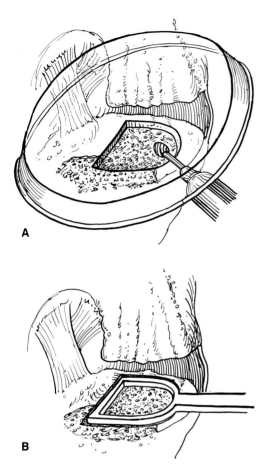

A

B

FIG. 10-65 Double compartment Marmor Modular Knee (continued). A. Trough cut in tibial plateau with air drill. Pyrex pie plate covers operative area. B. Tibial template inserted to test area cut out.

a high spot that should be removed, especially in the posterior aspect of the tibia (Fig. 10-66). Slight rocking when the knee is extended and flexed should be of no concern at this stage of the procedure. The plateau need not be inserted perfectly parallel to the intercondylar eminence, and the tibial component can toe in or out. In the lateral view, the plateau need not be horizontal for a good result. It can slope either anteriorly or posteriorly. Generally, the tibial plateau slopes posteriorly, and this position allows for better flexion postoperatively.

The medial tibial trial component should be removed at this stage to aid in exposure of the lateral compartment. Removal of the component allows the medial side to collapse, and the lateral side will open. The best position for obtaining exposure through the lateral incision is to flex the knee between 30° to 45° and to adduct the leg which tends to open the lateral compartment (Fig. 10-67). At times it is difficult to gain exposure if there is some remaining articular surface. This should be removed from the femoral condyle as well as the tibial plateau. It is not necessary to remove $\frac{1}{4}$ inch of the femoral condyle on the lateral side to gain exposure for

up to the blue line and deepened approximately 5 mm for insertion of the trial plateau. How deep one inserts the plateau is not critical because varying thicknesses are available. The tibial marking template can be used to check the dimensions of the standard plateau, and when the area has been drilled out properly, the template will fit easily within the confines of the bone trough (Fig. 10-65B).

A 9-mm tibial trial plateau is then inserted, but a tight fit is not necessary because the cement to be used later in the procedure will hold the components in place (Fig. 10-63C). If the trial tibial component tends to rock, there is usually

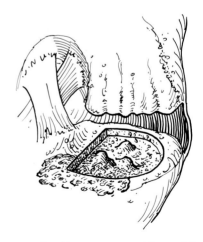

FIG. 10-66 Double compartment Marmor Modular Knee (continued). High spots that will cause tibial trial component to rock.

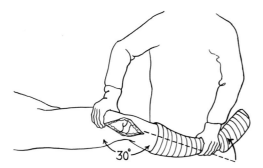

FIG 10-67 Double compartment Marmor Modular Knee replacement (continued). Knee being flexed approximately 30° and adducted by the assistant surgeon to expose lateral compartment.

replacement of the articular surface. Removal of the anterior lip of the tibia on the lateral side will often correct the flexion deformity and allow more working room.

On exposing the lateral plateau, it is sometimes an advantage to insert a lamina spreader from the medial side of the lateral incision in the intercondylar notch to gain exposure of the tibial plateau (Fig. 10-68). If the lateral plateau appears smaller than the medial, it is usually due to sloping of the intercondylar eminence toward the lateral side. An osteotome can be used to remove the slope, giving further exposure and a broader lateral plateau (Fig. 10-69). If the plateau is too small for the standard size, the extra small tibial plateau can be utilized.

The tibial marking template is coated with methylene blue and inserted on the lateral tibial plateau, leaving a rim. With a Pyrex pie plate as a cover, a power tool with a sharp 5-mm bur is used to cut out the area for insertion of the lateral tibial trial component. The 9-mm plateau is inserted in the lateral trough, and a similar trial is placed in the medial trough (Fig. 10-68B). The two tibial trial components may be inserted parallel to each other and the tibial spines, or they may toe in or out without interfering with the results. After the trial prosthesis has been inserted into the tibia, the knee is

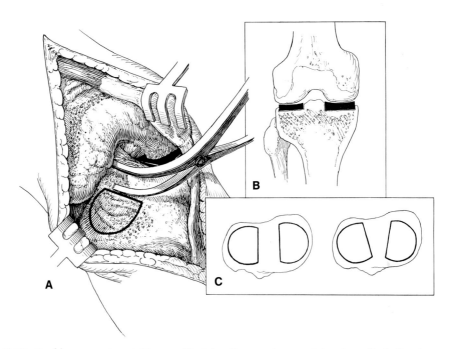

FIG. 10-68 Double compartment Marmor Modular Knee replacement (continued). A. Lamina spreader inserted in the intercondylar area. B. Tibial trial components inserted on the medial and lateral sides. C. Placement of the tibial components—parallel to the intercondylar eminence (left); toeing in (right). (Courtesy Richards Manufacturing Company.)

brought up into full extension to check the medial lateral stability. It is not necessary for these tibial components to be perfectly horizontal, and they may tilt away from the intercondylar spines to follow the normal slope of the tibia or they may be horizontal without interfering with the final result. If the knee is unstable because of a valgus deformity, a larger tibial trial plateau is placed on the lateral side. If a varus deformity is present, a larger trial is placed on the medial side to correct the deformity. This is only a rough determination at this time. The knee is then brought up into full extension with the tibial trials in place, and through the medial incision, the femoral condyle is marked with a thin methylene blue line where the tibial plateau

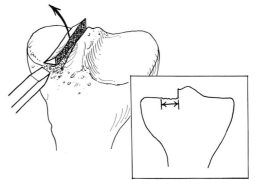

FIG. 10-69 Double compartment Marmor Modular Knee (continued). Removing sloping ridge from intercondylar eminence in lateral compartment.

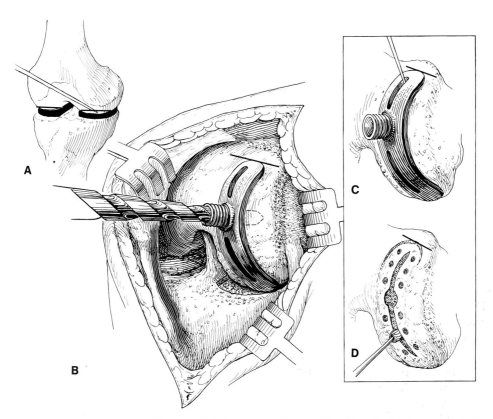

FIG. 10-70 Double compartment Marmor Modular Knee replacement (continued). A. The mark to indicate where the tibial trial component strikes the femoral condyle. B. The femoral template impacted on the femoral condyle. A $\frac{3}{8}$-inch drill is inserted. C. Marking the slot in the template for the fin of the prosthesis. D. Cutting out the slot. Note anterior depression for anterior edge of femoral component. A series of cement holes are made within the dimensions of the femoral template. (Courtesy Richards Manufacturing Company.)

component strikes the femur (Fig. 10-70). Through the lateral incision, a similar procedure is carried out to mark the femoral condyle and indicate the proper placement for the femoral template. The knee is then flexed 90° and the tibial trial components are removed. The medial component is removed from the medial incision, and the lateral tibial trial component from the lateral incision.

With the knee flexed 90°, the medial incision is opened widely to retract the patella laterally and expose the femoral condyles. A template for the medial femoral condyle is selected by measuring it alongside the medial condyle to obtain the correct size, or a trial-and-error method can be used to see which template fits the condyle the best. The femoral template is attached to the driver and impacted onto the femoral condyle with its anterior edge resting at the methylene blue line. The template is placed on the femoral condyle following its normal wear lines, and it may toe in or out, depending upon the patient's femoral condyle. The driver is removed from the femoral template, and the assistant holds the template in place. A $3/8$-inch drill bit is inserted into the hole where the driver came off, and a hole is drilled $1\frac{1}{2}$ inches deep to make room for the stem of the femoral component. The slot in the femoral template and the edges of the femoral template are marked with methylene blue.

The template is removed, and the power tool with a thin 2.3-mm carbide drill is used to cut a slot following the methylene blue line from the center drill hole distally. This slot is to accept the fin of the femoral component and should be drilled deeper toward the center hole than at the periphery because of the shape of the fin. The anterior edge near the methylene blue line limiting the anterior placement of the femoral condyle should be deepened so that the trial anterior edge will fit snugly and not protrude out from the bone and catch the patella on flexion. The necessity for a smooth fit is the reason femoral components should have thin anterior edges. Final components with blunt edges should be avoided. Holes are drilled within the outline of the template for cement fixation.

Then the femoral trial is inserted into place with the impactor. The knee should be flexed as much as possible by the assistant to aid in inserting the femoral trial, which should fit reasonably snug on the femoral condyle. If a good fit has been obtained, the trial should be removed.

The lateral condyle is prepared next through the medial incision. A blunt retractor is placed behind the lateral femoral condyle and a rake retractor on the patellar ligament to pull the patella over as far laterally as possible and expose the femoral condyle with the knee flexed.

Occasionally the patella will cause some difficulties in gaining exposure and will have to be cut around its periphery to allow retraction because of the existing osteophytes blocking the view of the lateral condyle. Removal of the fat pad gives adequate exposure of the lateral condyle in almost all cases. Any prominence on the tibial eminence due to arthritic changes may also block the view and should be removed.

The femoral template is impacted on the lateral condyle in a manner similar to that for the medial femoral condyle. It is not necessary to use the same sized template on both condyles. If a larger or smaller size fits better, it may be selected for the lateral condyle. One can look through the lateral incision and make sure a good fit is obtained. The femoral slots are marked in a similar manner, and the template is removed. With the power tool, a slot is cut for the fin, and a center hole for the stem of the component.

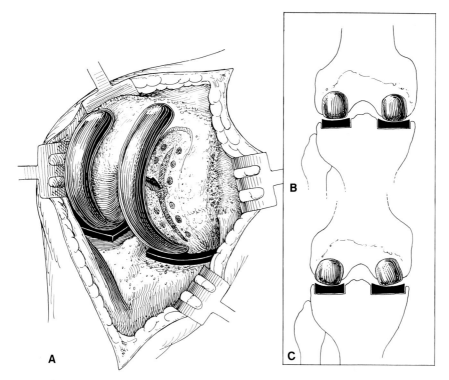

FIG. 10-71 Double compartment Marmor Modular Knee replacement (continued). A. Insertion of all four components. B. Position of femoral components—parallel (top) or toeing in (bottom). (Courtesy Richards Manufacturing Company.)

At this stage all four trial components are inserted (Fig. 10-71). The tibial components are generally put in first, one from the medial side and the other from the lateral side. Both femoral components are inserted through the medial incision and then are impacted into place (Fig. 10-72). The knee should be tested in full extension with all of the components in. If there is instability of the ligaments or persistent valgus or varus deformity, the tibial trial should be removed on the involved side, and a thicker one should be substituted. When the correct component is in place, the knee will be stable in full extension in both abduction and adduction (Fig. 10-73). The knee should flex smoothly, with the femoral condyle gliding over the tibial plateau. If the knee tends to rock open, then the components are too tight, and a thinner size of tibial com-

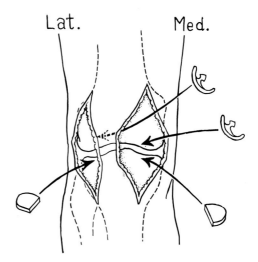

FIG. 10-72 Double compartment Marmor Modular Knee (continued). Drawing to show method of insertion of four components, through the two incisions.

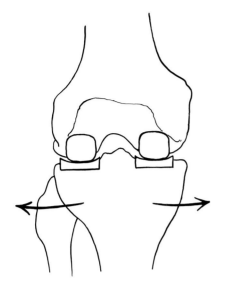

FIG. 10-73 Double compartment Marmor Modular Knee replacement (continued). Testing the knee in abduction and adduction in full extension after all four components have been inserted.

ponent should be substituted, or the trough should be deepened to allow better motion. It is better to err slightly on the looser side than to put the components in too tight. *Overcorrection* is not indicated in the Marmor Modular Knee replacement.

At this stage also, the intercondylar notch should be checked for encroachment on the tibial spine. Osteophytes in

the intercondylar area will often impinge and result in destruction of the anterior cruciate ligament (Fig. 10-74).

Any combination of trial components and femoral components can be used. If a satisfactory fit is obtained, all of the components are removed, and the proper sizes are ordered from the circulating nurse. The operating nurse should be informed as to where the components are to go so that the proper size will be given to the surgeon at the right time. The cement is mixed at this time by the assistant.

The patella is everted, and any osteophytes are removed from its edges. Any protruding area should be smoothed with a rasp, and the entire joint is thoroughly irrigated with antibiotic solution. With a 4-mm bur, holes about $\frac{1}{2}$ inch deep are drilled at varying angles in the tibial plateau for cement fixation (Fig. 10-75). The bone should be dried as thoroughly as possible to aid in fixation of the cement.

The nurse should prepare the proper instruments for insertion of the tibial components. The tibial components are put in first to prevent damage to the metal femoral components (Fig. 10-76). Either the lateral or medial tibial plateau component may be inserted first, de-

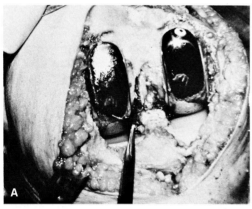
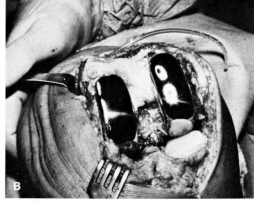

FIG. 10-74 Double compartment Marmor Modular Knee (continued). Surgical views after insertion of trial components. A. An osteotome is used to open the intercondylar eminence. B. The osteophytes have been removed to prevent impingement on the intercondylar eminence.

pending upon which is easier for the surgeon in each particular case. The lateral plateau is inserted through the lateral incision with the knee flexed 30° and adducted as much as possible. A small amount of cement is packed into the tibial trough and forced down into the cement holes. There should be no excessive cement in the posterior aspect of the joint. The nurse will coat the underside of the tibial component with a layer of cement, keeping a minimal amount posteriorly so that it will not well up behind the joint. The component is then seated against the posterior edge of the trough and pressed into place, compressing the cement. A periosteal elevator can be used to depress the plateau by rocking it against the femoral condyle and forcing the tibial component down into the trough (Fig. 10-77). All excess cement should be removed with a curette, and the area should be thoroughly cleaned. The opposite tibial component is then placed into its trough in a similar fashion. Then the knee

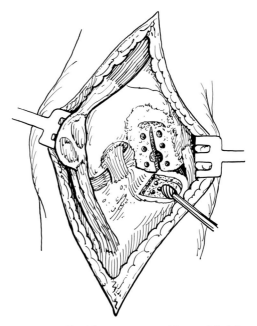

FIG. 10-75 Double compartment Marmor Modular Knee replacement (continued). Holes drilled in tibia for cement.

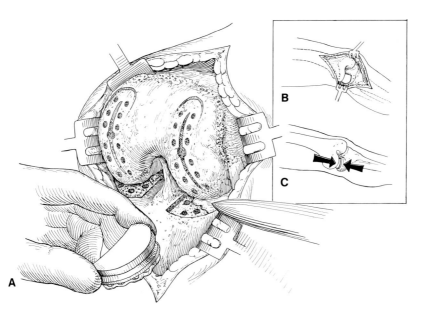

FIG. 10-76 Double compartment Modular Knee replacement (continued). A. Tibial plateau coated with cement on underside and ready for insertion. Cement has been forced into the tibial trough and the cement holes in the tibial plateau. B. The opposite tibial plateau cemented in place. C. Leg brought into full extension to lock tibial components into place. (Courtesy Richards Manufacturing Company.)

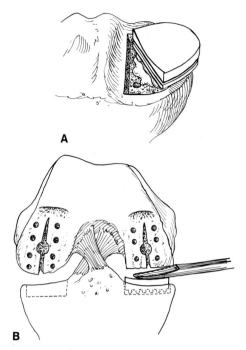

A

B

FIG. 10-77 Double compartment Marmor Modular Knee replacement (continued). A. The tibial component is forced into the trough in the tibia until it strikes the back ledge. B. A periosteal key elevator is used to force the tibial component into place.

should be carefully examined to be certain that the opposite component has not been displaced. The femoral trials are inserted with the knee flexed, and the knee is brought up into full extension, locking the tibial components into place against the femoral trials. This will tend to compress the cement and give better fixation.

At this stage there can be a slight adjustment for varus or valgus angulation by manipulating the leg toward the side where one would wish to squeeze out more cement and leaving more cement on the opposite side where the correction is deemed necessary. Any excess cement should be removed as it comes up. If cement has hardened, it should be removed with a small osteotome or rongeur. One has to be careful because there is a tendency for the hard cement chips to fly up out of the wound.

As the surgeon becomes more experienced, it will be possible to put all four components in with one batch of cement.

Another batch of cement is mixed for the femoral components once the tibial components are hardened and in place. The medial or lateral femoral component can be inserted first through the medial incision. Cement is forced into the center hole with a curette, and cement is also smoothed along the femoral condyle with the gloved finger. The nurse should check the size of the femoral component, coat the underside with cement, and hand the component to the surgeon with the curve properly oriented posteriorly. With the knee flexed the component is pushed into place and is impacted with a femoral driver, being careful to compress the anterior edge to prevent it from sticking up and catching the patella (Fig. 10-78). The excess cement that oozes out along the margins should be removed with a plastic spatula to prevent scratching of the femoral condyle.

The opposite femoral component is inserted in a similar manner with cement, and then the knee is flexed and extended several times to compress out

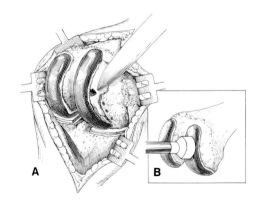

A　　　**B**

FIG. 10-78 Double compartment Marmor Modular Knee replacement (continued). A. The femoral components cemented into place. B. Impacting the components with the Femoral Condyle Driver. (Courtesy Richards Manufacturing Company.)

the extra cement. The excess cement is removed with the plastic spatula to prevent scratching the metal component, and the knee is then brought up into full extension to compress the femoral components. One can make minor corrections of varus or valgus at this stage also by compressing one component more than the other to force out additional cement. When the components are fixed in the hard cement, any excess cement that protruded out of the margins of the femoral components should be removed carefully with an osteotome to prevent scratching the femoral surface.

Suction tubes are brought out through the suprapatellar pouch for drainage postoperatively, the tourniquet is released, and hemostasis is secured (Fig. 10-79). The expansions are closed with 0 interrupted silk or chromic catgut sutures. The subcutaneous tissue is closed with 3-0 chromic sutures and the skin with 3-0 nylon continuous sutures. The skin incisions are covered with nonstick sterile gauze, and the knee is loosely wrapped with a 6-inch bias stockinette. A bulky Jones compression-type dressing is applied.

Postoperative Care. On the day of surgery, the patient is encouraged to flex and extend the knee joint and to do quadriceps exercises. It is important to be sure to tell the patient that there is nothing to fear by doing the exercises and the earlier he begins motion, the better the result will be. On the first postoperative day, the physical therapist will start the exercise program. The patient may be up in a wheelchair with the leg elevated. On the second postoperative day, the bulky dressing is changed, and the suction tubes are removed. A small dressing is placed on the wound, and the skin is painted with skin adherent to prevent the bias stockinette from sliding down during the postoperative exercises and after the swelling begins to decrease. On the third day, the

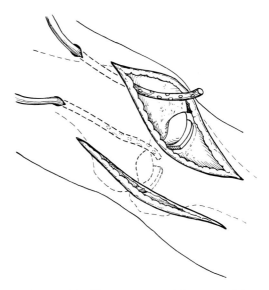

FIG. 10-79 Double compartment Marmor Modular Knee (continued). Drawing showing suction tubes.

patient may stand on the leg to get into the wheelchair and may also start dangling the leg over the bedside for further flexion. On the fourth postoperative day ambulation with full weight bearing is started with a walking aid if the bone is not osteoporotic; otherwise partial weight bearing is continued for 6 weeks. The patient continues to increase the exercise program until the sutures are removed on the tenth to the fourteenth day. The Hubbard tank or whirlpool may be used for hydrotherapy to aid in increasing the range of motion.

Manipulation of the knee is not recommended postoperatively to regain motion, even for patients who have limited motion. A painful knee may result because manipulation may compress the soft cancellous bone and loosen the cement from the tibia.

Patients must be encouraged to work within the first week after surgery to gain flexion. It has been noted that with the passage of time, even up to a year, the knees continue to improve and further motion can be expected to return (Fig. 10-80).

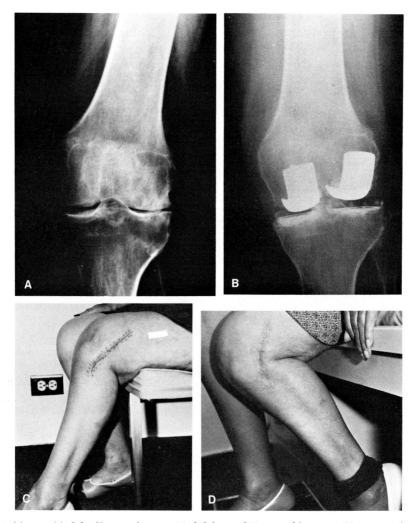

FIG. 10-80 Marmor Modular Knee replacement in left knee of 58-year-old woman. Her range of motion was 20° to 90° with 70° of actual motion. A. Preoperative roentgenogram showing a 15° valgus deformity with a 20° flexion contracture. B. Roentgenogram 9 months after correction of valgus deformity. C. Photograph 2 months after surgery reveals 60° of flexion. D. Photograph a year postoperatively shows patient had 105° of flexion. She is walking free of pain. At follow-up 1.5 years after operation, the patient's range of motion was 15° to 110°.

Allied Problems. Certain situations that arise in patients with advanced rheumatoid arthritis of the knee joint require discussion. At times several of these problems may be present in the same knee joint and can be managed by the replacement of the joint surfaces with the Marmor Modular Knee.

FLEXION CONTRACTURES. The patient with an advanced stage of rheumatoid arthritis of the knee joint tends to de-

velop a flexion contracture. This can be related to a severe flexion contracture of the hip, or it may be a primary problem arising from disease of the knee joint. In the past, wedging casts and preoperative traction were often utilized to aid in correcting the deformities. The deformity is not due to tightness of the posterior structures and posterior release in most cases is not necessary (Fig. 10-81). The femoral condyle tends to erode into the tibial plateau, and this erosion is often obvious in the lateral roentgenologic view. The anterior lip of the tibia strikes the front of the femoral condyle and prevents full extension.

Flexion contractures in patients with deformities of 15° to 20° and reasonably normal roentgenograms are usually due to muscle spasm and synovial proliferation. Simple synovectomy will relieve the flexion contracture in these cases but will be of no value in advanced disease.

The Marmor Modular Knee can be utilized for the correction of severe flexion deformities without the use of wedging casts or preoperative stretching (Fig. 10-82). The operative technique is similar to that for the usual Marmor Modular Knee replacement except that

the anterior lip of the tibia should be removed down to the grooved area in the tibial plateau. Removal of this bone allows the knee to come up into full extension on the operating room table despite the fact that a contracture may have been present for 10 years or longer. Although the flexion deformity can be corrected at the time of surgery, postoperatively the patient may develop spasm in the hamstring muscles and require muscle relaxants for a period of time. Gradually the flexion contracture will continue to stretch out and improve with the patient's use of the knee.

VARUS OR VALGUS DEFORMITIES. Rheumatoid arthritis can produce severe varus or valgus deformities of the knee joint. These are often associated with

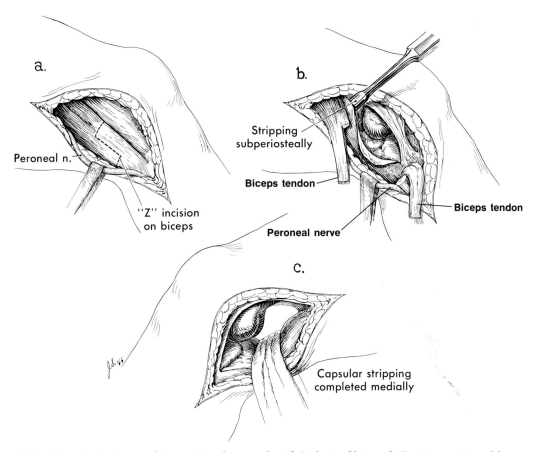

FIG. 10-81   a. Posterior capsulotomy. Lateral approach with Z-plasty of biceps. b. Periosteum stripped from femur. c. Medial exposure with posterior release of capsule.

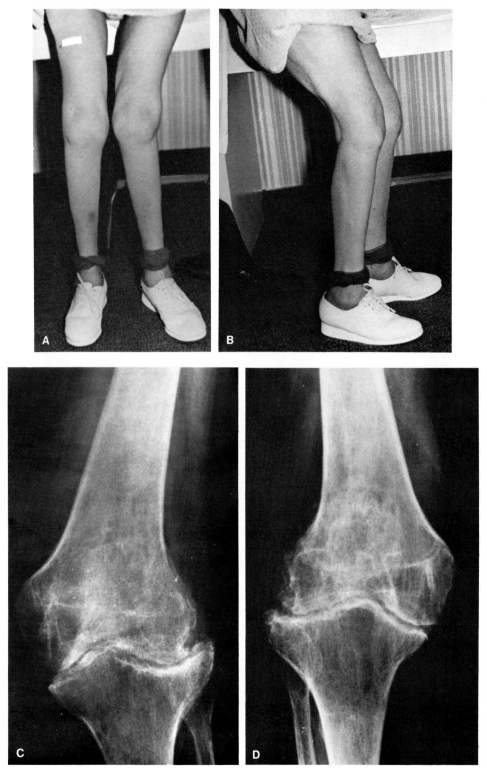

FIG. 10-82 Correction of flexion contractures of both knees. Preoperative studies: A. Anterior view. The patient is unable to stand without assistance. B. Lateral view. C. Roentgenogram of left knee. Severe destruction is seen in both joint surfaces. D. Roentgenogram of right knee also shows severe destruction of joint surfaces.

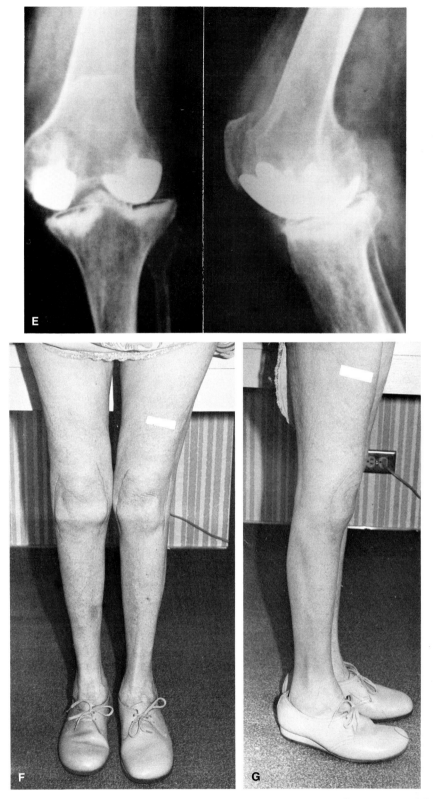

FIG. 10-82 (Cont'd.) Postoperative studies: E. Roentgenogram of left knee with Marmor Modular Knee units in place. F. Anterior view after replacement of both knee joints. There is no evidence of swelling and patient has no pain. G. Lateral view showing correction of flexion deformities. The patient can stand erect without assistance.

flexion deformities (Fig. 10-83). As the disease progresses in the knee joint, a varus or valgus deformity will develop with destruction of the tibial plateau. Once the deformity is established, it tends to progress quite rapidly with fragmentation of the rim of the tibial plateau. Deformities of 25° of varus or 50° of valgus can be corrected along with the flexion deformity by using the Marmor Modular Knee unit.

The slope of the tibia is removed with an osteotome to develop a new tibial plateau at a lower level so that it is again horizontal (Fig. 10-84). A trough is cut out for the tibial trial component, and the various thicknesses of the prosthesis are utilized to rebuild the lost tibia to its appropriate level. Cement should never be used to build up a deformity, as cement will tend to crack and break.

Overcorrection should be avoided in these cases to prevent excess tightening of the collateral ligaments which could

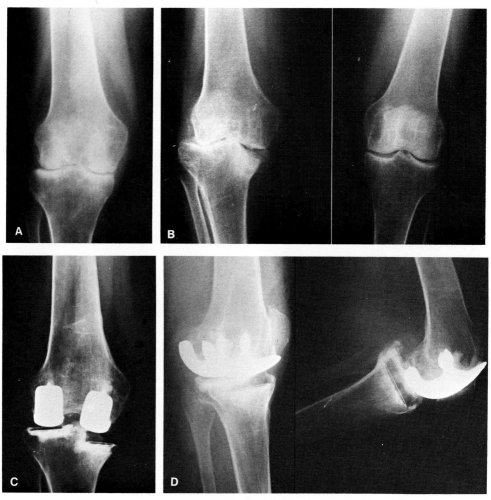

FIG. 10-83 Correction of varus deformity. Preoperative roentgenograms: A. Right knee revealing advanced rheumatoid disease. B. Two years later revealing destruction of right knee joint with subluxation and loss of medial tibial plateau. Left knee for comparison: C. After insertion of Marmor Modular Knee components in right knee. D. Lateral view of right knee in full extension and full flexion. The patella was shaved down to a wafer. The patient has excellent range of motion without pain.

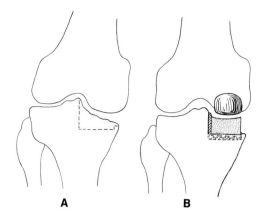

FIG. 10-84 Correction of varus deformity. A. Area of tibia to be removed to create horizontal tibial plateau. B. Tibial component filling the defect.

result in postoperative pain. In correcting severe valgus deformities that are fixed, it is always important to caution the patient about the possibility of a peroneal palsy. As long as overcorrection is avoided, peroneal palsy should not be a problem.

ANKYLOSIS. Ankylosis of the knee joint does occur spontaneously in rheumatoid arthritis. It can follow injury to the knee from trauma or surgical proce-

dures. In far advanced disease, frequently the joint will gradually lose motion, and bony union can occur through the pannus formation. The collateral ligaments usually remain intact, since these ligaments are outside of the knee joint. The cruciate ligaments, however, are frequently involved in the disease process.

Spontaneous fusion frequently occurs in a bad position for ambulation. When deformities interefere with walking, one can at least consider a replacement of the joint surface and the taking down of an ankylosed knee. If it is fused in an excellent position for walking, it would not be advisable to replace the joint. However, if joint replacement is carried out in a badly positioned knee, and the prosthesis fails, one can always fuse the knee in a much better position for walking and correct the severe deformities.

At the site of the fusion the roentgenogram will often reveal the cleavage plane that will indicate the correct area for taking the joint apart (Fig. 10-85). If there is no evidence of a cleavage plane,

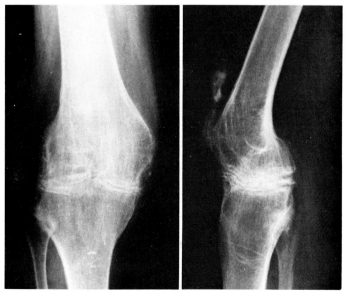

FIG. 10-85 Roentgenogram of ankylosed knee joint showing the cleavage line.

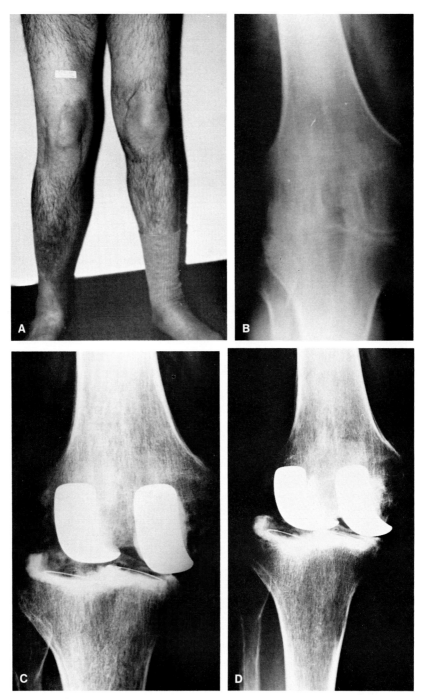

FIG. 10-86 Marmor Modular Knee replacement for ankylosis in 36-year-old patient who had had a synovectomy of the right knee followed by a spontaneous hemorrhage one week later, resulting in bony ankylosis of the knee. A. Preoperative photograph. The ankylosed right knee is fixed in 15° of valgus and 30° of flexion. B. Roentgenogram of right knee 5 years after spontaneous fusion reveals a solid bony ankylosis. After Marmor Modular Knee replacement: C. Roentgenogram reveals subluxation of femur medially. Both tibial plateaus are sloped toward medial side. D. Roentgenogram 3 years later. There is no change in the subluxation, and the patient is free of pain.

one again should hesitate to take the joint apart because the exact level of the old joint will be hard to find. During the surgical procedure it is important not to use force but to use an osteotome or a similar instrument to divide the bones in the proper plane. Force may result in an avulsion fracture through the osteoporotic bone. Patients who have had spontaneous fusions will often have severe osteoporosis, and the bone will be soft and fatty at the site of the osteotomy. If the knee is fused in full extension, the quadriceps mechanism will be contracted, and it will be difficult to regain motion postoperatively; however, if the knee has fused in flexion of 45° or 50°, this position will aid considerably in obtaining postoperative motion (Fig. 10-86).

When inserting the tibial plateau prostheses in the ankylosed knee it is

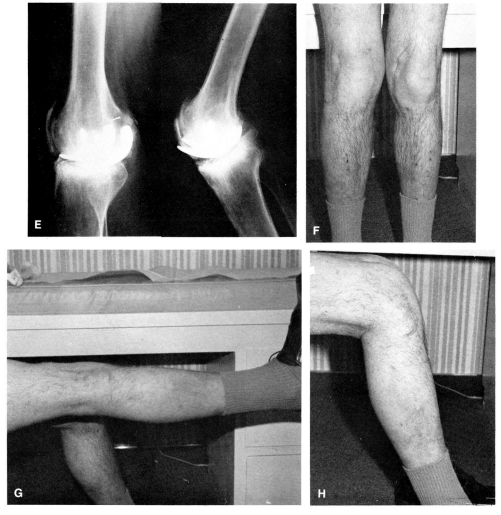

FIG. 10-86 (Cont'd.) E. Lateral view showing range of motion. Note that the patella has been shaved to a small wafer. F. Clinical photograph 2 years after replacement. The valgus deformity has been corrected and there is no swelling. G. Clinical photograph showing full extension of knee joint. H. Clinical photograph showing amount of flexion.

advisable not to tilt *both* plateaus either medially or laterally because the femoral components will be going downhill and the knee may sublux. They should be either placed horizontally or tilted slightly away from the intercondylar eminence. In the preparation of the femoral condyles, it is advisable to widen the slot for the fin so that there is a looser fit in the bone. When the final femoral components are cemented in, they will assume the shape to match the tibial components and present a broad surface for articulation.

Complications. Some of the complications that follow total knee replacement are specific for knee surgery because of the anatomy of the knee, and others are a result of the disease process. The insertion of the Marmor Modular Knee in the arthritic patient with thin skin carries with it a greater risk than in the average patient with normal skin.

INFECTIONS. Superficial infections are much more common in the total knee replacement than in the total hip replacement. The thin skin and poor subcutaneous layer tend to give minimal protection to the joint. In fact, the skin suture line in many patients lies right on the joint capsule because of the thin layers between the tendinous expansion of the vastus muscle and the skin. Skin sutures that are not put in loosely enough can cut the skin during early motion and cause cellulitis.

The use of a suction tube or tubes to drain the knee joint for 48 hours has helped considerably in decreasing the swelling and the appearance of the skin incision. Small doses of antibiotics postoperatively have been of value in preventing cellulitis and septicemia. At the first dressing change 48 hours after surgery, the suction tubes are removed along with the bulky Jones dressing, the skin incisions are coated with a layer of local antibiotic, and a sterile dressing is applied. Since exposure of the wound could lead to contamination, it has been helpful to paint the skin above and below the incision with a skin adherent to prevent the dressing from slipping down as the swelling in the knee recedes, especially during the night when the patient is asleep. The incidence of skin problems has decreased with the use of suction tubes and adherent dressings.

Draining sinuses occur occasionally because of the poor tissue and the inability to close the capsule tightly. Secondary infection through a draining sinus should be of concern to the surgeon. If drainage occurs in the hospital, it would be advisable to use a bulky dressing and stop all mobilization of the knee joint for 5 to 7 days to see if the draining sinus will seal off. If it does not seal off, it is probably advisable to excise the sinus under sterile conditions in the operating room and do a primary closure.

Deep infections usually occur in any series. The infection rate in 332 cases has run approximately 3.5 percent since we began using a laminar flow room and space suits. Seven of the infections occurred early in the operative series. Three of these responded to antibiotics, and the Modular Knee components are still in. One patient maintained 90° of motion, and the other two patients, 30° of motion postoperatively. Four of the infections were due to pseudomonas, and all of the knee replacements in these patients failed. Pseudomonas generally will not respond to antibiotic therapy, and arthrodesis is indicated. Arthrodesis has been carried out by the Charnley technique, despite the fact that there was active infection. The components were removed at the time of arthrodesis, and the infections subsided. Immobilization of the knee following arthrodesis will aid considerably in controlling the infection.

LOOSENING OF COMPONENTS. Loose components have been one of the major causes of pain after the Marmor Modular Knee replacement. There has been no evidence of loosening of the femoral components inserted by the procedure described in this chapter, but the tibial components have come loose from the bone. So far, though, only 4 tibial components in our series have been displaced (Fig. 10-87), and in general the loose component tends to stay in place. The 6-mm tibial plateaus have bent and show evidence of loosening in 12 patients, and 5 patients have had replacements with thicker plateaus.

The thin 6-mm tibial plateau, which in reality is only 4 mm thick because of the small locking legs on the undersurface, tends to buckle under pressure and has a high incidence of loosening, especially in the heavy patient. Replacement with a 9-mm component, or one thicker, and careful cementing have solved the problem. It is recommended that the thicker components be used initially in most patients.

Patients with loose tibial components will complain of tenderness at the joint line or pain radiating down into the tibia. The pain is generally related to weight bearing and may increase during walking. The roentgenograms will reveal a definite radiolucent line and sclerosis developing beneath the cement (Fig. 10-88).

In the long-term follow-up of the cases, a radiolucent line has developed after 6 to 12 months between the cement of the tibial component and the bone. The line is not associated with pain nor do the components appear loose. Sclerosis does not occur beneath the cement.

Infection is an obvious cause of loosening of the tibial component. Poor cementing is another. Careful drying of the bone before inserting the cement is essential to obtain adequate fixation of a cement bond. The holes drilled into the

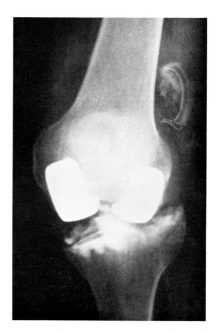

FIG. 10-87 Roentgenogram 9 months after a Marmor Modular Knee replacement when patient began to have severe pain and increased valgus deformity. The tibial plateau has come loose and is floating in the suprapatellar pouch.

cancellous bone to aid in fixation must be placed at varying angles, and the cement must be forced into them.

The arthrogram does not appear to be of much value in determining loosening of the component. The radiopaque material will not penetrate beneath the component because the space is filled with fibrous tissue (Fig. 10-89).

THROMBOPHLEBITIS. Thrombophlebitis has not been a problem when anticoagulants and dextran have not been used. All patients who can tolerate the medication are placed on two buffered aspirin, four times a day, for one week before the operation and for one week postoperatively. There has been no unusual bleeding related to aspirin, and the incidence of phlebitis has been less than 1 percent. In most series of operative procedures the incidence of thrombophlebitis is less in patients with rheumatoid arthritis. There were 4 cases of

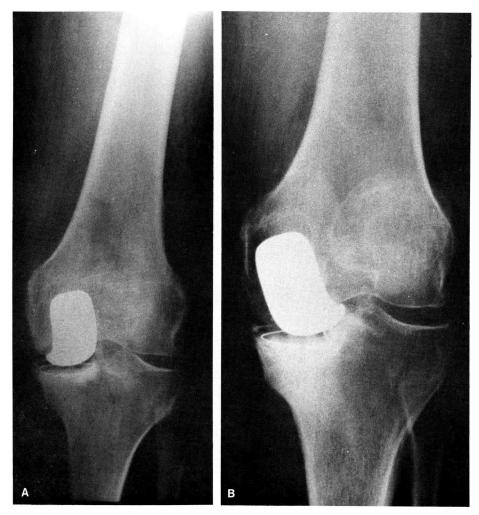

FIG. 10-88 Roentgenograms after Marmor Modular Knee replacement. The patient continued to have pain in the area of the tibial plateau. A. Immediately after the operation. B. Eight months later, showing sclerosis of the tibia beneath the cement.

thrombophlebitis and 1 case of pulmonary embolism in patients with osteoarthritis.

LOSS OF MOTION. Patients who are started on early motion postoperatively and are motivated have had few problems in regaining motion. The majority of patients will have over 90° of flexion and as much as 135° of flexion and will continue to improve up to a year or longer.

Manipulation is not recommended. It is my feeling that forced manipulation postoperatively may crush the cement interface of the bone and lead to loosening of the tibial components. Patients with severe osteoporosis certainly should not have manipulation postoperatively and should be placed on partial weight bearing for at least 6 weeks.

Patients with limited motion preoperatively should not be promised a great deal more motion after a total knee replacement. Patients who are stiff in extension have a contracture of the quadriceps mechanism. A second operation may be necessary to lengthen the quadriceps.

URINARY RETENTION. A high percentage of elderly patients tend to have urinary retention postoperatively. This has been recognized in men with prostate problems but has been overlooked in women. A history of frequency of urination or nocturia should alert the physician to the possibility of poor bladder tone or urethral stricture. In the postoperative period, patients will frequently be uncomfortable and just not feel well but will not indicate that they have not voided. Nurses often overlook difficulty with voiding. It is extremely important to insert a catheter early to prevent stretching of the bladder and loss of tone. A culture should be obtained at the time of insertion of the indwelling catheter, and proper antibiotic therapy should be instituted for protection. Every attempt is made to avoid catheterization to prevent septicemia and hematogenous infection of the joint.

POSTOPERATIVE ANEMIA. Although the operation is performed under tourniquet control, it is surprising how much blood loss occurs postoperatively. The drainage from the suction tube will be between 200 to 400 cc in 36 hours. Postoperative examination of the patient's hemoglobin will reveal a drop of 2 to 4 gm on the first postoperative day. Therefore, iron can be given postoperatively to treat this anemia.

PATELLAR IMPINGEMENT. Patellar impingement can occur in the rheumatoid patient with the development of severe

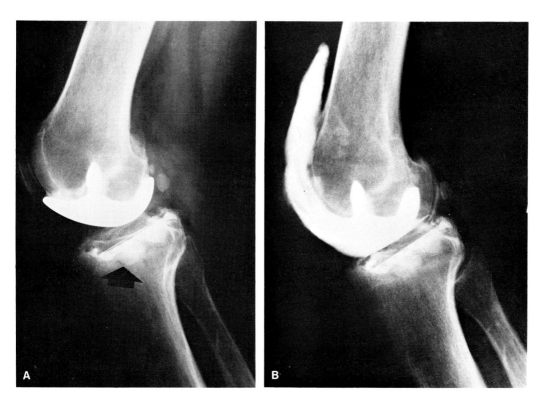

FIG. 10-89 A. Lateral roentgenogram of knee joint with a Marmor Modular Knee unit in place. The radiolucent line (arrow) beneath the cement may be an indication of loosening of the component. B. Arthrogram does not reveal loosening of component because dye does not go into the radiolucent area, which is filled with fibrous tissue.

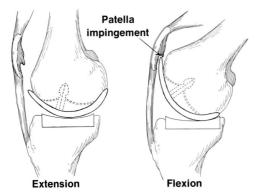

FIG. 10-90 Patellar impingement. The protruding anterior edge of the femoral condyle catches the patella on flexion.

pingement occurs, it is due to a protrusion of the femoral component, the anterior end of which sticks above the femoral condyle and catches the patella on flexion (Fig. 10-90). At the time of reoperation it may be noted that grooves are cut into the undersurface of the patella. Cineradiography may be of value in confirming this diagnosis, and in most cases replacement of the component will solve the problem.

pain postoperatively. The major cause of patellar impingement is a mismatch in the templates and components used in the insertion of the Marmor Modular Knee. It is important that the template, trial, and final component are all the same size. Therefore, the components from one manufacturer should not be used with the instruments of another unless all of the components and instruments are the same size. If patellar im-

Arthrodesis

Arthrodesis of the knee is not indicated very often in rheumatoid arthritis because of the severe involvement of the other joints in the lower extremities. Arthrodesis will tend to increase the stress upon the ankle and the hip joint, and the loss of knee motion can be a severe handicap to the rheumatoid patient. Since the disease is progressive, other joints may gradually become involved with the passage of time, and it may be impossible for the patient to reach the foot in order to dress. Stiffness

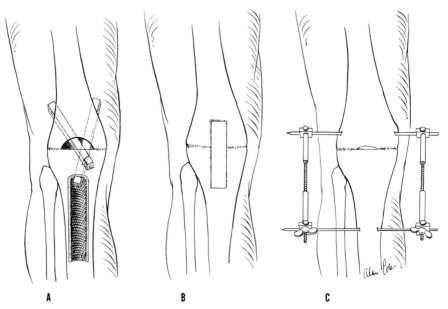

FIG. 10-91 Techniques for arthrodesis of the knee. A. Sliding bone grafts removed from femur and inserted across joint space. B. A bone graft inserted anteriorly as a block. C. Charnley compression type.

in both knees is a severe handicap that will make it difficult for the patient to arise from a sitting position. Motorized chairs that allow the patient to rise from a sitting position can be of great value for this type of patient.

Arthrodesis is probably the procedure of choice for patients with severe destruction of one knee joint. The failure of a hinge prosthesis or other type of total knee replacement due to infection may require an arthrodesis to salvage the knee joint.

Operative Technique. A number of techniques using internal fixation have been described for arthrodesis of the knee (Fig. 10-91). The method of choice for arthrodesis of the knee is a compression technique described by Charnley.

A transverse incision is made over the knee joint, and the patella may be excised or left in place, depending on the surgeon's choice. It can be excised from the patellar ligament and used as a bone graft if necessary to fill the defect in the tibia (Fig. 10-92). All diseased tissue should be removed from the articular surface of the joint, and the superior aspect of the tibia can be flattened with an osteotome or a power saw transversely to the shaft. A similar amount of bone is removed from the femur so that the surfaces fit together with the knee in approximately 15° of flexion to full extension, depending on the cosmetic appearance. The more flexion present, the less the cosmetic improvement. The varus or valgus deformity should be corrected by altering the plane of the femoral saw cut or osteotomy line.

A heavy Steinmann pin is inserted transversely across the proximal tibia, and the compression clamps are used as a guide for insertion of the Steinmann pins through the distal femur. The clamps are tightened, putting a compression force on the raw bony surfaces. It may be advisable to insert a Steinmann pin from the femur down into the tibia to

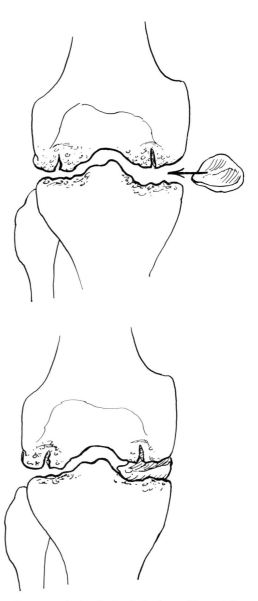

FIG. 10-92 Arthrodesis of the knee. The patella excised and used as a bone graft.

prevent anterior-posterior sliding of the fragments (Fig. 10-93). The wound is closed, and the leg is encased in a plaster splint for 4 to 6 weeks. If the patient had an infection at the time of the arthrodesis, it is advisable to leave the pins in place for at least 6 weeks. Following this, the pins are removed, and the patient is placed in a walking cylinder cast for another 4 to 6 weeks.

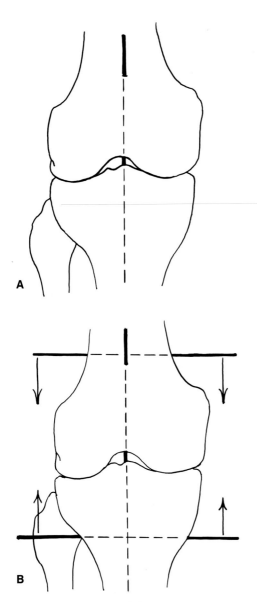

The large effusions and synovial hypertrophy associated with active rheumatoid disease produce high intracapsular pressures and tend to rupture through the posterior capsule into the popliteal fascia. The connection of the cyst with the joint can be demonstrated by an arthrogram using contrast media.

Excision of the popliteal cyst is not indicated in most patients. The operation of choice for a popliteal cyst is to remove the synovium through the anterior approach. When the synovial disease has been removed, the popliteal cyst will gradually disappear. The large cyst in the calf will persist for a considerable length of time after the operative procedure but generally subsides. Pinder reported on 16 cases of popliteal cysts treated by anterior synovectomy alone with disappearance of the posterior cyst.

Numerous bursae are located in the popliteal space between the hamstring muscles, the collateral ligaments, and the heads of the gastrocnemius muscle. A cyst can arise in the semimembranosus bursa and the head of the medial gastrocnemius. If symptoms warrant, excision of the bursa is indicated.

Frequently popliteal cysts may be confused with a deep vein phlebitis because of the swelling and pain.

FIG. 10-93 Arthrodesis of the knee. A. Dislocation is prevented by drilling a Steinmann pin vertically from the femur into the tibia. B. Compression applied to transverse pins.

Popliteal Cyst (Baker's Cyst)

Patients with rheumatoid arthritis with active involvement of the knee joint frequently develop a popliteal cyst. These cysts can grow to a large size and dissect down into the calf of the leg to produce a massive swelling (Fig. 10-94).

Osteoarthritis

The knee joint is affected more often by osteoarthritis than any other joint in the body. With the advent of the tibial osteotomy and then the total joint replacement, there has been a great deal of interest in osteoarthritis of the knee joint. Compared with the hip, shoulder, and spine the pattern of pathologic changes within the osteoarthritic knee has received relatively little study until recent years. It has become apparent that osteoarthritis of the knee is often associated with a varus or valgus deformity which produces an overloading of the compartment of the knee involved. The disease process may start when the patient is in the early 40's and is often due to preexisting trauma such as a torn meniscus, fracture of the patella with involvement of the joint surface, and healed fractures of the femur or tibia with malposition. Obesity also seems to play a role in some patients, with destruction of the articular cartilage being accelerated because of the additional weight.

Primary osteoarthritis of the knee joint is generally associated with either a varus or valgus angulation. The early

changes noted in the knee joint involve the articular cartilage which shows damage to the ground substance and fibrous lamellae. The normal basophilic ground substance becomes eosinophilic. With the loss of articular cartilage the varus or valgus deformity tends to increase (Fig. 10-95). In most athletic men who develop osteoarthritis a varus deformity with loss of the medial joint space seems to be most commonly found.

As the disease process continues, the joint cartilage begins to grind down to the bony surface, probably because of overloading of the joint surface and wear (Fig. 10-96). It is possible that hypermobile menisci may be a cause of early osteoarthritic change. Vascularization and ossification of the articular

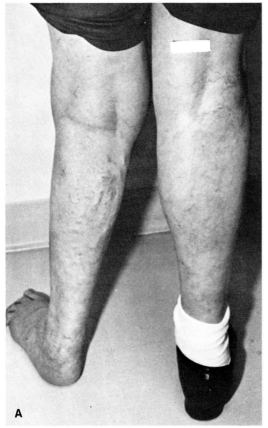 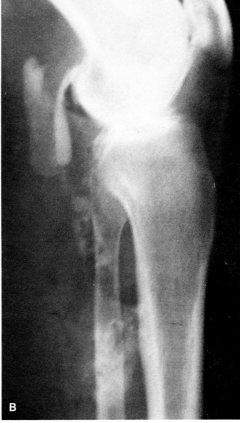

FIG. 10-94 Popliteal cyst. A. Clinical view. The right calf is enlarged. B. Arthrogram.

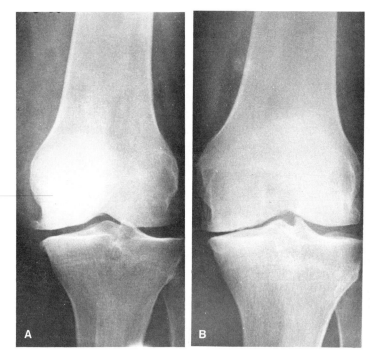
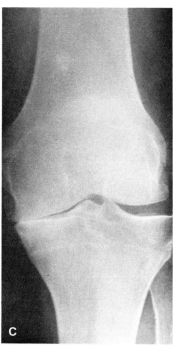

FIG. 10-95 Development of varus deformity in osteoarthritis of the knee. A. Early osteoarthritis with osteophyte formation. B. One year later. With narrowing of joint space, there is an increase in varus deformity. C. Two years later. The narrowing of the joint space and the varus deformity have increased substantially.

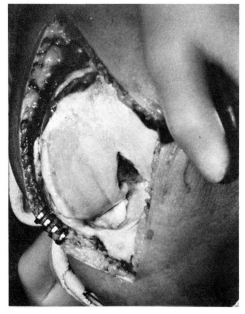

FIG. 10-96 Surgical view showing loss of articular cartilage of the medial femoral condyle. A remnant of the meniscus is present in the joint space. The intercondylar notch is narrowed.

cartilage increase the density of the cancellous bone near the joint margins (Fig. 10-97). Fibrosis of the marrow and marginal osteophytes develop (Fig. 10-98). With additional weight bearing there is gradual subluxation of the femoral condyle medially on the tibia. This allows the intercondylar eminence to strike the medial side of the lateral femoral condyle (Fig. 10-99A). This area becomes eroded, and the disease, if allowed to continue unabated, will proceed to the lateral joint compartment. Advanced disease of the lateral compartment may take many years unless it is associated with trauma. Many patients with far-advanced disease of one compartment still have an excellent opposite compartment of the knee joint (Fig. 10-99B). Chondromalacia of the patella may also develop with osteophyte formation around its periphery (Fig. 10-99C). In these advanced cases, the

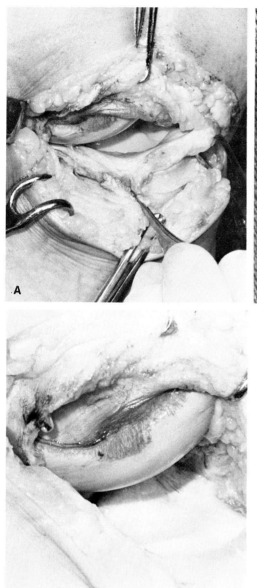

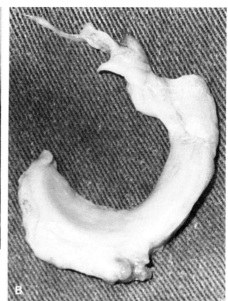

FIG. 10-97 Pathologic changes in osteoarthritis of the knee joint. A. Irritation of joint surface and vascularization along the subchondral margin. B. Meniscus originally diagnosed as hypermobile after removal. Few changes are seen. C. Vascular changes and early destruction of articular cartilage on femoral condyle visible after removal of meniscus.

medial meniscus is generally ground down, and a remnant of the posterior horn may still be present in the joint (Fig. 10-99D). In some patients diffuse white fibrous tissue is scattered throughout the joint from the grinding up of the medial or lateral meniscus. This tends to resemble steroid deposits from previous intra-articular injections that have not been absorbed, but it is much more diffuse throughout the joint.

Meniscectomy for a torn meniscus should not be considered innocuous and may be the first stage in the development of osteoarthritis of the knee joint. Varus deformity associated with a meniscectomy often is followed within 5 to 10 years by degenerative arthritis of the knee joint. A meniscectomy should not be considered for patients over 50 years of age with evidence of a torn meniscus without considering the state of the

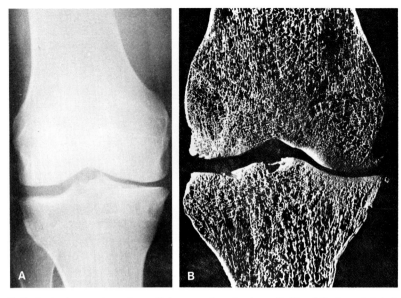

FIG. 10-98 Pathologic changes in early medial compartment osteoarthritis of the knee joint. A. Roentgenogram revealing narrowing of the joint space. B. Cross section through the gross specimen showing fibrosis of the marrow, osteophyte formation along the margins, sclerosis and thickening of the cortex on the medial side.

articular surface. Loss of the articular surface and a varus deformity in patients with osteoarthritis lead to tearing and injury to the meniscus. The meniscus tear is usually secondary to the osteoarthritis in these older patients (Fig. 10-100).

Generally the patient with osteoarthritis of the knee is in the 50- to 60-year age group and may be overweight. Trauma, of course, or a previous meniscectomy can accelerate the arthritic process and the age group may be much younger. The patients will complain of aching pain on motion, stiffness in the joint after rising from sitting, and difficulty in going up and down stairs. Pain increases with the passage of time and is generally related to weight bearing. As the disease process progresses, the patient may note the development of a bowleg or knock-knee deformity and a feeling of instability in the knee joint (Fig. 10-101). The older patient often expresses a fear of falling or of the knee giving away.

On physical examination in the early stages of osteoarthritis the patient may only have an occasional effusion in the knee joint and some tenderness along the medial joint line. Early varus or valgus may be noted on clinical examination. As the disease progresses, there is evidence of increased angulation of the joint with osteophyte formation palpable along the femoral condyle and tibial plateau. Crepitation may become noticeable, and there will be medial-lateral instability in full extension due to loss of articular cartilage and bone. Generally the collateral ligaments are intact in osteoarthritis, and the ligamentous instability is due to bone loss rather than to ligament stretching. In advanced bicompartment disease the anterior cruciate ligament may be destroyed.

The earliest change in osteoarthritis generally seen on the roentgenogram is slight narrowing of the joint space. Occasionally there will be a small osteophyte along the margin of the femoral condyle or tibial plateau and perhaps on the pole of the patella. Although the changes seen on roentgenograms appear to be minor, an extensive loss of the articular cartilage has been found in some patients at the time of surgical intervention (Fig. 10-102). As the disease process continues, narrowing of the joint space becomes obvious, and there are sclerosis of the opposing surfaces, evidence of osteophyte formation (Fig. 10-103), gradual subluxation, and changes around the periphery of the opposite compartment. In advanced cases, both compartments may be severely involved with no joint space remaining on either side (Fig. 10-103B). Patients who have evidence of subluxation generally will have destruction of the anterior cruciate from osteophytes in the intercondylar notch.

The roentgenogram of a patient with traumatic arthritis due to tibial plateau fracture or intra-articular fractures involving the knee joint may often show

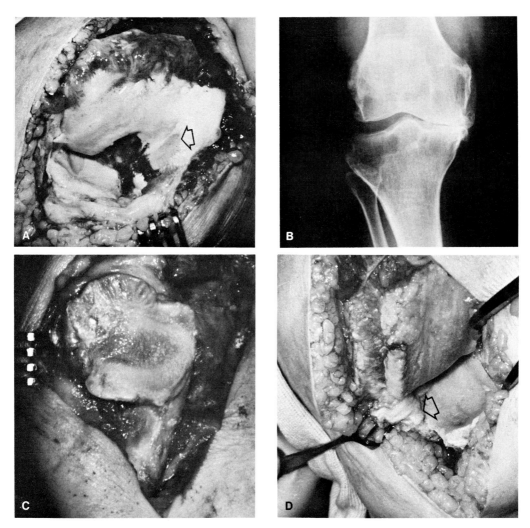

FIG. 10-99 Pathologic changes in osteoarthritis of the knee. A. Surgical view showing erosion on the medial side of the lateral condyle produced by tibial spines (arrow). B. Roentgenogram showing advanced disease in medial compartment but no involvement in lateral compartment. C. Chondromalacia of the patella with osteophyte formation around its periphery. D. Large posterior horn (arrow) retained in joint.

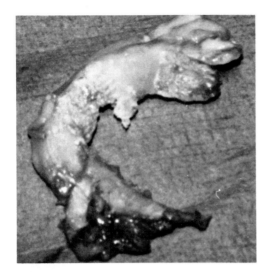

FIG. 10-100 A meniscus showing evidence in the medial portion of having been trapped in the knee joint because of degeneration of the articular cartilage.

what appears to be a good joint surface on the opposite side. However, at the time of surgery fibrous adhesions are often found within the joint and loss of the normal articular cartilage (Fig. 10-104). One should always be suspicious of the opposite compartment in traumatic arthritis because the disease is often more advanced than what appears in roentgenograms.

Conservative Treatment

The patient with osteoarthritis of the knee joint in the early stages can be treated conservatively unless symptoms are so severe that they interfere with the daily activities of living. The patient with an acute effusion or chronic swelling of the knee joint due to osteoarthritis should be advised to restrict activities such as walking and jogging which would increase the wear of the articular surface. The use of salicylates, two tablets, four times a day, often will reduce the symptoms and irritation within the knee joint. The overweight patient should be advised to lose weight to decrease the loading of the joint surface

which may help alleviate his symptoms. Indomethacin (Indocin) or phenylbutazone (Butazolidin) can be utilized also or added to the salicylate therapy when symptoms persist.

Physical therapy may be of value in developing a strong quadriceps muscle, and isometric exercises will allow muscle strengthening without additional grinding of the joint surface. All quadriceps and weight-lifting exercises should

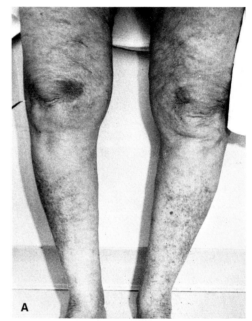

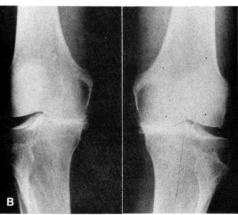

FIG. 10-101 Osteoarthritis of the knee. A. Clinical view showing varus deformities. The one on the left is especially severe. B. Roentgenograms revealing narrowing of the medial compartments.

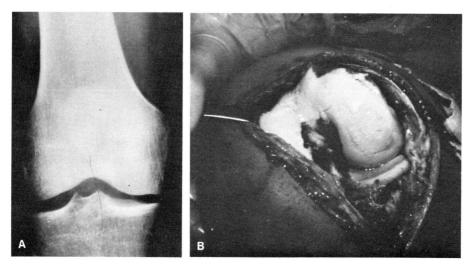

FIG. 10-102 Early osteoarthritis of the knee. The patient had severe pain in the joint. A. Roentgenogram (patient standing) reveals minimal changes. B. Surgical view reveals degenerative changes in the articular surface of the femoral condyle.

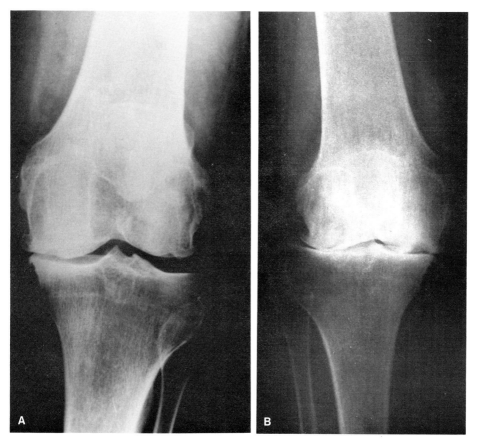

FIG. 10-103 Roentgenograms of advanced osteoarthritis of the knee. A. Narrowing of medial compartment and osteophyte formation around the periphery of the joint. B. Narrowing of both compartments with subluxation indicates destruction of anterior cruciate ligament from osteophytes in the intercondylar notch.

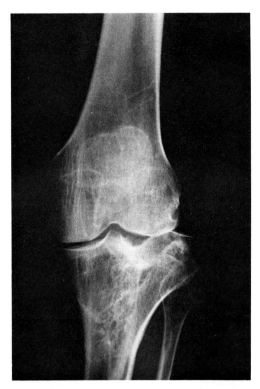

FIG. 10-104 Roentgenogram of knee joint with traumatic arthritis. The medial compartment appears to be normal, but extensive destruction of the articular cartilage was found when the knee was operated on.

be carried out with the *knee in full extension*. The use of an exercise boot with the knee flexed and then brought up into full extension tends to grind the articular surface and increase the patient's symptoms.

In many cases the acute episode will subside, and the patient will be able to function reasonably well. If symptoms persist, the local injection of steroids into the joint may reduce the patient's symptoms. Most patients will not use a cane, although it is a valuable aid in reducing the stress on the joint, especially for the elderly patient. If all conservative therapy fails, surgical intervention will be necessary to relieve the patient's symptoms.

Surgical Treatment

A number of surgical procedures have been advised for the treatment of the patient with osteoarthritis of the knee. There has been a gradual sorting out of these operations, and although at times a good result can be obtained with some of them, the average results have been fair but they were the best operations that were available in the past. With the development of joint replacement, it is now possible to correct the arthritic area and replace it with these new devices. This has made many of the operations previously performed obsolete.

It is important to realize that, since osteoarthritis is primarily a degeneration of the articular surface of the joint with secondary involvement of the synovium, synovectomy is not a procedure of choice in osteoarthritis. There is no indication for synovectomy as a primary procedure, and it should only be performed in patients with rheumatoid arthritis where the synovium is primarily involved. Repeated synovectomies have been performed in patients with osteoarthritis, but the swelling and other symptoms have recurred (Fig. 10-105). The reason is obvious. Synovectomy does not treat the articular surface which is the primary problem.

Joint debridement originally proposed by Magnuson was an early attempt at trying to salvage the knee of the patient with advanced osteoarthritis. This procedure is no longer recommended for patients with a loss of articular cartilage. Osteotomy or replacement of the joint surface is a much better operative procedure.

The role of patellectomy is extremely limited in osteoarthritis and should be reserved for patients who have primary involvement of the patella with no evidence of narrowing of the joint surface on roentgenograms from the standing position and no evidence of articular disease involving the femoral condyles or tibial plateau. Patients with evidence of articular damage on the weight-bearing surface of the femur or tibia should have replacement of the joint surfaces that are involved and not a patellectomy. This is a trap to be avoided in the patient with osteoarthritis.

Meniscectomy

There is no doubt that meniscectomy is an excellent procedure in patients with torn menisci related to trauma. However, in patients with degeneration of the meniscus and osteoarthritis of the knee, meniscectomy should be under-

taken only after careful evaluation of the patient. Patients who develop osteoarthritis of the knee joint involving a medial or lateral compartment also tend to develop changes in the meniscus. Degenerative changes in the meniscus have been very specifically described by Smillie. The horizontal or cleavage lesion occurs in a high percentage of patients above the age of 40. Since the joint space tends to narrow due to loss of the articular surface, increased pressure is applied to the weight-bearing surface of the meniscus and gradual tearing and grinding away of the meniscus often occurs, especially the anterior aspect of the joint. In most cases of osteoarthritis that have been explored the meniscus is badly degenerated or

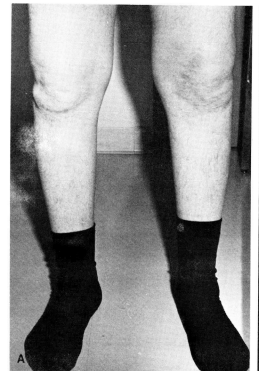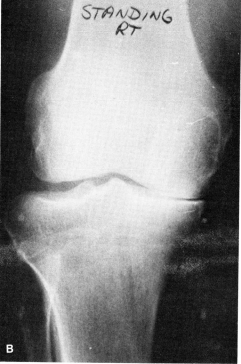

FIG. 10-105 Synovectomy for treatment of osteoarthritis of the knee. A. Clinical view after three synovectomies shows recurrence of swelling. B. Roentgenogram of the right knee reveals narrowing of the medial compartment. No further effusions occurred after an osteotomy to shift the weight to the lateral side, despite the fact that the synovium was not removed.

torn. In many cases it is completely nonexistent except for the posterior horn. If the roentgenogram taken with the patient standing shows minimal involvement of the joint space and the patient has evidence of locking or symptoms suggestive of a bucket handle tear, meniscectomy may be indicated. If there is narrowing of the medial joint space with osteoarthritis, meniscectomy will give limited improvement postoperatively, and generally the patient will have to be subjected to another procedure such as a tibial osteotomy or single compartment replacement with a total knee unit. It is advisable in patients with osteoarthritis to obtain permission to replace the joint surface, if necessary, at the time meniscectomy is being performed if there is extensive articular destruction. If the surgeon is adverse to single joint replacement or not familiar with this technique, osteotomy may be a better primary procedure than meniscectomy for the patient with degenerative changes of the meniscus. Many orthopaedic surgeons recommend that when unicompartment arthritis exists with a varus or valgus deformity, osteotomy should be the first step in treatment, even when joint debridement may seem indicated. The pain relief obtained with the osteotomy often eliminates the need for meniscectomy.

Operative Technique. A tourniquet may be used in the removal of the meniscus. A transverse curved incision paralleling the rim of the medial femoral condyle is utilized to obtain access to both the anterior and posterior joint cavities and frequently prevents division of the infrapatellar branch of the saphenous nerve. The vertical parapatellar incision or a transverse incision passing along the joint line may also be used.

The capsule is generally incised in the line of its fibers from the midpoint of the patella down to the tibia. This incision generally exposes the anterior half of the meniscus and the infrapatellar fat pad. After inspection of the joint, the articular surface of the femoral condyle, and the cruciate ligament, the appearance of the opposite femoral condyle should be noted. The meniscus is detached at its anterior horn by sharp dissection, and is grasped with a strong clamp. The meniscus knife then is passed gently beneath the medial collateral ligament and along the rim of the articular surface of the tibia, slipping the meniscus into the intercondylar notch where it is detached and removed. It is important to remove the posterior segment of the meniscus. If there is any problem, a posterior incision can be made in the capsule behind the medial collateral ligament to allow for easy removal of this posterior segment.

The synovium may be closed with 3-0 chromic catgut, the expansion with 0 interrupted chromic catgut sutures, and the skin with 3-0 nylon. In some situations the injection of a steroid into the joint on closure may reduce some of the inflammatory response postoperatively. A soft bulky Jones dressing is applied, and the patient is started on early motion in this dressing. At the end of 2 days the bulky dressing is removed, and the patient is started on further motion, quadriceps exercises, and gradual weight bearing. Instead of early motion, some surgeons advocate the use of a splint or cast for 1 or 2 weeks to rest the joint and prevent chronic effusions.

Osteotomy

Tibial osteotomy has been a valuable adjunct to the treatment of patients with unicompartment osteoarthritis of the knee. The object of the osteotomy is to shift the weight-bearing axis of the knee joint from the damaged compartment to the opposite side (Fig. 10-106). Review of numerous papers published on the results of osteotomy indicate that approxi-

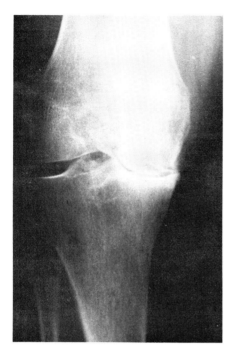

FIG. 10-106 Roentgenogram of single compartment disease. The lateral compartment is normal. Osteotomy relieved the patient's symptoms for 5 years.

mately 70 to 80 percent of the patients will be improved by the operation. However, osteotomy is becoming a much less valuable operation than the single compartment knee joint replacement for the management of unicompartment osteoarthritis.

It is apparent that the immediate success of the single compartment replacement far exceeds the results that can be obtained with an osteotomy, but long-term results are not yet available. Excellent results are being obtained with single compartment replacement in 90 to 95 percent of these operations. For patients who are 60 or more years old, the single compartment replacement is becoming the operation of choice.

The criteria for the selection of the patient for osteotomy have become more established, but with the advent of single compartment knee joint replacement indications for osteotomy will be passing through a state of flux. The indications

now for an osteotomy would depend upon the age of the patient and the amount of disease noted on the roentgenogram. Osteotomy is definitely indicated for the young, vigorous patient who wishes to maintain an active athletic life and who has minimal deformity with advanced symptoms. Osteotomy in a young woman should be considered carefully, because of the deformity it produces in overcorrecting to shift the weight to the opposite compartment (Fig. 10-107). Patients with over 15° of valgus angulation or 10° of varus angulation generally are not considered for an osteotomy because the chances for success are much less as the angulation increases (Fig. 10-108). According to the literature, however, osteotomy is the operation of choice for patients with a varus or valgus deformity, even in the older age group. An osteotomy also can be used to relieve the symptoms in osteonecrosis (Fig. 10-109). At the present time the medial compartment would be replaced if the patient is in the older age group.

The surgeon must weigh very carefully whether to do the operation proximal to the tibial tubercle or distal because of the advantages inherent in each operation. Coventry proposes these advantages for the high tibial osteotomy:

1. The osteotomy is close to the site of the deformity.
2. It is in cancellous bone which has the ability to heal rapidly.
3. Staples give adequate fixation to maintain compression.
4. Postoperative immobilization is less.
5. The danger of delayed union or nonunion is eliminated.
6. Compression at the osteotomy site is aided by contraction of the muscles.
7. The collateral ligaments can be placed under physiologic tension.

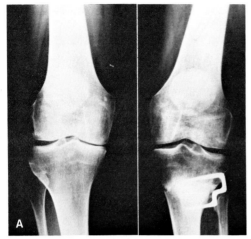

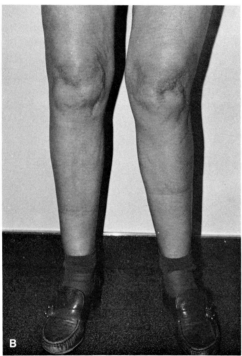

FIG. 10-107 Comparison of osteotomy and single compartment replacement. A. Preoperative roentgenogram revealing high tibial osteotomy shifting weight of left knee to opposite compartment and narrowing of medial compartment of right knee. B. Medial compartment knee replacement on the right knee is cosmetically more acceptable than the osteotomy in the left knee.

A fair number of complications have been associated with most series of high tibial osteotomies. The disadvantages of this procedure are:

1. Once the operation has been carried out, there is no opportunity postoperatively to change the angulation or position to gain further correction.
2. If the osteotomy is performed too high, splitting into the articular surface of the joint can occur.
3. Severe deformities can be created by the high tibial osteotomy.

The osteotomy performed below the tibial tubercle in the area where the cancellous bone is still present can also give excellent results. Stapling is not required. By impacting the distal fragment into the proximal and accepting a small amount of shortening, deformity can be corrected and fixation is adequate to allow early weight bearing in a walking cast. There is no question that healing will be slower than for the high tibial osteotomy, but the angulation can be corrected by wedging casts postoperatively to gain further correction. Delayed union or nonunion can occur at this level and may require future bone grafting.

The indications for either a high or low tibial osteotomy are disabling pain due to osteoarthritis and roentgenograms that reveal degenerative changes in either the medial or lateral compartment associated with a varus or valgus deformity.

Operative Technique—High Tibial Osteotomy. Before attempting a high tibial osteotomy, roentgenograms should be obtained while the patient is standing as an aid in determining the amount of bone to be resected to obtain a correction. Bauer and his associates recommend removing 1 mm of bone for every 1° of angular correction desired. Torgerson, however, feels that this formula tends to remove more bone than is re-

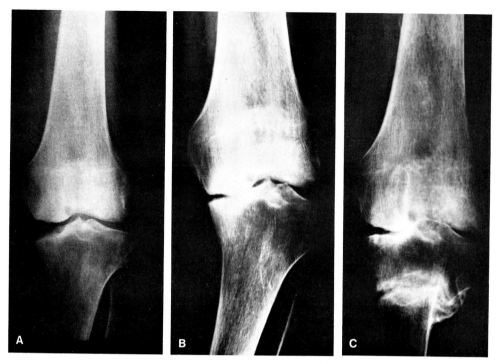

FIG. 10-108 Osteotomy in 74-year-old patient with severe varus deformity. A. Preoperative view (non-standing) showing destruction of the medial plateau. B. Preoperative view (standing) showing varus deformity of the medial compartment. C. Postoperative view showing weight shift to lateral side. Patient had developed teeter-totter effect, which was relieved by replacement of the medial compartment.

quired. In general, the consensus is to use a procedure similar to that described by Gariepy, Coventry, and Torgerson.

The operation for a varus deformity is often done under tourniquet control after wrapping the leg with a Martin bandage. The knee is flexed nearly 90°, and an incision is made through the distal iliotibial band parallel and anterior to the lateral collateral ligament and extending proximally to the level of the joint space. The biceps femoris tendon and the lateral collateral ligament are removed by sharp dissection from the head of the fibula. The fibular head is excised with an osteotome, and during this step, the peroneal nerve should be identified and protected. An incision is made in the capsule of the knee to see the lateral lip of the tibia for orientation. The soft tissue is removed from the front of the tibia as far as the patellar tendon

and posteriorly the full width of the posterior surface of the tibia. One should be able to visualize both the anterior and posterior tibial cortex.

The osteotomy is then carried out under direct vision with a wide osteotome. The upper limb of the wedge to be removed should be marked out first along a plane approximately 2 cm below and parallel to the articular surface. The appropriate wedge is marked distal to this area, and the wedge of bone is removed. Following the removal of the wedge, the medial cortex of the tibia should be perforated to aid fracture of the medial cortex. The knee is extended at this stage, and the bone ends are brought together and held securely with a staple. The tourniquet should be released and hemostasis should be secured. With the knee flexed approximately 45°, the biceps tendon and lateral

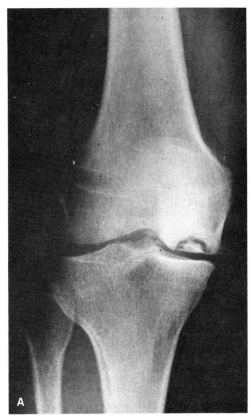 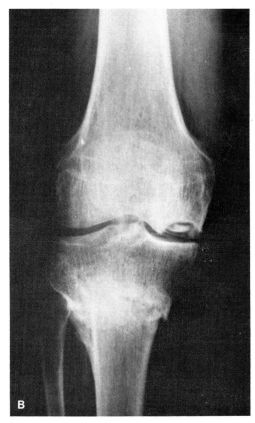

FIG. 10-109 Indication for osteotomy. A. Roentgenogram showing large area of osteonecrosis on the medial condyle. B. Postoperative view after osteotomy to shift weight to the lateral side of the joint. At the present time joint replacement would be considered in this 66-year-old man.

collateral ligament are reattached with a suture through a hole drilled in the neck of the fibula. The fascia lata is then repaired and suction drainage is used.

In the patient with a valgus deformity, a medial approach to the tibia is required. The knee is flexed 90°, and a skin incision is made from the joint surface distally, parallel to the medial collateral ligament. The medial collateral ligament and pes anserinus are retracted posteriorly. The wedge of the tibia is removed by a procedure similar to that taken for the lateral approach. Fragments are closed and secured with a staple, and the same postoperative management is carried out. It would be advisable for those who do not do osteotomies frequently to take a

roentgenogram at the time of surgery before final stapling to be sure of the correction. Undercorrection or overcorrection, will result in failure and continued symptoms postoperatively.

Postoperative Care. Postoperatively, a soft dressing of the Jones type is used with or without a protective posterior plaster splint. Approximately 8 to 10 days after the operation, a cylinder cast should be applied and weight bearing with crutches can be allowed for another 5 weeks. Generally after removal of the cast, the patient will have symptoms for several months, but gradually his knee motion and symptoms will improve.

Complications. Osteotomies in patients with severe deformities generally have a poor chance of success (Fig.

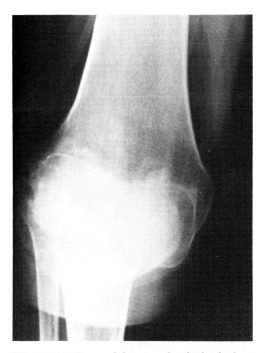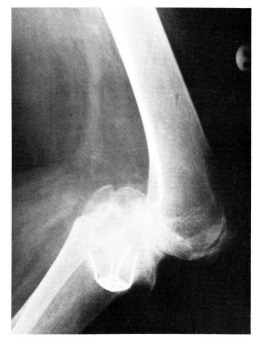

FIG. 10-110 Severe deformity after high tibial osteotomy.

10-110). It has been stated in the literature that patients with over 10° of varus angulation and 15° of valgus angulation have a poor chance of success by tibial osteotomy. After an osteotomy patients with severe bone loss tend to have a teeter-totter effect, and the femoral condyles will seesaw back and forth over the intercondylar eminence. The knee of the patient who has had an osteotomy that has failed can still be salvaged with the Marmor Modular Knee. The deformity of the osteotomy itself must be considered, and overcorrection is not indicated with the knee replacement.

One of the main problems with the high tibial osteotomy with internal fixation is that if overcorrection of the tibia into the opposite deformity is not carried out, the patient will continue to have symptoms (Fig. 10-111). It is important to overcorrect an osteotomy and to shift the weight to the opposite side of the joint which has the normal articular cartilage. Nonunions also occur with high tibial

osteotomies and it is possible to split the proximal tibia resulting in further complications (Fig. 10-112).

Younger patients, especially young women, with single compartment disease should be carefully evaluated prior to considering osteotomy. Osteotomy tends to create a deformity of the leg that may be cosmetically unacceptable to many women (Fig. 10-107B).

Operative Technique—Low Tibial Osteotomy. The technique for the low tibial osteotomy was described on page 350.

Complications may occur with low tibial osteotomy, also. Nonunion is more common in low tibial osteotomies, especially when correcting varus angulation to valgus angulation. The fibula may heal rapidly if a segment is not removed resulting in distraction of the tibia with delayed or nonunion. Reoperation with removal of a segment of the fibula and bone grafting of the tibia may be necessary (Fig. 10-113).

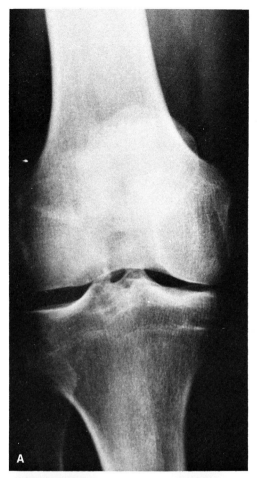
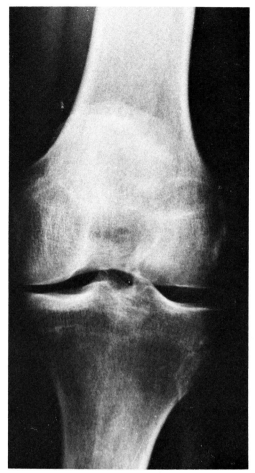
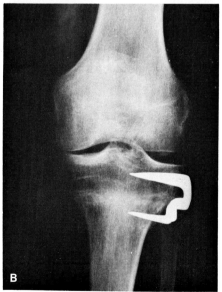

FIG. 10-111 Complication after undercorrected high tibial osteotomy. A. Roentgenogram showing medial compartment disease in both joints. B. Postoperative view showing tibia still in varus and narrowing of medial compartment. Internal fixation prevents change of angulation to relieve pressure on medial compartment where pathologic changes persist.

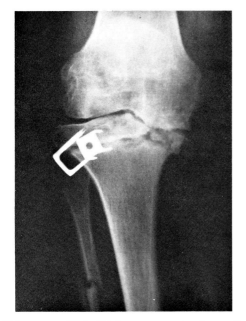

FIG. 10-112 High tibial osteotomy that has split into the joint space.

Tibial Plateau Prosthesis

The metal tibial plateau prostheses of MacIntosh and others have been in use for a number of years. Some of these prostheses were described on page 361. The metal tibial plateau was a step forward in an attempt to restore loss of tibial height due to arthritis. It has the disadvantage of any hemiarthroplasty because it replaces only one of the degenerated surfaces of the knee joint. In osteoarthritis both the femoral and tibial surfaces are severely involved (Fig. 10-114). The problem with this type of prosthesis is that the results are not consistently good. In over 100 cases of my own, the results were 50–50 with no excellent result (Fig. 10-115). MacIntosh and Hunter reported 80 percent excellent or good results for 41 cases of osteoarthritis. In my experience, the results have remained somewhat stable over the passage of years. The advantage of the tibial plateau prosthesis is that it does not burn any bridges that can be utilized if it does fail. At the present time, I am

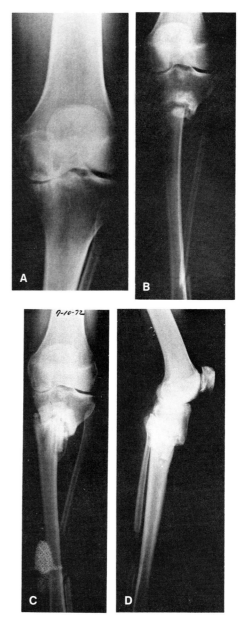

FIG. 10-113 Complication of a low tibial osteotomy. A. Preoperative roentgenogram showing osteoarthritis in the medial compartment. B. Postoperative view showing nonunion. C. Anterior view after removing bone graft from fibula and placing sliding grafts across the osteotomy site. D. Lateral view showing bone graft across tibia.

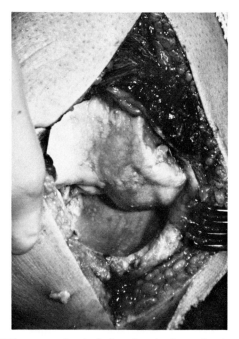

FIG. 10-114 Surgical view showing loss of articular cartilage down to the raw bone in the medial compartment.

no longer using tibial plateau prostheses but have switched completely to total knee replacement with the Marmor Modular Knee unit. However, in patients with good articular cartilage on the femoral condyle good results may be obtained if the surgeon desires a much more conservative procedure. The advantage of the tibial plateau prosthesis is that the total knee replacement can be done later if the prosthesis fails. The major contraindications to the use of the plateau prosthesis are medial or lateral tibial subluxation, flexion contractures greater than 30°, large subchondral cysts, previous sepsis, Charcot joints, and muscular weakness.

MacIntosh Operative Technique. The operation is performed under tourniquet control and through a medial parapatellar incision with complete lateral displacement of the patella (Fig. 10-116). The meniscus is excised if still present within the joint. A level bed is cut for the prosthesis on one or both tibial plateaus.

The osteotomy cuts are vertical to protect the intercondylar area, and then the plateau is shaped with a power drill or saw to provide a level bed. In the MacIntosh technique no lateral or posterior ridge is left to stabilize the prosthesis. Varus or valgus angulation is corrected by the insertion of the prosthesis of the appropriate thickness and diameter. Trimming of the osteophytes from the patella can also be carried out at this stage. Excision of the patella should be avoided. The tourniquet is released before closure, and hemostasis secured.

Postoperative Care. Postoperatively the knee is kept in extension for 5 days in a massive compression dressing. Quadriceps exercises are started immediately. The patient is allowed up on crutches after 2 days, and active flexion is encouraged after 5 days.

Marmor Operative Technique. The Marmor technique for implanting the tibial plateau prosthesis was described on pages 361–364. A synovectomy will not be needed, however, for the patient with osteoarthritis. If a single compartment is being replaced, either a medial or lateral incision is made, depending on the side of the joint to be replaced. If both compartments are to be replaced, both incisions are used for exposure. The single compartment incision is made one finger breadth medial to the patella on the medial side and two finger breadths lateral to the patella on the lateral side. When both incisions are used simultaneously, they should be kept apart to prevent interference with the circulation to the intervening skin flap.

Patellectomy

Patellectomy is seldom required in osteoarthritis of the knee. Isolated patellofemoral disease is an indication for patellectomy if only the patella is involved with no evidence of osteoarthritis involving the knee joint surface on

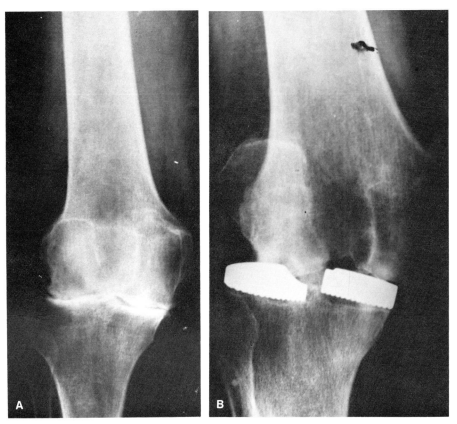

FIG. 10-115 Tibial plateau prostesis. A. Preoperative view revealing osteoarthritis in both compartments. B. Postoperative view after insertion of MacIntosh prostheses. There is evidence of subluxation and the patient continued to have pain.

weight bearing (Fig. 10-117). In patients with advanced osteoarthritis of the joint, replacement of the joint has generally relieved the patient's symptoms and the patella does not seem to be a source of problems during the recovery period. Occasionally patellectomy will be required following a total knee replacement, but this should not be performed at the same time as the total knee or other intra-articular procedure because of the possibility of stiffness due to immobilization of the knee.

Marmor Modular Knee—Single Compartment

Total knee replacement in osteoarthritis is somewhat a misnomer because the entire joint is not replaced in this procedure. Although the insertion of some bicondylar replacements requires removal of both femoral condyles and tibial plateaus, this procedure is not indicated in unicompartment osteoarthritis. It is not advisable to sacrifice a good compartment to install the bicondylar components. Single compartment disease does exist in osteoarthritis, and single compartment replacement is possible if a grooved unit is not used. The Polycentric unit and other types that have a groove into which the femoral condyle fits are, I believe, contraindicated in osteoarthritis with single compartment disease. The normal knee joint during flexion and extension rotates between 8° to 25° with an average rotation of approximately 13°. If one com-

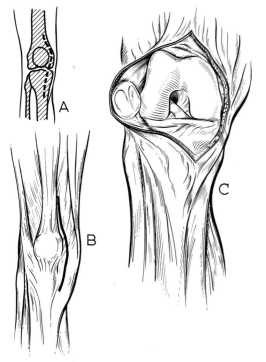

FIG. 10-116 MacIntosh technique for tibial plateau prosthesis. A. Parapatellar incision. B. Line for opening the expansion. C. Retraction of patella laterally to expose entire anterior aspect of the knee joint.

partment is fixed and cannot rotate, the stress on the replaced single compartment will be tremendous. It has been estimated that the force on a joint that does not rotate is approximately 200 kg in the soft tissue when rotation is prevented. The grooved units have tended to fail in single compartment disease because of this problem. The Marmor Modular Knee was designed as an articular resurfacing and has no grooves or ridges to prevent rotation (Fig. 10-118). Therefore, single compartment disease can be easily handled with this unit with a minimum of bone removal. Patients with single compartment replacements have done exceedingly well postoperatively and tend to regain their preoperative motion with reasonable ease.

An indication for unicompartment or single compartment replacement is narrowing of the joint space in the involved compartment (Fig. 10-119). The opposite compartment should look reasonably normal on the roentgenogram taken while the patient is standing. Stress films

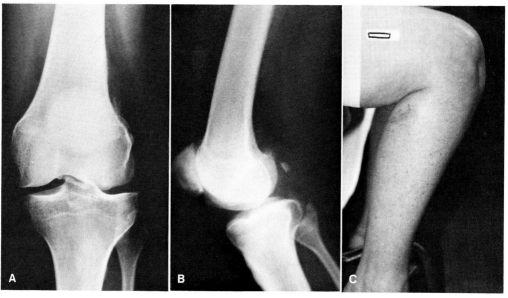

FIG. 10-117 Patellectomy in patient who had pain in knee on rising or sitting or climbing stairs. A. Preoperative anteroposterior roentgenogram revealing no evidence of narrowing of the joint space. B. Lateral view showing evidence of patellofemoral arthritis. C. Postoperative clinical view showing flexion with no pain.

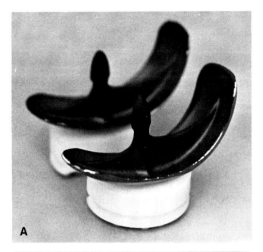

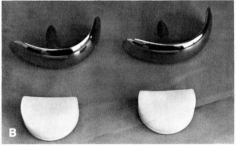

FIG. 10-118 Marmor Modular Knee components. A. Side view of metal condyles and high density polyethylene tibial plateaus. B. View of flat surfaces of tibial components which articulate with the smooth, rounded femoral condyles.

contraindication to replacement (Fig. 10-120A)., nor is severe bone loss of the tibia (Fig. 10-120B).

Varus deformity of 25° and valgus deformities of 45° can be corrected quite easily. Preoperative flexion deformities of 40° can also be corrected at the time of surgery. However, in single compartment disease, flexion deformity is generally less than 20°. If at the time of single compartment repair the flexion deformity does not improve, one *must* make a lateral incision and inspect the anterior aspect of the lateral compartment or the opposite compartment from the one being operated upon. Prior infection should be a contraindication to joint replacement. There may be a good deal of ligamentous laxity due to bone loss of the tibia, but this is not a contraindication to repair. The use of high density polyethylene in varying thicknesses allows for correction of the bone loss and tightening of the ligaments (Fig. 10-121). Bone loss should not be compensated for

have been utilized to try to see if the opposite side would close down, but they have not been very valuable. It is always wise to caution the patient preoperatively that the opposite side will be observed through the incision and if there is extensive disease present the compartment will be replaced. A certain amount of disease process can be accepted in the older patient. The cartilage in someone 70 or 80 years of age may show some discoloration and softening, but if there is a reasonable cartilage layer on the weight-bearing surface of the femur, the joint should not be replaced. Preoperative subluxation of the femur medially on the tibia is not a

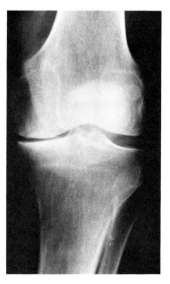

FIG. 10-119 Indication for single compartment replacement. Roentgenogram reveals narrowing of the medial side and a varus deformity. The lateral compartment is free of osteophytes, sclerosis and subchondral bone changes.

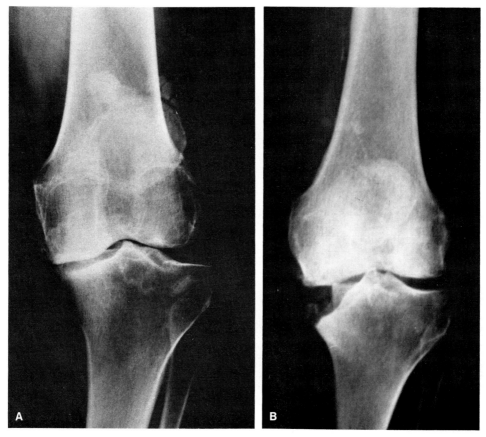

FIG. 10-120 Marmor Modular Knee replacement. A. Subluxation of the femur on the tibia is not a contraindication. B. Severe bone loss can be corrected with tibial component.

by the use of methyl methacrylate cement because it is brittle and will tend to crack if left unsupported by bone.

Operative Technique. The operative technique to be described is that recommended for replacing a single compartment in osteoarthritis or traumatic arthritis of the knee joint. It is possible to replace either the medial compartment or the lateral compartment through a single incision placed on the proper side of the knee joint. The medial approach is much easier than the lateral approach and if any problem is encountered in inserting the femoral component in the lateral approach, a medial incision can be made to aid in the surgical approach to the femoral condyle.

The operation is performed under tourniquet control, and a median parapatellar incision is made for approximately 5 inches (Fig. 10-122). The incision is usually placed one finger breadth medial or lateral to the patella, depending on the compartment involved. The expansion and synovial layer are opened, exposing the joint space. A small portion of the infrapatellar fat pad is excised from the medial side of the joint carefully to prevent damage to the lateral compartment. The joint is examined, and a check is made to determine if the cruciate ligaments are present (Fig. 10-123). By carefully lifting the patella with a blunt retractor, the surgeon can inspect the opposite femoral

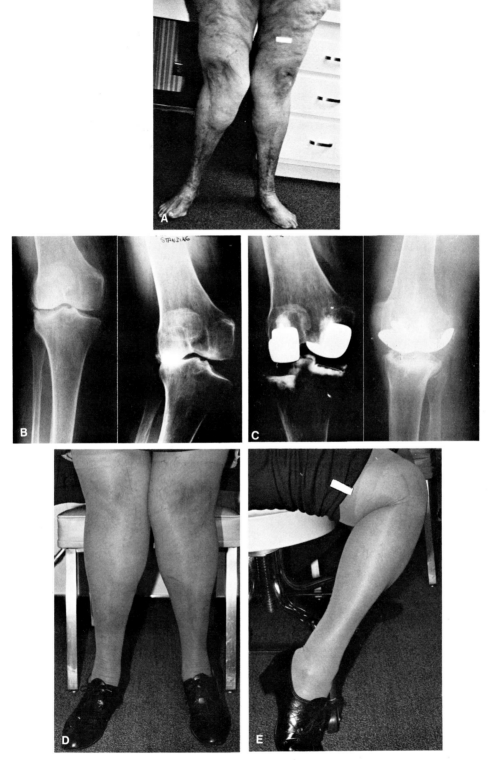

FIG. 10-121 Marmor Modular Knee replacement to correct ligamentous laxity and severe valgus deformities. A. Clinical preoperative view. Patient had difficulty walking. B. Roentgenograms, standing and nonstanding, revealing severe depression of lateral compartment, widening of the medial compartment, and ligamentous instability. C. Postoperative roentgenogram showing varying heights of tibial components cemented in to increase ligamentous stability. D. Clinical view 2 years postoperatively showing excellent stability. E. Lateral view revealing flexion of 100°.

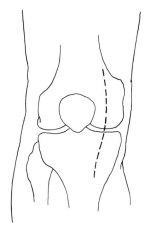

FIG. 10-122 Skin incision for single compartment Marmor Modular Knee replacement.

condyle to observe the articular surface. The knee is gradually flexed for further exposure of the weight-bearing surface of the opposite femoral condyle. If the articular cartilage is in relatively good condition, one can assume that the tibial side is also normal and no further surgery on the opposite side is contemplated. The meniscus on the damaged side is now removed from the anterior aspect of the joint space. If any osteophytes protrude anteriorly on the tibial plateau, these should be removed with

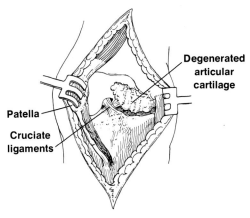

FIG. 10-123 Single compartment Marmor Modular Knee replacement. Retraction of the patella and synovial layer to expose the degenerated joint space. The lateral compartment is normal.

an osteotome. The knee is flexed 90°, and an osteotome is used to remove one-fourth inch of the posterior aspect of the femoral condyle parallel to the tibial plateau (Fig. 10-124). If this is not removed, the template cannot be inserted and visualization of the tibial plateau is not possible. After removing this portion of bone, the posterior recess of the joint, including the posterior capsule of the knee joint, should be clearly seen. If the capsule is not visible, a portion of the posterior horn of the meniscus remains. This should be removed to gain further exposure of the tibial plateau (Fig. 10-125). With the knee flexed 90°, a lamina spreader is inserted into the intercondylar notch for further exposure of the tibial plateau if needed. The tibial plateau is then marked with the tibial marking template which is coated with methylene blue and placed on the plateau so as to leave a posterior rim of at least 2 mm and as much bone as possible around the periphery (Fig. 10-63). If the tibial plateau is very small, the inner aspect of the marking template can be used to outline the tibial plateau for the smaller plastic component. A power tool turning at 100,000 rpm should be used with a steel bur to remove the bone within the methylene blue outline down to approximately 4 to 6 mm deep (Fig. 10-126). An attempt should be made to preserve the periphery of the rim of the tibia to aid in locking the tibial component into place (Fig. 10-63). A sterilized Pyrex pie plate, 9 to 10 inches in diameter, is held over the area to prevent bone dust and bone chips from contaminating the air. When an adequate amount of bone has been resected with the power tool, the tibial marking template can be inserted into the depression if a standard size is being used to check the dimensions of the prepared cavity (Fig. 10-127). When a satisfactory depth has been reached and an adequate fit is possible, a 9 mm tibial component should

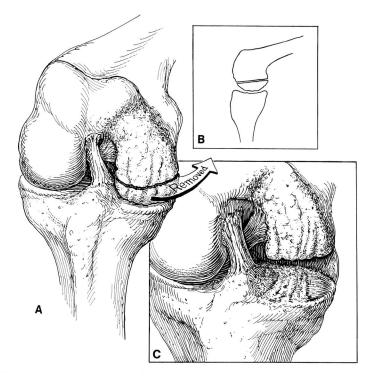

FIG. 10-124 Single compartment Modular Knee (continued). A. Knee flexed 90° for removal of ¼ inch of femoral condyle. B. Lateral view to show portion to be removed. C. After removal the entire tibial plateau and posterior capsule of the knee joint should be visible. (Courtesy Richards Manufacturing Company.)

be selected and impacted into place. If there has not been much bone loss, the trough should be deep enough so that only 1 or 2 mm of the component should protrude above the joint surface. A tight fit in the tibia is not necessary because the cement will give adequate final fixa-

tion of the component. The component may be horizontal or tilted slightly toward the periphery because the normal tibia does slope away from the intercondylar notch (Fig. 10-128). A posterior slope is

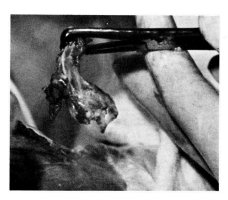

FIG. 10-125 Single compartment Marmor Modular Knee (continued). Posterior horn of the meniscus removed to gain more exposure of tibial plateau.

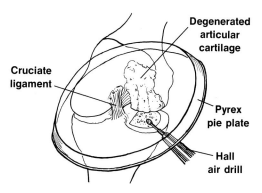

FIG. 10-126 Single compartment Marmor Modular Knee (continued). Removing bone within methylene blue outline on tibial plateau with a power tool. A sterilized Pyrex plate covers the operating field to prevent dust and bone chips from arising.

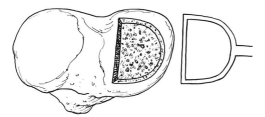

FIG. 10-127 Single compartment Marmor Modular Knee (continued). Checking the dimensions of the prepared cavity.

also advisable to aid in gaining flexion postoperatively. For the patient with a severe varus or valgus deformity with a loss of the tibial plateau bone, it will be necessary to use the increased thickness of the tibial component to restore the lost bone.

When the tibial plateau component has been satisfactorily inserted, the knee is brought up into full extension and the femoral condyle is marked with a thin methylene blue line at the point where the anterior edge of the tibial trial component strikes the femoral condyle (Fig. 10-129). This is the landmark for positioning the femoral template. It is important to have the knee in full extension when this is carried out. The knee is again flexed 90°, and the tibial trial

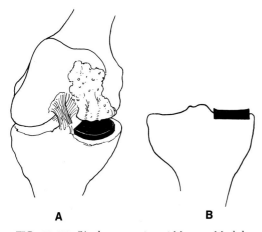

FIG. 10-128 Single compartment Marmor Modular Knee (continued) A. The trial tibial prosthesis in place. B. Drawing shows protrusion above the joint surface and slight tilt.

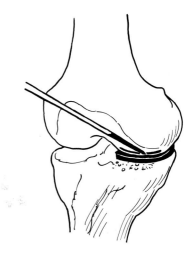

FIG. 10-129 Single compartment Marmor Modular Knee (continued). Marking the line where the anterior edge of the trial tibial component strikes the femoral condyle.

component is removed and set aside for later use. The proper size of femoral template is selected and screwed onto the driver and impacted into the femoral condyle with its leading edge placed against the methylene blue line (Fig. 10-130). The template is inserted so that in full extension it will cover the middle of the tibial component and also will have adequate placement on the femoral condyle. The femoral template driver is removed from the template, and a $\frac{3}{8}$-inch twist drill is employed to make a center hole, approximately $1\frac{1}{2}$ inches deep, right through the template into the femoral bone for the main cement anchoring hole. The outline of the femoral template is traced onto the femoral condyle with methylene blue. The slots in the template are also marked with methylene blue, and the template is then removed. With a high speed carbide bur approximately 2.3 mm in diameter, the slot is cut through to the center hole that had been drilled previously (Fig. 10-131). This slot is made to accommodate the fin of the femoral component and should be cut perpendicular to the articular surface of the femoral condyle to prevent

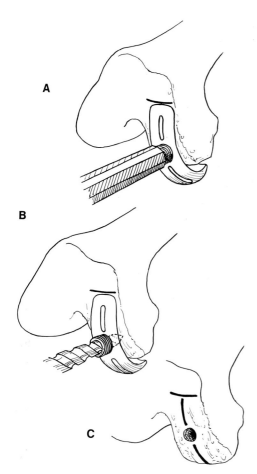

FIG. **10-130** Single compartment Marmor Modular Knee (continued). A. The femoral template placed on the driver for impaction onto the femoral condyle. The anterior edge is against the methylene blue line. B. Using a ⅜-inch drill to make a hole for the spike of the femoral component. C. The slot in the template outlined in methylene blue.

patella. If a satisfactory fit has been obtained, the component is removed, the tibial trail component is inserted first, and then the femoral trial component is reinserted. When properly placed, the femoral trial component will protrude slightly beyond the anterior edge of the tibial trial plateau and will glide smoothly on flexion and extension of the knees (Fig. 10-132). If the tibial trial

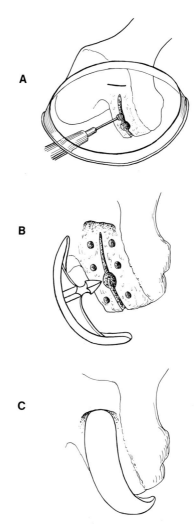

FIG. **10-131** Single compartment Marmor Modular Knee (continued). A. Drilling the slot. B. Series of small cement holes on either side of the main channel. C. Impacting the femoral trial prosthesis. Note depression cut in condyle near methylene blue line.

angulation of the prosthesis. The outline within the perimeter of the femoral marking template is cleaned of all soft tissue and remaining cartilage down to the cortical bone. A series of small cement holes are drilled on either side of the main slot.

The appropriate femoral trial component is now impacted into place to test its fit. The front end of the bone should be undercut near the methylene blue line to accommodate the prosthesis so that there is no protrusion to catch the

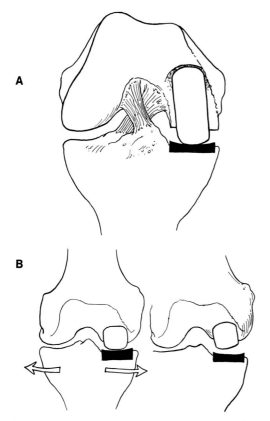

FIG. 10-132 Single compartment Marmor Modular Knee (continued). A. The knee flexed to check fit of components. The femoral condyle prosthesis should glide smoothly over the tibial plateau prosthesis. B. The knee in full extension to test if the joint rocks open (right).

component tends to flip out of the joint or lift up anteriorly, there may be a high spot in the trough that should be removed or the posterior portion of the trough should be deepened. The knee is then brought up into full extension and abducted and adducted to see if the joint rocks open. If there is instability, the next larger tibial component should be inserted. At this stage the 9-mm tibial trial plateau should be the thinnest one used for single compartment disease. The 6-mm one is too thin as a final component and may tend to buckle in heavy patients.

In osteoarthritis with a varus or a valgus deformity, it is important to note

that the knee should not be overcorrected by putting in too large a component. Overcorrection as one would do with an osteotomy can lead to pain postoperatively.

If the patient has had varus or valgus angulation all his life, the collateral ligaments will allow correction to whatever is normal for that patient. If the surgeon tries to overcorrect the joint, the fit will be too tight, and the knee will rock open rather than glide easily over the tibial component. It is usually better to err on the side of looseness rather than making the components too tight. The cement will take up some of the space and correct any loosening. When the proper size has been selected, it is important to note that the anterior edge of the femoral component is not protruding upward above the bony or cartilaginous surface of the condyle. If it protrudes too high, it is better to undercut the anterior edge so that the femoral prosthesis can be impacted smoothly with the surface of the femoral condyle and will not catch the patella on flexion of the knee.

If the joint functions satisfactorily, the trial components should be removed. The joint is thoroughly irrigated with antibiotic solution and dried. At this time, cement holes are made in the tibial plateau at varying angles, and the assistant surgeon or nurse should start to mix the bone cement (Fig. 10-133). The patella, the femoral condyle, and the tibial plateau are examined, and any osteophytes should be removed. When the cement has reached its proper consistency, the surgeon should line the bed of the tibia with cement and force cement down into the cement holes that have been drilled in the bone (Fig. 10-134). The tibial component is coated with a thin layer of cement, and the surgeon will place the posterior edge of the tibial component against the posterior wall of the tibial plateau and press the component down into place. The tibial

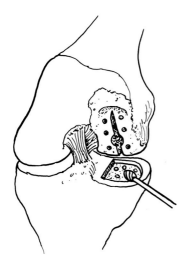

FIG. 10-133 Single compartment Marmor Modular Knee (continued). Drilling cement holes in the tibial plateau.

impactor can be used to tap it in securely. All excess cement should be removed at this time. The knee is then flexed 90°, and the assistant will hold the tibial plateau component in place with his finger while cement is placed into the femoral condyle with a curette.

In the meantime the nurse will coat the undersurface of the femoral component, being sure that the component is the proper size, and then hand it to the surgeon who will place it into the femoral condyle. It is finally tapped in lightly with the impactor, and the knee is brought up into extension and flexed and extended several times to compress the component and force out any excess cement. The excess cement is removed from the femoral condyle with a plastic spatula, and then the knee is brought up into full extension and held until the cement hardens (Fig. 10-135). At this point, suction tubes are inserted through the suprapatellar pouch and brought out through the skin of the front of the thigh above the knee. Two medium-sized tubes are generally required. When the cement has hardened, the joint is inspected, and any excess cement is carefully removed to avoid scratching the

femoral component with an osteotome and a mallet. The joint is thoroughly irrigated, and the tourniquet is released and removed from the extremity. Hemostasis is secured, and then the expansion is carefully closed with 0 interrupted silk sutures. When there is an excellent layer

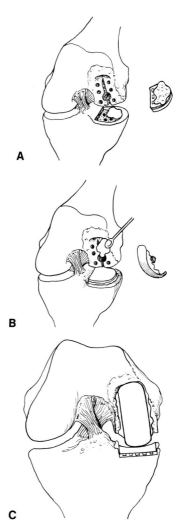

A

B

C

FIG. 10-134 Single compartment Marmor Modular Knee (continued). A. Bed of the tibia and underside of the tibial plateau component are lined with cement. B. The tibial component has been impacted into place. Cement is placed in the femoral holes and on the underside of the final femoral component. C. The knee is flexed and extended after insertion of both components to force out excess cement.

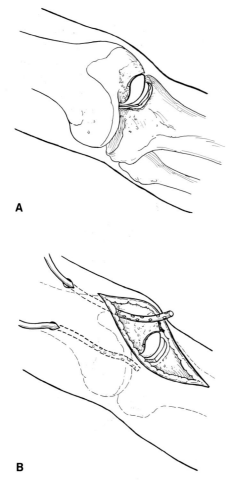

A

B

FIG. 10-135 Single Compartment Marmor Modular Knee (continued). A. The knee is held in full extension to force cement down into tibia. B. Two suction tubes are brought out through the suprapatellar pouch.

of synovium, it may be repaired with a separate layer of 3-0 chromic catgut. Because it is extremely important not to catch the suction tubes with the sutures on closure, the tubes are generally pushed into the opposite compartment. The subcutaneous tissue is closed with 3-0 chromic suture and the skin with a continuous 3-0 nylon suture. A bulky Jones dressing is applied for compression.

Postoperative Care. Postoperatively, the patient is started immediately on motion and exercises in the bulky dress-

ing. On the second postoperative day, the bulky dressing is removed and the suction tubes are taken out. The suture line is covered with an antibiotic ointment, and a small dressing is applied. The patient is generally placed on an oral antibiotic on the first postoperative day and kept on it for 5 to 7 days. The patient is allowed out of bed the first postoperative day, and by the fourth postoperative day is allowed to ambulate with a walker or crutches, using full weight bearing as tolerated. Patients should be encouraged to flex their knees to about 90° by the first week if possible.

In some patients the knee joint will swell, with cutting in of the suture line. In these patients it is advisable to remove the sutures early. The sutures can be removed at 6 or 7 days postoperatively if the skin is coated on each side of the incision with a skin adherent followed by the application of butterfly tapes that will stick to the adherent and prevent separation of the wound.

The results of patients having single compartment replacements have been excellent in most cases, and return of motion is quite rapid (Fig. 10-136). Age is no contraindication to the single compartment replacement (Fig. 10-137).

Double Compartment

Double compartment replacement in osteoarthritis is indicated where there is destruction of the articular surface of the medial and lateral compartments of the knee joint. It is not always possible preoperatively to determine whether a single or double compartment replacement will be required because the roentgenograms frequently do not reveal the true picture of the knee joint. At the time of single compartment exploration, one always should look across to the opposite compartment to be sure that it is normal or reasonably so in the elderly patient. If there is any doubt, the oppo-

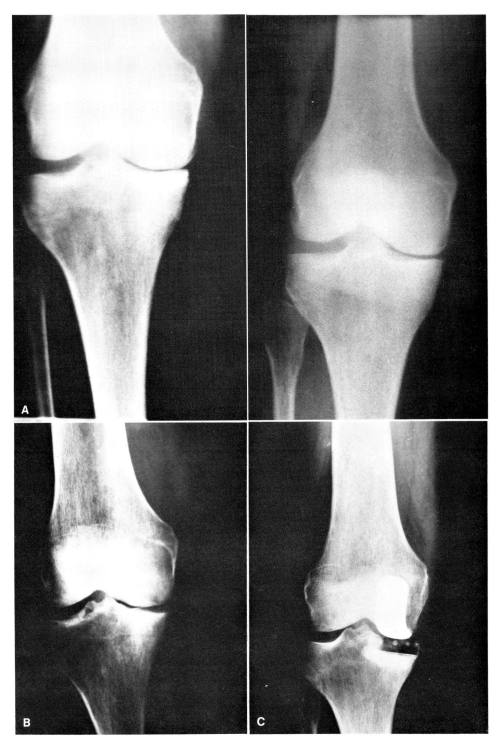

FIG 10-136 Single compartment Marmor Modular Knee replacement. A. Preoperative roentgenograms. Beginning narrowing of the medial compartment is seen on the right. One year later (left) narrowing has increased. B. Roentgenogram 18 months later reveals evidence of destruction of tibial plateau and development of varus deformity. C. Anteroposterior view after insertion of Modular Knee reveals excellent fixation of the components, correction of the varus deformity, and an excellent lateral compartment.

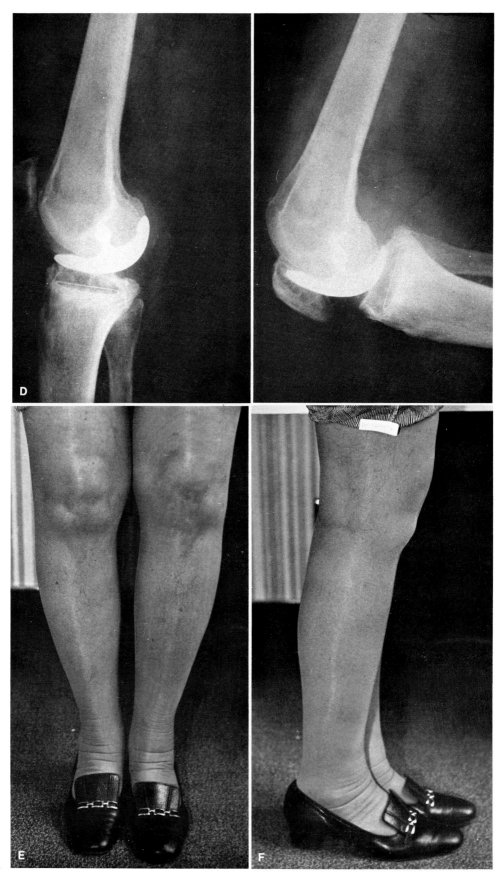

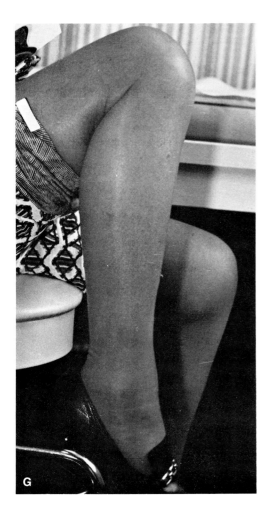

G

FIG. 10-136 (Cont'd) D. Lateral roentgenogram 2 years postoperatively shows full extension (left) and the flexion possible (right). E. Photograph 2 years postoperatively. F. Lateral view showing slight loss of extension. G. Lateral view showing flexion of 120° with no pain.

site compartment should be opened and explored. In patients who have had a single compartment replacement that still maintains some evidence of flexion contracture, it is advisable to open the opposite compartment to inspect the tibial plateau and intercondylar area because frequently osteophytes projecting from the tibial spines may prevent full extension.

In patients with severe medial compartment disease, there is a tendency for the femur to sublux medially on the tibia, resulting in encroachment of the intercondylar eminence against the medial aspect of the lateral femoral condyle. This is sometimes obvious on the preoperative roentgenogram revealing a lytic area in the lateral condyle. This, however, is not an indication for replacement of the lateral compartment if the main articular surface appears normal at the time of surgery.

Intercondylar osteophytes are quite common in osteoarthritis, and in severe disease can narrow the intercondylar area so that the osteophytes gradually will impinge against the anterior cruciate ligament. These osteophytes can be extremely sharp and gradually will erode through the anterior cruciate ligament and destroy it. Complete destruction has been noted in severe osteoarthritis, and in various stages of the

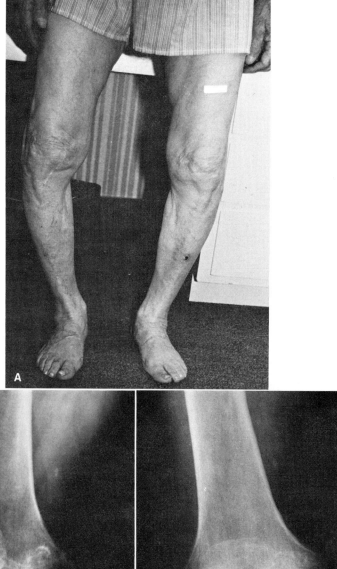

FIG. 10-137 Results of single compartment Marmor Modular Knee replacement in 84-year-old man. A. Preoperative photograph of varus deformities in both knees accompanied by incapacitating pain. B. Preoperative roentgenogram of right knee showing subluxation and collapse of the medial compartment. C. Postoperative roentgenogram showing Marmor Modular Knee components in the medial compartment. The lateral compartment is still good. The patient is free of pain and able to walk long distances.

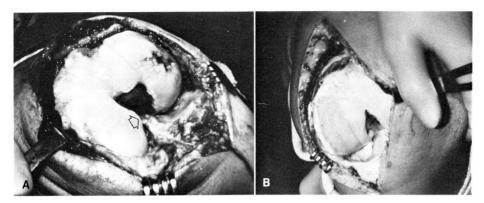

FIG. 10-138 Surgical views of pathologic changes in knee joints from osteoarthritis. A. A sharp osteophyte encroaches on the anterior cruciate ligament (arrow). B. The intercondylar notch has been narrowed to a triangular shape by osteophyte formation, the anterior cruciate ligament has been destroyed, and only a remnant of the meniscus is present in the depressed tibial plateau.

disease partial to complete destruction of the anterior cruciate has been noted (Fig. 10-138). Since osteoarthritis is not a synovial disease, the anterior cruciate is not destroyed in the same way as in rheumatoid arthritis. Loss of the anterior cruciate ligament in no way deters the surgeon from doing a Marmor Modular Knee replacement. In preoperative subluxation, it is advisable not to slope the tibial components in the same direction medially, as there is a tendency for the femoral condyles to slide down the slope. It is much better to tilt the plateaus slightly away from the intercondylar eminence to aid in the prevention of medial-lateral subluxation.

Patellectomy is not recommended at the time of articular surface replacement and should be reserved for patients who have severe problems 6 to 12 months postoperatively. When a patient has an extremely wide arthritic patella with numerous osteophytes around the periphery, it is advisable to cut away the osteophytes and narrow the patella considerably. The articular facet is maintained in the center of the patella, and the lateral and medial facets are undercut like a gull wing so that only a small portion of the patella articulates with the surface of the femoral condyle. This

technique has been called the "Jonathan Livingston Seagull" procedure and has been utilized in a number of cases of severe osteoarthritis of the knee (Fig. 10-139). The patella has been less of a

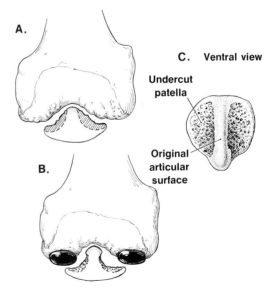

FIG. 10-139 A. Tangential view of the patella revealing the area to be removed in patients with severe patellofemoral arthritis to produce a Jonathan Livingston Seagull patella. B. Drawing illustrating the area removed to give a gull wing effect maintaining the thickness of the patella but preventing it from articulating with the femoral component. C. Ventral view of the patella illustrating the area removed from the original surface.

problem since this procedure has been carried out.

Operative Technique. The operative technique for the double compartment replacement with the Marmor Modular Knee was described on page 371. In the procedure for the patient with osteoarthritis there is of course no need for a synovectomy first. After the medial parapatellar incision has been made, however, a portion of the infrapatellar fat pad should be excised to improve exposure. Any scar tissue should be released to allow flexion of the knee to 90°. The cruciate and the medial collateral ligaments should be inspected, and the anterior portion of the medial meniscus should be detached and excised from the joint. The remainder of the infrapatellar fat pad is detached and excised from the joint through the lateral incision (Fig. 10-140).

The procedures for fitting the trial components and inserting the final com-

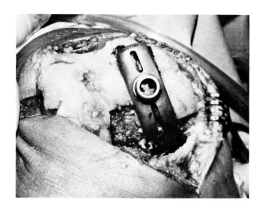

FIG. 10-141 Correct placement of the femoral template toward the intercondylar notch so that the template will line up over the tibial component. The overhanging medial bone will be removed.

ponents are the same as those in the operation for rheumatoid arthritis in the knee. An error in centering the femoral template must be avoided in the patient with severe osteoarthritis. This patient often has a wide femoral condyle because of osteophyte formation. The tendency is to place the template too far medial so that it will not be centered over the tibial plateau (Fig. 10-141).

Complications. Infection, loosening of the components, thrombophlebitis, loss of motion, patellar impingement, urinary retention, and postoperative anemia—all complications following implantation of the Marmor Modular Knee in the patient with rheumatoid arthritis—are also seen following operation on the patient with osteoarthritis.

Charcot Joints. The Modular Knee should not be considered for patients with Charcot joints. The patient with minimal pain and severe joint destruction may have a neuropathic joint. In some cases bone fragments in the joint can be a clue, but this is not true in all situations. The components tend to come loose in neuropathic joints, and cement does not seem to hold to the bone.

Overcorrection. The problem of overcorrection should be considered to prevent postoperative pain. If, in uni-

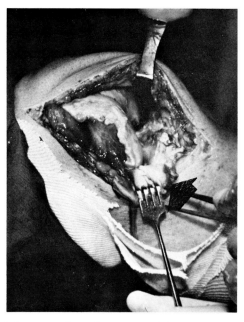

FIG. 10-140 Lateral exposure of knee joint after removal of infrapatellar fat pad allows excellent visualization of front of tibia. The lateral meniscus (arrow) should be excised.

compartment disease, the tibial prosthesis is not inserted deep enough, there will be overcorrection of the compartment, producing postoperative pain. The medial collateral or lateral collateral ligament will be stretched to its maximum, and the patient may even be forced into weight bearing on the opposite compartment as in an osteotomy (Fig. 10-142). It is better to put the component in slightly loose than too tight. In patients with minimal bone loss but loss of the articular cartilage, the tibial component should be seated almost flush with the bony surface because the femoral component will take up several millimeters of thickness in the joint. This fact is often overlooked.

Subluxation. Subluxation can occur after the operation in patients with severe osteoarthritis who have this problem preoperatively because of destruction of the anterior cruciate ligament and laxity of the collateral ligaments. In correcting this type of knee, it is important to insert a thick enough tibial component to tighten the collateral ligaments and reduce the tendency for subluxation (Fig. 10-143). It is also worthwhile to be sure not to tilt both tibial plateaus in the same direction of the subluxation because the femoral components will then

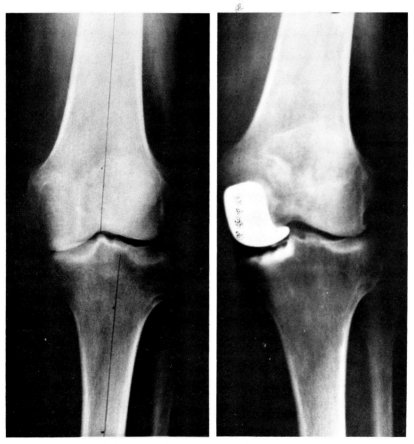

FIG. 10-142 Overcorrection of deformity with Marmor Modular Knee unit. Preoperative view (left) of varus deformity with medial compartment disease. Postoperative view (right) reveals overcorrection on the medial side so that the knee is in valgus position.

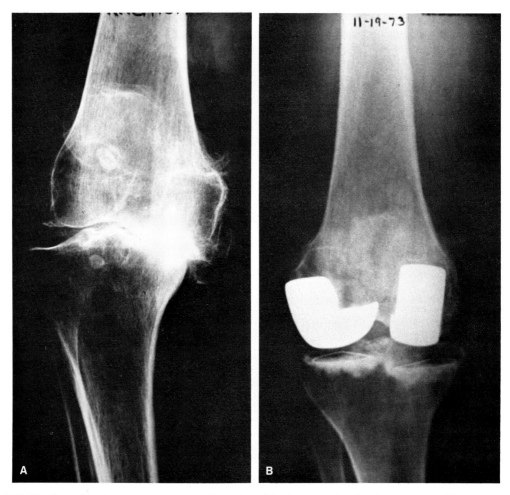

FIG. 10-143 A. Roentgenogram showing subluxation of the femur on the tibia in an 82-year-old woman. B. Roentgenogram 1½ years after total knee replacement. The anteroposterior view reveals toeing in of the femoral components and correction of the subluxation.

slide toward their original subluxation deformity (Fig. 10-144). A slight tilt of the components the opposite direction from the intercondylar eminence may reduce this tendency. The patient whose knee joint has a tendency toward subluxation should be immobilized for a longer period to allow scar tissue to form and increase the stability.

It is recommended that reconstruction of the knee be carried out early before severe destruction of the joint and instability. Stability can be obtained in patients with severe fixed valgus deformities by bony interlocking of the femur and the tibial. Replacement with a smooth surface will result in subluxation (Fig. 10-145). A hinge joint or a knee joint replacement with inherent stability should be inserted in these patients.

Allied Problems. FLEXION CONTRACTURES. The patient with osteoarthritis of the knee joint may develop a flexion contracture in the late stages of the disease. The femoral condyle tends to erode into the tibial plateau, and the anterior lip of the tibia strikes the front of the femoral condyle and blocks full extension. The lateral roentgenogram may reveal this anterior bony block (Fig.

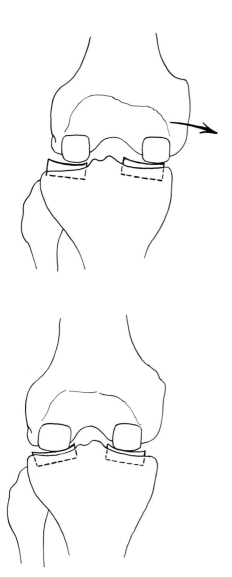

FIG. 10-144 Subluxation after double compartment replacement. Both tibial plateaus are sloped the same way (top). Tibial plateaus are tilted slightly away from the intercondylar eminence to prevent subluxation (bottom).

10-146). Until the bony block is removed, complete extension is not possible.

It is no longer recommended that wedging casts or preoperative traction be carried out to correct flexion deformities. Wedging only tends to compress the femoral condyle or the anterior edge of the tibia.

Posterior capsulotomy has been used for the treatment of flexion contractures, but in the patient with arthritis the deformity is usually caused by a bony block, not by tightness of the posterior structures. This release is indicated only when there is a soft tissue contracture (Fig. 10-81).

The correction of severe flexion deformities with the Marmor Modular Knee unit is not extremely difficult. The operative technique is similar to that for the usual Marmor Modular Knee replacement, except that the anterior ledge of the tibia is removed with an osteotome down to the grooved area in the tibial plateau (Fig. 10-147). Removal of this bone allows the knee to come into full extension on the operating room table, despite the fact that a contracture may have been present for 10 years or longer. A residual 15° contracture from muscle spasm usually corrects itself gradually later on, and will not interfere with reasonable function of the knee postoperatively (Fig. 10-148). The greater the contracture, the easier the return of flexion and motion postoperatively. If full correction of a contracture in a patient with single compartment disease is not apparent at the time of operation, the opposite compartment should be opened to see what is blocking full extension.

Postoperatively the patient may develop spasm in the hamstring muscles and require muscle relaxants for a period of time. Gradually the contracture will stretch out, and extension will improve as the patient uses the knee.

VARUS OR VALGUS DEFORMITIES. Arthritis can produce severe varus or valgus deformities of the knee joint. These are often associated with flexion deformities. As the disease progresses and destroys the tibial plateau, varus or valgus deformity will develop. Once the deformity is established, it tends to progress rapidly and to fragment the rim of the tibial plateau. These deformities may

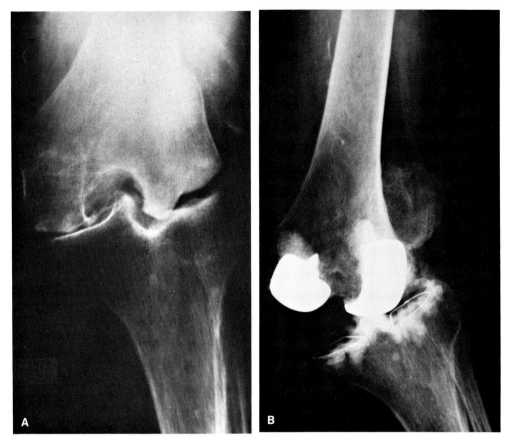

FIG. 10-145 A. Roentgenogram of patient with severe valgus deformity associated with bone destruction. B. Dislocation of the joint after insertion of a Marmor Modular Knee. The Marmor Modular knee should not be used in patients with gross instability and bone destruction.

be corrected by the Marmor Modular Knee. The varying heights of the tibial plateau component allow correction of valgus deformities up to 40° and varus deformities of 25° or more (Figs. 10-149; 10-150).

The operative procedure to correct a varus or valgus deformity consists of removing the slope of the tibia that has been eroded away by the arthritic process (Fig. 10-84). The slope parallel to the intercondylar eminence is carefully removed with an osteotome. Once the new level of the tibial plateau has been developed, the tibial marking template is used to outline the area to be cut out for the new trough. The correct thickness of

the tibial trial component is selected to rebuild the tibia back to the appropriate level. Cement should never be used to build up a deformity because the cement tends to crack and break. It is important not to overcorrect the deformity as is usually done when performing an osteotomy. It should be remembered that most patients have some bowleg or knock-knee deformity. Overcorrection of the deformity will result in tightening the collateral ligaments and will prevent the components from gliding easily. They will tend to rock open and bind posteriorly (Fig. 10-151). This can severely limit flexion postoperatively and also create pain by stretching of the soft

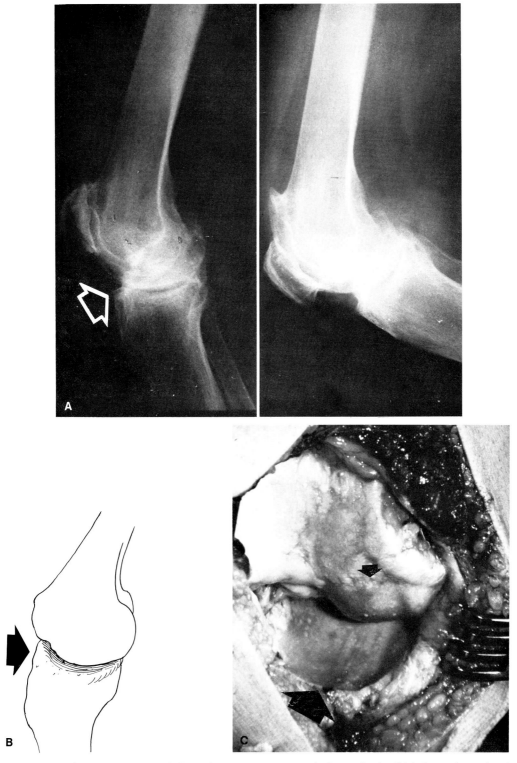

FIG. 10-146 Flexion contracture. A. Lateral roentgenogram reveals depression in tibial plateau (arrow) and bony ledge that blocks full extension. B. Diagram of depression in tibia and anterior bony ledge (arrow). C. Surgical view of depression and anterior ledge. A ridge in the femoral condyle corresponds with the anterior edge of the tibia.

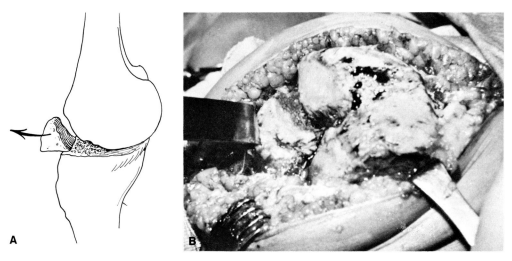

FIG 10-147 Correction of flexion contracture with Modular Knee unit. A. Diagram showing anterior ledge of the tibia to be excised. B. Surgical view showing anterior ledge being excised with an osteotome.

tissues. It is important in correcting severe valgus deformities to caution the patient about the possibility of a peroneal palsy. As long as overcorrection is avoided, peroneal palsy should not be a problem.

MACINTOSH PLATEAU. Patients with unsatisfactory MacIntosh or similar tibial plateau prostheses are also candidates for the Marmor Modular Knee. The prosthesis should be removed, and the layer of fibrous tissue beneath the plateau should be cleaned away with a curette (Fig. 10-152). The remaining tibial plateau is marked with the template, and the trough is cut out with a power tool. The procedure is similar to that for a varus or valgus deformity. Both compartments may be corrected at the same time to salvage the knee (Fig. 10-153).

LIGAMENTOUS INSTABILITY. Patients with osteoarthritis develop ligamentous instability because bone destruction will result in relaxation of the ligaments. The anterior cruciate ligament may be destroyed by osteophyte formation in the intercondylar notch. In advanced osteoarthritis sharp osteophytes tend to erode through the anterior cruciate ligament as medial-lateral subluxation occurs with a

varus or valgus deformity. The collateral ligaments are always intact in osteoarthritis unless trauma has been superimposed upon the arthritis.

Ligamentous stability is obtained by inserting tibial components which tend to tighten the ligaments by lifting the femoral condyle up similar to jacking up a car (Fig. 10-154). In some patients it has been necessary to repair the medial collateral ligament by overlapping the ligament after dividing it if it still remains loose following the insertion of a thick plateau. Following repair of the medial collateral ligament, a soft dressing is applied and flexion is retarded for about one week, and then gradually the same postoperative course is used as for any Marmor Modular Knee replacement (Fig. 10-155).

TIBIAL PLATEAU FRACTURES. The Marmor Modular Knee is useful also in patients with depressed tibial plateau fractures. It is important to wait until the fracture has healed before considering a total knee replacement of this compartment (Fig. 10-156). The bone will usually be extremely soft from the fracture, and the patient who had a normal knee will not appreciate a total knee if he has

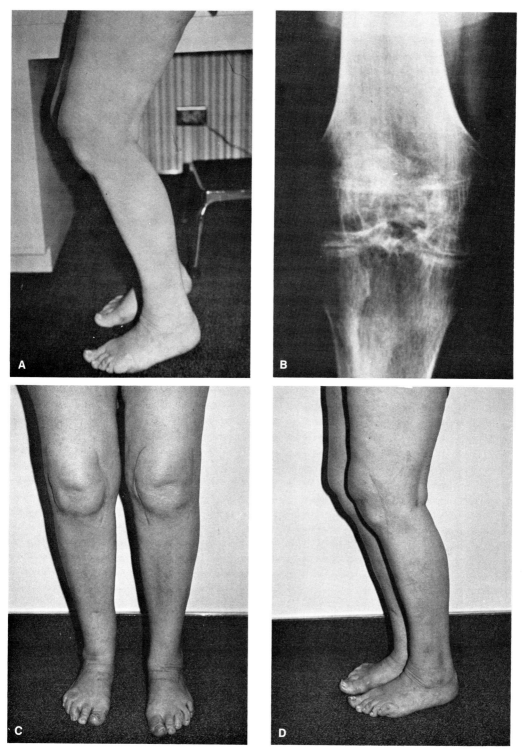

FIG. 10-148 Correction of flexion contractures of 45°. A. Preoperative lateral view. Patient can stand only on her toes and can walk only short distances. B. Preoperative roentgenogram reveals destruction of the joint space. C. Photograph 6 months after Marmor Modular Knee replacement. D. Lateral view. There is a slight flexion deformity, but patient can stand and walk flat on her feet and is able to take care of her home and family.

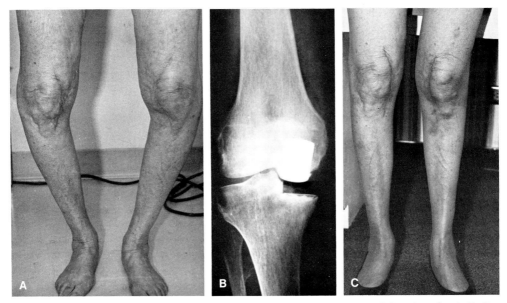

FIG. 10-149 Varus deformities. A. Preoperative photograph showing varus deformity of 25°. B. Postoperative roentgenogram of medial compartment replacement. C. Postoperative photograph following replacement of medial compartments of both knee joints.

symptoms postoperatively. It is better to allow the wound to heal and the bone to solidify before considering total knee replacement. Many patients with severe depression of the tibial plateau can manage for a number of years without any symptoms whatsoever. Therefore, one cannot always determine from the roentgenogram whether reconstruction is necessary.

The medial collateral ligament should always be checked because in some lateral tibial plateau fractures the collateral ligament is ruptured (Fig. 10-157). If there is any concern about the condition of the medial collateral ligament, a stress roentgenogram would be of value. If the ligament has been ruptured, surgical repair will have to be considered at the time of Marmor Modular Knee replacement of the lateral compartment.

Patients with limited range of motion with a tibial plateau fracture should be investigated in regard to the opposite compartment. Although the compart-

ment looks perfectly normal on the preoperative film, a severely damaged compartment may be found at the time of surgery. Frequently this compartment must be replaced, and it is wise to caution the patient preoperatively. This is seen most often in traumatic arthritis where the knee joint has been markedly involved and motion is limited. The articular cartilage of the side that is not severely involved often is destroyed, or there will be adhesions that prevent motion. In traumatic arthritis, the femoral condyles may be distorted and will require remodeling at the time of operation (Fig. 10-158). Patients who have limited motion in extension will have limited motion postoperatively because usually the quadriceps mechanism is adherent to the femur or contracted. These patients may at a subsequent time require a quadricepsplasty to regain further motion.

HEMOPHILIA. Blood dyscrasia such as hemophilia can produce severe destruction within the knee joint. Progression is

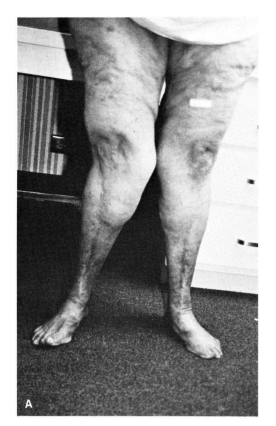

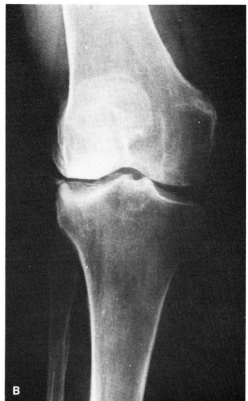

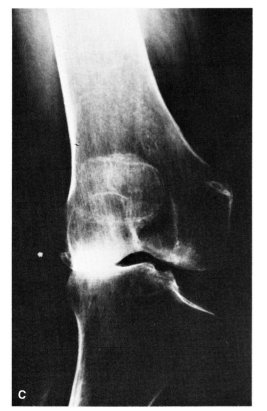

FIG. 10-150 Valgus deformities. A. Preoperative photograph of severe deformity in right leg. The 72-year-old patient was unable to walk. B. Roentgenogram (nonstanding) revealing some pathologic change in the lateral compartment. C. Roentgenogram (standing) revealing narrowing of the lateral compartment and widening of the medial side.

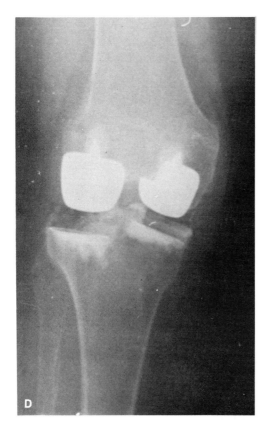

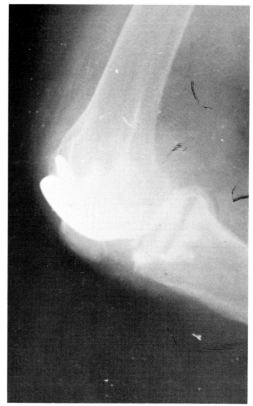

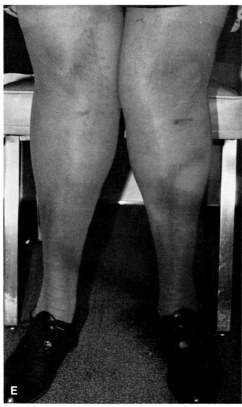

FIG. 10-150 (Cont'd.) D. Postoperative roentgenograms of Marmor Modular Knee units in place. Anterior view reveals correction of valgus deformity of 30°. E. Photograph 1 year postoperatively. The patient can walk without difficulty and has excellent correction of the valgus deformity with over 90° of motion and no pain.

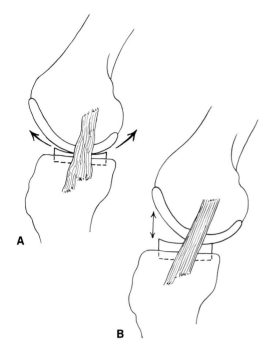

FIG. 10-151 Correction of varus or valgus deformity. A Gliding motion on flexion and extension with relaxed collateral ligament. B. Overcorrection with stretched ligament binding of posterior portion, and opening of the anterior portion.

gradual, and the repeated hemorrhages produce severe synovitis with loss of the articular cartilage. These patients frequently are addicted to drugs because of the severe pain or very close to addiction. After proper medical evaluation and regulating their blood preoperatively under the care of a hematologist, surgery can be performed in a routine manner. Synovectomy is advised to remove the villous diseased synovium which may be trapped in the joint and cause postoperative bleeding. These patients tolerate surgery well and are improved by the replacement of the articular surface of their knees. The pain relief is dramatic and the surgery is extremely worthwhile.

PATELLOFEMORAL ARTHRITIS. Patellofemoral arthritis, frequently seen in advanced osteoarthritis, is often discussed in total knee replacement. Many authors believe that if the articular surface of the patella is not replaced at the time of total knee replacement, the prosthesis is not a true total knee but a partial knee replacement. If the roentgenograms of a patient reveal patellofemoral arthritis along with narrowing of the joint space, the operation of choice is not patellectomy but replacement of the joint surfaces of the compartment involved.

It is surprising how often patients will continue to have pain on weight bearing after a patellectomy for this type of problem. Patients with specific patellofemoral arthritis have most of their symptoms on flexing the knee. When

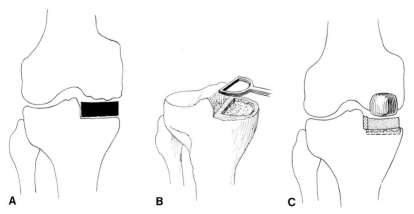

FIG. 10-152 Replacement of the MacIntosh plateau prosthesis. A. Prosthesis to be removed. B. Development of new trough for Marmor Modular Knee unit in tibial plateau. C. Defect built up with tibial plateau component opposite femoral unit.

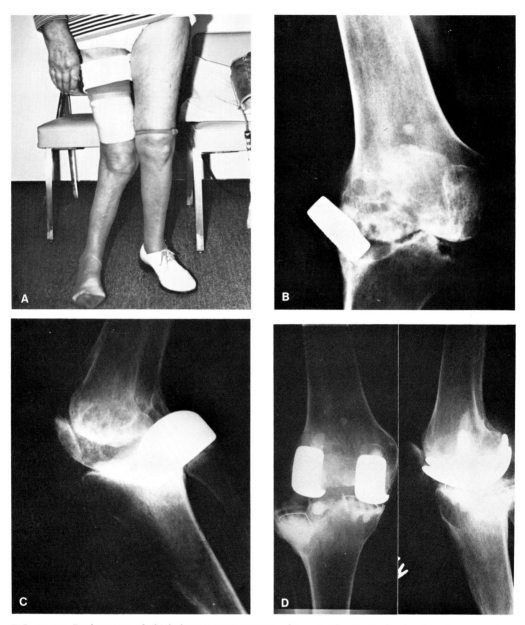

FIG. 10-153 Replacement of tibial plateau components in rheumatoid patient who developed severe valgus deformity requiring use of long-leg brace. A. Preoperative photograph. B. Roentgenogram showing plateau protruding obliquely out of the joint. C. Lateral view showing plateau had completely migrated from its tibial position. Destruction of femoral condyle is evident. D. Roentgenograms after replacement with Marmor Modular Knee unit.

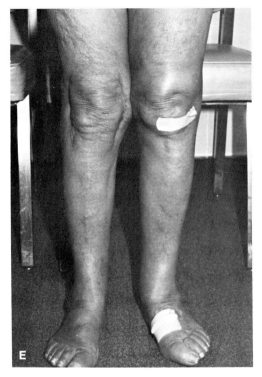
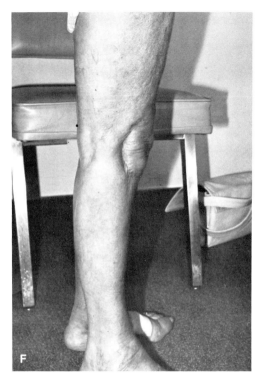

FIG. 10-153 (Cont'd.) E. Clinical view 2 years after replacement. The patient is ambulatory and has minimal discomfort. F. Lateral view revealing excellent correction in full extention. The patient had 110° flexion.

they are getting up from a sitting position or sitting down, the patella grates against the articular surface of the femoral condyles. The only indication, then, for patellectomy in patients with arthritis is localized patellofemoral arthritis with a normal standing anteroposterior roentgenogram (Fig. 10-159). This does occur occasionally and in those patients patellectomy or patelloplasty is indicated. The patella should not be removed at the time of a total knee replacement, regardless of its condition. The patella in patients with unicompart-

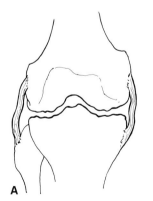
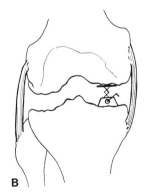
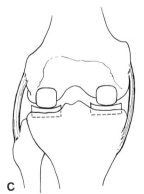

FIG. 10-154 Correction of ligamentous instability. A. Relaxation of the ligaments. B. The effect of jacking the femur up to increase distance between femur and tibia. C. Tightening of ligaments by replacing articular surfaces with Marmor Modular Knee unit.

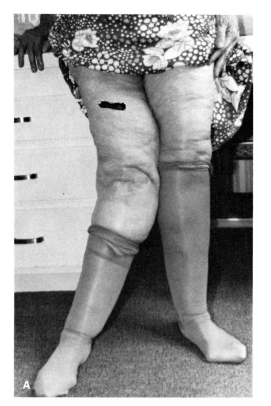

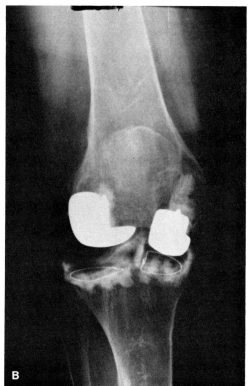

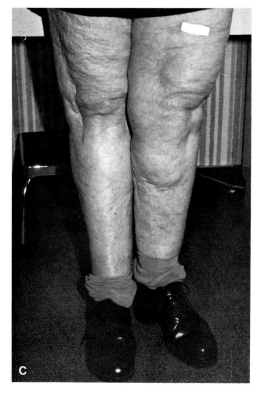

FIG. 10-155 Ligamentous instability. A. Preoperative photograph of 70-year-old patient with severe valgus deformity of the right knee and gross instability. B. Roentgenogram 1 year after insertion of Marmor Modular Knee unit. C. The patient has 90° of motion and walks without a brace.

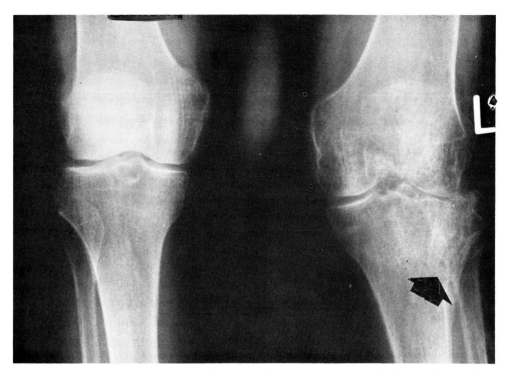

FIG. 10-156 Tibial plateau fracture in left knee (arrow). For 3 years patient had been able to ambulate without difficulty.

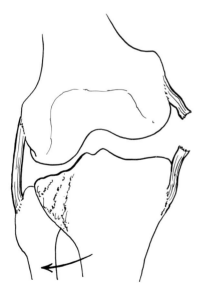

FIG. 10-157 Drawing showing rupture of medial collateral ligament that often accompanies lateral tibial plateau fracture.

ment disease generally is in reasonable condition but may have some osteophytes that can be cut away around the periphery, especially at the lower pole. If the femoral component is well seated anteriorly, it will not catch the patella and should not cause symptoms. In some patients the patella may be shaved down to a wafer, but in general my procedure has been to undercut the patella away from the center in a gull-wing fashion to allow only a small articular surface to touch the femoral condyles. (We have called it the "Jonathan Livingston Seagull" procedure.) This gull-wing effect lifts the edges of the patella away from the femoral components and maintains the thickness of the patella so that the quadriceps mechanism is not interfered with. It is not unusual for some patients to have patellar symptoms that gradually disappear within a year.

It is important also to remove any osteophytes along the superior aspect of

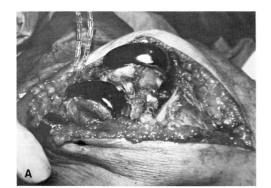
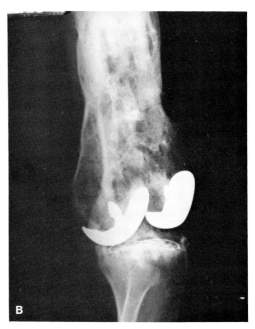

FIG. 10-158 Remodeling femoral condyles distorted by traumatic arthritis. A. Surgical view showing 90° rotation of femoral condyles and positioning of the femoral components. B. Postoperative roentgenogram revealing comminuted femoral shaft and the position of the components.

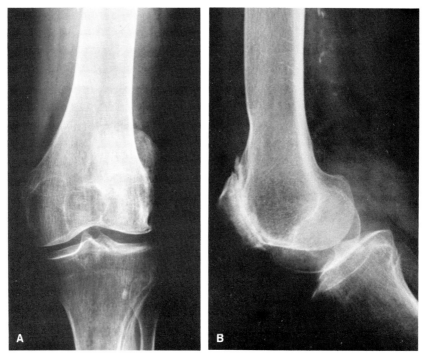

FIG. 10-159 Indication for patellectomy. A. Anteroposterior roentgenogram (standing). The joint appears normal. B. Lateral roentgenogram revealing isolated patellofemoral arthritis.

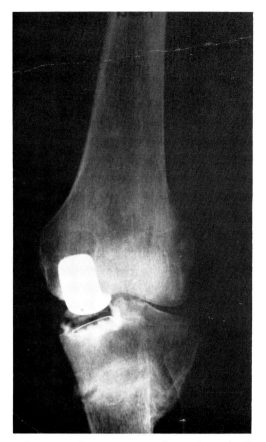 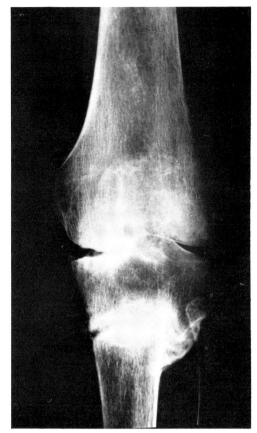

FIG. 10-160 Roentgenogram of a patient who has had a previous osteotomy of the left knee with a recurrence of severe disease in the medial aspect of the joint (right). The left view shows the replacement of the medial compartment by a Marmor Modular Knee. The patient was free of pain.

the femoral condyles where the patella will pass back and forth. The rough surfaces should be cut away with a rongeur and then smoothed down flush with the shaft of the femur with a rasp. This procedure will prevent some of the postoperative symptoms related to the patella.

Previous Osteotomy. Patients who have had unsuccessful osteotomies for severe deformities from rheumatoid or osteoarthritis in the knee or after a number of years have pain from wearing out of the joint surfaces may have the knee salvaged by the Marmor Modular Knee. The deformity from the previous osteotomy must be considered and cannot be corrected by the knee replacement be-

cause the deformity is distal to the knee joint. If the opposite compartment still has good articular cartilage, only the diseased compartment needs to be replaced (Fig. 10-160). If both compartments are involved, both should be replaced.

Bibliography

Rheumatoid Arthritis

Adams, R.: Rheumatic arthritis of the knee joint. Dublin, J. Med. Science, 17:520, 1840.

Aidem, M. P., and Baker, L.D.: Synovectomy of the knee joint in rheumatoid arthritis. J.A.M.A., *187*:4, 1964.

Baker, W. M.: Chronic disease of the knee joint—large cyst of the calf. St. Bart. Hosp. Reports, *13*:254, 1877.

Benjamin, A.: Double osteotomy for the painful knee in rheumatoid arthritis and osteoarthritis. J. Bone Joint Surg., *51-B*:694, 1969.

Bernstein, M. A.: Synovectomy of the knee joint in chronic arthritis. Ann. Surg., *98*:1096, 1933.

Boon-Itt, S. B.: A study of the end results of synovectomy of the knee. J. Bone Joint Surg., *12*:853, 1930.

Boyd, H. B., and Hawkins, B. L.: Patellectomy; a simplified technique. Surg., Gynecol., Obstet., *86*:357, 1948.

Brown, J. E., McGraw, W. H., and Shaw, D. T.: Use of cutis as an interposing membrane in arthroplasty of the knee. J. Bone Joint Surg., *40-A*:1003, 1958.

Brown, P. W., and Urban, J. G.: Early weight-bearing treatment of open fractures of the tibia. An end-result study of sixty-three cases. J. Bone Joint Surg., *51-A*:59, 1969.

Burleson, R. J., Bickel, W. H., and Dahlen, D. C.: Popliteal cyst. J. Bone Joint Surg., *38-A*:1265, 1956.

Carruthers, F. W.: Debridement and synovectomy of the knee joint. Western J. Surg., *68*:382, 1960.

Carruthers, F. W.: Synovectomy of the knee joint. South. Med. J., *33*:550, 1940.

Charnley, J., and Lowe, H. G.: A study of end results of compression arthrodesis of the knee. J. Bone Joint Surg., *40-B*:633, 1958.

Childress, H. M.: Popliteal cysts associated with undiagnosed posterior lesions of the medial meniscus. J. Bone Joint Surg., *36-A*:1233, 1954.

Convery, F. R., Conaty, J. P., and Nickel, V. L.: Flexion deformities of the knee in rheumatoid arthritis. Clin. Orthop., *74*:90, 1971.

Cooper, R. R.: Orthopedic surgery in arthritis of the knee and foot, J. Am. Phys. Ther. Assoc., *44*:614, 1964.

Coventry, M. B., et al.: A new geometric knee for total knee replacement. Clin. Orthop., *83*:157, 1972.

Dehne, E., et al.: Non-operative treatment of the fractured tibia by immediate weight-bearing. J. Trauma, *2*:514, 1961.

DePalma, A. F.: Diseases of the Knee. Philadelphia, J. B. Lippincott Co., 1954.

Eyring, E. J.: The therapeutic potential of synovectomy in juvenile rheumatoid arthritis. Arthritis Rheum., *11*:688, 1968.

Geens, S.: Synovectomy and debridement of the knee in rheumatoid arthritis. J. Bone Joint Surg., *51-A*:617, 1969.

Geens, S., et al.: Synovectomy and debridement of the knee in rheumatoid arthritis. J. Bone Joint Surg., *51-A*:626, 1969.

Ghormley, R. K.: End results of synovectomy of the knee joint. Am. J. Surg., *53*:455, 1941.

Goldie, I., and Schlossman, D.: Radiologic changes in rheumatoid knee joints. Clin. Orthop., *64*:101, 1969.

Gunston, F. H.: Polycentric knee arthroplasty. J. Bone Joint Surg., *53-B*:272, 1971.

Hall, A. P., and Scott, J. J.: Synovial cysts and rupture of the knee joint in rheumatoid arthritis. Ann. Rheum. Dis., *25*:32, 1966.

Harvey, J. P., Jr., and Corcos, J.: Large cysts in lower leg originating in the knee joint occurring in patients with rheumatoid arthritis. Arthritis Rheum., *3*:218, 1960.

Heyman, C. H.: Synovectomy of the knee joint. Surg. Gynecol. Obstet., *46*:127, 1928.

Hughes, G. R., and Pridie, R. B.: Acute synovial rupture of the knee—a differential diagnosis from deep vein thrombosis. Proc. R. Soc. Med., *63*:587, 1970.

Inge, G. A. L.: Eighty-six cases of chronic synovitis of the knee joint treated by synovectomy. J.A.M.A., *111*:2451, 1938.

Johansen, P. E., and Sylvest, O.: Synovial fluid changes in degenerative joint disease, rheumatoid arthritis and traumatic arthritis. Acta Rheum., *7*:240, 1961.

Jones, W. N.: Mold arthroplasty of the knee joint. Clin. Orthop., *66*:82, 1969.

Kay, N. M., and Martins, H. D.: The MacIntosh tibial plateau hemiprosthesis for the rheumatoid knee. J. Bone Joint Surg., *54-B*:256, 1972.

Kettlekamp, D. B., and Chao, E. Y.: A method for quantitative analysis of medial and lateral compression forces at the knee during standing. Clin. Orthop., *83*:202, 1972.

Key, J. A.: The reformation of synovial membrane in the knees of rabbits after synovectomy. J. Bone Joint Surg., *7*:793, 1925.

London, P. S.: Synovectomy of knee in rheumatoid arthritis, J. Bone Joint Surg., *37-B*:392, 1955.

Lucas, D. B., and Murray, W. R.: Arthrodesis of the knee by double plating. J. Bone Joint Surg., *43-A*:795, 1961.

MacIntosh, D. L.: Hemiarthroplasty of the knee using a space occupying prosthesis for painful varus and valgus deformities. J. Bone Joint Surg., *40-A*:1431, 1958.

MacIntosh, D. L., and Hunter, G. A.: The use of the hemiarthroplasty prosthesis for advanced osteoarthritis and rheumatoid arthritis of the knee. J. Bone Joint Surg., *54-B*:244, 1972.

Magnuson, P. B.: Technic of debridement of the knee joint for arthritis. Surg. Clin. North Am., *26*:249, 1946.

Marmor, L.: Surgery of rheumatoid knee, synovectomy and debridement. J. Bone Joint Surg., *55-A*:535, 1973.

Marmor, L.: Salvage of the rheumatoid knee by osteotomy. J. West, Pacific Assoc., *11*:3, 1974.

Marmor, L.: Surgery of the rheumatoid knee. Am. J. Surg., *111*:211, 1966.

Marmor, L.: Synovectomy of the rheumatoid knee. Clin. Orthop., *44*:151, 1966.

Maudsley, R. H., and Arden, G. P.: Rheumatoid cysts of the calf and their relation to Baker's cyst of the knee. J. Bone Joint Surg., *43-B*:87, 1961.

McKeever, D.: Patellar prosthesis. J. Bone Joint Surg., *37-A*:1074, 1955.

McKeever, D.: Tibial plateau prosthesis. Clin. Orthop., *18*:86, 1960.

McMaster, M.: Synovectomy of the knee in juvenile rheumatoid arthritis. J. Bone Joint Surg., *54-B*:263, 1972.

Milch, H.: Juxta-articular partial tibial osteotomy. Surg. Gynecol. Obstet., *59*:87, 1934.

Milch, R. A.: Rationale and technique for radical surgical debridement in the treatment of chronic arthritis of the knee joint. Minerva Med., *2*:1514, 1961.

Mori, M., and Ogawa, R.: Anterior capsulotomy in the treatment of rheumatoid arthritis of the knee joint. Arthritis Rheum., *6*:130, 1963.

Pap, K., and Krompecher, S.: Arthroplasty of the knee, J. Bone Joint Surg., *43-A*:523, 1961.

Pardee, M. L.: Synovectomy of knee joint. J. Bone Joint Surg., *30-A*:908, 1948.

Perri, J. A., Rodnan, G. P., and Mankin, H. J.: Giant synovial cysts of the calf in patients with rheumatoid arthritis. J. Bone Joint Surg., *50-A*:709, 1968.

Pinder, I. M.: Treatment of the popliteal cyst in the rheumatoid knee. J. Bone Joint Surg., *55-B*:119, 1973.

Platt, G., and Pepler, C.: Mold arthroplasty of the knee. J. Bone Joint Surg., *51-B*:76, 1969.

Potter, T. A.: Arthroplasty of the knee with tibial metallic implants of the McKeever and MacIntosh design. Surg. Clin. North Am., *49*:903, 1969.

Ranawat, C. J., Ecker, M. L., and Straub, L. R.: Synovectomy and debridement of the knee in rheumatoid arthritis. Arthritis Rheum., *15*:571, 1972.

Shiers, L. G. P.: Arthroplasty of the knee. J. Bone Joint Surg., *42-B*:31, 1960.

Shorbe, H. B., and Dobson, C. H.: Patellectomy, repair of extensor mechanism. J. Bone Joint Surg., *40-A*:1281, 1958.

Somerville, E. W.: Flexion contractures of the knee. J. Bone Joint Surg., *42-B*:730, 1960.

Speed, J. S.: Synovectomy of the knee joint. J.A.M.A., *83*:1814, 1924.

Steindler, A.: Synovectomy and fat pad removal in the knee. J.A.M.A., *84*:16, 1925.

Swett, P.: Review of synovectomy. J. Bone Joint Surg., *20*:68, 1938.

Swett, P.: Synovectomy in chronic infectious arthritis, J. Bone Joint Surg., 5:110, 1923.

Taylor, A. R., and Ansell, B. M.: Arthrography of the knee before and after synovectomy for rheumatoid arthritis. J. Bone Joint Surg., 54-B:110, 1972.

Torppi, P., and Heikkinen, E.: Partial synovectomy as a therapeutic method for rheumatoid and non-specific synovitis of the knee. Ann. Chir. Gynaecol. Fenn., 54:29, 1965.

Townley, C. O.: Articular plate replacement arthroplasty for the knee joint. Clin. Orthop., 36:77, 1964.

Walldius, B.: Arthroplasty of the knee using an endoprosthesis. Acta Orthop. Scand., 30:137, 1960.

West, F. E.: End results of patellectomy. J. Bone Joint Surg., 44-A:1089, 1962.

Wilson, P. D.: Posterior capsulotomy in certain flexion contractures of the knee. J. Bone Joint Surg., 11:40, 1929.

Wolcott, W. E. Regeneration of synovial membrane following synovectomy. J. Bone Joint Surg., 9:67, 1927.

Young, H.: Use of a hinged Vitallium prosthesis for arthroplasty of the knee. J. Bone Joint Surg., 45-A:1627, 1963.

Osteoarthritis

Bauer, G. C. H., Insall, J., and Koshino, T.: Tibial osteotomy for gonarthrosis. J. Bone Joint Surg., 51-A:1545, 1969.

Brady, T. A., and Garber, J. N.: Knee joint replacement using Shiers knee hinge. J. Bone Joint Surg., 56-A:1610, 1974.

Charnley, J.: Positive pressure in arthrodesis of the knee joint. J. Bone Joint Surg., 30-B:478, 1948.

Chrisman, O. D., and Snook, G. A.: The role of patelloplasty and patellectomy in the arthritic knee. Clin. Orthop., 101:40, 1974.

Coventry, M. B.: Osteotomy of the upper portion of the tibia for degenerative arthritis of the knee. J. Bone Joint Surg., 47-A:984, 1965.

Coventry, M. B., et al.: A new geometric knee for total knee arthroplasty. Clin. Orthop., 83:157, 1972.

Devas, M. B.: High tibial osteotomy for arthritis of the knee. J. Bone Joint Surg., 51-B:95, 1969.

Engelbrecht, E.: The "sledge" prosthesis: A partial prosthesis for destructions of the knee joint. Chirurg (Berlin), 42:510, 1971.

Frymoyer, J. W., and Hoaglund, F. T.: The role of arthrodesis in reconstruction of the knee. Clin. Orthop., 101:82, 1974.

Gariepy, R.: Genu varum treated by high tibial osteotomy. J. Bone Joint Surg., 46-B:783, 1964.

Gariepy, R.: Genu varum treated by high tibial osteotomy. Paper read at the fourth combined meeting of the American, British, and Canadian Orthopaedic Associations, Vancouver, British Columbia, Canada, June 18, 1964.

Harris, W. R., and Kostuik, J. P.: High tibial osteotomy for osteoarthritis of the knee. J. Bone Joint Surg., 52-A:330, 1970.

Helal, B.: The pain in primary osteoarthritis of the knee. Its causes and treatment by osteotomy. Postgrad. Med. J., 41:172, 1965.

Insall, J., Shoji, H., and Mayer, V.: High tibial osteotomy. J. Bone Joint Surg., 56-A:1397, 1974.

Jackson, J. P.: Osteotomy for osteoarthritis of the knee. J. Bone Joint Surg., 40-B:826, 1958.

Jackson, J. P.: The treatment of osteoarthritis of the knee. Physiotherapy, 52:244, 1966.

Jackson, J. P. and Waugh, W.: Tibial osteotomy for osteoarthritis of the knee. J. Bone Joint Surg., 43-B:746, 1961.

Johnson, R. J., et al.: Factors affecting late results after meniscectomy. J. Bone Joint Surg, 56-A, 719, 1974.

Magnuson, P. B.: Joint debridement. Surg. Gynecol. Obstet. 73:1, 1941.

Magnuson, P. B.: Technique of debridement of the knee joint for arthritis. Surg. Clin. North Am., 26:249, 1946.

Marmor, L.: Osteoarthritis of the knee. J.A.M.A., 218:213, 1971.

McKeever, D. C., and Elliot, R. B.: Tibial plateau prosthesis. Clin. Orthop., *18*:86, 1960.

Milch, R. A. (editor): Surgery of Arthritis. Baltimore, Williams and Wilkins, *13*:241, 1964.

Murray, D. G., and Barranco, S.: Femoral condylar hemiarthroplasty of the knee. Clin. Orthop., *101*:68, 1974.

Potter, T. A.: Arthroplasty of the knee with tibial metalic implants of the McKeever and MacIntosh design. Surg. Clin. North Am., *49*:903, 1969.

Shiers, L. G. P.: Arthroplasty of the knee. J. Bone Joint Surg., *42-B*:31, 1960.

Smillie, I. S.: The changing pattern and pathology of internal derangements of the knee. J. Bone Joint Surg., *46-B*:775, 1964.

Torgerson, W. R.: Tibial osteotomy in the treatment of osteoarthritis of the knee. Surg. Clin. North Am., *45*:779, 1965.

Walldius, B.: Arthroplasty of the knee using an endoprosthesis. Acta Orthop. Scand., *30*:137, 1961.

Arthritis in the ankle joint leads to loss of motion and increasing pain. Trauma to the ankle joint tends to be one of the precipitating causes of arthritis and is often associated with fractures that involve the articular surface. This results in gradual loss of the articular cartilage over the years because of incongruity of the joint surfaces.

Rheumatoid arthritis can also involve the ankle joint but is not frequently a cause of severe disability in most patients. The treatment of arthritis of the ankle joint will depend upon the stage of the disease and the patient's symptoms.

Anatomy

The problems in the ankle may be divided anatomically into the areas within the joint and the areas adjacent to the joint capsule. The ankle joint is composed of the talus which is set into a mortise formed by the tibia and fibula enclosing the talus within the medial and lateral malleoli. This type of articulation forms a hinge joint which allows the talus to move upward and downward but does not allow rotation or pronation and supination. The latter motions take place in the subtalar joint. The upper surface of the talus, which is convex, is so firmly supported by the mortise that lateral mobility will not occur at any point in the range of ankle motion. The synovial tissue that lines the capsule of the ankle joint is attached to the borders of the articular surface. As compared to the knee joint, the ankle joint has a minimal amount of synovial tissue. The deltoid ligament, which is attached above to the medial malleolus and below to the navicular, sustentaculum tali of the calcaneus, and the talus, tends to enclose the ankle joint in a firm, fibrous capsular attachment. On the lateral aspect of the ankle, the lateral collateral ligaments perform a similar duty (Fig. 11-1). These ligaments tend to enclose the capsule and synovial tissue so that swelling of the ankle will be obvious only anteriorly or posteriorly. Any swelling noted on the medial or lateral border of the ankle will be associated with the tendon sheaths in these areas. Each of the tendons crossing the ankle joint is enclosed partially in a synovial sheath for approximately 8 cm (Fig. 11-2). These tendon sheaths are particularly prone to become involved in rheumatoid arthritis.

The neurovascular bundle supplying

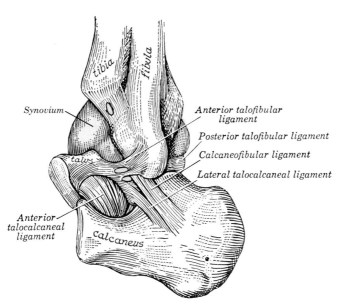

FIG. 11-1 Lateral aspect of the left ankle showing the synovial membrane of the capsule (distended) and the collateral ligaments. (From Gray's Anatomy of the Human Body, 29th edition. C. M. Goss, editor, Philadelphia, Lea & Febiger, 1973.)

the foot tends to pass posterior to the medial malleolus through a tarsal tunnel. Swelling in this area can frequently lead to symptoms similar to those seen in a carpal tunnel syndrome in the wrist. Injections in this area should be made cautiously because of the proximity of the neurovascular bundle to the posterior tibial tendon.

A large bursa located between the calcaneus and the Achilles tendon can become involved in rheumatoid arthritis, occasionally interfering with the motion of the ankle joint.

Physical Examination

The patient should be observed walking, standing, and sitting down.

Inspection

While the patient is standing, the observer should check the relationship of the ankle joint and subtalar joint. In most patients severe pronation of the rheumatoid foot is due to involvement of the subtalar joint and not the ankle joint (Fig. 11-3). Occasionally destruction of the ankle can produce some pronation because of instability within the ankle joint.

Localized swelling along the medial or lateral side of the ankle is usually due to involvement of the tendon sheaths (Fig. 11-4). Localized swelling on the anterior aspect of the ankle joint is observed in patients with synovial hyperplasia involving the ankle. The synovium can swell only anteriorly because of the strong collateral ligaments and capsule about the medial and lateral sides of the ankle joint. Swelling noted in the posterior aspect of the ankle may often be due to involvement of the Achilles bursa. Extensive swelling and

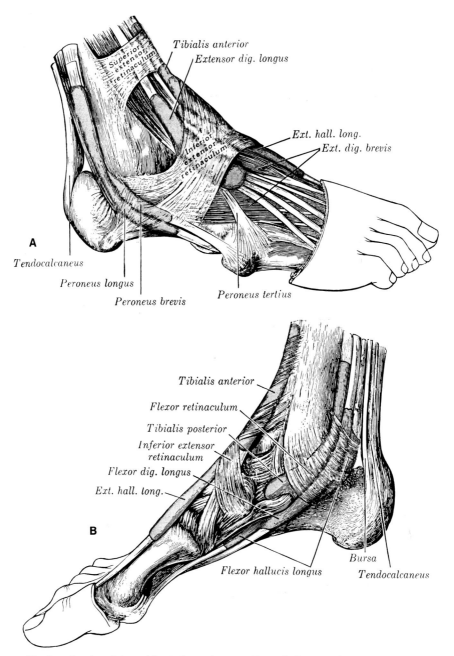

FIG. 11-2 Tendon sheaths of the ankle. A. Lateral aspect. B. Medial aspect. (From Gray's Anatomy of the Human Body, 29th ed. C. M. Goss, editor. Philadelphia, Lea & Febiger, 1973.)

enlargement of the entire ankle joint are indications of osteoarthritis as a result of previous trauma. Scars from surgical incisions may be related to internal fixation of severe fractures of the ankle joint, which may lead to traumatic arthritis.

Palpation

Palpation can be valuable in the diagnostic evaluation of the ankle. Localized tenderness over the peroneal tendon sheaths and thickening are signs

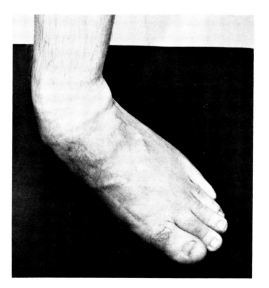

FIG. 11-3 Severe pronation of the foot.

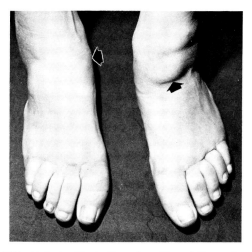

FIG. 11-5 An illustration of swelling of the posterior tendon of the right ankle (arrow) and of a large synovial mass protruding from the left ankle (arrow).

of tenosynovitis. Tenderness of the posterior tibial tendon sheath on the medial side of the ankle on palpation and on inversion and eversion of the foot is another indication of tendinitis. Tenderness over the anterior aspect of the ankle joint and thickening of the synovial membrane will give a doughy feeling on palpation and tend to localize the pathologic condition to the ankle joint (Fig. 11-5). Palpation of the Achilles tendon should be carried out to determine its continuity because ruptures do occur in rheumatoid arthritis without severe pain.

Range of Motion

Since the ankle joint is primarily a hinge joint with the talus fitting in the mortise, the only movements possible are flexion (plantar-flexion) and extension (dorsiflexion). The normal range of motion is approximately 85° for extension and to 155° for flexion. Loss of motion is noted in patients with advanced rheumatoid arthritis of the joint. Limited range of motion and swelling of the joint are frequently seen in advanced osteoarthritis of the ankle joint.

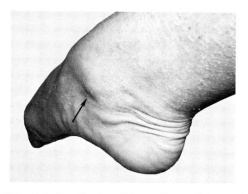

FIG. 11-4 Localized swelling on the medial aspect (arrow) of the ankle.

Rheumatoid Arthritis

Pain and loss of motion are the major problems in rheumatoid arthritis of the ankle joint. The disease process primarily affects the synovial tissue within the ankle joint and the synovial sheaths surrounding the tendons about the joint. The various bursae, especially the

Achilles bursa, can also be involved early in rheumatoid arthritis. Both ankles tend to be involved simultaneously, but frequently to a different extent. Severe ankle disease tends to occur late in the course of rheumatoid arthritis, except in young patients who may have primary involvement of the ankle joint. The disease of the ankle is often associated with rheumatic symptoms in multiple other joints in the lower extremity.

Stress Fractures of the Fibula

The rheumatoid patient may develop stress fractures of the fibula within several inches of the ankle joint. The patient will often complain of pain in the ankle on weight bearing and difficulty in walking.

A stress fracture is easy to overlook during diagnosis. On physical examination of the ankle there may be slight swelling at the lower end of the fibula and localized tenderness over the area of the stress fracture. Roentgenologic examination may be delayed because the physician may believe that the pain is due to arthritis of the ankle joint. Roentgenograms will reveal evidence of periosteal changes and even a stress fracture line at the site of localized tenderness found clinically (Fig. 11-6).

Treatment is symptomatic, and cast immobilization is not necessary for this problem. It is better to avoid casts in patients with rheumatoid arthritis to prevent the development of stiffness in the ankle joint that will delay their rehabilitation. Occasionally crutches or a posterior splint may be necessary.

Achilles Bursitis

The Achilles bursa or retrocalcaneal bursa is located between the Achilles tendon and the calcaneus; it is lined with

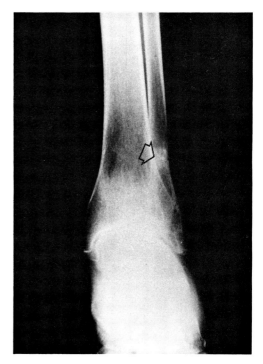

FIG. 11-6 Roentgenogram revealing a healing stress fracture of the lower end of the fibula (arrow), pathologic changes from rheumatoid arthritis, and loss of the normal mortise in the ankle.

synovial tissues which can become inflamed due to rheumatoid arthritis. The patient will experience pain and swelling behind the ankle and difficulty in dorsiflexion of the foot. On examination the normal depression on either side of the Achilles tendon will be found to be lost due to the enlargement of the bursa.

Treatment

Injection of the bursa with a local steroid may frequently relieve the pain and limitation of motion. If severe symptoms persist, surgical excision of the bursa is indicated. The lateral approach to the bursa through a 3-inch incision parallel to the Achilles tendon is safe and adequate. Early motion is advised to allow early return of function of the ankle joint.

Achilles Tenosynovitis

Frequently the patient will complain of pain and swelling on the medial or lateral side of the ankle beneath the malleoli. Since, anatomically, the joint capsule cannot distend the medial or lateral aspect of the ankle, owing to the strong deltoid ligament on the medial side and the collateral ligament on the lateral side, swelling is due to a tenosynovitis of the tendons about the ankle joint.

The peroneal tendon sheath can become inflamed and thickened. Pronation or supination of the foot does not tend to accentuate the symptoms as it usually does in a traumatic tenosynovitis. The persistent swelling in the region of the sheath beneath the lateral malleolus is the best clue (Fig. 11-7). On palpation this area can be quite tender and crepitation can be felt.

Involvement of the posterior tibial sheath may produce pain and swelling on the medial side of the ankle joint behind and below the medial malleolus. The anterior tibial tendon and the extensor tendon sheaths may also be involved with a proliferative rheumatoid synovitis. Swelling occurs beneath the cruciate ligament over the anterior aspect of the ankle.

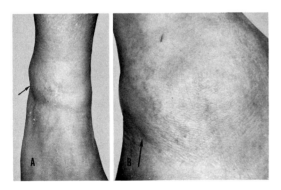

FIG. 11-7 Peroneal tenosynovitis. A. Anterior view of ankle showing swelling (arrow). B. Lateral view of swelling beneath the lateral malleolus.

Treatment

Injection of the sheath with Xylocaine and a local steroid will often bring considerable relief of symptoms. If symptoms are recurrent, surgical release of the tendons and excision of the synovial tissue will bring more lasting relief.

Nerve Entrapment

Occasionally the deep peroneal nerve can become entrapped beneath the annular ligament due to the swelling of the tendon sheaths (Fig. 11-8). The patient will complain of pain over the dorsum of the foot and a feeling of numbness or tingling. Tinel's sign may be elicited over the nerve at the annular ligament.

Treatment

Injection of lidocaine (Xylocaine) and a steroid into the tendon sheaths may relieve the symptoms as the synovitis subsides. If symptoms persist, division of the anterior annular ligament will relieve them permanently.

Tarsal Tunnel Syndrome

The posterior tibial nerve also may be entrapped in the space between the medial malleolus and the Achilles tendon beneath the ligament. The nerve divides beneath the ligament into the medial and lateral plantar nerves to the foot. The median branch supplies sensation to the great toe, to the second and third toes, and to the medial side of the fourth toe. The lateral nerve supplies the lateral aspect of the fourth and fifth toes and the lateral plantar surface of the foot.

The space in the tarsal tunnel between the Achilles tendon and the medial malleolus is occupied by the posterior tibial tendon and sheath, the flexor digitorum longus tendon and sheath, the

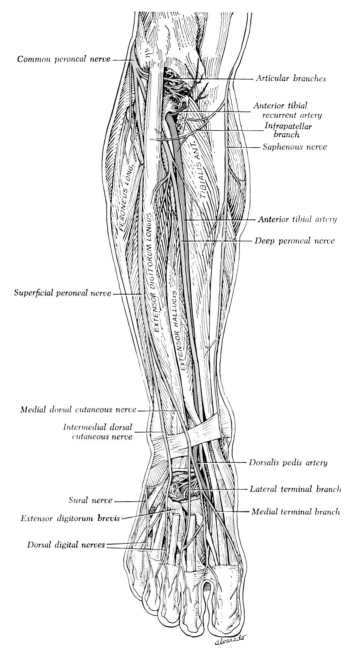

FIG. 11-8 Deep nerves of the anterior leg. (From Gray's Anatomy of the Human Body, 29th ed. C. M. Goss, editor. Philadelphia, Lea & Febiger, 1973.)

posterior tibial artery and veins, the posterior tibial nerve, and the flexor hallucis longus. Swelling of the tendon sheaths in this tunnel can easily lead to compression of the posterior tibial nerve.

The tarsal syndrome resembles the carpal tunnel syndrome. The symptoms consist of pain or paresthesia in the sole of the foot with some radiation into the ankle and calf. Tinel's sign may be present over the nerve in the tarsal tunnel.

Sensory loss may be demonstrated by pinprick or light touch over the sole of the foot.

Treatment

Surgical release of the entrapped nerve is the best therapy. The posterior tibial nerve may be approached through a 3-inch incision parallel to the leg between the Achilles tendon and the medial malleolus. The crural ligament should be divided to release the posterior tibial nerve, and the tendon sheath of the posterior tibial tendon should be opened and any thick synovium removed.

Tendon Ruptures

The proliferative synovium tends to invade the tendon and to interfere with its nutrition leading to necrosis. Therefore, rupture of the tendons about the ankle and foot is not too rare in rheumatoid arthritis. The most frequent tendons to rupture are the Achilles tendon and the posterior tibial, respectively.

Achilles Tendon Rupture

The Achilles tendon is susceptible to rupture because of the frequent involvement of the Achilles bursa by synovial proliferation. The synovium infiltrates the tendon, which will rupture under minimal stress (Fig. 11-9). Bilateral rupture is not uncommon in rheumatoid arthritis, and occasionally both tendons will rupture simultaneously. The patient usually does not complain of pain but experiences difficulty in walking and cannot push off on or rise up on his toes (Fig. 11-10).

On examination a defect may be obvious in the Achilles tendon about 1 inch from the calcaneus since this is the common site of rupture of the tendon. The defect will not be obvious if the patient is seen several weeks after the

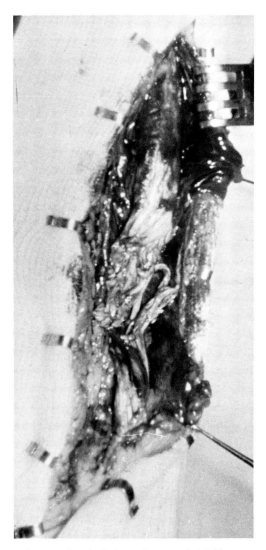

FIG. 11-9 Surgical view of ruptured Achilles tendon.

rupture because of organization of the blood clot and proliferation of fibrous tissue. The patient may have some plantar flexion of the foot, but this is not due to partial rupture of the tendon since rupture is usually complete. The patient will be unable, however, to stand on his toes and raise his heel from the ground. If the reaction to the test described by Thompson for Achilles rupture is positive, this is pathognomic of complete rupture. The patient is asked to kneel on a table or chair with the leg to be tested

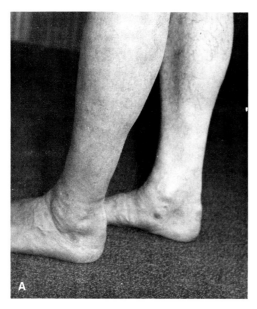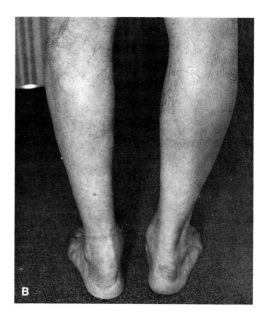

FIG. 11-10 Clinical views of patient with rupture of the left Achilles tendon. A. Lateral view. Note the depression in the area of the Achilles tendon. B. Posterior view. Note flattening of Achilles tendon in left ankle and atrophy of the calf.

extending beyond the edge (Fig. 11-11). The calf is grasped by the examiner's hand and squeezed. A normal tendon will shorten, moving the foot into plantar flexion. A ruptured tendon will not produce plantar flexion.

Soft-tissue roentgenograms may also demonstrate the rupture of the Achilles tendon.

The conservative management of this

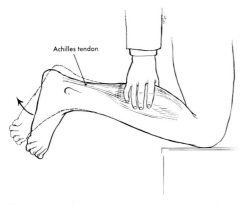

Achilles tendon

FIG. 11-11 Thompson test for rupture of the Achilles tendon. Note position of examiner's hand.

injury, placing the foot in the equinus position in a cast, has not always been successful, and early operative repair may be indicated. A number of techniques are available for repair of the early and late injury.

Lindholm Technique. In the early case, in which the muscle has not contracted, the degenerated tissue should be excised to normal tendon and an end-to-end repair made. If this is not possible with the knee and ankle flexed, the technique described by Lindholm may be used. A flap of proximal tendon is turned down and sutured to the distal end (Fig. 11-12). The leg is then immobilized in a plaster cast with the foot in plantar flexion for 4 to 6 weeks. It is advisable not to immobilize the arthritic patient too long in this position. Having the patient wear a shoe with a heel higher than its mate on the affected foot for about 6 additional months to protect the repair is of value.

McLaughlin Technique. The Mc-Laughlin method of repair may also be

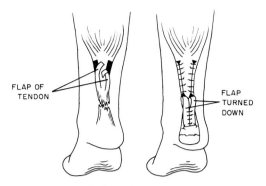

FIG. 11-12 Lindholm technique for repairing rupture of Achilles tendon.

utilized for early or late repair. Internal fixation is employed; this requires a shorter period of immobilization in a cast than does the method described by Lindholm. A bolt is placed through the calcaneus, and a wire is woven through the musculotendinous junction and pulled down to each side of the bolt (Fig. 11-13). This tends to remove the stress on the suture line, allowing a relaxed repair. A "pull-out" wire is placed subcutaneously to aid in the removal of the wire 6 weeks postoperatively. Immobilization with plaster may be used for several weeks after surgery.

Two-pin Technique. Lavine, Kara, and Warren described a two-pin technique for repair of a ruptured Achilles tendon. This method is quite effective in keeping the tendon ends together without tension. Two Steinmann pins ($\frac{1}{8}$ inch in diameter) are inserted in the following manner. One pin is placed through the calcaneus below the insertion of the tendon, and the other pin is placed through the proximal musculotendinous junction. A Charnley clamp is applied and tension is exerted until the ends are coapted (Fig. 11-14). The Steinmann pins may be incorporated in a long leg-cast with the knee flexed and the ankle in an equinus position. Then the Charnley clamp may be removed, if desired. At 4 weeks the cast may be changed and the Steinmann pins removed. A short leg-cast is applied for 3 more weeks. This method may be of value to overcome a large defect in patients with a chronic rupture.

Posterior Tibial Tendon Rupture

The posterior tibial tendon usually ruptures at the medial malleolus within the tendon sheath. The patient will experience weakness of the foot and develop a pronated, painful foot with loss of the longitudinal arch.

Repair. Repair of the tendon is indicated when possible. A free graft or tendon advancement may be necessary to span the area of the degenerated ten-

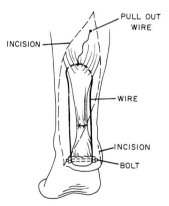

FIG. 11-13 McLaughlin technique for repairing rupture of the Achilles tendon.

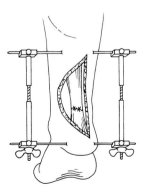

FIG. 11-14 Two-pin technique for repairing rupture of the Achilles tendon.

don. If surgery is not possible or the patient does not desire correction, an arch support will be of value. The arch support should be molded to the foot when it is not bearing weight so that the arch is restored.

Synovitis

The ankle joint itself may be involved by the rheumatoid disease, and the synovial tissue hypertrophy produces pain and swelling of the joint. The thickened synovium limits the range of motion in the joint, and the swelling is obvious in the anterior aspect of the joint. Roentgenograms usually reveal narrowing of the joint space with adjacent sclerosis (Fig. 11-15). It is important to examine the subtalar joint carefully before considering any surgical procedure on the ankle, because frequently both are involved (Fig. 11-16).

Frequently the medial and lateral tendon sheaths may be affected when the ankle joint is involved. It is advantageous to release these sheaths at the time of an ankle synovectomy.

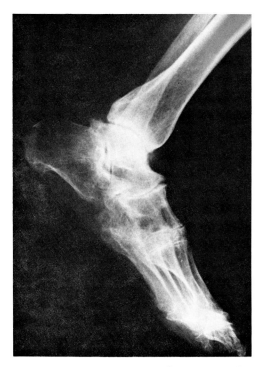

FIG. 11-16 Roentgenogram revealing severe pathologic changes in the subtalar, talonavicular joints, and ankle.

Synovectomy

If the ankle joint alone is affected and the disease has not destroyed the joint, synovectomy may relieve the symptoms due to the active inflammation of the synovium. The joint may be approached through an anterior incision between the extensor hallucis longus and the common extensors (Fig. 11-17). The neurovascular bundle should be carefully retracted. The synovium is excised from the joint and its recesses. The posterior aspect of the joint may be approached through a lateral incision parallel to the Achilles tendon to remove the proliferative synovium in the back of the joint. The lateral incision avoids the neurovascular bundle located on the medial side.

Postoperatively a bulky compression dressing is used for a few days, and early

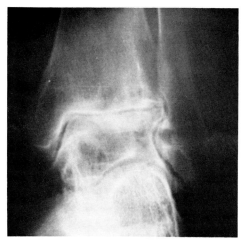

FIG. 11-15 Roentgenogram revealing narrowing of joint space, erosions, and sclerosis of rheumatoid arthritis in the ankle.

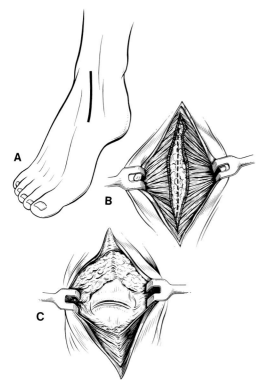

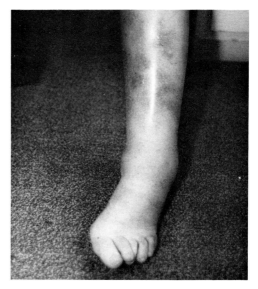

FIG. 11-18 Clinical view of results of articular destruction. Note the severe varus deformity.

FIG. 11-17 Synovectomy of the ankle. A. Anterior incision between the extensor hallucis longus and the common extensor tendons. B. Opening of the capsule of the joint. C. Exposure of the joint surface. (Redrawn from Campbell's Operative Orthopaedics, 5th ed. H. H. Grenshaw, editor. St. Louis, C. V. Mosby, 1971.)

surface and sclerosis of the joint margins (Fig. 11-19).

Conservative Treatment

If local injections of steroids do not control the patient's symptoms, arthrodesis of the ankle is indicated. This may also be necessary if the joint becomes markedly unstable.

motion is started in this dressing. Weight bearing may be instituted as soon as tolerated by the patient.

Articular Destruction

The ankle joint functions mainly in weight bearing; stability is more important than motion, especially if the tarsal joints are normal. A great deal of destruction may occur in the ankle joint before the patient has severe disability (Fig. 11-18). Pain is usually the presenting complaint and can seriously limit the patient's ambulation. Roentgenograms of the ankle will reveal loss of the joint

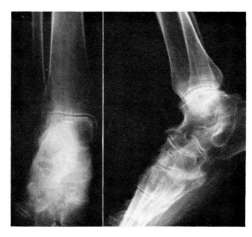

FIG. 11-19 Roentgenograms revealing loss of joint space and sclerosis in the ankle.

Arthrodesis

There a number of methods for arthrodesis of the ankle joint. Most of them are satisfactory for the rheumatoid patients, whose joints ankylose readily, especially when denuded of cartilage and pannus.

For several reasons it is not advisable to use the Charnley method of compression arthrodesis and cutting of the tendons and vascular bundle in the rheumatoid patient. Many rheumatoid patients have moderate osteoporosis because of disuse and steroid therapy. Under compression the pins would have a tendency to cut through the soft bone. Secondly, these patients have some vascular disease and it is better to preserve the vessels if possible.

An ankle joint replacement has been developed but is still somewhat experimental. Since stability is more important than motion in the ankle joint, especially if the tarsal joints are normal, arthrodesis remains the operation of choice.

Operation Technique. The anterior approach to the ankle joint gives adequate exposure of both the medial and lateral aspects of the joint. A longitudinal incision is made over the anterior aspect of the ankle joint between the anterior tibial tendon and the extensor hallucis longus for 3 inches above the joint and 2 inches beyond (Fig. 11-20). The anterior annular ligament is divided, and the neurovascular bundle is carefully retracted to one side. The capsule of the ankle joint is opened and stripped off the tibia along with the periosteum. The exposure is developed to permit access to the medial and lateral malleoli. Plantar flexion of the talus exposes the articular surface. The synovium and articular cartilage are scraped from the joint with curettes, and the remainder of the cartilage is removed with an osteotome. The talus and the tibial surfaces are then "fish-scaled" with a gouge to

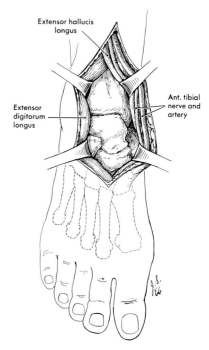

FIG. 11-20 Arthrodesis of the ankle. Retraction of the extensor hallucis longus, the anterior tibial tendons, along with the neurovascular bundle, and the extensor digitorium longus to expose the joint.

improve the surface area for fusion. A sliding bone graft may be developed from the lower tibia and slid into a trough made in the talus, locking the foot in the desired position (Fig. 11-21), ap-

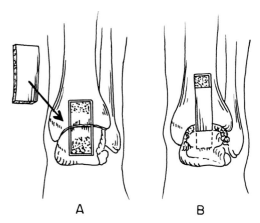

FIG. 11-21 Arthrodesis of the ankle. A. A trough made in the talus (arrow). B. A bone graft slid into the trough.

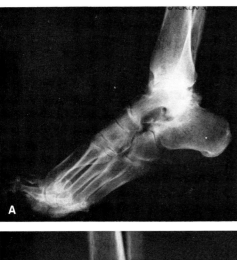

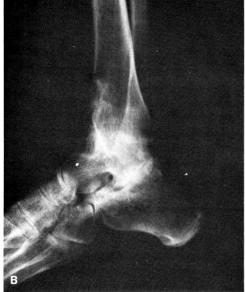

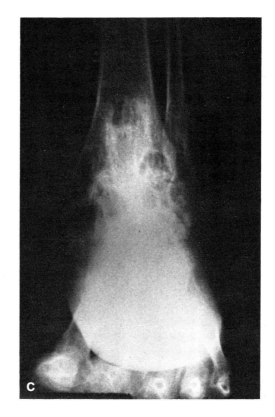

FIG. 11-22 Arthrodesis of the ankle. Roentgenograms: A. Preoperative view revealing pathologic changes in the ankle from rheumatoid arthritis. B. Postoperative lateral view revealing sliding anterior bone graft that has united with the talus. C. Postoperative anterior view showing solid fusion of the joint.

proximately 90° to 95° for a male patient and about 100° to 105° for a woman who desires to wear a higher heel (Fig. 11-22).

Postoperative Management. It is advantageous to use postoperative suction to prevent hematoma formation and pressure on the poor skin of the arthritic. A long-leg plaster of Paris cast is applied for 6 weeks, and then a short-leg walking cast for 4 weeks. If the fusion appears solid clinically and roentgenographically, no further immobilization is necessary.

Osteoarthritis

Osteoarthritis of the ankle joint is rare. It is generally secondary to trauma disrupting the articular surface of the ankle joint and producing a traumatic arthritis (Fig. 11-23) or to deformity of the tibia or the knee joint that has produced excessive angulation resulting in varus or valgus stress on the ankle joint. With a severe varus position of the tibia, the

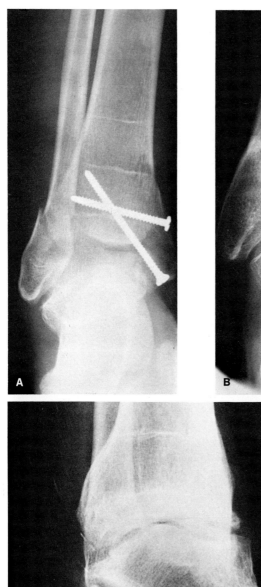

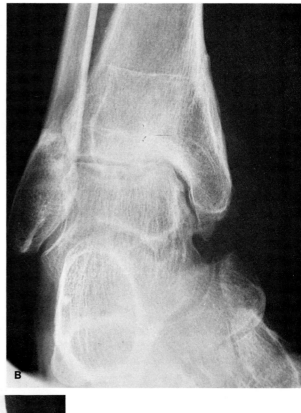

FIG. 11-23 Roentgenograms of pathologic changes from traumatic arthritis in the ankle. A. Anterior view revealing severe disruption of the joint. B. Anterior view of articular destruction due to previous trauma. C. Lateral view revealing deformity of the talus and loss of the joint space.

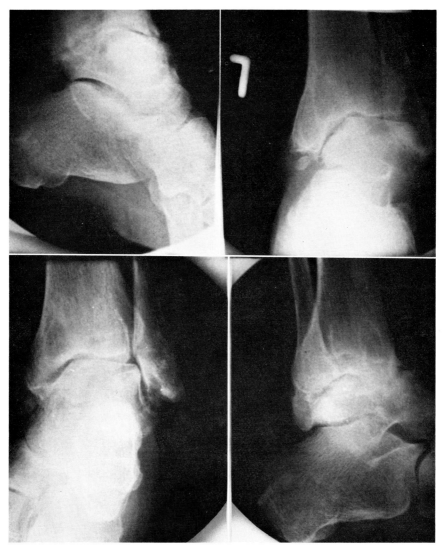

FIG. 11-24 Roentgenograms of severe varus deformity of the ankle joint due to osteoarthritis. No history of trauma was obtained.

ankle joint is forced into a valgus position with excessive stress on the lateral aspect of the talus (Fig. 11-24). This can produce the development of osteoarthritis with symptoms in the ankle joint. Involvement of the tendon sheaths seen in rheumatoid disease does not occur in osteoarthritis.

Conservative Treatment

The patient with osteoarthritis of the ankle joint can frequently be treated conservatively for long periods of time by the local injection of steroids. It is important to realize that there is no correlation between the appearance of the roentgenogram and the patient's clinical symptoms. Many patients with severely disrupted ankle joints and advanced osteoarthritis have minimal symptoms for 10 years or more. In some cases, however, symptoms may become severe soon after the injury and may require surgical intervention. If the patient responds to conservative treatment with

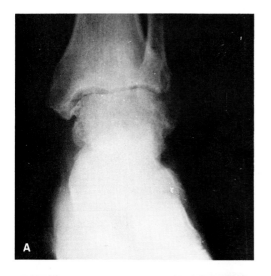

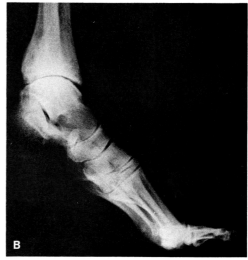

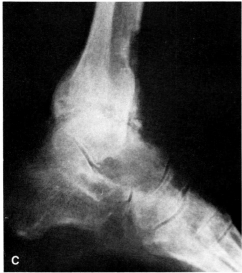

FIG. 11-25 Traumatic arthritis of the ankle as a result of an injury 10 years earlier. A. Pre-operative anterior view. B. Lateral view revealing loss of joint space and sclerosis. C. Post-operative lateral view after arthrodesis. Note the sliding bone graft extending from the tibia into the talus.

local injections of steroids and in-domethacin (Indocin) surgery is not indicated.

Surgical Treatment

Arthrodesis at the present time is still the operation of choice in osteoarthritis of the ankle. Various types of ankle fu-sions can be performed, and the tech-nique we prefer is described in the rheu-matoid arthritis section (Fig. 11-25).

Bibliography

Rheumatoid Arthritis

DiStefano, V. J., et. al.: Achilles tendon rupture. J. Trauma, *12*:671, 1972.

Keck, C.: The tarsal-tunnel syndrome. J. Bone Joint Surg., *44-A*:180, 1962.

Kopell, H. P., and Thompson, W. A. L.: Peripheral entrapment neuropathies of the lower extremity. N. Engl. J. Med., *262*:56, 1960.

Kristensen, J. K., et. al.: Rupture of the Achilles tendon. J. Trauma, *12*:794, 1972.

Lam, S. J. S.: A tarsal-tunnel syndrome. Lancet, *2*:1354, 1962.

Lam, S. J. S.: Tarsal tunnel syndrome. J. Bone Joint Surg., *49-B*:87, 1967.

Lavine, L. S., Karas, S., and Warren, R. F.: Two pin technic for Achilles tendon repair. Clin. Orthop., *40*:137, 1965.

Lindholm, A.: A new method of operation in subcutaneous rupture of the Achilles tendon. Acta Chir. Scand., *117*:261, 1959.

McLaughlin, H. L.: Trauma. Philadelphia, W. B. Saunders Co., 1959, p. 366.

McLaughlin, H. L., and Francis, K. C.: Operative repair of injuries to quadriceps extensor mechanism. Am. J. Surg., *9*:651, 1956.

Moloney, S.: Tarsal-tunnel syndrome. Calif. Med., *101*:378, 1964.

Thompson, T. C.: Spontaneous rupture of the tendon Achilles: A new clinical diagnostic test. J. Trauma, *2*:126, 1962.

Osteoarthritis

Baker, P. L.: SACH. heel improves results of ankle fusion. J. Bone Joint Surg., *52-A*:1485, 1970.

Thomas, F. B.: Arthrodesis of the ankle. J. Bone Joint Surg., *51-B*:482, 1969.

Wilson, H. J., Jr.: Arthrodesis of the ankle. A technique using bilateral hemimalleolar onlay grafts with screw fixation. J. Bone Joint Surg., *51-A*:904, 1969.

Surgical treatment of the foot can relieve pain, improve function and the appearance of the foot, and give a great psychologic lift to the patient (Fig. 12-1). If man can walk on the moon, he should at least be able to walk on earth.

The success rate for operations on the foot is high, and the patient need not exercise to achieve a good result. In patients who do not seem to be motivated to cooperate in postoperative therapy, foot surgery gives the surgeon a good chance to evaluate the patient for future surgery.

Anatomy

The problems of the foot may be divided anatomically and clinically into those of the forefoot and the hindfoot. The hindfoot is composed of the talus, calcaneus, navicular, cuboid, and cuneiform bones (Fig. 12-2). The forefoot is composed of the metatarsal bones and the phalanges. Since all of these joints contain articular cartilage with movable joints surrounded by a synovial layer, rheumatoid arthritis can affect any of the joints of the foot, as well as the tendons that pass through the synovial tendon sheaths in the region of the hindfoot.

The longitudinal axis of the foot passes through the subtalar joint where the motions of inversion and eversion of the foot take place. The motion of flexion and extension takes place in the ankle joint and was discussed in Chapter 11.

The hindfoot containing the subtalar joint contributes to the longitudinal arch of the foot. Destruction of this arch leads to a severe pronation deformity and flat foot (Fig. 12-3). Located between the talus and calcaneus is the tarsal sinus which contains synovial tissue from the anterior talocalcaneal and talonavicular joints. This can be a site of chronic inflammation and pain.

The plantar calcaneal-navicular ligament is an important ligament in the foot. It tends to maintain the position of the head of the talus and to support it. The ligament is aided in maintaining the position of the head of the talus by the support of the posterior tibial tendon. Destruction of this ligament leads to pronation and loss of the arch of the foot (Fig. 12-4).

The plantar aponeurosis extends from the tuberosity of the calcaneus anteriorly into the transverse metatarsal ligament at the base of the metatarsals. This structure bolsters the arch of the foot and inflammation at its attachment to the calcaneus frequently can give rise to symptoms.

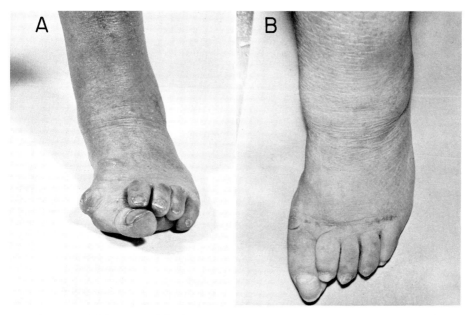

FIG. 12-1 Rheumatoid deformities of the foot. A. Preoperative view. B. Appearance one year after Clayton resection of the forefoot.

There are two longitudinal arches in the foot. The most important one is composed of the calcaneus, talus, navicular bones, the three cuneiforms, and the first, second, and third metatarsals. The key joint in this arch is the joint between the talus and the navicular, and destruction of this joint tends to lead to collapse of the longitudinal arch of the foot (Fig. 12-5).

There are several important bursae about the foot which can become involved in rheumatoid disease. A large bursa is located between the Achilles tendon and the calcaneus and another between the skin and Achilles tendon.

The foot functions as a support for the body in weight bearing. Joints of the foot have to change their positions constantly on walking to adjust to the irregular surfaces the foot is placed on. As the patient progresses forward, the entire weight of the body is raised from the ground and propelled forward by the muscles attached to the joints of the foot.

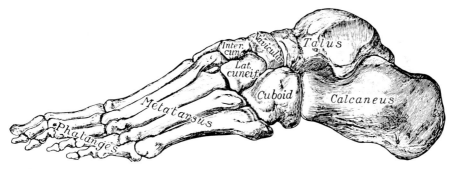

FIG. 12-2 Skeleton of the foot. Lateral aspect. (From Gray's Anatomy of the Human Body, 29th ed. C. M. Goss, editor. Philadelphia, Lea & Febiger, 1973.)

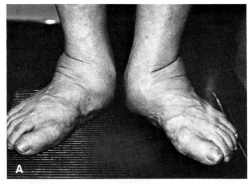

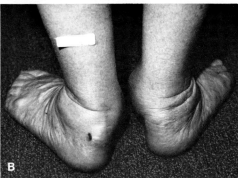

FIG. 12-3 Pronation deformity from destruction of the longitudinal arch of the foot. A. Anterior view. B. Posterior view. Note the valgus position of the heels. The talus has slipped off the calcaneus and is pointing medially.

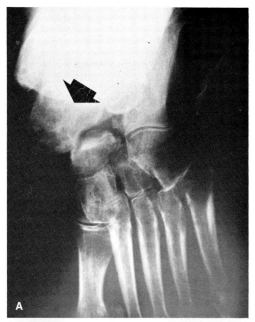

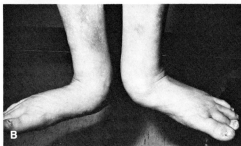

FIG. 12-5 Complete collapse of the subtalar joint with pronation of the forefoot. A. Roentgenogram. Note the medial deviation of the talus on the calcaneus (arrow). B. Clinical view.

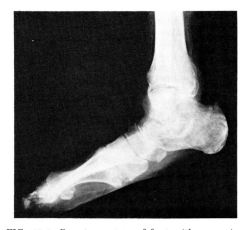

FIG. 12-4 Roentgenogram of foot with pronation deformity from destruction of plantar calcaneonavicular ligament. The subtalar joint has collapsed and the talus is deviated medially on the calcaneus.

Physical Examination

The foot must be examined in respect to the entire function of the lower extremity. The function of the foot can be altered considerably by deformity of the knee joint. Severe valgus or varus deformities of the knee can lead to varus or valgus deformities of the foot in order to

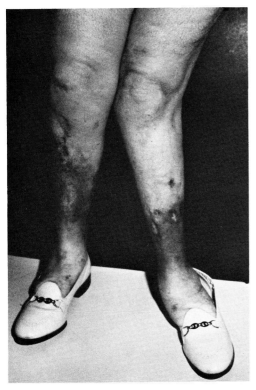

Fig. 12-6 Multiple deformities of lower extremities from rheumatoid arthritis. The patient has a severe valgus deformity of the left knee and involvement of the ankle and subtalar joint.

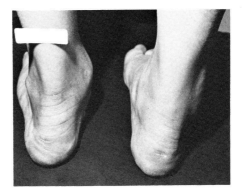

FIG. 12-7 Posterior view. The patient has a valgus deformity of the left heel and a varus deformity of the right heel.

compensate for the angulation at the knee. This must be taken into consideration when evaluating the problems of the foot or knee (Fig. 12-6).

Inspection

The patient should be usually examined standing and nonstanding to determine the deformities of the foot. Frequently when the foot is examined with the patient sitting or without weight bearing, deformities will not be obvious. The surgeon should note whether there is a varus or valgus deformity of the heel in inspecting the hindfoot and the appearance of the longitudinal arch of the foot (Fig. 12-7). Severe pronation may be obvious on standing and should be noted. In severe pronation the talus will

often be resting upon the surface of the floor, and a large callus may be obvious in this area. In equinus deformities or a tight heel cord syndrome, the foot will be pronated and the calcaneus will be in valgus because of the tight Achilles tendon. The only way that the heel can come down to the floor is by producing the valgus and pronation deformity. The appearance of the toes should also be examined for clawing and for calluses (Fig. 12-8). A bunion deformity will also be more prominent with weight bearing than when the patient is lying or sitting

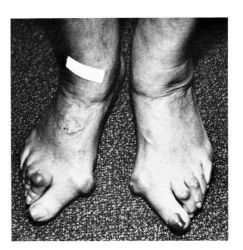

FIG. 12-8 Anterior view of patient with large bursae over proximal interphalangeal joints of the toes and over the first metatarsal heads on the medial aspect.

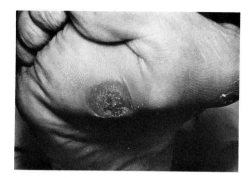

FIG. 12-9 The underside of a patient's foot. A large bunion and a prominent metatarsal head have resulted in ulceration.

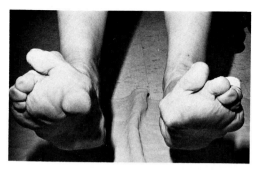

FIG. 12-10 Large rheumatoid bursae due to synovial masses beneath the metatarsal areas of the foot.

down. The undersurface of the foot or sole should be examined carefully for large bony prominences as well as calluses (Fig. 12-9).

Palpation

The various joints and callused areas of the foot should be palpated for tender spots. The tendon sheaths distal to the malleoli should also be examined by palpation to determine if there is thickness of the tendon sheath or localized tender areas. The sinus tarsi is frequently the site of tenderness, and palpation may reveal this area as a source of discomfort. The various joints in the foot may also be palpated and manipulated to see if they are fixed in a deformity or are freely movable. Palpation will also reveal if a thickened callused area is due to pressure from a synovial mass beneath the skin or from a bony prominence (Fig. 12-10).

It is important to check the circulation of the foot at this stage of the examination to be sure that there are a dorsalis pedis pulse and a posterior tibial pulse. Patients with vascular disease will often have loss of the hair about the foot as well as discoloration and even stasis dermatitis of the leg (Fig. 12-11).

Good pulses are generally present in the early stages of rheumatoid arthritis.

The sensation of the foot should be tested with pin prick and light touch to rule out neurologic disease of the foot.

Range of Motion

The range of motion should be examined in the patient by checking the inversion and eversion of the heel which are related to the subtalar joints as well as the motion possible in the metatarsal-phalangeal joints. Loss of motion in the first metatarsal-phalangeal joint is frequently seen with arthritis.

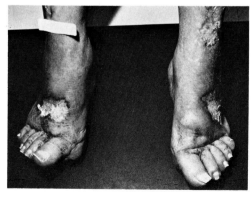

FIG. 12-11 Severe vasculitis of the legs and feet.

Rheumatoid Arthritis

Many patients note the onset of their rheumatoid arthritis as a disability arising in the foot. The disease can result in severe destruction of the forefoot that limits the activity of the arthritic patient. Because of the severe deformities patients have great difficulty obtaining suitable shoes and even custom-made molded shoes are neither comfortable nor fashionable. Patients will often complain of severe pain beneath the metatarsals and the inability to walk with or without shoes. Often they will describe the situation as feeling as though they were walking on marbles or stones in their shoes. These painful deformities may severely limit the ability to earn a living and to take care of household responsibilities (Fig. 12-12).

The Hindfoot

The hindfoot is involved in rheumatoid arthritis but not as frequently as the forefoot. Destruction of the subtalar joint or the talonavicular joint severely limits motion and can produce pain on walking, especially on uneven ground. Severe involvement of this joint may lead to a spastic flat foot due to peroneal muscle spasms. This should be differentiated from the peroneal spasm due to a talonavicular or calcaneonavicular bridge or bar due to a congenital deformity. Roentgenograms of the foot, as suggested by Harris, should aid in the differential diagnosis (Fig. 12-13). Another differential point is that spastic flat foot is most common in young children. The roentgenogram of the foot in hindfoot disease will reveal narrowing of the joint space between the talus and the navicular or the subtalar joint (Fig. 12-14). Cystic formation occurs late in this condition. As the subtalar joint is destroyed, the calcaneus will rotate laterally, and the talus will point toward the medial side of the foot.

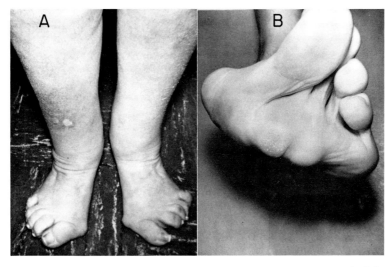

FIG. 12-12 Deformities of the foot from rheumatoid arthritis. A. Dorsal view reveals dislocations of the metatarsophalangeal joints and severe valgus position of the great toe. B. Plantar view of the deformity of the great toe and the prominent metatarsal heads.

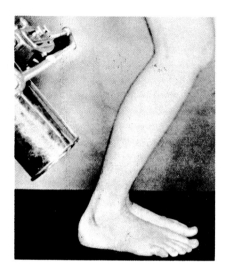

FIG. 12-13 Projection necessary to demonstrate a talocalcaneal bridge. The angle of projection is from behind, forward and downward. (Permission of E. and S. Livingstone Ltd., from Harris, R. I., and Beath, T.: Etiology of peroneal spastic flat foot. J. Bone Joint Surg., *30-B*:625, 1948.)

Conservative Treatment

The treatment at the onset of symptoms due to rheumatoid arthritis of the subtalar joints should be conservative. The use of local injections of steroids into the sinus tarsi or talonavicular joint will give prolonged relief in many cases. The use of a custom arch support protecting the longitudinal arch of the foot is extremely worthwhile. Molded shoes can also give prolonged relief of the patient with early involvement of the subtalar joint.

Arthrodesis

When the joint of the hindfoot is severely involved with rheumatoid disease and symptoms are pronounced, arthrodesis is the operation of choice. Only the diseased joint should be fused.

Occasionally the talonavicular joint alone will be involved by rheumatoid arthritis. In these situations the patient may be treated by arthrodesis of the talonavicular joint. Disease of this joint can produce severe pain on weight-bearing and limit the patient's ability to walk. Bony spurs may often be palpated at the site of the arthritic change in the talonavicular joint.

In a number of cases of far-advanced rheumatoid disease the foot is extremely pronated and multiple joints are affected (Fig. 12-15). This type of patient will not benefit from a subtalar or talonavicular arthrodesis alone. The best operation for this type of foot is a triple arthrodesis, which should be performed before the disease process has completely destroyed the foot (Fig. 12-16).

The skin of the arthritic patient, especially if he has been on prolonged steroid therapy, is generally thin and poor in quality. Therefore, great care should be utilized in retraction of the skin to prevent complications with wound healing.

Subtalar Joint. The subtalar joint should be approached through a lateral incision placed over the sinus tarsi (Fig. 12-17). Soft tissue should be removed from the area located between the talus and calcaneus with a rongeur and curettes. A small lamina spreader inserted in the joint will allow visualization of the articular cartilage between the talus and calcaneus in the subtalar joint. This cartilage should be removed with a broad osteotome if any is remaining. The area should be cleared to cancellous bone, and chips should be turned up from both surfaces for an excellent bed for fusion. It is extremely important not to place the heel in a varus position in fusing the subtalar joint. About 5° of valgus of the heel is adequate. The sinus tarsi should be packed with bone chips or bank bone, if available, to increase the chance of fusion. If the joint is unstable and the position is difficult to maintain, a staple may be used between the talus and calcaneus. It is important when using staples to spread the prongs slightly to produce a compression force rather than a distracting force when the staple is inserted. In some cases a Steinmann pin also can be used to maintain

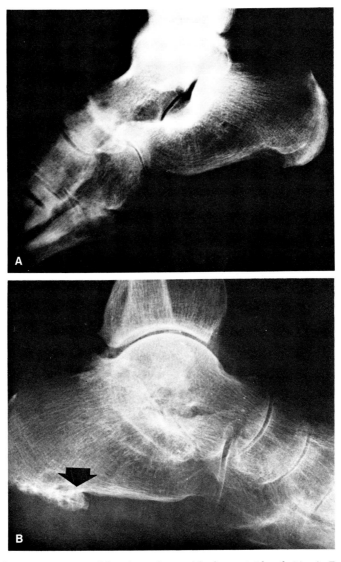

FIG. 12-14 Lateral roentgenograms of feet in patients with rheumatoid arthritis. A. Far-advanced talonavicular disease. B. Severe subtalar joint disease, with a large heel spur (arrow).

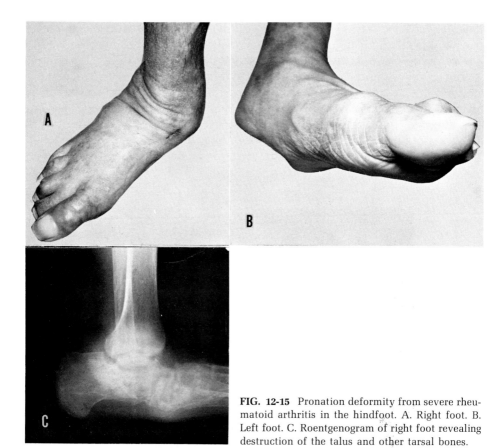

FIG. 12-15 Pronation deformity from severe rheumatoid arthritis in the hindfoot. A. Right foot. B. Left foot. C. Roentgenogram of right foot revealing destruction of the talus and other tarsal bones.

the position. The pin is drilled from the heel into the talus and is then incorporated in a cast.

A short-leg cast should be used for 6 weeks and then a walking cast for 4 weeks more. It should be stressed that in order to prevent a contracture of the Achilles tendon, it is important to place the ankle in a neutral position of 90° to avoid equinus.

Talonavicular Joint. A small horizontal incision placed over the talonavicular joint on the medial side of the foot will often give adequate exposure of the joint. The posterior tibial tendon should be protected. The capsule should be turned back, exposing the articular surface, and all of the sclerotic bone should be removed with a small gouge to freshen the areas for a good bony fusion. The foot should be placed postopera-

tively in a short-leg cast for 6 weeks without weight bearing and then in a walking cast for approximately 4 to 6 weeks more (Fig. 12-18).

Multiple Joints. In these severe deformities, it is recommended that both a lateral and a small medial incision be used to gain exposure of the various joints involved. The sinus tarsi is the key to the anatomy of the lateral incision, and the peroneal tendons must be protected. The incision should extend from the talonavicular joint down toward the lateral side of the foot. The sinus tarsi should be cleaned of all synovial tissue, and the ligaments between the talus and calcaneus should be cut. The extensor tendons of the foot are retracted medially to expose the talonavicular joint. The extensor brevis muscle covers the calcaneocuboid joint, and its origin must

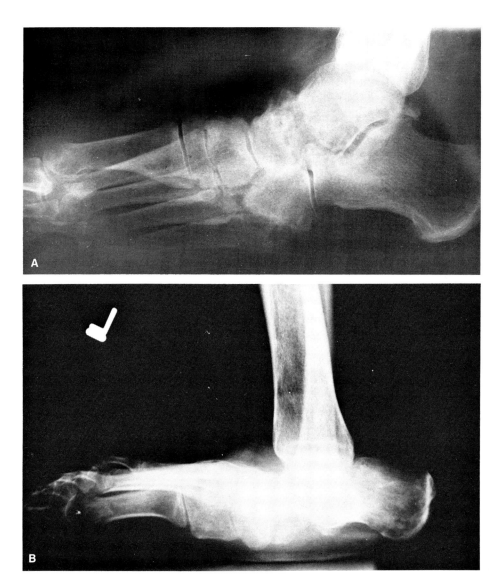

FIG. 12-16 Progression of rheumatoid arthritis of the hindfoot. A. First roentgenogram was taken during early stages. B. Roentgenogram 7 years later shows severe destruction and collapse of the joints.

be elevated from the calcaneus to expose the joint. The articular cartilage should be carefully excised from the subtalar, the calcaneocuboid, and the talonavicular joints, and appropriate small wedges should be removed to allow for repositioning of the foot in either a neutral or a slightly valgus heel position. Care should be exercised not to pronate or supinate the forefoot. Staples may be used to maintain the position of the foot until the cast is applied (Fig. 12-19). In some patients the joints and the bone will be badly destroyed by the rheumatoid process, and it may be difficult to obtain fixation. Occasionally bone from the ilium or from a bone bank will aid considerably in obtaining stability and fusion of the joints (Fig. 12-20), but may not improve the appearance of the foot.

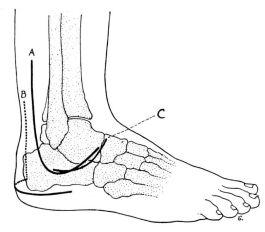

FIG. 12-17 Various approaches to the foot and ankle. A. Kocher approach to the ankle. B. Kocher approach to the calcaneus. C. Ollier approach to the subtalar joint (From Campbell's Operative Orthopaedics, 5th ed. H. H. Grenshaw, editor. St. Louis, C. V. Mosby, 1971.)

Heel Nodules

Nodules frequently develop in rheumatoid arthritis, especially in areas where there is a fair amount of pressure (Fig. 12-21). Although they are most common in the region of the elbow, nodules do develop beneath the calcaneus and can be quite large and painful. These nodules are hard and feel like a movable stone beneath the thin part of the heel, between the skin and the calcaneus. In some patients, the nodules are not obvious and can be quite soft. When the patient stands without a shoe, the nodules will protrude considerably from the surface of the foot, producing large, soft swellings. These nodules may be extremely thick and at times contain a good deal of yellow necrotic material (Fig. 12-22). These large, soft tissue masses make wearing of a shoe difficult and sometimes require surgical attention (Fig. 12-23).

If the symptoms warrant, the mass can be excised from the heel, but the dissection may be quite extensive and a portion of the heel pad may have to be excised (Fig. 12-24). Loss of the pad does not seem to produce a painful area on weight bearing, and the postoperative results generally are satisfactory.

Plantar Fasciitis

The patient with rheumatoid arthritis may also at times complain of severe pain in the region of the heel. The patient will notice most of the discomfort on arising in the morning, but after a few steps the pain often tends to lessen. However, in some cases the pain can be severely disabling and prevent the patient from walking. Usually only one foot is involved at a time. On examination there is no evidence of a hard nodule in the region of the bottom of the heel. There will be localized tenderness at the insertion of the plantar fascia into the calcaneus. At times the roentgenogram in the lateral view will reveal a heel spur which is a small osseous projection at the site of insertion of the plantar fascia (Figs. 12-14B; 12-25).

Conservative Treatment

In the past, surgical excision has been performed for plantar fasciitis, but the treatment of choice at the present time is

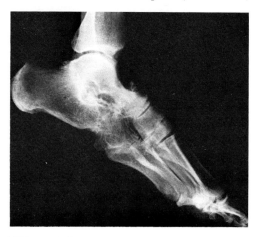

FIG. 12-18 Roentgenogram 8 years after arthrodesis of talonavicular joint to relieve pain and improve walking. Spontaneous fusion of the calcaneocuboid joint is almost complete.

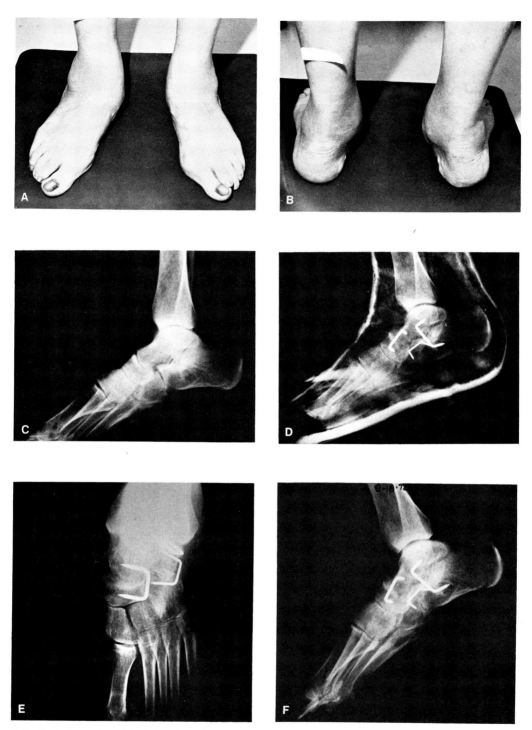

FIG. 12-19 Pronation of both feet from rheumatoid arthritis in the hindfeet. Photographs: A. Anterior view. B. Posterior view. Valgus deformities are seen in the heels. Roentgenograms: C. Lateral view of left foot. The subtalar joint is beginning to collapse and there is destruction of the calcaneocuboid joint. D. After triple arthrodeses to restore the longitudinal arch. Staples have been inserted to maintain the position of the foot. E. Dorsal view. F. Lateral view showing stabilization of subtalar joint.

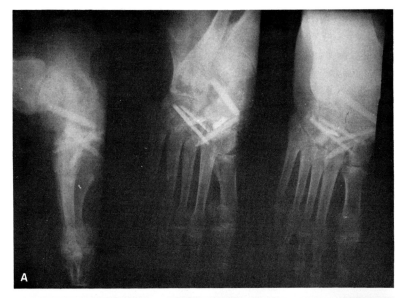

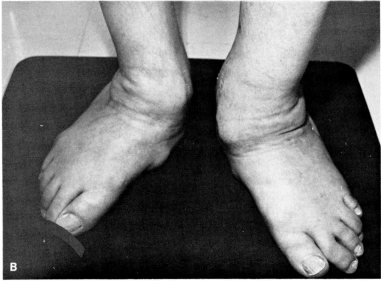

FIG. 12-20 Use of bone graft with arthrodesis for severe disease of the hindfoot. A. Roentgenogram of bone grafts drilled through various joints of the foot. B. Seven years later. Despite severe pronation, the joints are stabilized and the patient can walk without pain.

local injection of the area with Xylocaine and cortisone. The area should be prepared carefully, and with sterile technique the tender area is injected with a mixture of 3 cc lidocaine (Xylocaine) and 1 cc of a local steroid. The needle should be inserted deeply until it strikes the calcaneus near the area of tenderness, which is usually at the site of the insertion of the fascia. Constant movement of the needle while injecting the medication spreads the mixture throughout the area and should give dramatic relief of the symptoms. The patient should be advised that pain will return in several hours as the local anesthetic wears off. However, within 1 to 2 days, the patient usually will be

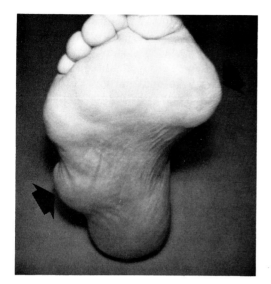

FIG. 12-21 Large rheumatoid nodules along the lateral border of the foot (arrow) and beneath the metatarsal heads.

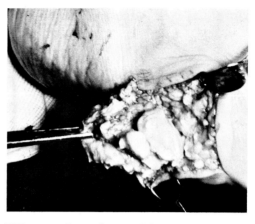

FIG. 12-22 Surgical view of thick nodule containing necrotic material.

symptom free. If symptoms return or are not completely relieved, a repeat injection will often be of value in about 1 to 2 weeks.

The Forefoot

Crippling deformities from rheumatoid arthritis occur more often in the

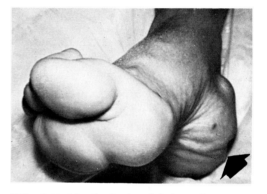

FIG. 12-23 Massive heel nodule (arrow).

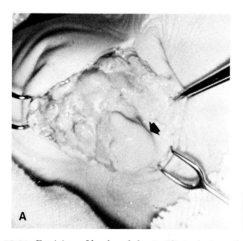

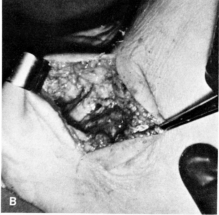

FIG. 12-24 Excision of heel nodule. A. Clinical view of yellow necrotic material (arrow). B. Clinical view of defect after excision of the heel pad.

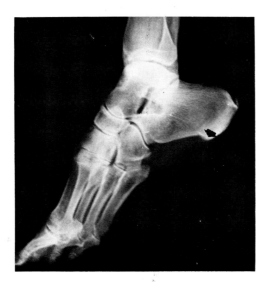

FIG. 12-25 A bony spur at the insertion of the plantar fascia (arrow).

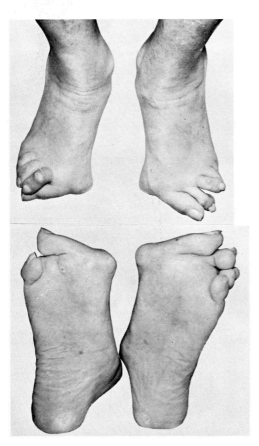

FIG. 12-26 Deformities of the forefoot from rheumatoid arthritis. Top, dorsal view. Bottom, plantar view.

forefoot than in the hindfoot (Fig. 12-26). The ratio is approximately 20 to 1. The symptoms of the majority of rheumatoid patients with foot problems are produced by the mechanical deformities, rather than by the inflammation of the arthritis itself. Early in the onset of the disease in the foot, the metatarsal-phalangeal joints are frequently affected, producing a synovitis with localized swelling in the ball of the foot. The progression of the disease in this area produces crippling deformities such as clawing of the toes, bunions, and dislocations of the metatarsal-phalangeal joints. The patient with deformed feet finds it impossible to obtain suitable shoes or to walk barefoot without pain due to the prominent metatarsal heads (Fig. 12-27). These deformities tend to be combined in the severe advanced case of rheumatoid arthritis and the foot may be extremely rigid. The abnormal pressure of the shoe on the deformed foot produces large, painful calluses and pain.

The deformities produced by rheumatoid arthritis in the forefoot are due to

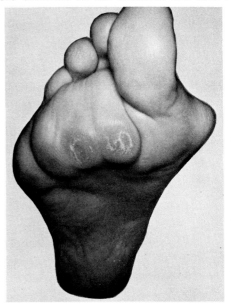

FIG. 12-27 Prominent metatarsal heads.

the proliferation of the synovial tissue in the metatarsal-phalangeal joints. The inflammatory swelling of the synovium distends the capsule and stretches the collateral ligaments. The synovium gradually invades the subchondral bone and destroys the articular surface of the metatarsal head. The pain in the foot produces spasm of the musculature about the foot with resultant contractures and deformities. The extensor tendons in the foot contract and produce clawing of the toes with subluxation of the metatarsal-phalangeal joints (Fig. 12-28). Finally, as the capsule and ligaments are destroyed, the extensor tendon pulls the phalanx dorsally, and the phalanx dislocates on top of the metatarsal head (Fig. 12-29). The displaced phalanx depresses the head down into the sole of the foot to produce the painful bony prominence.

Claw Toes. Two types of claw toes occur in rheumatoid disease, both of which can produce painful corns over the proximal interphalangeal joints. The first type is produced by hyperextension of the metatarsal-phalangeal joint due to contracture of the long extensor tendon. The patient will develop a subluxation of the proximal phalanx, producing clawing of the interphalangeal joint due

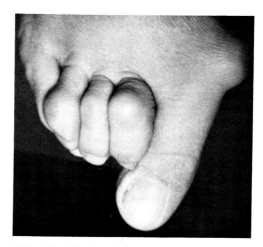

FIG. 12-28 Clawing of the toes, subluxation of the metatarsophalangeal joints, and a nodule on the medial aspect of the metatarsal head of the hallux.

to the pull of the flexor tendons. This is often associated with a synovitis of the metatarsal-phalangeal joint.

The second type of claw toe is associated with a normal metatarsal-phalangeal joint and severe clawing of the proximal interphalangeal joint. This type of claw toe is most satisfactorily treated by fusion of the proximal interphalangeal joint.

Bunions. The problem of the large painful bunion has been treated most successfully in our experience by the Keller procedure of excising the prom-

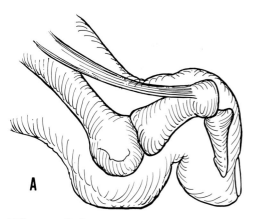
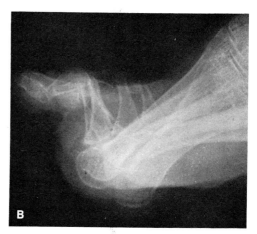

FIG. 12-29 Dislocation of the phalanx dorsally on top of the metatarsal head, forcing the head down into the sole of the foot and producing a bony prominence. A. Drawing. B. Roentgenogram.

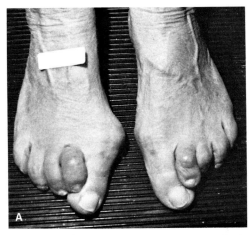 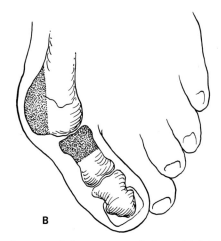

FIG. 12-30 Keller arthroplasty for bunions without involvement of the metatarsophalangeal joints. A. Preoperative view. Note also the clawing of the second toes. B. Drawing of Keller technique. Shaded areas indicate prominence on medial side and area of the proximal phalanx to be excised.

inence of the first metatarsal and the proximal half of the proximal phalanx (Fig. 12-30).

Multiple Deformities. A great number of arthritic patients have a combination of dislocated metatarsal-phalangeal joints, bunions, and depressed metatarsal heads (Fig. 12-31).

In 1912, Hoffman advised the excision of the metatarsal heads, and this operation gave relief and corrected the deformities. However, gradually the calluses returned as the base of the phalanx became prominent because of the pull of the extensor tendons.

Flint and Sweetnam in 1960 advised

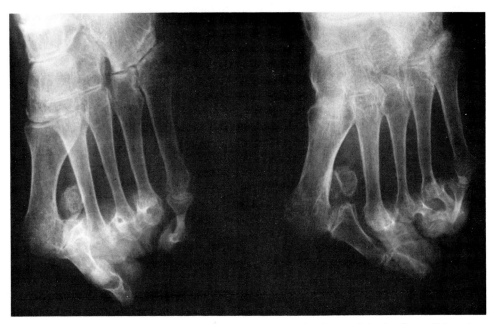

FIG. 12-31 Roentgenogram of multiple deformities of rheumatoid arthritis of the forefoot—dislocations of metatarsophalangeal joints, formation of bunions, and depression of the metatarsal heads.

amputation of the toes for severe deformities. This operation does not correct the prominent metatarsal heads and also is quite deforming and cosmetically very poor (Fig. 12-32).

Clayton recommended the resection of the metatarsal-phalangeal joints, including tenotomy of the extensor tendons, for the severe problems affecting the forefoot in rheumatoid arthritis.

Conservative Treatment

Conservative treatment of the forefoot in rheumatoid arthritis will be of some value in a number of patients. Paring down of the painful calluses and having the patient wear soft flexible shoes will give a certain amount of relief. The use of a metatarsal bar will relieve a good deal of pressure from weight bearing on the metatarsal heads. In the early stage of active synovitis the ball of the foot will swell and the local injection of steroids may be of value to decrease symptoms. Oxyphenbutazone (Tandearil used in appropriate doses may also help control the inflammatory process. Frequently, when the patient is examined, the deformities are fixed and conservative therapy has less to offer. Custom-made "space" shoes, which accommodate the deformities of the foot may help the patient to bear weight.

Soft Tissue Release

The surgical procedure for claw toes from contracture of the long extensor tendon is to perform a Z-plasty with a tenotomy of the extensor brevis tendon and a dorsal capsulotomy of the metatarsal-phalangeal joint (Fig. 12-33). Any hypertrophied synovium may be removed at this time from the joint. The reduction of the phalanx and release of the tight extensor will prevent or delay the development of complete dislocation of the proximal phalanx and depression

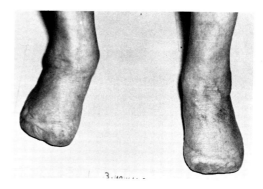

FIG. 12-32 Photograph of feet after amputation of the toes. The patient is able to walk, but feels unstable on her feet.

of the metatarsal head that leads to a severe, painful metatarsalgia.

Arthrodesis

Arthrodesis is the preferred surgical procedure for the second type of claw toes. An incision is made over the joint in either a transverse or longitudinal manner, and where possible the extensor tendon should be preserved over the interphalangeal joint. The tendon is carefully retracted out of the way, leaving it attached to the distal phalanx to prevent development of a hammer toe. The articular cartilage is removed from the surfaces of the joint, and a tunnel is

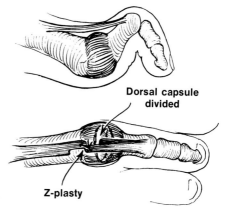

**Dorsal capsule
divided**

Z-plasty

FIG. 12-33 A Z-plasty and dorsal capsulotomy to relieve clawing of the toes due to subluxation at the metatarsophalangeal joint.

made in the base of the middle phalanx with a curette or with a small toe reamer. The head of the proximal phalanx may be rounded off with a rongeur or with a female reamer in a power tool. The two bones will then fit together with a good bony contact. A 0.045-inch Kirschner wire is drilled distally through the middle phalanx and the distal phalanx and is brought out beneath the pulp of the toenail (Fig. 12-34). The wire is then drilled back across the joint, and into the proximal phalanx to fix the joint in complete extension. The wire is cut off subcutaneously at the end of the toe and is tapped with a mallet so that it does not protrude through the skin. It is left in place for approximately 6 weeks until good bony union has occurred. The wire then may be removed under local anesthesia, as it is located just beneath the skin in most patients.

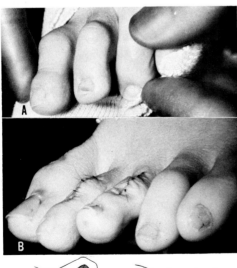

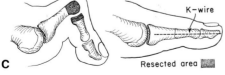

FIG. 12-34 Arthrodesis of the proximal interphalangeal joint. A. Preoperative photograph of claw toes due to subluxation of the joint. B. Postoperative view. C. Drawing of operative technique.

Keller Arthroplasty

The foot is carefully wrapped with a Martin elastic bandage, starting distally and just overlapping the bandage slightly up to the ankle. Four turns are overlapped at the ankle to produce a tourniquet. The bandage is then unrolled from the foot, starting with the distal end, up to the ankle leaving the foot free of blood.

A curved 2-inch incision is made over the medial-dorsal aspect of the joint and bunion. The long extensor tendon is retracted, and the joint capsule is opened. The collateral ligaments are divided, and the toe is flexed to expose the articular surface of the first metatarsal. The periosteum is stripped from the distal aspect of the metatarsal, and a nick is made in the medial aspect of the cortex proximal to the exostosis of the shaft. This will prevent splitting the shaft. An osteotome is then placed at the edge of the medial aspect of the remaining normal cartilage, and the exostosis is removed. The dorsal and medial edges are smoothed with a rasp. Then the proximal phalanx is grasped at its base with a towel clip or bone-holding clamp and is retracted dorsally. The capsule, collateral ligaments, and adductor tendon are carefully dissected from the base of the phalanx. The flexor tendon must be protected at this stage, since it lies close to the plantar capsule. The phalanx is then removed with an osteotome placed about one third to one half along the proximal portion of the phalanx. If the long extensor appears too tight, it may be lengthened by a Z-plasty and repaired with a simple suture of 3-0 chromic catgut. The excess synovium and bursal tissue are excised from the toe, and the tissues are sutured while the toe is held in an overcorrected position with traction by the assistant.

In the rheumatoid patient it is advisable not to put a bulky dressing between the first and second toes to overcorrect the valgus deformity of the great toe because such a dressing will displace the other toes laterally. A bulky dressing is applied to the foot with bias stockinette, and two tongue blades are incorporated into the dressing on the medial side. The great toe is then taped carefully to the tongue blade to correct the great toe without displacing the other toes. The patient is allowed to bear weight on the heels by the fourth or fifth postoperative day and is allowed to bear full weight by the seventh day.

If the preoperative roentgenogram reveals a severe primus varus deformity, a better result can be obtained in a younger patient by combining the Keller procedure with an osteotomy at the base of the first metatarsal (Fig. 12-35). A piece of bank bone or a portion of the exostosis may be inserted into the osteotomy opening to correct the varus deformity and maintain the position.

Care should be taken to maintain the normal relationship of the metatarsal head lest it be displaced up or down by the osteotomy, or the mechanics of the foot will be altered and painful symptoms arise. The foot should be placed in a slipper cast for 6 weeks to prevent displacement. This procedure requires more immobilization and would not be indicated usually in the older patient or in the patient with active disease.

Clayton Resection

The operative procedure for the correction of multiple deformities of the forefoot is performed under tourniquet control to allow visualization of the anatomic structures (Fig. 12-36). The claw toes are manipulated by hyperextending the proximal interphalangeal joints to correct any fixed contractures. A dorsal skin incision is made over the metatarsal heads just proximal to the web space of the toes from the medial to the lateral border of the foot. A heavy scissors is used to spread the skin flaps to gain adequate exposure. The common extensor tendon and brevis tendon are exposed to the second toe, and small

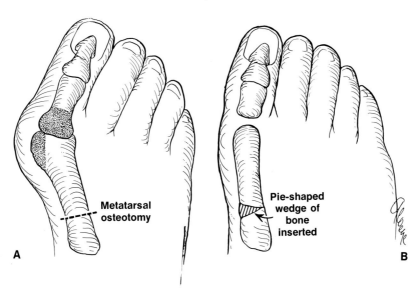

FIG. 12-35 Metatarsal osteotomy combined with Keller arthroplasty. A. Dotted line indicating base of first metatarsal. B. Pie-shaped wedge of bone inserted. (From Marmor, L.: Surgery of the rheumatoid foot. Surg. Gynecol. Obstet., *119:*1009, 1964. By permission of Surgery, Gynecology & Obstetrics.)

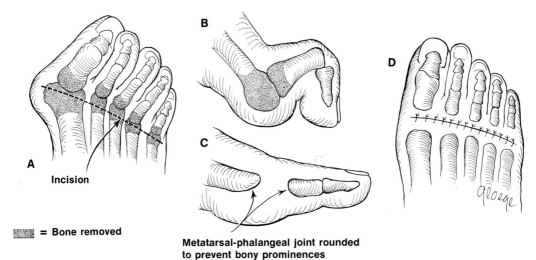

A
Incision

B

C

D

= **Bone removed**

**Metatarsal-phalangeal joint rounded
to prevent bony prominences**

FIG. 12-36 Clayton resection of the forefoot. A. Incision close to the web space of the toes. Shaded areas indicate bone to be removed. B. Lateral view of toe joint. Shaded area represents amount of bone to be resected to obtain a good correction without pressure under the metatarsal neck. C. Edges of bones rounded to prevent bony prominences. D. Skin sutures in place and toes held in corrected position. (From Marmor, L: Surgery of the rheumatoid foot. Surg. Gynecol. Obstet., *119*:1009, 1964. By permission of Surgery, Gynecology & Obstetrics.)

blunt retractors inserted. A Z-plasty tenotomy is performed to divide the common extensor, and a simple transverse tenotomy is used to divide the brevis tendon.

The base of the proximal phalanx is exposed by dividing the dorsal capsule, and the base is then dissected free from the surrounding soft tissue (Fig. 12-37). The flexor tendon is protected, and the proximal half of the phalanx is excised with a bone cutter. In a similar manner

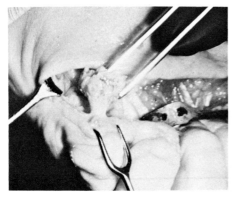

FIG. 12-37 Surgical view of destruction at the base of the phalanx due to rheumatoid disease.

the third, fourth, and fifth phalanges are exposed, their bases are excised, and a tenotomy is done on the extensor tendons.

Next, the second metatarsal head is exposed, and the periosteum is stripped from the neck. A bone cutter is inserted just proximal to the flare of the neck to divide the bone. The head is then excised from the capsule and soft tissue. The third metatarsal is then exposed and removed slightly proximal to the second metatarsal. The fourth and fifth metatarsals are also removed at their necks slightly proximal to the third metatarsal (Fig. 12-38).

The great toe is exposed last because it is easier to do after the small toes have been released. The extensor hallucis longus is exposed, and a Z-plasty tenotomy is performed. The capsule and collateral ligaments are divided to expose the proximal phalanx. The joint is forcibly flexed to gain better exposure of the first metatarsal head. The head can be removed with an osteotome even with the second metatarsal, or it may be re-

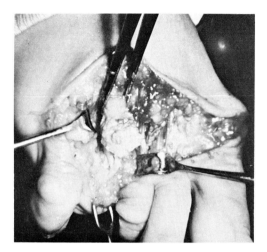

FIG. 12-38 Surgical view of rheumatoid destruction of metatarsal head.

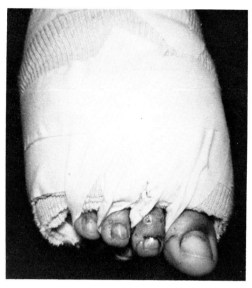

FIG. 12-40 Bulky dressing with tape folded between the toes to maintain correction.

moved piecemeal with a rongeur. The flexor tendon is protected while the base of the phalanx is dissected free, and the proximal half is excised.

The remaining ends of the metatarsals are then rounded off with a rongeur or with small cup reamers to remove any sharp points. The ball of the foot should be palpated to be sure that a metatarsal shaft is not left too long.

The common extensors may be approximated loosely with a simple suture. If the extensors are left intact, the toes generally will not come down to the floor. It is not necessary to approximate the extensors to the small toes, especially

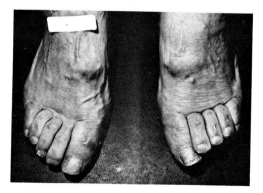

FIG. 12-39 Postoperative photograph after Clayton resection without division of the extensor tendons. The toes do not come down to the floor.

in a severely deformed foot (Fig. 12-39). The subcutaneous tissue is approximated with the toes held in a corrected position, and then the skin is closed.

A bulky pressure dressing is applied with bias stockinette, and the tourniquet is released. One-inch tape is folded between the toes to hold them in a corrected position (Fig. 12-40). The night of surgery the dressing should be split on the lateral border of the foot down to the skin. On the second postoperative day the dressing should be changed, and the patient can start dangling the feet. On the fifth day the patient is allowed to walk on the heels to the bathroom. A rubber sole from a Japanese zori (sandal) is applied to the bottom of the dressing, and the patient may start walking as soon as it feels comfortable. (Fig. 12-41).

The dressing is changed once a week for 3 additional weeks until the foot is healed so that the toes will maintain their corrected position. The sutures are removed if the incision is healed. The patient may then wear slippers or loose sandals until the swelling has disappeared and then may wear soft leather shoes until healing is complete (Fig.

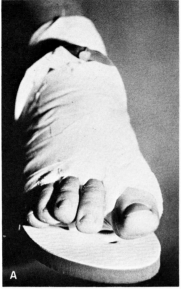
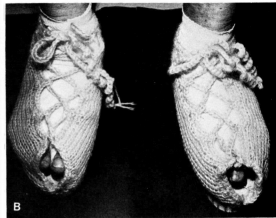

FIG. 12-41 A Japanese zori used as a sole for postoperative ambulation. A. Taped to the bottom of the dressing. B. Attached to a crocheted slipper.

12-42). The patient should be cautioned that swelling will persist for a long period of time.

Results. In our series of over 311 patients with resections of the metatarsal-phalangeal joints, 89 percent had good results from the operation in a follow-up from 1 to 10 years (Fig. 12-43). Most patients were able to wear regular shoes.

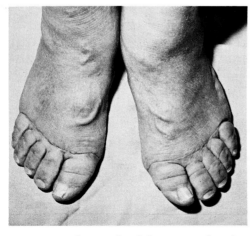

FIG. 12-42 Photograph of feet 6 months after Clayton resection.

Complications. Infection tends to occur in the foot quite frequently despite preparation with hexachlorophene (pHisoHex) and other antiseptic solutions for several days before surgery. Infections will gradually heal with minimal scarring. Antibiotics can be utilized to localize the infection and speed healing and are suggested for prophylactic use. The patient may be ambulated despite the infection because the incision is located on the dorsal surface of the foot. This incision is a decided advantage over the plantar incision when infection does occur.

Recurrence of a callus or deformity usually is due to an elongated metatarsal (Fig. 12-44), or to failure to lengthen or tenotomize the extensor tendons (Fig. 12-45). If only one or two metatarsals are involved, the problem may be solved by resecting a small portion of the metatarsal under local anesthesia and dividing the extensor tendon.

Resection of only a few metatarsal heads will lead to recurrence of symptoms under the remaining metatarsal

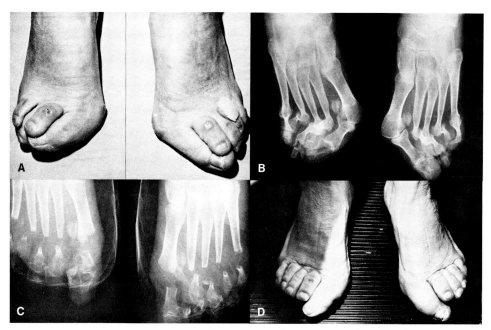

FIG. 12-43 Results of Clayton resection. A. Preoperative photograph of deformities of forefoot due to rheumatoid arthritis. B. Roentgenogram of the joint destruction. C. Postoperative roentgenogram of the amount of resection of the metatarsophalangeal joints. D. Photograph 5 years after the resections. Symptoms have not recurred, and the correction has been maintained.

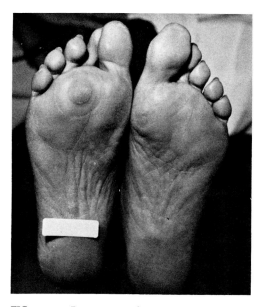

FIG. 12-44 Recurrence of a callus beneath the third metatarsal of the right foot due to an elongated metatarsal.

heads (Fig. 12-46). When prominent metatarsal heads are left behind, weight bearing during the next few years is almost certain to bring recurrences.

A patient with a relatively small foot may have problems from the resection of the metatarsal-phalangeal joints. It may be difficult to find a small enough shoe to wear. Patients should be made aware that the surgery will shorten the foot from one to two sizes.

Osteoarthritis

Osteoarthritis of the foot is generally localized to several small areas. The talonavicular joint is a frequent site of osteoarthritis, but the subtalar joint is not as often involved in osteoarthritis as it is in rheumatoid disease. The other

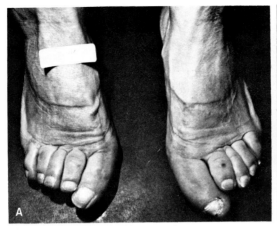
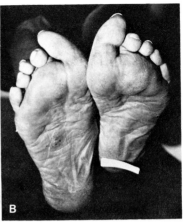

FIG. 12-45 Recurrence of deformities due to reattachment of the extensor tendons. A. Dorsal view. B. Plantar view. The metatarsals are prominent beneath the second and third toes of the left foot and beneath the second toe of the right foot. A bursa has formed from pressure from the metatarsal head.

most common site involves the forefoot and often is localized even further to the first metatarsal-phalangeal joint. Osteophyte formation, which is quite common in these areas and also at the first metatarsal cuneiform joint, can prevent the patient from comfortably wearing a shoe.

Pain is generally the most common complaint related to osteoarthritis.

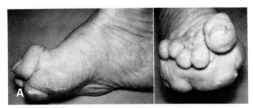

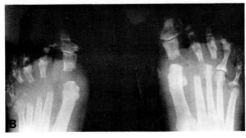

FIG. 12-46 Recurrence of deformities after partial resection of the forefoot. A. Photograph of prominences beneath the first and fifth metatarsals. B. Roentgenogram showing several prominent metatarsal heads remaining.

The Hindfoot

Osteoarthritis may be related to trauma of the joint surfaces of the foot. Athletic injuries can frequently produce osteoarthritic changes in the talonavicular joint. The patient will experience gradual increasing pain on weight bearing in the region of the arch of the foot, and a prominence will often develop over the area of this joint. Osteophyte formation and loss of the joint space can be seen frequently on the roentgenogram (Fig. 12-47).

Arthrodesis

In the early case removal of the osteophytes occasionally will relieve the patient's symptom. However, the disease process generally is progressive, and it is a loss of the articular cartilage that leads to the painful symptoms. In the advanced case arthrodesis is indicated.

Operative Technique. A tourniquet is generally applied at the upper thigh, the leg is wrapped with a Martin rubber bandage to the tourniquet, and the tourniquet is inflated. A small 2-inch incision is made over the talonavicular joint on the medial side of the foot. The posterior tibial tendon may be en-

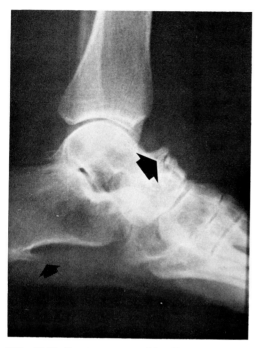

FIG. 12-47 Roentgenogram of hindfoot. An osteophyte is prominent on the talus (large arrow). The heel spur (small arrow) is not characteristic of osteoarthritis and is not the cause of the patient's complaints.

countered and should be carefully lifted away, leaving it attached distally. The joint capsule should be opened to expose the joint. The sclerotic bone present in osteoarthritis makes fusion more difficult. It should be removed with an osteotome to cancellous bone to obtain good bony contact. If good contact is available, a staple may be inserted across the joint. The joint should be compressed so that the staple will not be distracted when it is inserted. The foot should be in a neutral position to avoid pronation or supination of the forefoot with the hindfoot. In some patients a sliding bone graft can be taken from the talus and inserted into the navicular for good bony contact.

Postoperative Care. The patient should be placed in a short-leg cast for approximately 2 to 3 weeks without weight bearing. Then a walking heel may be applied, and the patient may be

allowed to ambulate for about a total of 12 weeks at which time the cast may be removed and roentgenograms should be obtained. If union has occurred, the patient is taken out of immobilization and given support stockings or an Ace bandage wrap. It is important to caution the patient that swelling will continue for a considerable amount of time and that the symptoms in the foot will gradually disappear.

The Forefoot

Osteoarthritis of the forefoot is a gradual progressive disease and may involve both feet. It is generally localized to the first metatarsal-phalangeal joint and in the advanced cases has been called hallux rigidus.

The clinical symptoms are the gradual onset of pain in the region of the first metatarsal-phalangeal joint on walking and the development of a small prominence in the region of the first metatarsal-phalangeal joint. Osteophyte formation may produce tender areas with calluses on the dorsum of the first metatarsal-phalangeal joint, and as the disease progresses, these areas become larger and tend to produce a bulky first metatarsal-phalangeal joint with evidence of minor bunion formation (Fig. 12-48). Gradual loss of the motion in the

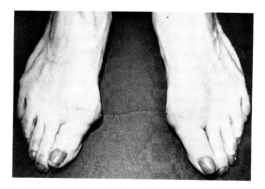

FIG 12-48 Osteoarthritis of the forefoot. The osteophytes of the metatarsophalangeal joint resemble a bunion and are related to hallux rigidus.

joint is experienced, and when this has become fixed, it is difficult for the patient to wear a normal shoe. The push-off of the first metatarsal-phalangeal joint is lost and symptoms may become severe, limiting the ability of the patient to walk. If the hallux rigidus or fusion occurs spontaneously in some extension, the patient has a much better gait and fewer symptoms. This condition is similar to that in patients who had an arthrodesis for a hallux valgus deformity.

Osteoarthritis of the first metatarsal-phalangeal joint tends to be related to osteoarthritis involving other joints, especially the carpal-metacarpal joint of the thumb and the distal phalangeal joints of

the fingers which may have Heberden's nodes. Cervical osteoarthritis is also extremely common in these patients.

The roentgenogram is a valuable aid in the diagnosis. Early in the disease process slight narrowing of the metatarsal-phalangeal joint is seen along with minor osteophyte formation. Gradually osteophyte formation increases until most of the joint space is lost and the joint is widened (Fig. 12-49).

Metatarsal-Cuneiform Joint

Some patients develop a prominence on the dorsum of the metatarsal-cuneiform joint as they get older. The

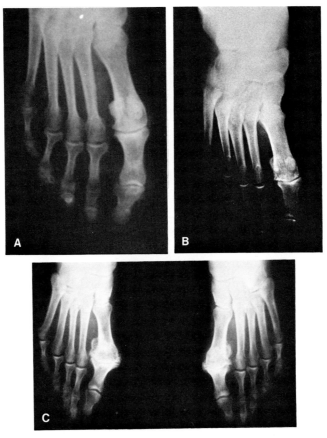

FIG. 12-49 Roentgenograms of osteoarthritis in the foot. A. Early stage with narrowing of joint space and small osteophytes along edges of the metatarsal and phalanx. B. Advanced stage with incongruity of the joint space, cystic formation, and narrowing of joint space. C. Late stage with severe deformity of metatarsophalangeal joint.

joint tends to become arthritic, and spurs that develop on the dorsum produce a bursa when the shoe rubs against this prominence. The pressure of the footwear on the osteophyte, not the joint itself, generally produces the symptoms. Under local anesthesia it is possible to excise the osteophytes with a rongeur, and generally the swelling will disappear gradually over a period of months and the patient can then wear appropriate footwear.

Keller Arthroplasty

When symptoms are severe, operative intervention may be necessary. The operation of choice in osteoarthritis of the first metatarsal-phalangeal joint is a Keller arthroplasty (page 492). This may be combined with a Swanson Silastic insert in the base of the phalanx to maintain the joint space because these patients tend to develop stiffness. The major problem with a Silastic implant in the foot is infection. If infection occurs and does not respond to local antibiotics, the prosthesis can be removed and a satisfactory result generally can be obtained.

Bibliography

Rheumatoid Arthritis

Barton, N. J.: Arthroplasty of the forefoot in rheumatoid arthritis. J. Bone Joint Surg., *55-B*:126, 1973.

Benson, G. M., and Johnson, E. W.: Management of the foot in rheumatoid arthritis. Orth. Clin. North Am., *2*:733, 1971.

Brattstrom, H.: Surgery of metatarsalphalangeal joints. II-V, in rheumatoid arthritis. Acta Orthop. Belg., *58*:107, 1972.

Calabro, J. J.: A critical evaluation of the diagnostic factors of the feet in rheumatoid arthritis. Arthritis Rheum., *5*:19, 1962.

Clayton, M. L.: Surgery of the forefoot in rheumatoid arthritis. Clin. Orthop., *16*:136, 1960.

Clayton, M. L.: Surgical treatment of the rheumatoid foot. In Foot Disorders, 2nd ed. N. J. Giannestras, editor. Philadelphia, Lea & Febiger, 1973, p. 444.

Flint, M., and Sweetnam, R.: Amputation of all toes. J. Bone Joint Surg., *43-B*:90, 1960.

Fowler, A. W.: A method of forefoot reconstruction. J. Bone Joint Surg., *41-B*:507, 1959.

Harris, R. J.: Rigid valgus foot due to talocalcaneal bridge. J. Bone Joint Surg., *37-A*:169, 1955.

Hoffmann, P.: An operation for several grades of contracted or clawed toes. Am. J. Orthop., *9*:441, 1911.

Keller, W. L.: Surgical treatment of bunions and hallux valgus. N. Y. Med J., *80*:741, 1904.

Key, J. A.: Surgical revision of arthritic feet. Am. J. Surg., *79*:667, 1950.

Kuhns, J. G.: The foot in chronic arthritis. Clin. Orthop., *16*:141, 1960.

Marmor, L.: Resection of the forefoot in rheumatoid arthritis. Clin. Orthop., *108*:223, 1975.

Marmor, L.: Rheumatoid deformity of the foot. Arthritis Rheum., *6*:749, 1963.

Marmor, L.: Surgery of the rheumatoid foot. Surg. Gynecol. Obstet., *119*:1009, 1964.

Thomas, F. B.: Arthrodesis of the subtalar joint. J. Bone Joint Surg., *49-B*:93, 1967.

Thompson, T. C.: The management of the painful foot in arthritis. Med. Clin. North Am., *21*:1785, 1937.

Osteoarthritis

Giannestras, N. J.: Foot Disorders, Medical and Surgical Management, 2nd. ed. Philadelphia, Lea & Febiger, 1973.

Keller, W. L.: Further observations of the surgical treatment of halix valgus or bunions. N. Y. J. Med., *95*:696, 1912.

Morris, H. D.: Arthrodesis of the foot. Clin. Orthop., *16*:164, 1960.

Thomas, F. B.: Arthrodesis of the subtalar joint. J. Bone Joint Surg., *49-B*:93, 1967.

Wilson, J. N.: Cone arthrodesis of the first metatarsal-phalangeal joint. J. Bone Joint Surg., *49-B*:98, 1967.

Arthritis tends to involve the spine in different areas depending upon the disease process. Osteoarthritis, which is a natural progression of the wear and tear of the normal activities of life, frequently results in disease of the cervical and lumbar spine. In contrast, rheumatoid arthritis occasionally will affect the cervical spine, especially in juvenile rheumatoid patients.

Rheumatoid spondylitis, which is a different disease, affects the lower lumbar spine early with gradual involvement of the entire spine. Back pain, regardless of the etiology or type of arthritis, can produce severe disability.

Anatomy

The human spine is made up of twenty-four movable segments that are supported upon the five fused segments of the sacrum. The intervertebral disks comprise approximately one fourth of the length of the spinal column, and the vertebral bodies make up the additional three-quarters. There are seven cervical, twelve thoracic, and five lumbar vertebrae in the spinal column. The cervical and lumbar vertebrae have a normal lordotic curve in contrast to the reverse curve of the thoracic vertebrae. Because of these curves the spine has an elasticity that takes up the shocks and strains of daily activities.

The seven cervical vertebrae are the smallest of the true vertebrae (Fig. 13-1). The first cervical vertebra is called the atlas because it supports the globe or head (Fig. 13-2). It is peculiar because it has no body; its body has become the dens (odontoid process) of the second vertebra. The second cervical vertebra is called the axis or epistropheus because it is the pivot upon which the atlas and the head rotate. The most outstanding feature is the large (dens) odontoid process (Fig. 13-2B, C). This process forms a synovial joint anteriorly with the atlas and posteriorly with the transverse ligament (Fig. 13-3). The transverse ligament is a strong band upon which the atlanto-odontoid articulation depends for stability. It tends to hold the odontoid process against the posterior aspect of the anterior surface of the atlas. Several bursae lined with synovium may be found about the odontoid process and the ligaments in this region. Rheumatoid changes in these bursae lead to subluxation and destruction in this area of the cervical spine.

The thoracic vertebrae each have a facet on the body for articulation with a

503

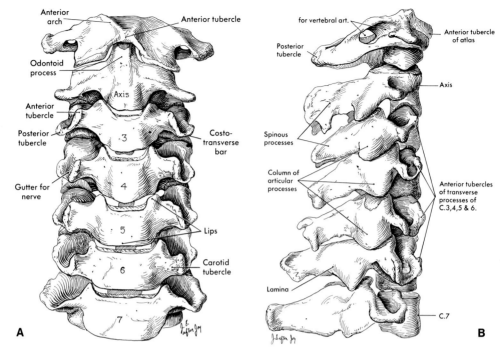

FIG. 13-1 The cervical spine. A. Visualized from the anterior surface. B. Lateral view.

rib. These costovertebral joints tend to move with respiration and can be affected in ankylosing (rheumatoid) spondylitis that will result in loss of thoracic motion (Fig. 13-4).

The five lumbar vertebrae are the largest in the body and frequently are involved in osteoarthritis rather than rheumatoid disease (Fig. 13-5).

Physical Examination

The patient with arthritis should be examined for spinal disease. For an adequate examination the patient should disrobe to expose the spine and the entire trunk.

Inspection

The patient should be examined standing, if possible, and also sitting. The spine should be observed from the lateral view to see whether there is a normal curvature with a cervical and lumbar lordosis and in the anteroposterior view to determine whether there is a deviation producing scoliosis. Any operative scars and gross deformity should be noted at this time. If scoliosis does exist, the patient should be asked to bend over to a 90° angle if possible. If the scoliosis is due to a short leg, there will be no deformity of the thoracic or lumbar areas of the trunk. If there is a structural deformity due to rotation of the vertebrae in true scoliosis, there will be a prominence of one or the other side of the thoracic cage, posteriorly, or of the lumbar region, depending upon the location of the curve.

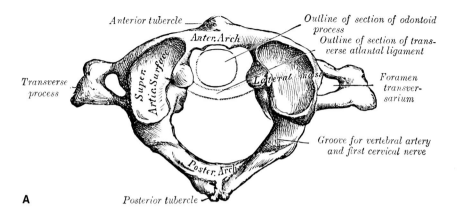

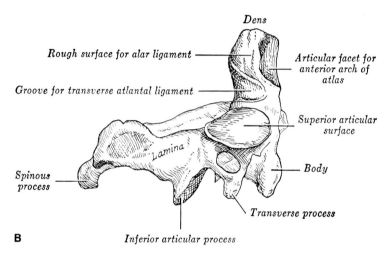

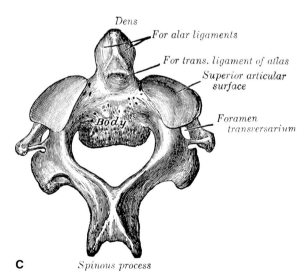

FIG. 13-2 The cervical spine. A. First cervical vertebra, or atlas. B. Second cervical vertebra viewed from the side. C. Second cervical vertebra viewed from above. (From Gray's Anatomy of the Human Body, 29th ed. C.M. Goss, editor. Philadelphia, Lea & Febiger, 1973.)

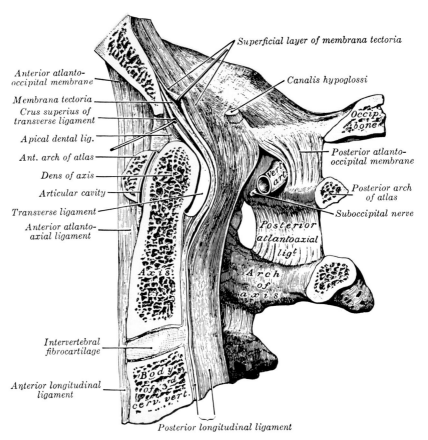

FIG. 13-3 Midsagittal section of the upper cervical spine and foramen magnum showing the relationship of the synovial tissue, ligaments, odontoid process, and anterior arch of the atlas. (From Gray's Anatomy of the Human Body, 29th ed. C. M. Goss, editor. Philadelphia, Lea & Febiger, 1973.)

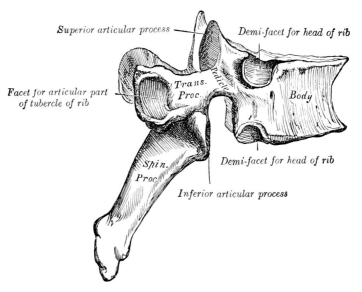

FIG. 13-4 A thoracic vertebra viewed from the side. Note the facet for articulation with the rib. (From Gray's Anatomy of the Human Body, 29th ed. C. M. Goss, editor. Philadelphia, Lea & Febiger, 1973.)

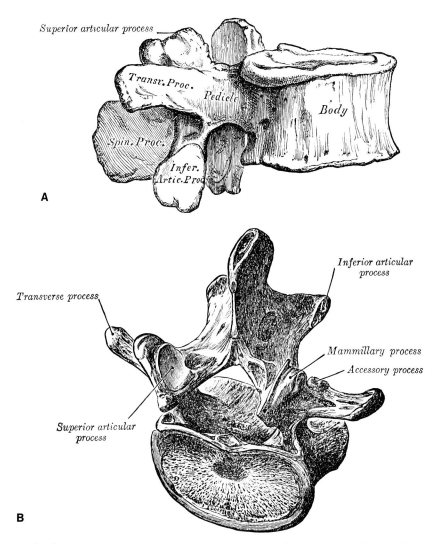

Superior articular process

Transv. Proc.

Pediclc

Body

Spin. Proc.

Infer.
Artic.Proc

A

Inferior articular
process

Transverse process

Mammillary process

Accessory process

Superior articular
process

B

FIG. 13-5 A lumbar vertebra. A. Viewed from the side. B. Viewed from above and behind. (From Gray's Anatomy of the Human Body, 29th ed. C. M. Goss, editor. Philadelphia, Lea & Febiger, 1973.)

Palpation

The neck and back should be palpated along the joints of the spine to determine if there is any tenderness. Muscular spasm may be also noted by palpation.

Range of Motion

The range of motion in the cervical spine should be noted and recorded for flexion, extension, lateral bend, and rotation. In some patients with arthritis there will be severe limitation of motion of the cervical spine that must be considered in selecting the anesthesia to be administered during the operative procedure. It may be impossible to pass an airway because of limitation of the temporomandibular joint as well as the cervical spine. It is well to alert the anesthetist to such complications in advance of the scheduling of the surgery.

Motion of the thoracic spine is related to inspiration and expiration of the thoracic cage. The vertebrae themselves are rigidly fixed and do not move. It is important to observe the respiratory motion of the thorax. The circumferential measurement of the lower third of the adult chest normally expands by 7 cm or more. This expansion may be decreased by rheumatoid involvement of the costovertebral joints in ankylosing spondylitis.

The lumbar spine should be observed in flexion and extension, as well as lateral bend, to determine the range of motion possible. In severe muscular spasm the normal lordosis may be absent and in patients with severe hip disease, there may be a marked lordosis due to the flexion contractures of the hip.

Neurologic Evaluation

If during the examination or the clinical history there is evidence of involvement of the spinal nerves, a neurologic examination should be carried out.

Rheumatoid Arthritis

The upper cervical spine is much more frequently affected by rheumatoid arthritis than by osteoarthritis. Weiss and Freehafer reported in 1964 that the spine is involved in 50 percent of the patients with rheumatoid arthritis and that the cervical spine is affected in 80 percent of this group. Subluxation of the atlantoaxial joint is being recognized much more frequently by the medical profession (Fig. 13-6). Conlon, Isdale, and Rose found an incidence of approximately 25 percent in patients hospitalized with rheumatoid arthritis. Mathews noted

that of 76 consecutive patients treated as outpatients, 25 percent had 3 mm of separation or more in lateral tomographs of the neck taken in flexion. In Rana, Hancock, Taylor, and Hill's series it was noted that 36 of 41 patients were taking a corticosteroid daily.

Cervical Spine

Although atlantoaxial subluxation is quite well known in rheumatoid arthritis, upward translocation of the dens or odontoid process has also been reported to occur without any evidence of platybasia (Fig. 13-7). McGregor's baseline described in 1948 is utilized in diagnosing this condition. McGregor's line is drawn from the upper surface of the posterior edge of the hard palate to the most caudal point on the occipital curve. The distance between the tip of the odontoid process (dens) is measured in millimeters, with 4.5 mm being considered the upper limit of normal displacement of the odontoid above the McGregor's line. This condition is believed to be caused by destruction and collapse of the joints in the upper cervical region.

The synovial (apophyseal) joints and the bursae about the upper cervical spine can frequently be involved by synovial proliferation and swelling in rheumatoid arthritis. The pannus formation and destruction of the subchondral bone along with the loss of the ligamentous structures leads to a loss of stability. Granulomatous lesions in the bodies of the vertebrae lead to their destruction and collapse (Fig. 13-8). Various degrees of destruction of the transverse ligament can occur. The atlantoaxial joint is involved most often in rheumatoid disease and subluxation, therefore, is common at this level. Hauge reported a case of complete destruction of the first and second vertebrae by rheumatoid arthritis. Destruction of the

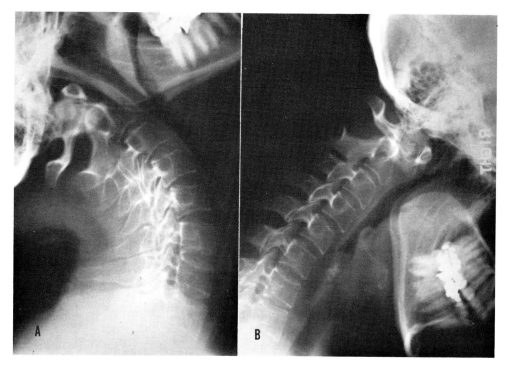

FIG. 13-6 Subluxation of the atlantoaxial joint. A. Extension film reveals relationship of the odontoid process to the axis. B. Flexion film reveals separation of the axis ring from the odontoid process.

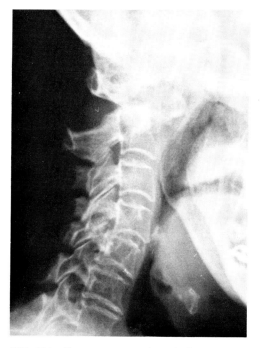

FIG. 13-7 Roentgenogram of cervical spine. Note the collapse of the relationship between the axis and the odontoid process.

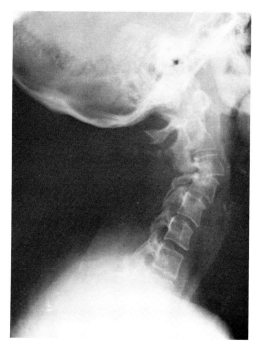

FIG. 13-8 Roentgenogram of cervical spine. Granulomatous lesions have destroyed the disk spaces and the bodies and caused collapse of adjacent vertebrae, C3-C4.

axis leads to herniation of the odontoid process (dens) into the foramen magnum without trauma. Vertebral subluxation may occur in rheumatoid arthritis at varying levels and can be multiple throughout the cervical spine (Fig. 13-9). Subluxation through a narrowed disk space may be pathognomonic of rheumatoid subluxation (Fig. 13-10).

The majority of patients with rheumatoid arthritis of the cervical spine have no symptoms whatsoever. However, patients with subluxation at the atlantoaxial joint have a history of having had rheumatoid arthritis for a number of years. Generally patients with active disease or problems in the cervical spine will have severe pain with radiation into the head. Occasionally complaints such as pain behind the eye or in the ear will be noted. Neurologic involvement generally does not occur unless subluxation is severe.

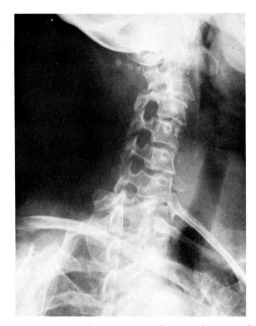

FIG. 13-10   Roentgenogram of cervical spine of patient with advanced rheumatoid disease. Narrowing of the foramen is seen in C3 and C4 and loss of disk space in C2 and C3.

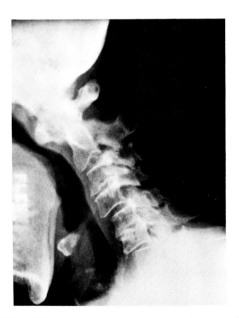

FIG. 13-9   Roentgenogram of cervical spine of patient with rheumatoid arthritis. Note the subluxation of C1 on C2, narrowing of C3-C4 disk space, subluxation of C4 on C5, spontaneous fusion and loss of disk space in C5-C6, and subluxation of C6 on C7.

On physical examination, loss of neck motion is observed frequently. Flexion and extension should be recorded carefully because of subluxation. Cervical spine disease may be suspected if the patient's complaints of pain in the head and neck are relieved, when the patient is lying down and increased when the patient is standing. Roentgenograms of the cervical spine, including those taken during flexion and extension, are of value in the rheumatoid patient who has any neck symptoms. Tomograms may also be of value in evaluating the cervical spine in these patients. The characteristic roentgenographic findings in rheumatoid arthritis patients with involvement of the cervical spine are (1) narrowing of the intervertebral disk spaces, (2) change of the vertebral plate, (3) involvement of the apophyseal joints, and (4) subluxation. The most common disk spaces involved in rheumatoid arthritis are C2-C3 and

C3-C4. Usually there is narrowing of the disk space without osteophyte formation. In osteoarthritis it is less common to have involvement of C2-C3 or C3-C4, and there is usually severe sclerosis with extensive osteophyte formation. In rheumatoid arthritis the vertebral plates commonly show erosion that may even simulate that due to tuberculosis.

It is difficult to demonstrate roentgenographically early changes of destruction in the apophyseal joints. Rheumatoid arthritis may produce a good deal of destruction that will not be obvious on the roentgenogram.

Roentgenograms of the cervical spine should include lateral views of the neck in full flexion and extension. These should be examined for abnormal distance between the odontoid process and the atlas. The normal distance is 3 mm. Anything beyond this generally is considered to be abnormal.

Rheumatoid arthritis can severely affect the transverse ligament and cause instability and increased motion at this joint. Herniation of the atlas into the foramen magnum may also occur in rheumatoid arthritis.

Conservative Treatment

Treatment of the rheumatoid patient with cervical arthritis in most cases is conservative. Medical therapy to control the active rheumatoid disease may aid considerably in reducing the symptoms of the cervical spine. A soft collar and light cervical traction may relieve the muscular spasm and reduce the patient's pain.

Patients with severe pain in the upper cervical spine due to subluxation of C1 on C2 and active rheumatoid disease generally will improve with conservative care. The use of a brace may be worthwhile during the acute phase, but gradually the symptoms will disappear.

Symptoms may last as long as a year without abatement. The patient may be frantic. However, surgical procedures in these patients with severe osteoporosis and active disease should be avoided because of the numerous complications and the severity of the operation.

Anterior Cervical Fusion

The cervical spine may require fusion when there is subluxation of C1 on C2 with neurological findings or localized impingement of a nerve root due to collapse of the disk space and the adjacent foramen.

The cervical spine may be operated on through an anterior approach with a minimum amount of surgical dissection and blood loss. The technique of employing a dowel plug of bone in an interspace may be used if only one joint is severely involved. For patients with multiple joint and disk involvement, the longitudinal bone graft technique described by Bailey and Badgley is the method of choice. The anterior approach, however, is not recommended generally for the atlantoaxial subluxation. When planning an anterior fusion in a patient with long-standing rheumatoid arthritis, the surgeon must take into consideration that the donor site from the ilium may be extremely osteoporotic and soft. Bank bone may be a necessity in performing this type of procedure.

Operative Technique. A folded towel or sheet is placed beneath the interscapular region to extend the patient's neck. It is advisable to use intranasal intubation for administration of anesthetics. A transverse skin incision is made on the right or left side of the neck, depending upon the approach desired. In approaching the upper cervical spine, care must be exercised to prevent perforating the pharynx above the glottis. A vertical

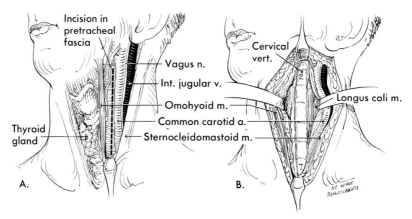

FIG. 13-11 Anterior cervical fusion, operative approach. A. Vertical incision. B. Retraction of muscles.

incision is then made on the medial side of the sternocleidomastoid muscle, and the strap muscles are retracted medially.

The carotid sheath is visualized, and another vertical incision is made through the pretracheal fascia just medial and parallel to the carotid sheath (Fig. 13-11). The carotid sheath and sternocleidomastoid muscle are retracted laterally; the sternohyoid, sternothyroid, and omohyoid muscles, the esophagus, trachea, and thyroid gland are retracted medially.

The anterior longitudinal ligament overlying the cervical vertebrae is evident. The prevertebral fascia is divided in the midline, and the anterior surface of the vertebrae is exposed (Fig. 13-12).

The vertebrae to be fused are identified, a trough is cut on the bodies, and the intervertebral disk space is cleaned out. A large slab graft of iliac bone or bone from the bank is mortised into place in the trough (Fig. 13-13). Autogenous bone chips are packed into the disk space and about the large graft.

When a single disk space is to be fused, the dowel technique can be used cutting out a plug of disk with the adjacent vertebrae, and a bone graft cut in the shape of the dowel is inserted into the disk space. The prevertebral fascia is sutured over the graft to hold it in place. It is wise to insert a large drain for 48 hours. The patients in whom the Bailey

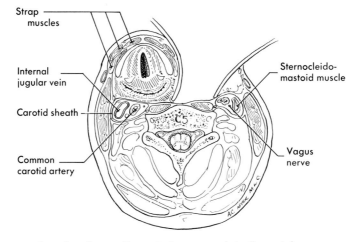

FIG. 13-12 Cross section of neck revealing anterior approach to the vertebrae.

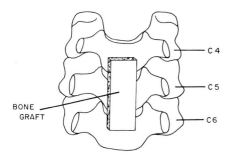

FIG. 13-13 Anterior fusion of cervical spine with a large bone graft.

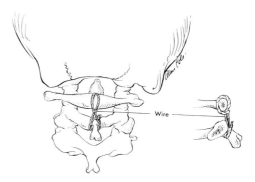

FIG. 13-14 Method of Mixter and Osgood for internal fixation of the atlas and axis.

technique is used should be kept in traction until the wound has healed, and then a leather or plastic brace can be used for 3 to 6 months until fusion is obvious on the roentgenogram.

Posterior Cervical Fusion

The posterior approach should be used for the atlantoaxial subluxation because the anterior approach does not allow adequate exposure of the region. It is advisable to use wire for internal fixation of the vertebrae. The posterior approach may also be used in place of the anterior approach for fusion of any of the cervical vertebrae.

Operative Technique. After the patient is intubated, 10 pounds of cervical traction are applied. The patient is placed in a prone position with his head supported on a cerebellar head rest. The spinous processes of C1-2-3 are approached through the midline. Care should be exercised not to damage the vertebral artery which lies approximately 1 to 1.5 inches from the midline. The spinous processes and laminae are decorticated with a rongeur, avoiding trauma to the neck. A heavy wire is passed beneath the atlas in a loop and fastened to the axis (Fig. 13-14). Matchstick grafts are placed from C1 to C3 over the decorticated laminae, and the wound is closed.

The patient is kept in traction until the wound heals and then is allowed out of bed. A brace is worn for 4 to 6 months until fusion occurs.

Ankylosis

In the adult patient with rheumatoid arthritis of the cervical spine, the disease is generally destructive and ankylosis is rare. In contrast, however, Still's disease or juvenile rheumatoid arthritis tends to produce ankylosis of the joints, and the cervical spine is frequently involved, but ossification of the anterior and posterior longitudinal ligaments seen in rheumatoid spondylitis does not occur. Fusion tends to take place in the apophyseal joints (Fig. 13-15). Patients with Still's disease tend to have involvement of the cervical spine and limitation of motion. If the temporomandibular joint is also affected, it becomes difficult to intubate these patients when giving a general anesthesia (Fig. 13-16). Tracheostomy is generally not necessary in management of these patients but may in some cases be a necessity.

Thoracic and Lumbar Spine

The thoracic spine seldom is involved in rheumatoid disease. The major pathologic change is generally due to osteoporosis which can be associated with steroid medications or with disuse

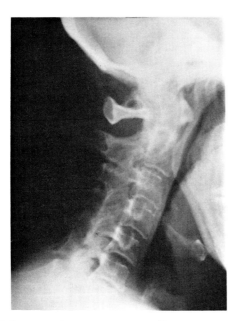

FIG. 13-15 Roentgenogram revealing spontaneous fusion of the apophyseal joints.

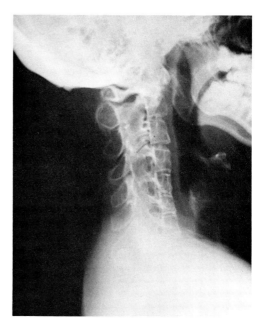

FIG. 13-16 Roentgenogram to show rheumatoid changes in cervical spine and temporomandibular joint of patient who had Still's disease as a child.

in elderly patients. Compression fracture with collapse of the thoracic spine does occur and is the most common cause of severe pain in the upper back in these patients. Gradual kyphosis with beginning wedge formation of the anterior portion of the vertebrae may develop from softening of the thoracic vertebrae.

The roentgenogram is a valuable aid in diagnosing compression fracture and osteoporosis of the thoracic spine (Fig. 13-17).

Rheumatoid arthritis is also rare in the lumbar spine. Rheumatoid spondylitis is more frequently seen in this area of the spine and in the sacroiliac joints (Fig. 13-18).

Treatment

The use of a corset or Taylor back brace may be of value in the treatment of the patient with a compression fracture of the thoracic spine. In general, these fractures will heal and it is advisable to keep these patients, especially those in

the elderly age group, active to prevent other complications. The use of vitamin D and calcium has never been proven as a valuable treatment in the management of osteoporosis.

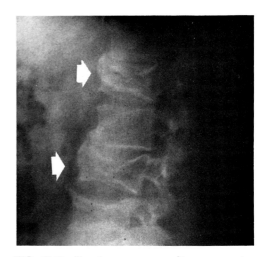

FIG. 13-17 Roentgenogram revealing compression fractures and osteoporosis of spine.

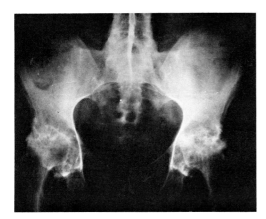

FIG. 13-18 Roentgenogram of lumbar area of the spine and the hip joints of a patient with rheumatoid spondylitis. The patient has a bamboo spine and loss of the sacroiliac joints, as well as pathologic changes in both hip joints.

Osteoarthritis

Osteoarthritis of the spine is a natural progression of wear and tear due to activities of life that frequently produce symptoms in the cervical spine and in the lower back. Although degenerative changes from osteoarthritis occur in the thoracic spine, symptoms are rare. The site of involvement tends to differ in osteoarthritis from that in rheumatoid arthritis because osteoarthritis is not a synovial disease.

Cervical Spine

The site of osteoarthritis in the cervical spine is more frequently observed in the lower cervical spine at C5-C6 and the two adjacent joints than in the upper site at C2-C3 and C3-C4 seen in rheumatoid arthritis, especially in juvenile rheumatoid disease (Fig. 13-19). Subluxation of C1 on C2 is not seen in osteoarthritis unless associated with severe trauma. The excess of motion of the cervical spine and the lordosis tend to contribute

to degenerative changes occurring in the disk space with settling of the apophyseal joints posteriorly. Wearing of the articular cartilage produces osteophytes and limits motion.

The joints of Luschka, or co-vertebral joints, which are found only in the cervical spine, are frequently involved in osteoarthritis. They are small synovial-lined joints adjacent to the intervertebral foramina along the posterior lateral margin of the vertebral bodies. A vertical lip that extends from the side of each vertebral body is located at the junction of the vertebral body and the base of the spinal arch or lamina. A small joint cavity lies between this lip and the adjacent rim of the body of the intervertebral disk. The spinal nerve passing through the foramina lies directly over the joint as it exits. Degenerative changes in these joints produce spurs that can compress the foramina and the spinal nerve root and cause radiculitis (Fig. 13-20).

The clinical findings in cervical osteoarthritis are pain of an aching or nagging type in the region of the neck and occasionally radiating to the back of the head or behind the eye. The pain may also be referred down the shoulder or to the back or down the arm. The patient may state that symptoms are aggravated by motion. The onset is usually gradual, and the disease is most common in adults after the age of forty. When the joints of Luschka are involved, radiculitis can produce radiating symptoms of pain into the arm and paresthesia.

On physical examination, the patient may have a loss of the normal lordosis and occasional spasm of the paraspinal muscles. The range of motion may be limited in flexion, extension, and rotation. The compression test of pushing down on the head to compress the cervical spine may be positive if a radiculitis exists due to involvement of the foram-

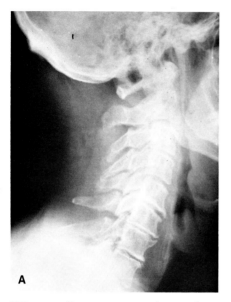 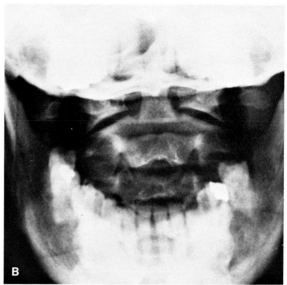

FIG. 13-19 Roentgenograms of cervical spine. A. Lateral view. Spur formation anteriorly and narrowing of the disk space are obvious in the degenerative arthritis at C5-C6 and C6-C7. B. Open mouth view of patient with cervical arthritis at C5-C6. Note the upper cervical spine is normal.

ina. Traction on the cervical spine will generally relieve the symptoms if they are due to cervical arthritis. Occasionally changes can be observed in the reflex of the upper extremity and the sensation to the forearm and hand.

The roentgenogram is of great value in the diagnosis of cervical arthritis. A routine neck series should be taken with an antero-posterior, a true lateral, and an oblique view. Osteophyte formation in the joints of Luschka can best be ob-

served in the oblique view showing encroachment on the foramina. Degeneration of the cervical disk may produce osteophyte formation of the anterior and posterior aspects of the vertebral bodies (Fig. 13-21). A large posterior osteophyte

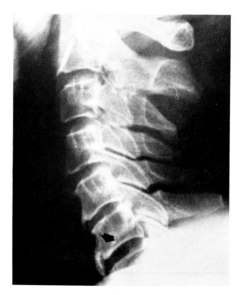

FIG. 13-20 Roentgenogram of degenerative changes in joints of Luschka. Bony spurs (arrow) encroach on the foramina.

FIG. 13-21 Roentgenogram of cervical spine revealing anterior osteophyte formation (arrow).

may produce involvement of the spinal cord with symptoms related to the lower extremities. The anterior osteophyte at times can be so large as to involve the esophagus and cause dysphagia. Fluoroscopic examination while the patient swallows barium may show the indentation of the esophagus by this bony spur or ridge. The most common site of osteophyte formation tends to be at C5-C6 and C6-C7.

Conservative Treatment

Patients with osteoarthritis of the cervical spine often become extremely uncomfortable and concerned about the cause of the pain. Reassurance about the cause and conservative management will bring dramatic relief in most cases. Only a small percentage will require surgical intervention.

Salicylates, hot packs, and massage to the neck frequently relieve the symptoms. In selected cases, indomethacin (Indocin) 25 mg three times a day, can also aid in relieving the pain.

Cervical traction can be utilized if it is kept between 5 to 7 pounds to prevent irritation of the jaw and the cervical spine itself. The most common error is to use 10 or 20 pounds of traction which frequently increases symptoms. The purpose of the traction is to relax the muscle spasm associated with the cervical arthritis by a gradual pull until the muscle tires and relaxes. In the beginning, the traction should be used for short periods of 15 to 30 minutes several times a day until the patient becomes accustomed to it. This may be done at home with an over-the-door traction, but it is important to remind the patient not to hyperextend the neck with traction. Hyperextension will increase symptoms. Traction in slight flexion tends to open the apophyseal joints and relieve the patient's symptoms.

A neck pillow that can be purchased at many department stores may be used at night to prevent tossing and turning of the neck. A soft cervical collar can be worn at times to accomplish the same thing.

Surgical Treatment

At one time anterior cervical fusion was extremely popular, and a number of patients were operated upon for cervical pain. With the passage of time, however, it has become apparent that only a small percentage of patients requires anterior body spinal fusion to open the foramina and to relieve the symptoms related to cervical arthritis.

Foraminotomy has been advised in some cases at the time of anterior body fusion to relieve the compression of the cervical spinal nerves and remove the osteophytes from the joints of Luschka. Robinson and others have stated that it is not necessary to remove these osteophytes and that they gradually disappear once solid fusion has been accomplished (Fig. 13-22).

When multiple areas are involved, it is not advisable to do multiple levels of anterior body fusion because the incidence of pseudarthrosis tends to increase. For patients with multiple joint involvement with severe symptoms, occasionally posterior spinal fusion can produce dramatic results.

Thoracic Spine

Osteoarthritis affects the thoracic spine but generally does not produce symptoms. The most common finding is osteophyte formation on the anterior aspect of the vertebral bodies (Fig. 13-23). These osteophytes may even overlap and join together anteriorly, but are most often asymptomatic.

The costovertebral joints tend to immobilize the thoracic spine and therefore the apophyseal joints are seldom a

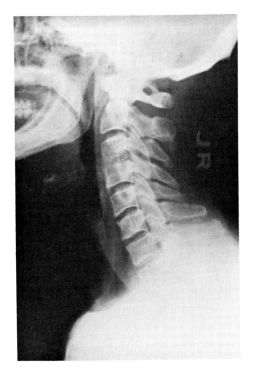

FIG. 13-22 Roentgenogram after anterior body fusion for cervical arthritis at C3-C4.

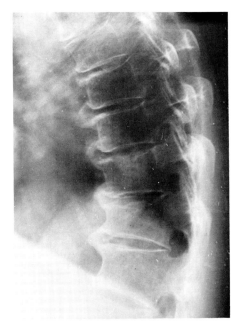

FIG. 13-23 Roentgenogram of thoracic spine with narrowing of disk space and anterior spur formation. This patient actually has bridging across the anterior aspect of the vertebral bodies.

source of pain. However, arthritis can affect the first costovertebral joint and could produce radiating thoracic and abdominal pain. The anatomic arrangement of the thoracic spine is such as to allow this to occur. The head of the first rib articulates with a single vertebral body by a full-facet synovial joint. The other ribs, 2 through 10, articulate by two hemifacets through the two adjacent vertebrae and the intervertebral disk located between them. A second rib is attached to the first and second vertebrae; therefore, the first two ribs are closer together and the first intercostaal space is narrower than the others. The first thoracic nerve emerges from its intervertebral foramina posterior to the first and second costovertebral joints. It tends to arch upward, passes laterally close to the joints in front of the neck and the internal border of the first rib, and joins the lower trunk of the brachial plexus. Roentgenograms taken directly anteroposteriorly in an oblique direction parallel to the plane of the first rib may reveal changes in this joint.

Treatment

Weinberg, et al. recommended the injection of 10 cc of 0.5 percent lidocaine (Xylocaine). In most cases, not more than four injections were necessary to relieve the patients' complaints.

Lumbar Spine

The apophyseal joints of the lumbar spine and the intervertebral disks are common sites of degenerative arthritis (Fig. 13-24). Generally the L4-L5 and L5-S1 apophyseal joints are involved. Osteophytes form anteriorly off the vertebral body and in the apophyseal joint region. Osteoarthritis is the most common cause of nagging backache and low back pain that radiates into the back and

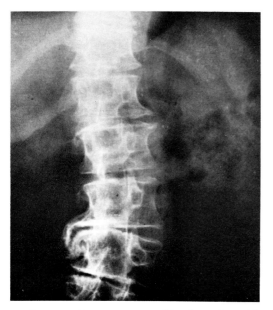

FIG. 13-24 Roentgenogram of lumbar spine with severe osteoarthritis of disk space between L2 and L3. Spur formation is noted between T12 and L1. Bony bridging has occurred along the lateral border of the vertebral bodies.

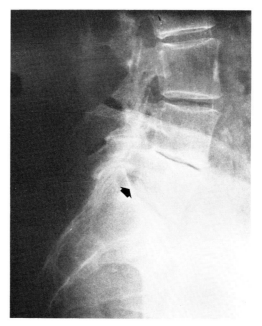

FIG. 13-25 Roentgenogram of lumbar spine. Note narrowing of disk spaces and sclerosis of apophyseal joints. A spondylolisthesis is present at L5-S1 due to collapse of the disk space (arrow).

thighs. Sclerosis, irregular bony margins, and osteophyte formation from the apophyseal joints may be seen on the roentgenograms (Fig. 13-25).

Conservative Treatment

The patient with osteoarthritis of the lower lumbar spine, especially one in the older age group, can usually be treated conservatively. With the passage of time nature tends to produce stiffness and ankylosis that result in loss of motion and a decrease of symptoms in these joints. In the active, young adult or middle-aged patient with intractable symptoms interfering with daily activities, it may be necessary to consider posterior spine fusion. Most patients tend to improve with the use of flexion exercises, analgesics, and physical therapy. Occasionally the wearing of a low back support will give considerable re-

lief in these patients. Analgesics and anti-inflammatory drugs may be of value in the acute case.

Surgical Treatment

The operative treatment of the lumbar spine should not be taken lightly. In the past, many operative procedures were performed for the patient with low back pain. The results of surgery have not been spectacular in a number of series, and pseudarthrosis is reasonably common when more than one joint is involved. Patients must be carefully evaluated for functional overlay and other causes of low back pain. Referred pain to the back can occur with disease located elsewhere in the abdominal cavity and this should be carefully ruled out as well as metastatic disease. Severe pain arising in the elderly patient at night should always raise the suspicion of a

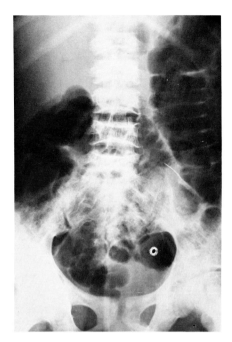

FIG. 13-26 Roentgenogram showing widespread degenerative changes in the lumbar spine and pelvis due to Paget's disease.

possible metastatic lesion. Roentgenograms, including a bone scan, may help to rule out metastatic disease, especially since anemia and an elevated sedimentation rate are common in the elderly patient. Paget's disease may also be a cause of low back pain (Fig. 13-26).

Bibliography

Rheumatoid Arthritis

Bailey, R. W., and Badgley, C. E.: Stabilization of the cervical spine by anterior fusion. J. Bone Joint Surg., 42-A:565, 1960.

Baggenstoss, A. M., Bickel, W. H., and Ward, L. E.: Rheumatoid granulomatous nodules as destructive lesions of vertebrae. J. Bone Joint Surg., 34-A:60, 1952.

Conlon, P. W., Isdale, I. C., and Rose, B. S.: Rheumatoid arthritis of the cervical spine. An analysis of 333 cases. Ann. Rheum. Dis., 25:120, 1966.

Crellin, R. Q., Maccabe, J. J., and Hamilton, E. B. D.: Severe subluxation of the cervical spine in rheumatoid arthritis. J. Bone Joint Surg., 52-B:244, 1970.

Davis, F. W., Jr., and Markley, H. E.: Rheumatoid arthritis with death from medullary compression. Ann. Intern. Med., 35:451, 1951.

DeBlecort, J. J., and Veenstra, S. M.: Transverse lesion in a patient with juvenile rheumatoid arthritis. Acta Rheum. Scand., 6:251, 1960.

Finger, H., and Kikillus, B.: Luxation of the atlanto-axial joint, a complication of chronic rheumatic diseases. Dtsch. Med. Wochenschr., 89:1546, 1964.

Gleason, I. O., and Urist, M. R.: Atlanto-axial dislocation with odontoid separation in rheumatoid disease. Clin. Orthop., 42:121, 1965.

Hauge, T.: So-called spontaneous cervical dislocations. Acta Chir. Scand. Suppl., 232:5, 1958.

Hopkins, J. S.: Lower cervical rheumatoid subluxation with tetraplegia. J. Bone Joint Surg., 49-B:45, 1967.

Kornblum, D., Clayton, M. L., and Nash, H. H.: Nontraumatic cervical dislocations in rheumatoid spondylitis. J.A.M.A., 149:431, 1952.

Lawrence, J. S., et al.: Rheumatoid arthritis of the lumbar spine. Ann. Rheum. Dis., 23:205, 1964.

Lindquist, P. R., and McDonnell, D. E.: Rheumatoid cyst causing extradural compression. J. Bone Joint Surg., 52-A:1235, 1970.

Lorber, A., Pearson, C. M., and Rene, R. M.: Osteolytic vertebral lesions as a manifestation of rheumatoid arthritis and related disorders. Arthritis Rheum., 4:514, 1961.

Margulies, M. E., Katz, I., and Rosenberg, M.: Spontaneous dislocations of the atlanto-axial joint in rheumatoid spondylitis. Neurology, 5:290, 1953.

Martel, W.: The occipito-atlanto-axial joints in rheumatoid arthritis and ankylosing spondylitis. Am. J. Roentgenol., *86*:223, 1961.

Martel, W., and Page, J. W.: Cervical vertebral erosions and subluxations in rheumatoid arthritis and ankylosing spondylitis. Arthritis Rheum., *3*:546, 1960.

Nathan, F. F., and Bickel, W. H.: Spontaneous axial subluxation in a child as the first sign of juvenile rheumatoid arthritis. J. Bone Joint Surg., *50-A*:1675, 1968.

Page, J. W.: Spontaneous tendon rupture and cervical vertebral subluxation in patients with rheumatoid arthritis. J. Mich. Med. Soc., *60*:888, 1961.

Pratt, T. L. C.: Spontaneous dislocation of the atlanto-axial articulation occurring in ankylosing spondylitis and rheumatoid arthritis. J. Fac. Radiologists, *10*:40, 1959.

Seaman, W. B., and Wells, J.: Destructive lesions of the vertebral bodies in rheumatoid disease. Am. J. Roentgenol., *86*:241, 1961.

Sharp, J., Purser, D. W., and Lawrence, J. S.: Rheumatoid arthritis of the cervical spine in the adult. Ann. Rheum. Dis., *17*:303, 1958.

Weiss, L. S., and Freehafer, A. A.: Atraumatic subluxation and dislocation of the cervical spine in rheumatoid arthritis. Clin. Orthop., *34*:53, 1964.

Werne, S.: Studies in spontaneous atlas dislocation. Acta Orthop. Scand. Suppl., *23*:1, 1957.

Osteoarthritis

Bishara, S. N.: The posterior operation and treatment of cervical spondylosis with myelopathy: A long-term follow-up study. J. Neurol. Neurosurg. Psychiatry, *43*:393, 1971.

Friedenberg, Z. P., Edeiken, J., and Spencer, H. N.: Degenerative changes in the cervical spine, J. Bone Joint Surg., *41-A*:61, 1959.

Jackson, R.: The cervical syndrome. Clin. Orthop., *5*:138, 1955.

Julkunen, H., Heinonen, O., and Pyorala, K.: Hyperostosis of the spine in an adult population. Ann. Rheum. Dis., *30*:605, 1972.

Meeks, L. W., et. al.: Vertebral osteophytosis and dysphagia. Two case reports of the syndrome recently termed ankylosing hyperostosis. J. Bone Joint Surg., *55-A*:197, 1973.

Newman, P. H.: Surgical treatment for derangement of the lumbar spine. J. Bone Joint Surg., *55-B*:7, 1973.

Nordby, E. J., and Lucas, G. L.: A comparative analysis of lumbar disk disease treated by laminectomy or chemonucleolysis. Clin. Orthop., *90*:119, 1973.

Orofino, C., Sherman, M. S., and Schecter, D.: Luschka's joint-A degenerative phenomena. J. Bone Joint Surg., *42-A*:853, 1960.

Robinson, R. A., et al.: The results of anterior interbody fusion of the cervical spine. J. Bone Joint Surg., *44-A*:1569, 1962.

Schlesinger, E. B., and Taveras, J. M.: Syndromes of cervical root compression: Neurologic and roentgenologic aspects. Med. Clin. North Am., *37*:451, 1953.

Spilberg, I., and Lieberman, D. M.: Ankylosing hyperostosis of the cervical spine. Arthritis Rheum., *15*:208, 1972.

Waldron, R. L. II., and Wood, E. H.: Cervical myelography. Clin. Orthop., *97*:74, 1973.

Weinberg, H., et al.: Arthritis of the first costovertebral joint as a cause of thoracic outlet syndrome. Clin. Orthop., *86*:159, 1972.

Wilfling, F. J., Klonoff, H., and Kokan, P.: Psychological, demographic and orthopaedic factors associated with prediction of outcome of spinal fusion. Clin. Orthop., *90*:153, 1973.

14 | Juvenile Rheumatoid Arthritis

Juvenile rheumatoid arthritis is a systemic rheumatoid disease that was originally described by Still in 1896 and has been called Still's disease. There are approximately over 250,000 children suffering from this disease in the United States alone. Therefore, the orthopaedic surgeon should be familiar with this disease because frequently these patients are referred to him first because of their joint symptoms. Juvenile rheumatoid arthritis should not be considered as the same disease occurring in the adult. It is a distinct entity requiring a team approach in order to achieve optimal care for the patients.

The onset of juvenile arthritis occurs at two peaks during childhood, but before the age of 17 years. The first peak occurs between 1 and 3 years of age, and the second tends to occur just before puberty. The disease is slightly more frequent in girls, but not as severe as that seen in the adult.

Calabro and his associates have described three modes of onset of juvenile rheumatoid arthritis. In approximately 20 percent of the cases, there are high fever and widespread systemic involvement. There may or may not be articular involvement in this type of onset. The second type is polyarticular and is seen in 50 percent of the children who have moderate systemic involvement and arthritis in four or more joints. The third type is called pauciarticular and occurs in about 30 percent of the children. Systemic features are minimal, and swelling occurs in one to three joints.

The American Rheumatism Association has delineated two classes of the disease. Class I consists of a polyarthritis or monoarthritis present for 3 months or more associated with swelling of the joint. If swelling is not present, the patient must exhibit at least two of the three following criteria:

1. Pain and tenderness.
2. Limitation of motion.
3. Heat in the joint.

The class II group consists of patients who have had arthritis for 6 weeks, but less than 3 months. These patients should show at least one of the following manifestations:

1. Rash of rheumatoid arthritis.
2. Iridocyclitis.
3. Rheumatoid factor in the blood.
4. Cervical vertebral involvement.
5. Tenosynovitis.

6. Pericarditis.
7. Intermittent fever.
8. Morning stiffness.

However, it is obvious that these symptoms can be related to other disease and a careful workup is required to differentiate juvenile rheumatoid arthritis from rheumatic fever, sickle cell anemia, hemophilia, leukemia, and other neoplastic diseases, as well as infection, trauma, and allergic reactions.

There are several characteristic differences between juvenile rheumatoid arthritis and adult rheumatoid disease. In juvenile rheumatoid arthritis, frequently there are a high fever, a characteristic rash, infrequent rheumatoid nodules, lack of rheumatoid factor, and the complication of iridocyclitis. Any patient complaining of tearing or photophobia in juvenile rheumatoid arthritis should be checked for iridocyclitis because of its high incidence in juveniles. Juvenile iridocyclitis is most frequently associated with the pauciarticular type of monoarticular arthritis and occurs in approximately 29 percent of the cases. It is rare in the acute febrile type of disease, as well as in the polyarticular type.

A report of the seminar on the role of the orthopaedist in the management of juvenile rheumatoid arthritis in 1972 listed the characteristic differences and the specific kind of joint involvement in juvenile rheumatoid arthritis and adult rheumatoid arthritis (See table at bottom of page).

Diagnosis

Diagnosis is difficult in juvenile rheumatoid arthritis because there are no specific laboratory tests of value. The development of high fever, rash, iridocyclitis, or other characteristic symptoms may be of value. A specific rheumatoid rash which may present as a salmon-pink macula with a pale center is pathognomonic of this disease. The most frequent error in diagnosis of juvenile rheumatoid arthritis in children is that of mistaking the disease for rheumatic fever. The disease can be suspected and diagnosed when the modes of onset are recognized. The three modes, as mentioned previously, are acute febrile response in 20 percent of the patients, monoarticular in 30 percent, and polyarticular in 50 percent. The patients with the acute febrile mode of onset clinically exhibit irritability, anorexia, weight loss, and acute illness. They may have an intermittent high fever, a characteristic

Comparison of Juvenile and Adult Rheumatoid Arthritis

Joint	JRA	ARA
Shoulder	Loss of motion	Pain
Elbow	Stiffens and deteriorates	Loosens and deteriorates
Wrist	Stiffens and may fuse or sublux	Painful, swollen, angulates and dislocates
Metacarpophalangeal	Rare ulnar drift, significant loss of motion	Significant ulnar drift and early loss of extension
Proximal interphalangeal	Generalized swelling and stiffness	More swan neck and boutonnière deformities
Hip	Dislocation	
Knee	Growth disturbances, especially with pauciarticular disease	
Tendons	Adhesions and tenosynovitis with loss of extension	Hypertrophic synovitis without serious loss of extension

rash associated with a myocarditis, splenomegaly, and minimal joint involvement.

The polyarticular type of juvenile rheumatoid arthritis involves four or more joints and has an abrupt onset in about half of the cases. These patients also are acutely ill and have low fever, weight loss, and anorexia. Many of the symptoms—polyarthritis, pain in the neck, headache, and rash—not only resemble those in adult rheumatoid arthritis but may easily be confused with rheumatic fever.

The monoarticular arthritis generally involves one joint, and occasionally several. It is usually insidious and frequently attacks the knees. The patient may begin to walk with a limp and have minimal swelling with pain and stiffness in the joints. The pain however, may, play a prominent role in the child with rheumatoid disease in the hip.

Laboratory Findings

Laboratory findings in the three modes of onset vary slightly. In the acute phase, the hemoglobin may be 9 to 11 gm, an indication of anemia. The white blood count is generally elevated to between 15,000 to 25,000 and the sedimentation rate is increased. In the polyarticular type of disease, the hemoglobin may be 10 to 12 gm, the white count between 10,000 to 20,000, and the sedimentation rate increased. In the monoarticular type of disease, the hemoglobin, white count, and sedimentation rate are normal. Rheumatoid factor in the juvenile arthritis patient is usually negative and is only positive in approximately 15 percent of the children. The immunoglobulins may be elevated in the active disease, and hip disease is often correlated with high titers of immunoglobulins. The antistreptolysin O titer can be elevated in 30 to 50 percent of the patients, but it is usually nonspecific.

The C-reactive protein is usually present in active disease and is also nonspecific.

Roentgenograms

Some characteristic clinical findings of juvenile rheumatoid arthritis may be obvious in the roentgenogram. The growth centers are usually affected by inflammatory changes due to arthritis, and premature closure of the epiphyseal plate may cause cessation of growth. The early signs of juvenile rheumatoid arthritis in the roentgenogram are soft tissue swelling osteoporosis, and periosteal bone apposition (Fig. 14-1). Evidence of joint destruction and erosions occurs late in juvenile rheumatoid arthritis. Spontaneous subluxation of large joints such as the hip is not infrequent. Involvement of the cervical spine occurs often with fusion of the apophyseal joints leaving the disk space uninvolved (Fig. 14-2). Subluxation of C1 on C2 is common. Ankylosis of involved joints occurs early in this disease (Fig. 14-3). Involvement of the jaw and premature closure of the mandibular epiphysis are also common in juvenile rheumatoid arthritis.

Treatment

The basic logic of treatment is to allow the child to live as normal a life as possible. In evaluating the child, it is often of great value to have a team approach consisting of a rheumatologist, a pediatrician, and an orthopaedic surgeon. It is important for the physician to realize that anxiety is often associated with this disease in the child. Emotional problems can become manifest at the time of deciding upon a minor medical procedure. Therefore, it is important for the physician and the patient to understand the disease and for the physician to explain the prognosis in terms the family will understand. In general, the

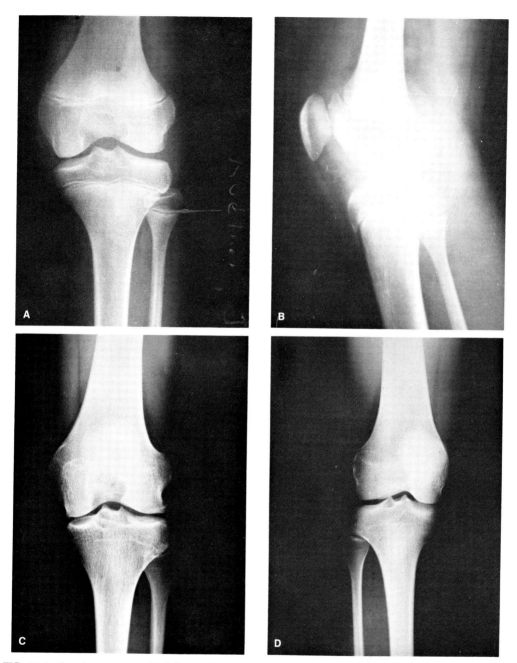

FIG. 14-1 Roentgenograms of left knee of patient with juvenile rheumatoid arthritis. A. Anterior view at age of 8 years. Note the erosion of the femoral condyle. B. Lateral view showing massive swelling of soft tissue. C. Anterior view of same patient at 16 years of age. Note the good joint space, evidence of old arthritis changes in the lateral femoral condyle, and a small bony spur on the medial femoral condyle. The epiphyseal plate has closed. D. Anterior view of the right knee.

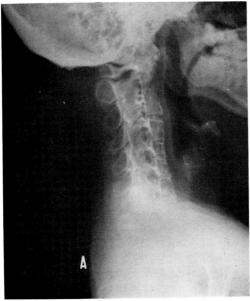
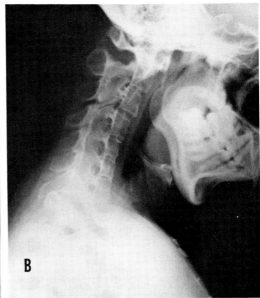

FIG. 14-2 Roentgenograms of cervical spine of patient with juvenile rheumatoid arthritis. A. In extension. B. In maximum flexion. There are marked limitation of motion and small vertebral bodies.

treatment program should be carried on as much as possible in the home and should be designed to prevent as much joint damage as possible.

The treatment must be individualized because of the wide variety of clinical manifestations. Two goals are (1) suppression of severe life-threatening symptoms, and (2) prevention of systemic and articular disease in order to allow nor-

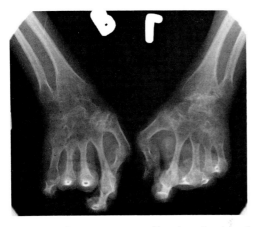

FIG. 14-3 Roentgenograms of hands and wrists of patient with juvenile rheumatoid arthritis.

mal growth and development without deformities.

Conservative Treatment

General supportive treatment should be given to keep the child in good health. It is advisable to avoid long periods of bed rest because physical activity will stimulate normal growth.

Frequently children with juvenile rheumatoid arthritis do not grow to full stature because of premature closure of the epiphysis or lack of physical activity (Fig. 14-4). Rest periods during the day in the active phase of the disease are important as well as daily physical therapy. Deep heat or cold therapy tends to relieve the pain associated with inflamed joints. Joints should be put through a full range of motion to prevent the development of flexion contractures. Passive exercise and active assisted exercise can aid in regaining motion in the joints and also preserve motion that would otherwise be lost.

Positioning of the patient in bed and

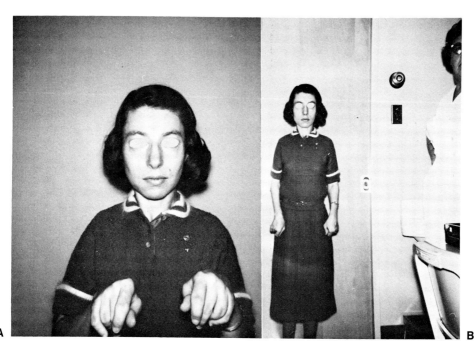

FIG. 14-4 Photographs of young patient with juvenile rheumatoid arthritis. A. The small jaw is due to premature closure of the mandibular epiphysis. B. Premature closure of the epiphyseal plates caused the small stature.

body alignment are extremely useful to prevent deformities. Night splints are recommended during the active phase of the disease when the joints are hot and painful, but rigid splinting or immobilization should be of short duration. It is important to realize that braces can prevent contractures, but braces should not be used to correct deformities.

The basic medical treatment is similar to that in the adult, but drug therapy should be instituted cautiously because of the toxity of most of the drugs in the growing child. Aspirin is an excellent drug and will tend to suppress the inflammation of the disease. Children may be maintained at fairly high doses of aspirin for long periods. On the average, 40 mg per pound of body weight divided into six doses are required. Corticosteroids should be used only when the disease is life threatening. They do not seem to alter the natural remission or the prognosis of the disease.

Surgical Treatment

Surgical treatment can be effective in relieving pain when medical treatment has failed. Surgical procedures, however, are performed much less frequently in juvenile patients than in the adult. Eyring and his associates have stated that less than 50 percent of the children with juvenile rheumatoid arthritis will need surgery. Since active disease in many of the joints in children can have a spontaneous subsidence after several years, synovectomy in the juvenile should not be considered until the symptoms have persisted for 18 to 24 months unless signs of rapid destruction within the joint are seen in the roentgenogram. Kampner and Ferguson feel that the most successful results of synovectomy occur in children over 7 years of age and that success may be related in part to the patient's cooperation. Failures in general were related to loss of motion

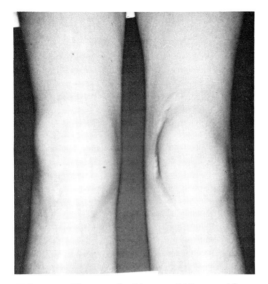

FIG. 14-5 Photograph of knees of 16-year-old patient who had a synovectomy of the left knee at the age of seven, with no recurrence of rheumatoid disease. The right knee is swollen and has evidence of rheumatoid disease.

following synovectomy. The best results with synovectomy tended to occur in patients with monarticular involvement rather than in to patients with polyarticular involvement. Synovectomy appears

to be much more effective in the large joints such as the knees, hips, elbows, and ankles than in the smaller joints of the fingers and wrists (Fig. 14-5). The synovitis can recur, but generally the incidence of recurrence is low.

Release of soft tissue can produce improved results and may be indicated. Release of the iliotibial band combined with synovectomy of the knee and posterior knee capsulotomy may relieve knee flexion contractures and prevent valgus and external rotation deformities of the knee. Release of the hip flexors and adductors with progressive hip disease may also be of value and can be combined with synovectomy of the hip. Contraindications to surgery are dry synovitis of the joint, especially in the region of the hand, and the uncooperative patient and parent.

Arthrodesis is occasionally of value in correcting deformities of the wrist and foot. A triple arthrodesis can correct a severe varus deformity of the foot and improve the function. Arthrodesis of the hip or knee is seldom indicated in rheu-

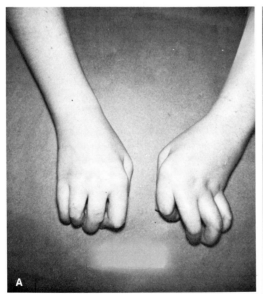

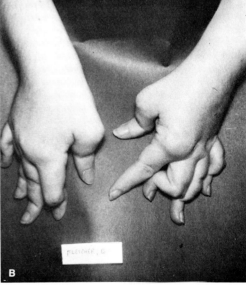

FIG. 14-6 Photographs of hands of young patients after surgical treatment of juvenile rheumatoid arthritis. A. After an arthroplasty of metacarpophalangeal joints of the right hand. Ankylosis has made the proximal interphalangeal joints stiff. B. Deformities after surgical procedures in another patient.

matoid arthritis in the child, and the development of total joint replacement for the hip or knee may aid considerably in the management of the older juvenile rheumatoid patient.

It is important to remember that it is difficult to obtain cooperation from young patients and therefore surgery should be undertaken with great caution (Fig. 14-6). Without the cooperation of the patient in postoperative exercises, there is a tendency for stiffness to develop. Poorly advised or ill-conceived surgical intervention in a patient with juvenile rheumatoid arthritis can produce severe deformities.

Bibliography

Arden, G. P., Ansell, B. M., and Hunter, M. J.: Total hip replacement in juvenile chronic polyarthritis and ankylosing spondylitis. Clin. Orthop., 84:130, 1972.

Bache, C.: Mandibular growth and dental occlusion in juvenile rheumatoid arthritis. Acta Rheum. Scand., 10:142, 1964.

Bywaters, E. G. L., and Ansell, B. M.: Monarticular arthritis in children. Ann. Rheum. Dis., 24:116, 1965.

Calabro, J. J., Katz, R. M., and Maltz, B. A.: A critical reappraisal of juvenile rheumatoid arthritis. Clin. Orthop., 74:101, 1971.

Cassidy, J. T., Brody, G. L., and Martel, W.: Monarticular juvenile rheumatoid arthritis. Arthritis Rheum., 7:298, 1964.

Colver, T.: The prognosis in rheumatoid arthritis in childhood. Arch. Dis. Child., 12:253, 1937.

Coss, J. A., Jr., and Boots, R. H.: Juvenile rheumatoid arthritis. A study of fifty-six cases with a note on skeletal changes. J. Pediat., 29:143, 1946.

Edström, G.: Rheumatoid arthritis and Still's disease in children—a survey of 161 cases. Arthritis Rheum., 1:497, 1958.

Eyring, E. J., Longert, A., and Bass, J.: Synovectomy in juvenile rheumatoid arthritis. J. Bone Joint Surg., 53-A:638, 1971.

Grokóest, A. W.: Juvenile rheumatoid arthritis. Am. J. Occup. Ther., 19:152, 1965.

Grossman, B. J., Ozoa, N. F., and Arya, S. C.: Problems in juvenile rheumatoid arthritis. Med. Clin. North Am., 49:33, 1965.

Johnson, N. J., and Dodd, K.: Juvenile rheumatoid arthritis. Med. Clin. North America, 39:459–487, 1955.

Kampner, S. L., and Ferguson, A. B., Jr.: Efficacy of synovectomy in juvenile rheumatoid arthritis. Clin. Orthop., 88:94, 1972.

Kelley, V. C., and Limbeck, G. A.: Management of arthritis in children. Mod. Treat., 1:1270, 1964.

Lindbjerg, I. F.: Juvenile rheumatoid arthritis. Arch. Dis. Child., 39:576, 1964.

Lockie, L. M., and Norcross, B. M.: Juvenile rheumatoid arthritis. Pediatrics, 2:694, 1948.

Miller, D. S.: Monarticular arthritis of children. Med. Clin. North Am., 49:49, 1965.

Pickard, N. S.: Rheumatoid arthritis in children, a clinical study. Arch. Int. Med., 80:771, 1947.

Powell, B. H.: Arthritis in childhood. Clin. Pediat., 4:25, 1965.

Scala, M., Raganati, M., and DeCicco, N.: The significance of the Latex fixation test in children. Pediatria (Napoli), 72:1252, 1964.

Still, G. F.: On a form of chronic joint disease in children. Trans. R. Med. Chir. Soc. (London), 62:47, 1897.

15 | Fractures in the Arthritic Patient

Fractures that occur in patients with arthritis may present special problems because of the preexisting arthritis. Arthritic patients tend to develop joint stiffness rather easily following injury, and although the fracture can be reduced, reduction may lead to a poor result because of the subsequent stiffness of the adjacent joint produced by the immobilization during healing of the fracture. The bones of arthritic patients are often osteoporotic, especially if patients have been on steroids which tend to contribute to the osteoporosis and softening of the bone. The osteoporosis may prevent internal fixation where it is often necessary in order to obtain a good result.

The key to successful treatment of fractures in the arthritic patient hinges upon early motion of the involved joint to prevent stiffness. If these basic principles are followed, better results can be obtained in the arthritic patient who sustains a fracture.

Fractures of the Wrist

The most common fracture that occurs at the wrist is the Colles' fracture. Even in the patient without arthritis, this fracture can be a problem in management. The most common cause of this fracture is a fall upon the outstretched hand, producing dorsiflexion of the wrist. The radius becomes shortened because of impaction of the fracture and reverse of the normal volar tilt of the distal radius. If the fracture is comminuted, especially on the volar surface, the fracture may be assumed to be unstable and will tend to collapse with the loss of the cortex, resulting in shortening and deformity of the wrist (Fig. 15-1). In the aged patient or the patient with osteoarthritis or rheumatoid arthritis of the hand, the surgeon must weigh the possibility of a deformity of the wrist versus the ability to regain a reasonably normal hand function. Patients with osteoarthritis tend to have Heberden's nodes on their distal finger joints, and these are an excellent clue to the fact that the patient may develop stiffness of the hand if immobilization is carried out for a long period of time. Closed reduction may be carried out in some cases following the local aspiration of the hematoma and the injection of lidocaine (Xylocaine) into the hematoma. This will give adequate anesthesia for manipulation of the fracture to improve its posi-

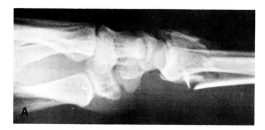

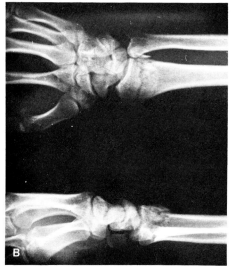

FIG. 15-1 Roentgenograms of fractures of the wrist. A. Colles' fracture with comminution of the volar surface. B. Anterior and lateral views of a fracture with no comminution of the volar surface.

tion. It is extremely important that the cast should not pass beyond the distal palmar crease and that the dorsal part of the cast is removed far enough back to allow good finger motion at the metacarpophalangeal joints.

In the older patient or the patient with advanced arthritis, it may even be necessary to accept the deformity and to utilize just a volar splint for protection of the wrist, without closed reduction. If this form of treatment is chosen, the patient should be advised of the fact that the deformity is present and that if symptoms become severe the ulnar head may have to be removed in the future. If the hand is allowed to get stiff by either improper immobilization or lack of use of the hand, recovery may be delayed for

a year or more, and mobility may never return in some patients. Numerous deformities of the wrist are usually seen in the patient with rheumatoid arthritis, but it is surprising how well the patient can continue to function despite the destruction of the wrist joint. Therefore, repeated reductions until a satisfactory position is seen in the roentgenogram should be discouraged in the elderly patient or the patient with advanced osteoarthritis. Subluxation and ulnar deviation of the carpal bones are commonly seen in rheumatoid arthritis, and shortening of the radius due to erosion and destruction from the rheumatoid process may occasionally give rise to discomfort in the radioulnar joint. This deformity is frequently treated by excision of the ulnar head, and this procedure can be kept in mind for the patient with a malunited Colles' fracture.

The arthritic patient with a fracture of the carpal navicular that is extremely displaced, involves the proximal one third, or goes on to nonunion may be a candidate for excision of the navicular and replacement with a Silastic prosthesis. The advantages of this procedure are early mobilization of the hand and the prevention of prolonged cast treatment that is often required with this type of fracture to obtain a union.

Fracture of the Elbow

The patient with fracture of the radial head and with arthritis is an ideal candidate for excision of the head because a diseased head can still produce symptoms after union. The radial head should be removed through a posterolateral approach. After the head has been removed from the rheumatoid patient, a synovectomy of the elbow joint can easily be carried out. All of the synovial tissue that can be reached easily with a rongeur or curette should be excised. In the patient with osteo-

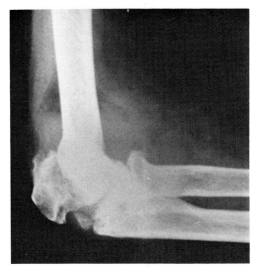

FIG. 15-2 Roentgenogram of elbow joint before excision of olecranon fragment and a synovectomy in a patient with rheumatoid arthritis.

arthritis, it is not necessary to perform a synovectomy. The radial head can be replaced with a Swanson Silastic radial head. This replacement will allow early pronation and supination without pain and maintain the length of the radius. The arthritic patient does not do well with immobilization of the joint after a surgical procedure or a recent fracture, and it is important to start early motion. Splinting is not necessary, and a soft dressing may be utilized to encourage the patient to flex and extend the elbow immediately after surgery. Dressings should be reduced to a minimum several days after the operation so as not to interfere with motion of the joint. Pronation and supination should be started immediately to regain as much function as possible. If the patient is immobilized in a cast or a posterior splint for several weeks, it will be difficult to regain motion after that period of time. Generally the golden period in the arthritic to regain motion is during the first week or so after the operative procedure or injury.

Comminuted fractures of the olecranon can also occur in the arthritic patient and are best treated by excision

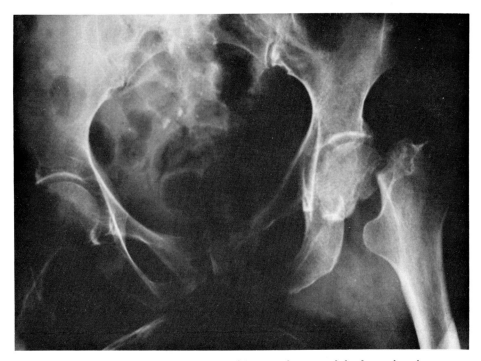

FIG. 15-3 Roentgenogram of hip showing a Pauwels' type 3 fracture of the femoral neck.

of the fragments and resuture of the triceps tendon to restore its continuity (Fig. 15-2). When there are arthritic changes in the humeral-ulnar joint, it is better to consider excision of the fragments rather than try to restore a rough joint surface. Generally very little articular cartilage is left, and the patient actually would benefit from excision of the portion of the joint that is involved. Early motion should be emphasized to regain as much function as possible.

Fracture of the Femoral Neck

The fracture of the femoral neck occurs frequently in the elderly patient. Many of these patients already have evidence of osteoarthritis of the hip or may have rheumatoid arthritis. If the fracture is displaced such as in a Pauwels' type 2 or 3, femoral nailing probably is not indicated if the patient is in the older age group (Fig. 15-3). The osteoarthritic patient with a good acetabulum and an arthritic femoral head may be considered for a hemi-arthroplasty with the removal of the femoral head (Fig. 15-4). This procedure, however, should not be considered in the patient with rheumatoid arthritis because of the osteoporosis and the involvement of the acetabulum. Cementing the shaft of the prosthesis into the femur with methylmethacrylate will allow the patient to bear weight early and will give an excellent fixation that will prevent distal migration of the prosthesis. It is advisable not to use a prosthesis of the Austin-Moore type because of the locking of the prosthesis into the cement. If removal of the prosthesis ever becomes necessary, it would be extremely difficult. For a fracture of the femoral neck in the patient with severe osteoarthritis involving the acetabulum or with severe rheumatoid arthritis, it would be advisable to consider a total hip replacement if the patient

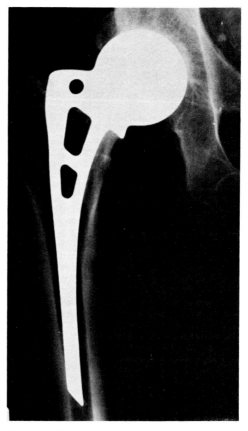

FIG. 15-4 Roentgenograms 10 years after Austin-Moore arthroplasty. There is no evidence of loosening.

is in reasonably good health. The cementing in of the components will relieve the patient of the arthritic pain, allow early ambulation, and solve not only the fracture of the hip but also the arthritic problem.

Intertrochanteric fractures or subtrochanteric fractures should be treated by internal fixation until union is established. Total hip replacement can be considered at a later date.

Supracondylar Fractures of the Femur

Supracondylar fractures of the femur occur with reasonable frequency in the patient with arthritis. They are more common in the rheumatoid patient because of the osteoporosis associated with the disease and often with the medical treatment. When the patient with a supracondylar fracture has arthritis involving the knee joint, special consideration must be given to the management to obtain a good result.

If the patient has osteoarthritis with narrowing of the medial or lateral aspect of the knee joint, it is possible to treat not only the supracondylar fracture but also the arthritis. Dual treatment is also possible in the patient with rheumatoid arthritis who has a varus or valgus deformity of the knee associated with a flexion contracture. The surgeon, in determining the mode of treatment of the fracture, can correct the deformity of

the knee joint at the same time. It is not unusual for the surgeon who is not familiar with fractures in the arthritic patient to treat the fracture without considering the arthritis in the knee joint. Failure to correct the deformity can lead to increased deformities or else leave the patient with a residual painful knee (Fig. 15-5). Fractures that extend into the knee joint should not be put in a cast for long periods of time because of the frequency of development of joint stiffness and increased symptoms in the arthritic patient. Open reduction is often necessary, and firm fixation should be sought so that early motion can be instituted in the knee joint (Fig. 15-6). If the patient has a varus or valgus deformity

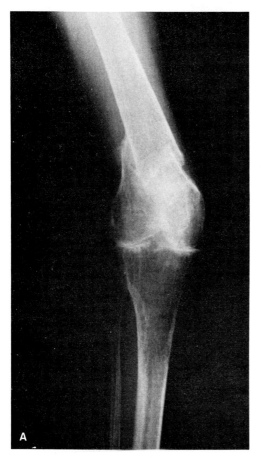
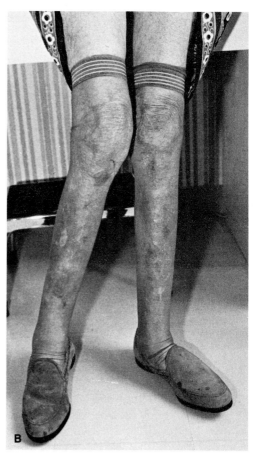

FIG. 15-5 A. Roentgenogram of supracondylar fracture of the femur reduced with valgus angulation. B. A clinical view of the deformity.

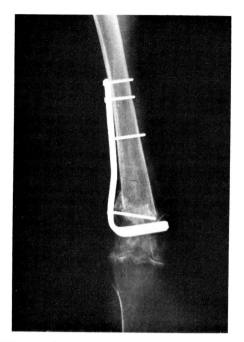

FIG. 15-6 Roentgenogram after osteotomy to correct varus deformity and shift weight to the medial compartment. Internal fixation was used to start early motion to prevent postoperative stiffness.

of the knee with narrowing of the joint space, overcorrection of the fracture into a valgus or varus position opposite to the arthritic joint narrowing will give a good postoperative result. As in an osteotomy, this shifts the weight to the better side of the joint and will relieve the patient's symptoms.

Fractures of the Proximal Tibia

The patient with osteoarthritis of the knee joint will often have a varus or valgus deformity with narrowing of either the medial or lateral side of the joint. If the proximal tibia is fractured in the region of the tibial tubercle in the patient with osteoarthritis involving a single compartment of the knee joint, a varus or valgus deformity can often be improved by the fracture treatment. Correction of the varus or valgus deformity through the proximal tibia is easily accomplished if there is a fracture,

and this procedure will shift the weight to the good side of the knee joint. It is similar to performing an osteotomy of the tibia at this level. Therefore, the surgeon who is familiar with this type of problem can easily correct the deformity. It is important to instruct the patient and his family preoperatively that the leg is being placed in this new position to overcorrect the preexisting osteoarthritic deformity. As long as the fracture line does not involve the joint surface, the cast may be used without fear of stiffness. Fractures extending into the joint or associated with bleeding into the joint may become stiff because of resulting adhesions. The arthritic patient may be allowed to ambulate in a long-leg plaster cast 2 weeks after treatment of the fracture, if the fracture is stable.

Bibliography

Bauer, G. C. H., Insall, J., and Koshino, T.: Tibial osteotomy in gonarthritis. J. Bone Joint Surg., *51-A:1545,* 1969.

Burgess, E. M., and Romano, R. L.: Fracture in the aged. Clin. Orthop., *11:21,* 1958.

Casagrande, P.A.: Surgical rehabilitation of shoulder and elbow in rheumatoid arthritis. Arthritis Rheum., *1:3,* 1971.

Charnley, J.: Arthroplasty of the hip: a new operation. Lancet, 1:1129, 1961.

Charnley, J.: Anchorage of the femoral head prosthesis to the shaft of the femur. J. Bone Joint Surg., 42-B:28, 1960.

Coventry, M. B.: Osteotomy of the upper portion of the tibia for degenerative arthritis of the knee. J. Bone Joint Surg., *47-A:984,* 1965.

Devas, M. B.: High tibial osteotomy for arthritis of the knee. J. Bone Joint Surg., *51-B:95,* 1961.

Gould, N.: Early mobilization of the joint in intra-articular fractures with special attention to the elbow joint. Surg. Gynecol. Obstet., *11*:575, 1962.

Harris, W. H.: Surgical management of arthritis of the hip. Sem. Arthritis Rheum., *1*:35, 1971.

Marmor, L.: Management of fractures in the arthritic patient. J. Trauma, *12*:847, 1972.

McLaughlin, H. L.: Trauma. Philadelphia, W. B. Saunders Co., 1959.

Stein, A. H., Jr., and Griz, J. R.: The treatment of femoral neck fractures by internal fixation or primary prosthesis. Surg. Gynecol. Obstet., *119*:1037, 1964.

Torgerson, W. R., and Leach, R. E.: Synovectomy of the elbow in rheumatoid arthritis. J. Bone Joint Surg., *52-A*:371, 1970.

Watson-Jones, R.: Fractures and Joint Injuries, Vol. II. London, E. & S. Livingstone Ltd., 1962.

Waugh, T. R.: Unreduced Colles fractures. J. Trauma, *3*:254, 1963.

Index

Italic numbers indicate pages with illustrations.
Numbers followed by t indicate pages with tables.